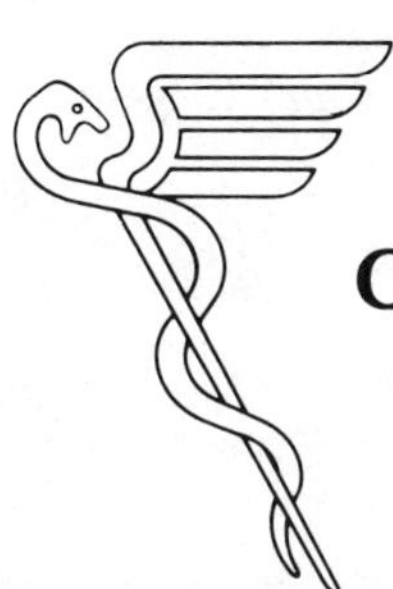

1982
YEAR BOOK OF

OBSTETRICS AND GYNECOLOGY

<h1 style="text-align:center">THE 1982 YEAR BOOKS</h1>

The YEAR BOOK series provides in condensed form the essence of the best of the recent international medical literature. The material is selected by distinguished editors who critically review more than 500,000 journal articles each year.

Anesthesia: *Drs. Kirby, Miller, Ostheimer, Saidman, and Stoelting.*

Cancer: *Drs. Clark, Cumley, and Hickey.*

Cardiology: *Drs. Harvey, Kirkendall, Kirklin, Nadas, Resnekov, and Sonnenblick.*

Dentistry: *Drs. Hale, Hazen, Moyers, Redig, Robinson, and Silverman.*

Dermatology: *Drs. Dobson and Thiers.*

Diagnostic Radiology: *Drs. Whitehouse, Adams, Bookstein, Gabrielsen, Holt, Martel, Silver, and Thornbury.*

Drug Therapy: *Drs. Hollister and Lasagna.*

Emergency Medicine: *Dr. Wagner.*

Endocrinology: *Drs. Schwartz and Ryan.*

Family Practice: *Dr. Rakel.*

Medicine: *Drs. Rogers, Des Prez, Cline, Braunwald, Greenberger, Bondy, and Epstein.*

Neurology and Neurosurgery: *Drs. De Jong, Sugar, and Currier.*

Nuclear Medicine: *Drs. Hoffer, Gottschalk, and Zaret.*

Obstetrics and Gynecology: *Drs. Pitkin and Zlatnik.*

Ophthalmology: *Dr. Ernest.*

Orthopedics: *Dr. Coventry.*

Otolaryngology: *Drs. Strong and Paparella.*

Pathology and Clinical Pathology: *Dr. Brinkhous.*

Pediatrics: *Drs. Oski and Stockman.*

Plastic and Reconstructive Surgery: *Drs. McCoy, Brauer, Haynes, Hoehn, Miller, and Whitaker.*

Psychiatry and Applied Mental Health: *Drs. Freedman, Kolb, Lourie, Meltzer, Nemiah, and Romano.*

Sports Medicine: *Drs. Krakauer, Shephard and Torg, Col. Anderson, and Mr. George.*

Surgery: *Drs. Schwartz, Najarian, Peacock, Shires, Silen, and Spencer.*

Urology: *Drs. Gillenwater and Howards.*

The YEAR BOOK of

Obstetrics and Gynecology

1982

Editor

ROY M. PITKIN, M.D.
*Professor and Head, Department of Obstetrics and Gynecology,
University of Iowa College of Medicine*

Associate Editor

FRANK J. ZLATNIK, M.D.
*Associate Professor and Vice-Chairman,
Department of Obstetrics and Gynecology,
University of Iowa College of Medicine*

YEAR BOOK MEDICAL PUBLISHERS, INC.
CHICAGO • LONDON

Table of Contents

The material covered in this volume represents literature reviewed up to August 1981.

Introduction

Special articles in the 1982 YEAR BOOK OF OBSTETRICS AND GYNE-COLOGY address two of the most common clinical problems in obstetrics and gynecology.

Postdate pregnancy often presents a dilemma for the obstetrician. Though Clifford is usually credited with the first recognition of the "postmaturity syndrome" in the early 1950s, the Scottish obstetrician Ballantyne, writing in the *Journal of Obstetrics and Gynaecology of the British Empire* a half-century earlier, gave as succinct and accurate description of the condition as has ever been written. When pregnancy extends beyond 42 weeks, the risk of antepartum and intrapartum death rises to a slight, albeit significant, degree. While aware of this risk, the obstetrician is also cognizant of the dangers of ill-timed intervention, inadvertent prematurity and prolonged induction of labor. Given the uncertainties and imponderables of dating gestation in the usual clinical situation, the major problem with postdate pregnancy involves establishing the diagnosis. Dr. Allan B. Weingold, of George Washington University, has prepared an excellent review of the topic in which he outlines his approach to this common and troublesome condition.

Among current controversies in gynecology, none is as prominent as that of menopausal estrogen replacement therapy. On the one hand, there are certain clear benefits—alleviation of vasomotor symptoms, correction of vaginal atrophy, and maintenance of normal bone metabolism. On the other hand, certain risks, chiefly an increased propensity to endometrial cancer, are established quite clearly. Dr. Stanley J. Birnbaum, of Cornell University, has prepared a thorough review, written from the point of view of an experienced and thoughtful clinician, of the risks and benefits of exogenous estrogen treatment. It should provide the basis for an informed decision, based on risk-benefit analysis, in the individual case.

ROY M. PITKIN, M.D.
FRANK J. ZLATNIK, M.D.

Current Literature Quiz

The questions below are an informal test of your knowledge before and/or after reading the YEAR BOOK. The questions are answered by locating the appropriate article in the text by its reference number, which appears in parentheses after each question. The reference numbers indicate the chapter in which the article appears and its numerical order within the chapter.

1. What hormones may be responsible for increased insulin resistance during pregnancy? (1–1)
2. What is the relationship between the maternal concentration of human chorionic gonadotropin and fetal sex? (1–5)
3. What is the biochemical basis for the observed sex difference in risk of respiratory distress syndrome? (1–10)
4. What happens to blood levels of anticonvulsant drugs during pregnancy? (1–19)
5. How might high maternal hemoglobin levels adversely affect the fetus? (1–21)
6. What is the treatment of choice of proliferative retinopathy accompanying diabetic pregnancy? (2–3)
7. Significant deterioration in renal function with pregnancy occurs in what proportion of gravidas with kidney transplants? (2–11)
8. What is the effect of pregnancy on viral hepatitis? (2–15)
9. What is the treatment of herpes gestationis? (2–21)
10. What blood magnesium levels may be anticipated with intravenous administration of 1 and 2 gm/hour? (3–3)
11. What happens to maternal blood levels of complement and C-reactive protein after premature rupture of the membranes? (3–8)
12. What are risk factors for group B streptococcal infections in infants? (3–10)
13. What proportion of infants with nonimmunologic hydrops have congenital malformations? (3–14)
14. Which technique of external cardiotocography gives the best results in terms of readable tracings? (4–1)
15. What treatment is indicated for fetal supraventricular tachycardia? (4–10)
16. What ultrasound measurement is most accurate in determining gestational age in the first trimester? (4–17)
17. What is the effect of blood, meconium, and vaginal secretion on phosphatidylglycerol levels? (4–24 and 4–25)
18. How soon after fetal death is amniotic fluid creatine kinase elevated? (4–27)
19. Do oral β-adrenergic drugs prevent or postpone the recurrence of threatened premature labor? (5–11)
20. What is the most significant maternal complication of β-adrenergic drug treatment of threatened premature labor? (5–13)
21. What is the effect of a distended bladder on uterine activity? (5–23)
22. How often is the volume of the intrapartum fetomaternal bleed larger

than that which one vial of Rh-immune globulin is designed to counteract? (5–26)

23. Is there a difference in prognosis with "thin" versus "thick" meconium staining? (5–28 and 5–29)
24. At what interval prior to delivery is meperidine administration to the laboring gravida most apt to be associated with neonatal depression? (6–1)
25. Is cimetidine effective prophylaxis against Mendelson's syndrome? (6–5 and 6–6)
26. Is the risk of genetic disease increased with increasing paternal age? (7–2 and 7–3)
27. What is the recurrence risk for neural tube defect when a couple has had a previous child who was affected? (7–6)
28. What amniotic fluid test may be helpful in intrauterine diagnosis of cystic fibrosis? (7–11 and 7–12)
29. Is Bendectin teratogenic? (7–17 and 7–18)
30. What are the effects of intrauterine diethylstilbestrol exposure on subsequent pregnancy outcome? (7–19)
31. What is the effect of nursing on maternal levels of oxytocin, prolactin, vasopressin, and prostanoids? (8–2 and 8–4)
32. What is the relationship between maternal diet and milk content of fat and protein? (8–6 and 8–7)
33. What constituent(s) of milk is associated with neonatal jaundice? (8–11)
34. How frequently do *Mycoplasma* organisms cause puerperal fever? (8–15)
35. What are the relative frequencies of *Chlamydia* organisms and gonococci as causes of neonatal ophthalmia? (8–17)
36. What is the relationship between time of onset of fetal growth retardation and later intellectual impairment? (9–3)
37. What are the effects of cesarean delivery on lung volumes and mechanics? (9–6)
38. What proportion of infants with brachial plexus injury at birth ultimately recover completely? (9–11)
39. Should exclusively breast-fed infants receive supplemental iron? (9–17)
40. Is the incidence of ectopic pregnancy increasing, decreasing, or staying about the same? (10–1)
41. What is the failure rate for sterilization by fibriectomy? (10–10)
42. What is the pathogenesis of tuboperitoneal fistulas after tubal sterilization procedures? (10–11)
43. What is the best means of closure of the abdomen to prevent wound disruption? (10–15)
44. Is obtaining a urine culture after the treatment of uncomplicated cystitis in women worthwhile? (11–1)
45. How can detrusor instability be distinguished from true stress incontinence? (11–10 and 11–11)
46. Describe the effects of estrogen therapy on the urethral pressure profile in postmenopausal women. (11–13)
47. What histopathologic finding in vulvar cancer best correlates with prognosis? (12–5)
48. What is the failure rate of cryotherapy of CIN III? (12–7, 12–8)
49. How does cell type (adenomatous, squamous, and adenosquamous) relate to prognosis in carcinoma of the cervix? (12–12)
50. In patients with endometrial cancer, what is the prognostic significance of prior estrogen usage? (12–18 and 12–19)
51. Does estrogen-progesterone receptor status correlate with the response of endometrial cancer to gestagens? (12–23)

52. What is the risk of associated malignancy in benign cystic teratomas after the menopause? (12–28)
53. Is in vitro chemotherapy testing more accurate in ovarian cancer when a favorable or an unfavorable response is predicted? (12–32)
54. What levels of pregnancy-specific placental proteins are found in gestational trophoblastic disease, and what do they mean? (12–39 and 12–40)
55. What causes thyrotoxicosis in choriocarcinoma? (12–42)
56. How often is the vagina involved in recurrent genital herpes infection? (13–1)
57. Why does metronidazole work in "nonspecific" vaginitis? (13–2)
58. What is the single-dose metronidazole regimen for treating vaginal trichomoniasis? (13–4)
59. Prepuberal gonorrhea infrequently is related to sexual assault. True or false? (13–5)
60. Are specimens for culture obtained at culdocentesis useful in managing acute salpingitis? (13–12)
61. How may endorphins be involved in the regulation of the menstrual cycle? (14–1 and 14–2)
62. Is 2-hydroxyestrone administration associated with an increase in serum prolactin levels? (14–4)
63. What is the effect of hyperprolactinemia on bone density? (14–5)
64. What is the relationship between obesity and serum sex steroid-binding globulin levels? (14–20)
65. What factors would suggest that acute adolescent menorrhagia might be a manifestation of an underlying coagulation disorder? (14–22)
66. Does gastrointestinal transit vary with the phase of the menstrual cycle? (14–24)
67. What is the correct dosage of danazol for the treatment of endometriosis? (14–29)
68. If estrogen is contraindicated, what can be used to treat menopausal symptoms? (14–44 and 14–45)
69. How well does laparoscopic recovery of sperm from the pouch of Douglas correlate with the postcoital test? (15–4)
70. How does the basal body temperature vary with the time of awakening? (15–6)
71. What role might the hamster egg serve in the evaluation of human infertility? (15–11)
72. Are there functional sequelae in the male to in utero diethylstilbestrol exposure? (15–12)
73. Why does "escape" ovulation not necessarily mean pregnancy in users of oral contraceptives? (16–3)
74. Why does rifampicin therapy decrease the efficacy of oral contraceptives? (16–7)
75. What is the rate of spontaneous abortion? (17–1)
76. Which pregnancy complications occur with increased frequency after induced abortion? (17–7)

OBSTETRICS

1. Maternal and Fetal Physiology

1-1 Correlation of Hyperprolactinemia With Altered Plasma Insulin and Glucagon: Similarity to Effects of Late Human Pregnancy. Pathologic increases in serum prolactin (PRL) levels have been associated with elevated plasma insulin levels. Anthony B. Gustafson, Michael F. Banasiak, Ronald K. Kalkhoff, Thad C. Hagen, and Hak-Joong Kim (Milwaukee) assessed plasma glucose and insulin responses to oral glucose and intravenous tolbutamide tolerance tests in 9 women with hyperprolactinemia and amenorrhea-galactorrhea syndrome (AGS) and in 9 controls matched for age and body weight. Nine women in the third trimester of pregnancy also were studied for their response to oral glucose tolerance tests.

Glucose tolerance curves, baseline insulin levels, and postchallenge plasma insulin responses to oral glucose tolerance tests were markedly higher in AGS subjects than in controls. Plasma glucagon levels were similarly suppressed in both AGS subjects and controls, though the suppression was more sustained in the AGS group. The response to oral glucose tolerance tests in the 9 pregnant women was similar to that for the AGS women. Intravenous tolbutamide produced a similar degree of hypoglycemia in controls and AGS women, though plasma insulin responses in the AGS group were significantly higher than in controls at 5 and 30 minutes.

The results suggest that hyperprolactinemia may contribute to the development of hyperinsulinemia and marked glucagon suppression in response to glucose that is characteristically found in the third trimester of pregnancy.

▶ [Resistance to the actions of insulin characterizes late pregnancy and, in order to maintain glucose tolerance, the gravida increases her insulin levels, both in the basal state and in response to a glycemic stimulus. Substances thought to be responsible for this physiologic hyperinsulinism include human placental lactogen estrogen, progesterone, and cortisol. To that list, prolactin apparently can now be added for, as indicated by this study, there are quite marked similarities in insulin release in response to an oral glucose challenge between women in late pregnancy and those with hyperprolactinemic amenorrhea. Because prolactin levels increase with gestation, perhaps prolactin may be responsible for insulin augmentation, but it is probably, at most, a contributory cause. Moreover, if prolactin calls forth an insulin response, perhaps a "borderline" diabetic might decompensate with development of hyperprolactinemia.] ◀

1-2 Bromocriptine Treatment During Early Human Pregnancy: Effect on Levels of Prolactin, Sex Steroids, and Placental Lactogen. During human pregnancy, the level of prolactin exceeds the nonpregnant level after 32–36 days from conception. It is not known whether this prolactin rise is crucial for the normal progress of preg-

(1–1)   J. Clin. Endocrinol. Metab. 51:242–246, August 1980.
(1–2)   Acta Endocrinol. (Copenh.) 95:412–415, November 1980.

nancy and the normal production of sex steroids and peptide hormones. O. Ylikorkala, S. Kivinen, and L. Rönnberg (Univ. of Oulu) studied the role of prolactin in the endocrinology of early pregnancy.

Of 50 healthy women admitted for abortion at 6 to 9 weeks' gestation, 28 were given 5.0 to 7.5 mg of bromocriptine daily for 2 weeks between weeks 6 and 9 of gestation; 22 served as controls. Blood samples were collected before and 1 and 2 weeks after the start of the trial for analysis of plasma prolactin, estradiol-17β, progesterone, testosterone, and human placental lactogen levels. All women then underwent uncomplicated abortions.

Bromocriptine treatment induced a prolactin depression at 1 week (7.3 vs. 23.7 ng/ml) and at 2 weeks (5.3 vs. 31.9 ng/ml). Estradiol-17β, progesterone, testosterone, and human placental lactogen levels were not significantly different between the two groups. Two women receiving bromocriptine (7.1%) and 1 control woman (4.5%) experienced spontaneous incomplete abortion during the study period, but these 3 already had a low estradiol-17β level and a low or undetectable placental lactogen level at the beginning of the study.

Neither maternal hypoprolactinemia nor bromocriptine treatment during early human pregnancy interferes with the normal progress of pregnancy or with the normal synthesis of sex steroids and human placental lactogen at this time.

▶ [These results indicate that bromocryptine administered during normal early gestation lowers prolactin levels but does not affect estradiol, progesterone, or placental lactogen values. Current labeling regulations, at least in the United States, require the statement that bromocriptine is contraindicated in patients wishing to conceive, but these results should provide some reassurance for the patient who does become pregnant while under therapy.] ◀

1–3 Plasma Prostaglandin F Metabolite Concentrations Following Cervical Encerclage. Rapid increases in plasma 13,14-dihydro-15-keto-prostaglandin $F_2\alpha$ (PGFM) concentrations after vaginal examination and amniotomy after the 37th week of pregnancy have been documented. P. S. Cocks, I. S. Fraser, R. Markham, M. Robinson, and R. P. Shearman (Univ. of Sydney) measured peripheral plasma concentrations of PGFM in 7 women having elective cervical encerclage in an otherwise normal pregnancy (gestation 12–16 weeks) to determine whether an increase in plasma PGFM levels occurred during this operation performed in the second trimester. To provide comparison, 2 patients having amniotomy at term and 4 patients having suction termination of pregnancy (2 under local and 2 under general anesthesia) also were studied. Ten ml of venous blood was collected prior to anesthesia, after anesthesia but before surgery, and at intervals during the 60 minutes from commencement of surgery. In group I (7 patients), a further specimen was collected at 24 hours. After addition of tritiated PGFM to monitor recovery, plasma samples were extracted, applied to microcolumns to separate PGFM from other prostaglandins, and then assayed with tritiated PGFM and a specific PGFM antiserum.

Only 3 women in group I showed a substantial rise in PGFM within

(1–3) Prostaglandins 20:493–502, September 1980.

60 minutes, and the others showed no change. All women showed a substantial fall by 24 hours, which was significantly less than both preoperative control value (t = 2.57, *P* <.05) and the 60-minute postoperative value (t = 8.78, *P* <.001). No other postoperative values were significantly different from either set of control values. Two patients at term had a substantial rise in plasma PGFM within 10 minutes of low amniotomy. There was a similar rise within 15 to 30 minutes of cervical dilatation and termination of first-trimester pregnancy.

Results suggest that most patients do not have a significant rise in PGFM levels following cervical encerclage. Since none of these subjects had any clinical evidence of uterine contractions, and since the safety of prostaglandin-inhibiting drugs in pregnancy has not been established, the authors conclude that routine administration of prostaglandin-inhibiting agents at the time of cervical encerclage is not justified. The extent of the rise in PGFM levels may be related to the degree of cervical manipulation, since the 4 first-trimester patients having elective termination of pregnancy with cervical dilatation to 9 mm showed significant rises in prostaglandin levels. It is not clear why there should be a statistically significant fall in PGFM from the preoperative to the 24-hour postoperative level.

▶ [Although elevated PGFM levels previously have been reported to result from cervical cerclage (1980 YEAR BOOK, pp. 163–164), the present study is not confirmatory. Most patients did not show an increase in metabolite concentration after the procedure.] ◀

1–4 **Decreased Prostacyclin Production: A Characteristic of Chronic Placental Insufficiency Syndromes.** Decreased production of vascular prostacyclin (prostaglandin I_2 or PGI_2) in maternal and placental circulation has been advanced as an etiologic factor underlying the pathophysiologic changes in preeclampsia. However, since fetal PGI_2 synthesis may be related to gestational age, it is questioned whether a deficiency in fetal prostaglandin metabolism is unique to preeclampsia or whether it occurs in other acute or chronic placental insufficiency syndromes.

Marie J. Stuart, Shirazali G. Sunderji, Thelma Yambo, David A. Clark, Judith B. Allen, Haim Elrad, and Jeffrey H. Slott (SUNY, Upstate Med. Center, Syracuse) measured production of 6-keto-PGF_1^α (stable end product of PGI_2) in the umbilical arteries of neonates born at various gestational ages from 28 weeks to term and compared that with PGI_2 levels in neonates born of pregnancies complicated by abruptio placentae, preeclampsia, intrauterine growth retardation (IUGR), or essential hypertension. The PGI_2 levels were reflected by conversion of ^{14}C-arachidonic acid (AA) to 6-keto-$PGF_{1\alpha}$. Uptake of AA was also measured to determine if this could account for differences in PGI_2 production.

Uptake of ^{14}C-AA was similar in all groups. Thus, the differences in conversion rates to 6-keto-$PGF_{1\alpha}$ were not the result of differences in uptake, nor were they related to gestational age. The amounts of conversion of ^{14}C-AA to 6-keto-$PGF_{1\alpha}$ were similar in neonates born

(1–4) Lancet 1:1126–1128, May 23, 1981.

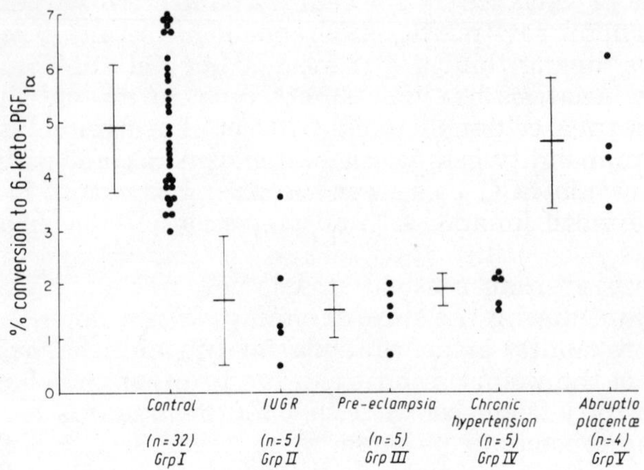

Fig 1–1.—Conversion of ^{14}C-arachidonic acid to 6-keto-PGF$_{1\alpha}$ in different groups of neonates. Results are expressed as the mean ± SD. (Courtesy of Stuart, M. J., et al.: Lancet 1:1126–1128, May 23, 1981.)

of normal pregnancies (mean, 4.9 ± 1.2%) and in those whose deliveries were complicated by abruptio placentae (mean, 4.6 ± 1.2%) (Fig 1–1). However, 6-keto-PGF$_{1\alpha}$ production was reduced markedly in pregnancies complicated by chronic placental insufficiency (P <.001). The percentage conversion was 1.7 ± 1.2% in neonates with IUGR, 1.5 ± 0.5% in neonates born to mothers with severe preeclampsia, and 1.9 ± 0.3% in neonates born to mothers with essential hypertension (Fig 1–1).

The results not only confirm that PGI$_2$ production is decreased in preeclampsia, but also demonstrate that a similar reduction occurs in pregnancies complicated by IUGR and essential hypertension.

▶ [Prostacyclin production by umbilical arteries was found to be lower than normal in IUGR, preeclampsia, and chronic hypertension in this study. The results are interesting, particularly in regard to preeclampsia. However, the relation between prostanoids and preeclampsia seems to us to be a bit of a chicken-egg problem. Since prostacyclin is a potent vasodilator, it is tempting to think of fetal prostacyclin deficiency as a primary cause. However, this conflicts with or leaves unexplained many known clinical correlates (such as primigravidity, improvement with fetal death, and occurrence with trophoblastic disease). Nevertheless, this area of research bears watching.] ◀

1–5 **Maternal Serum Human Chorionic Gonadotropin Concentrations and Fetal Sex Prediction.** It has been reported that during the third trimester of pregnancy, women bearing female fetuses have higher serum concentrations of human chorionic gonadotropin (hCG) than those bearing male fetuses. Hal Danzer, Glenn D. Braunstein, Joan Rasor, Alan Forsythe, and Maclyn E. Wade (Los Angeles) investigated the feasibility of using the absolute concentration of maternal serum hCG in a single third-trimester blood sample as a predictor of fetal sex. A total of 822 serum samples were obtained from 560 women with uncomplicated pregnancies and normal deliveries. Only single serum samples were taken after 17 weeks' gestation.

(1–5) Fertil. Steril. 34:336–340, October 1980.

Analysis of variance of the data by trimesters indicated a highly significant fetal sex–related difference in maternal serum hCG concentrations during the third trimester, but not the first and second trimesters. Analysis by lunar month revealed that the greatest sex difference appeared during weeks 37 to 40 of gestation. From the data obtained, probability graphs for fetal sex prediction based on a single maternal serum hCG measurement during the third trimester and during the tenth lunar month of pregnancy were developed (Fig 1–2). However, the utility of the graphs is limited: 57% of the women with fetuses of either sex had serum hCG concentrations between 4 and 15 IU/ml during the third trimester, which fall within the 40% and 60% probability areas, while during the tenth lunar month, more than 60% of the women had hCG concentrations with a greater than 60% probability factor for fetal sex prediction.

Fetal sex predictions based on maternal hCG determinations during late pregnancy are not as accurate as other methods such as amniocentesis with measurement of testosterone or follicle-stimulating hormone, fetoscopy, or third-trimester ultrasonic examination of external genitalia. At present, there are no medical or well-established social indications for third-trimester fetal sex determination.

▶ [Several reports over the past 15 years have noted that maternal hCG levels in late pregnancy are higher with a female than with a male fetus. This study is confirmatory and indicates further that the relationship becomes stronger with advancing pregnancy; levels during the first and second trimesters were not significantly different with respect to sex. There is sufficient overlap so that even during the last 4 weeks of gestation the majority of measurements will not be sufficiently discriminatory. However, as can be seen from Figure 1–2, levels of 20 IU/ml or more are 90% accurate in predicting a female infant and those of 3 IU/ml or less are 90% accurate in predicting a male. The explanation of this sex difference in maternal hCG levels is totally obscure, at least to us.] ◀

Fig 1–2.—Probability of a woman bearing a male or female fetus based on the hCG concentration in a single third-trimester serum sample. (Courtesy of Danzer, H., et al.: Fertil. Steril. 34:336–340, October 1980.)

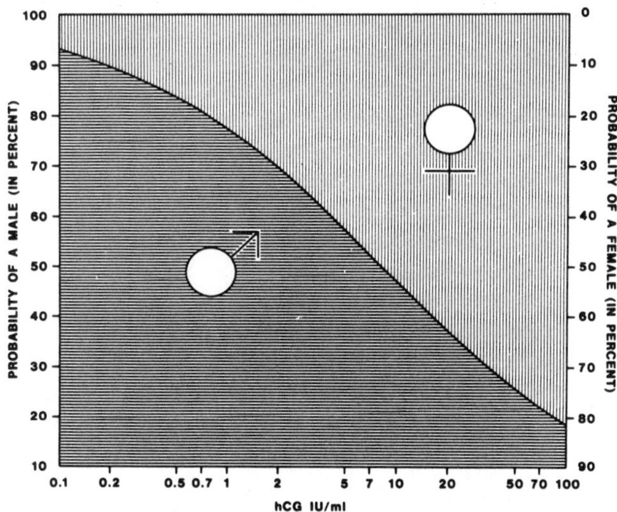

1–6 Maternal Plasma Adrenocorticotropin and Cortisol Relationships Throughout Human Pregnancy. Total serum cortisol concentrations increase during human pregnancy, but plasma ACTH concentrations have not been quantified in the same women throughout pregnancy. Bruce R. Carr, C. Richard Parker, Jr., James K. Madden, Paul C. MacDonald, and John C. Porter (Univ. of Texas Southwestern Med. School) measured plasma ACTH and cortisol concentrations prospectively in 5 pregnant women starting at 7 to 11 weeks' gestation. The women, aged 17 to 28 years, had normal pregnancies. Blood samples were obtained weekly, after overnight fast,

Fig 1–3.—Plasma concentrations of ACTH and cortisol during normal pregnancy. Blood samples were obtained weekly at 8 to 9 A.M. from 5 normal pregnant women and from 3 women during labor and on the second postpartum day. Umbilical cord plasma was also obtained from newborns of 3 subjects. Mean plasma concentrations of ACTH (picograms per milliliter) are denoted by solid circles, whereas plasma cortisol concentrations (nanograms per milliliter) are indicated by open circles. Vertical bars correspond to SEM. (Courtesy of Carr, B. R., et al.: Am. J. Obstet. Gynecol. 139:416–422, Feb. 15, 1981.)

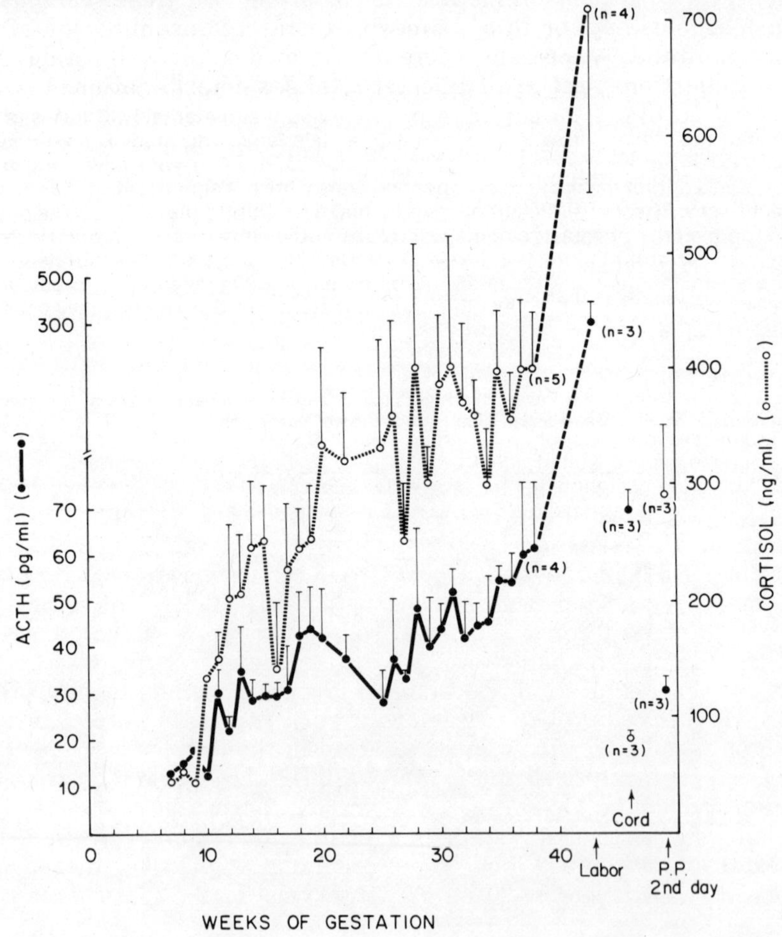

(1–6) Am. J. Obstet. Gynecol. 139:416–422, Feb. 15, 1981.

and in some cases during labor and delivery and 2 days post partum.

Concentrations of ACTH increased from a mean of 23 pg/ml at 12 weeks' gestation to 59 pg/ml at 37 weeks (Fig 1–3). Concentrations rose strikingly to a mean of 301 pg/ml during labor and delivery. Mean umbilical cord plasma ACTH values were 69 pg/ml. The maternal plasma ACTH concentration fell to a mean of 30.3 pg/ml on the second postpartum day. The mean plasma cortisol concentration rose progressively from 149 ng/ml at 11 weeks' gestation to 352 ng/ml at 26 weeks. The value then remained elevated but changed little until labor and delivery, when it rose to 706 ng/ml. Two days postpartum the mean maternal cortisol concentration was 296 ng/ml. The mean umbilical cord plasma cortisol concentration was 83 ng/ml. A diurnal rhythm of plasma cortisol was evident at all stages of pregnancy. A definite diurnal rhythm of plasma ACTH was less obvious, but it became more evident in the third trimester. Secretory spikes of ACTH were often, but not always, followed by increases in plasma cortisol concentrations.

Maternal plasma ACTH is suppressed during normal pregnancy, but a progressive rise in ACTH concentration occurs throughout pregnancy despite increasing plasma concentrations of cortisol, estrogen, and progesterone. Variations in plasma ACTH concentrations in these subjects were more marked than those in cortisol values. The cortisol feedback mechanism controlling ACTH secretion is probably not a one-to-one relationship. The central nervous system-hypothalamus appears to be central in controlling the episodic secretory activity of ACTH release.

▶ [This study indicates that levels of both ACTH and total cortisol in maternal blood increase more or less progressively throughout gestation. Assuming that total cortisol measurements reflect free cortisol levels, this relationship seems to contradict that of classic negative feedback. However, changes in total cortisol may well *not* reflect free cortisol during pregnancy, with its attendant estrogen-induced increase in corticosteroid-binding globulin. Or there may be an extrapituitary source of ACTH, specifically the placenta, during gestation.

In a related report, Nolten and Rueckert (*Am. J. Obstet. Gynecol.* 139:492, 1981) found that during gestation, the free cortisol index increased and that the responsiveness of the maternal adrenal gland to ACTH was enhanced.] ◀

1–7 **Diurnal Patterns and Regulation of Cortisol Secretion in Pregnancy.** Plasma levels of cortisol and corticosteroid-binding globulin have been shown to increase considerably during pregnancy. In addition, plasma free cortisol levels are consistently higher in pregnant than in nonpregnant women. This finding is difficult to reconcile with the absence of manifestations of hypercortisolism during pregnancy. Also, it would be expected that such increases in free cortisol would be associated with some alteration in the regulation of cortisol secretion. Wolfram E. Nolten, Marshall D. Lindheimer, Patricia A. Rueckert, Suzanne Oparil, and Edward N. Ehrlich investigated the physiology of cortisol secretion in 7 primigravid women in the third trimester of pregnancy and 3 nonpregnant women by measuring plasma cortisol levels at 20-minute intervals for 24 hours. Free cor-

---

(1–7) J. Clin. Endocrinol. Metab. 51:466–472, September 1980.

tisol levels were established by determining the free cortisol index and the rate of urinary cortisol excretion.

Plasma cortisol levels were persistently elevated in the pregnant women and showed nyctohemeral patterns qualitatively similar to those found in the nonpregnant controls. The mean plasma biologic half-lives and production rates of cortisol were significantly prolonged in pregnant subjects compared with nonpregnant controls. These differences may be explained by diurnal variations in the MCR of cortisol or by the possibility that cortisol secretion may not remain quiescent throughout the declining phase of the episode. Also, these increases in cortisol half-life and production rates would be expected to produce increases in plasma free cortisol. This was confirmed by determination of the free cortisol index and measurement of the rate of urinary free cortisol excretion.

The persistence of normal diurnal rhythmicity despite increased plasma free cortisol levels may be explained by decreased sensitivity of the maternal hypothalamic-pituitary regulatory mechanism to the suppressive influence of cortisol during pregnancy. The resetting of feedback regulation and the absence of manifestations of hypercortisolism during pregnancy may be explained by maternal tissue refractoriness to the action of cortisol in pregnancy.

▶ [Although the plasma free cortisol concentration is higher in the pregnant than in the nonpregnant state, the diurnal pattern is normal, suggesting a resetting of feedback regulation at the hypothalamic-pituitary level. Maternal tissues are apparently relatively refractory to cortisol during pregnancy. Is this related to the elevated levels of plasma progesterone?] ◀

1-8 **Direct Evidence of Sudden Rise in Fetal Corticoids Late in Human Gestation.** Glucocorticoids are known to stimulate fetal lung maturation in various mammals. In some species, the concentration of fetal cortisol increases dramatically near term, though studies of umbilical cord blood in humans have not revealed such an increase. Since much of the fetal cortisol is of maternal origin and its concentration at delivery is affected by maternal stress, Montserrat deM. Fencl, Robert J. Stillman, Jane Cohen, and Dan Tulchinsky (Boston) measured maternal plasma and urinary, umbilical cord blood, and amniotic fluid concentrations of corticosterone sulfate (BS), formerly referred to as compound B, during the course of pregnancy and labor in normal pregnant women, women pregnant with anencephalic fetuses, and a pregnant woman who had previously undergone complete adrenalectomy.

Plasma and urinary BS levels were higher in pregnant women than in nonpregnant controls and increased throughout pregnancy. Mean plasma concentrations increased from 6.7 ± 0.5 ng/ml^{-1} at midpregnancy to 16.0 ± 3.2 ng/ml^{-1} at term. During labor, plasma BS levels rapidly increased to a mean of 26.4 ± 6.3 ng/ml^{-1}. Urinary BS concentrations showed a similar pattern of increase. During labor, women with anencephalic fetuses had a significantly lower plasma BS than normal (8.3 ± 0.4 ng/ml^{-1}). In the woman without adrenals, the most pronounced increase in plasma BS occurred in the last week

(1–8) Nature 287:225–226, Sept. 18, 1980.

before labor began; there was no further increase during labor. In deliveries at midpregnancy, the concentration of BS in umbilical cord blood was only slightly lower than at term. Umbilical cord plasma BS concentrations in the woman with no adrenals were normal, while the concentrations in women with anencephalic fetuses at term were only 25% of normal values. Amniotic fluid levels of BS were also abnormally low in women with anencephalic fetuses.

The results indicate that at least 67% of maternal BS is derived from the fetus and that the production of BS by the fetal adrenal glands increases markedly near term.

▶ [Investigation of the role of the human fetal adrenal cortex in late pregnancy has been hampered by the fact that much of the measured fetal cortisol (e.g., in cord blood) is of maternal origin. This study suggests that corticosterone sulfate in maternal plasma or urine is largely of fetal origin. This compound (unfortunately abbreviated BS) can therefore serve as an indicator of fetal adrenal function. We are certain to see BS studies in association with changes in fetal lung maturity and with the onset of labor.] ◀

1–9 **Demonstration of Novel Compounds in Human Fetal Tissues and Consideration of Their Possible Role in Parturition.** Beverly E. Pearson Murphy (Montreal Gen. Hosp.) studied a new group of one or more compounds that behave chemically and chromatographically like steroids; these substances have been tentatively identified as analogues of 11-hydroxypregnenolone. The possibility of the compound being 11 β-hydroxy, 20-dihydropregnenolone is being pursued. Determined by radioenzymatic assay, the highest levels of the substance were found in the fetal zone of the fetal adrenal and were about 100 times those found in fetal serum. Concentrations were also high in the liver and were increased over serum concentrations in the lung, heart, and kidney. Umbilical cord levels were higher after spontaneous labor than after elective cesarean section or induced labor in premature and mature infants. The group with labor induced by oxytocin had intermediate values. The values of the total 11β-hydroxysteroids appeared to be more closely related to onset of labor than was the cortisol level or the nonglucocorticoid fraction alone.

The data suggest that the concentration of an 11-hydroxysteroid dehydrogenase (11-HSD) inhibitor, possibly an 11β-hydroxypregnenolone analogue, produced by the fetal zone of the fetal adrenal, rises in close association with onset of labor. The observation that the values in the group without labor fall into two categories, most being very low, but a few being high, suggests that the rise occurs before labor commences. It has not previously been recognized that 11-HSD has a much higher affinity for unusual steroids (11β-hydroxyprogesterone, 11β-hydroxypregnenolone, and their 20α-dihydro derivatives) than for cortisol. It seems possible that the fetal zone of the human fetal adrenal, under the influence of some fetal factor other than adrenocorticotropic hormone, may have as its primary function the production of an 11β-hydroxysteroid which, with its metabolites, passes directly to the placenta and via the urine and amniotic fluid to the membranes and decidua. There is evidence to suggest that, in the

(1–9) Am. J. Obstet. Gynecol. 139:353–358, Feb. 1, 1981.

decidua, it would be converted to a progesterone analogue, which might be expected to compete for progesterone receptors. Such competition could result in a decreased effective progesterone concentration in the decidua which, in turn, would result in increased sensitivity to oxytocin, increased prostaglandin production, and onset of labor.

▶ [A few years ago, it was thought that cortisol from the fetal adrenal might be important in the initiation of labor in human beings as it is in certain animals. Subsequent studies have not supported this view. The present report suggests that we should not give up on the fetal zone of the adrenal cortex. Although cortisol and corticosterone account for all of the 11-hydroxycorticosteroid (11-HCS) compounds measured in maternal serum, these two together account for less than half of the total 11-HCS in fetal serum. The speculation is that these other, as yet incompletely characterized, fetal 11-HCS compounds may have a role in parturition.] ◀

1–10 **Sex Differences in Fetal Lung Maturation.** It has long been recognized that male infants are at greater risk of respiratory distress syndrome (RDS). John S. Torday, Heber C. Nielsen, Montserrat DeM. Fencl, and Mary Ellen Avery (Harvard Med. School) retrospectively reviewed the lecithin-sphingomyelin (L/S) ratio and concentrations of saturated phosphatidyl choline (SPC) and cortisol in amniotic fluid from 73 male and 76 female fetuses between 28 and 40 weeks' gestation.

Analysis of covariance showed that female infants had higher indexes of pulmonary maturity; the difference in degree of fetal pulmonary maturity was 1.2 to 2.5 weeks. The L/S value generally used to indicate pulmonary maturity is 2.0/1; the predicted female mean reached this value at 32.4 weeks, whereas the predicted male mean reached it at 33.6 weeks. The predicted mean for female infants reached an SPC concentration highly predictive of fetal pulmonary maturity 1.4 weeks before the predicted male mean. For amniotic-fluid cortisol, the female mean reached maturity 2.5 weeks before the male mean.

It is concluded that there is a biochemical basis for the increased risk of RDS in male infants. It is possible that variables other than fetal sex were introduced by complications in these pregnancies (diabetes, Rh disease, toxemia, placenta previa, abruptio placentae, intrauterine growth retardation, hypertension, collagen vascular disease) to produce these results. The complications affect fetal development, but have not been shown to affect the factors measured. Analysis of covariance indicated that the regression lines for the logarithms of L/S and concentrations of SPC and cortisol were parallel between 28 and 40 weeks. Since there were very few points at the gestational extremes, it is difficult to be certain that the observed differences persist in the very immature of term/postterm fetus. Despite evidence that estrogens may play a role in fetal lung maturation, there is little evidence of a difference in estrogen concentrations in male and female fetuses. Therefore, it is postulated that differences in lung maturation are caused by the presence of androgens in the male infant. The finding that amniotic fluid cortisol concentration is significantly

(1–10) Am. Rev. Respir. Dis. 123:205–208, February 1981.

lower in the male fetus may indicate that a relative deficiency of cortisol, believed to regulate lung maturation, is the cause of the delay in male fetal lung maturation. However, this may merely reflect another aspect of pulmonary immaturity, because the lung has the capacity to metabolize cortisone to cortisol, and this is gestation dependent.

▶ [Female infants are less likely to develop RDS than are male infants of the same gestational age at birth. This study suggests a biochemical basis for the observed difference. At a given gestational age, the mean SPC levels and L/S ratios were higher in female than in male fetuses. The authors speculate that this may relate somehow to the presence of androgens in the male fetus. The spread of values at each week of gestation is large, and the dating of the pregnancies in this study is critical. The latter was based exclusively on the pediatric assessment of the newborn. Are we certain that there is no sex bias in this determination?] ◀

1–11 **Amniotic Fluid C-Peptide as an Index for Intrauterine Fetal Growth.** Insulin is a key regulator of fetal growth by stimulating the cellular uptake of amino acids and subsequent protein synthesis and enhancing deposit of glycogen and lipids in storage tissues. The mean concentration of glucose in fetal blood is the major determinant of the insulin concentration. Unlike insulin, C-peptide is minimally metabolized by the liver, and its concentration in amniotic fluid may reflect the amount of insulin secreted by the fetal pancreas. Chin-Chu Lin, Atef H. Moawad, Philip River, Petra Blix, Marilyn Abraham and Arthur H. Rubenstein (Univ. of Chicago) used an accurate, sensitive assay for C-peptide to determine amniotic fluid and cord blood concentrations in 103 nondiabetic infants, including 25 suspected prenatally of having intrauterine growth retardation. Concentrations of C-peptide in amniotic fluid obtained at 36 weeks' gestation or later were measured by radioimmunoassay.

Fetal plasma C-peptide concentrations were independent of maternal values. Neither amniotic fluid nor cord blood C-peptide concentrations correlated with placental weight, but both correlated signifi-

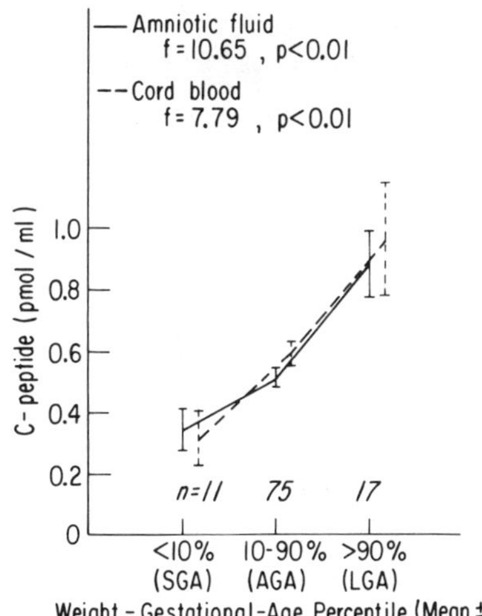

Fig 1–4.—Relation between amniotic fluid and cord blood C-peptide concentrations and infant weight-gestational age percentile classification. Statistical comparison by one-way analysis of variance. (Courtesy of Lin, C.-C., et al.: Am. J. Obstet. Gynecol. 139:390–396, Feb. 15, 1981.)

(1–11) Am. J. Obstet. Gynecol. 139:390–396, Feb. 15, 1981.

cantly with birth weight. Relations between the concentrations and the infant weight-gestational age percentile are shown in Figure 1–4. Differences between the average-gestational age and both small- and large-gestational age groups were significant. Neither the amniotic fluid insulin concentration nor the glucose-insulin ratio correlated significantly with infant birth weight or the weight-gestational age percentile. Mean C-peptide concentrations were lower in infants with an immature lecithin-sphingomyelin ratio.

The amniotic fluid C-peptide concentration is a reliable indicator of intrauterine fetal growth. High values are present in large for gestational age infants and low values in small for gestational age infants at term. Low insulin secretion in the small for gestational age fetus, secondary to chronic fetal hypoglycemia, may lead to retarded somatic growth, deficient glycogen storage in the liver and heart, and lack of subcutaneous fat. Helpful measures may include bedrest, infusion of hypertonic dextrose, administration of β-sympathomimetic agents such as ritodrine, or nutritional supplementation.

▶ [According to prevalent theory, insulin is the major growth hormone during fetal life. The results of this study are consistent with that hypothesis, because C-peptide levels (an accurate index of endogenous insulin secretion) in amniotic fluid and cord blood were found to correlate quite closely with birth weight and particularly with size-gestational age relationships.] ◀

1–12 **Placental Size During Early Pregnancy and Fetal Outcome: Preliminary Report of Sequential Ultrasonographic Study.** Henk J. Hoogland, Jelte de Haan, and Chester B. Martin, Jr. (Nijmegen, The Netherlands) used serial gray-scale ultrasonography to measure placental area in 50 primigravid women with singleton pregnancies and placentas located anteriorly. Before the 9th to 11th weeks of gestation the boundaries of the placenta could not be distinguished from the decidua and chorion frondosum. The smallest placental area measurable was 40 sq cm at 71 days. Thereafter, placental area usually increased rapidly.

Of the 50 newborn infants, 38 had appropriate birth weights, 10 were small for gestational age (below the 10th percentile), and 2 were large for gestational age (above the 90th percentile). Mean ultrasonically determined placental area at a menstrual age of 150 days was 188 sq cm in the 10 infants who were small for gestational age and 235 sq cm in the 38 who were appropriate for gestational age. The 2 large infants had placental areas at 150 days of 210 and 296 sq cm. A "warning limit" of placental area at 150 days was calculated to be 187 sq cm. Small for gestational age babies were born to 6 of 9 women with a placental area equal to or smaller than this limit and to only 4 of 41 with larger placentas.

Ultrasonographic placental area measurement in midpregnancy appears to be of prognostic value in identifying pregnancies at high risk for the subsequent occurrence of fetal growth retardation.

▶ [The well-known association between fetal and placental size at term does not answer the question of which of the two is primary. The results of this interesting study, in which area of anteriorly located placentas was measured ultrasonographically, sug-

(1–12) Am. J. Obstet. Gynecol. 138:441–443, Oct. 15, 1980.

gest that placental size at midpregnancy correlates with fetal size at term. As fetal growth retardation is not usually recognizable clinically prior to the third trimester, it would seem that either placental growth in early gestation is the primary determinant of fetal growth or, perhaps more likely, some other influence controls growth of both placenta (early) and fetus (late).] ◄

1–13 Percentile Ranks of Sonar Fetal Abdominal Circumference Measurements. Serial sonar biparietal diameter (BPD) values are especially useful in defining gestational age and in establishing a cephalic percentile growth bracket, while fetal sonar abdominal circumference (AC) is more useful than either BPD or chest diameter (CD) for estimating fetal weight. Ralph K. Tamura and Rudy E. Sabbagha (Northwestern Univ. Chicago) prospectively obtained serial ultrasonic BPD and AC fetal measurements in 200 women with low-risk pregnancies from weeks 18 to 42 of gestation to define the percentile ranks of sonar fetal ACs. Gestational age was defined by menstrual data in 92 patients and by ultrasound data in 108.

The fetal ACs were derived from both longitudinal and cross-sectional ultrasonic scans. The AC measurements were reproducible within a range of 2% of the mean. This range in error included variations introduced by the digitizer. Abdominal circumference percentile ranks were arranged by weeks of gestation (table). The differences in AC measurements between those whose gestational age was defined by menstrual data and those whose gestational age was defined by ultrasound data were not statistically significant. There also were no significant differences on the basis of race.

The 2% range of reproducibility allowed discrimination between fetuses with small ACs (<25th percentile) from those with average

FETAL AC MEASUREMENTS (CM)*

Percentile

Weeks of gestation	2.5	5	10	25	50	75	80	95	97.5	No.
18	9.8	10.3	10.9	11.9	13.1	14.2	14.5	15.9	16.4	3
19	11.1	11.6	12.3	13.3	14.4	15.6	15.9	17.2	17.8	10
20	12.1	12.6	13.3	14.3	15.4	16.6	16.9	18.2	18.8	24
21	13.7	14.2	14.8	15.9	17.0	18.1	18.4	19.8	20.3	26
22	14.7	15.2	15.8	16.9	18.0	19.1	19.4	20.8	21.3	28
23	16.0	16.5	17.1	18.2	19.3	20.4	20.7	22.1	22.6	30
24	17.2	17.7	18.3	19.4	20.5	21.6	21.9	23.3	23.8	28
25	18.0	18.5	19.1	20.2	21.3	22.4	22.7	24.1	24.6	18
26	18.8	19.3	19.9	21.0	22.1	23.2	23.5	24.9	25.4	11
27	20.4	20.9	21.5	22.6	23.7	24.8	25.1	26.5	27.0	9
28	22.0	22.5	23.1	24.2	25.3	26.4	26.7	28.1	28.6	2
29	23.6	24.1	24.7	25.8	26.9	28.0	28.3	29.7	30.2	15
30	24.1	24.6	25.2	26.3	27.4	28.5	28.8	30.2	30.7	24
31	24.7	25.2	25.8	26.9	28.0	29.1	29.4	30.8	31.3	48
32	25.4	25.9	26.5	27.6	28.7	29.8	30.1	31.5	32.0	51
33	25.7	26.2	26.8	27.9	29.0	30.1	30.4	31.8	32.3	34
34	26.8	27.3	27.9	29.0	30.1	31.2	31.5	32.9	33.4	28
35	28.9	29.4	30.0	31.1	32.2	33.3	33.6	35.0	35.5	18
36	30.0	30.5	31.1	32.2	33.3	34.4	34.7	36.1	36.6	14
37	31.1	31.6	32.2	33.3	34.4	35.5	35.8	37.2	37.7	18
38	32.4	32.9	33.5	34.6	35.7	36.8	37.1	38.5	39.0	37
39	32.6	33.1	33.7	34.8	35.9	37.0	37.3	38.7	39.2	34
40	32.8	33.3	33.9	35.0	36.1	37.2	37.5	38.9	39.4	23
41	33.8	34.3	34.9	36.0	37.1	38.2	38.5	39.9	40.4	3

*Circumference measurements were obtained from the outer aspect of the fetal abdomen at the area of the liver that shows the umbilical vein.

(1–13) Am. J. Obstet. Gynecol. 138:475, Nov. 1, 1980.

(25th to 75th percentile) and large (>80th percentile) AC values. However, the accuracy of the sonar AC values when compared with actual ACs was not as precise and fell within a range of 5.2%. Nonetheless, the reproducibility of sonar fetal AC measurements demonstrates the usefulness of sonar AC in establishing antenatal diagnostic parameters and adds a new dimension to the interpretation of BPD growth. In addition to being useful in defining the chances for fetal survival in women who may have to be delivered early for obstetric reasons, sonar AC measurements can be useful in establishing the severity and progress of some fetal abnormalities such as hydrocephalus and fetal ascites.

▶ [Ultrasonographic measurement of the fetal abdominal circumference may be helpful in identifying asymmetric intrauterine growth retardation. The authors point out its potential usefulness in the evaluation of the fetus for hydrocephalus and in monitoring fetal ascites, as well.] ◀

1-14 **Amniotic Fluid Volume and Composition Following Experimental Manipulations in Sheep.** Barbara E. Lingwood, Kenneth J. Hardy, Jeffrey G. Long, Marion McPhee, and E. Marelyn Wintour (Univ. of Melbourne) measured changes in amniotic fluid composition and volume after experimentally induced disturbances in fluid composition in 17 ewes at 85–135 days' gestation whose fetuses chronically were cannulated. Surgical procedures for the cannulation of the fetal carotid artery, jugular vein, bladder, and amniotic cavity have been described previously. Special care was taken to avoid spillage of amniotic fluid during the operation and to obtain a watertight seal in the uterus. Experiments were performed only on fetuses in a healthy unstressed condition, at least 5 days following surgery. The volume of amniotic fluid was measured by a dye dilution technique using ^{125}I-labeled γ-globulin. Samples were collected from both amniotic cannulas at various times after injection. After amniotic fluid volume was estimated, 20% to 30% of the fluid volume was replaced by isotonic solutions of saline, mannitol, or dextrose. Samples of fluid were then taken at various times from the opposite cannula and were analyzed for osmolality, sodium, potassium, chloride, urea, creatinine, and glucose.

In all cases of replacement of fluid, the sodium, potassium, and chloride concentrations returned to control values in 3–6 hours. Urea and creatinine behaved similarly in the saline and mannitol experiments, but rose above control values within 1 hour of dextrose replacement. Amniotic fluid volume rose significantly above control values after replacement in all 3 types of experiments; no further increases occurred after 1 hour. Fetal urine drainage to the exterior abolished the rapid return of urea and creatinine concentrations in the dextrose experiments, although no changes in renal function occurred in any experiments.

These studies attempted to imitate closely the normal variations in fetal or maternal fluid and electrolyte balance. Results suggest that some mechanism acts to control closely the composition of amniotic

(1–14) Obstet. Gyncol. 56:451–458, October 1980.

fluid in sheep. Probably this control is the result of normal regulatory processes in the amniotic fluid. The observed increase in fluid volume may be the result of the entry of water into the cavity to maintain a constant total solute concentration or with return of solute. The effect of urine removal on urea and creatinine concentrations during dextrose experiments was more dramatic than for other solutes; the rapid return and overshoot of urea and creatinine concentrations stopped almost completely. This result suggests that fetal urine is an important source of urea and creatinine entering the amniotic fluid, at least in dextrose replacement experiments.

Perinatal death in infants of diabetic mothers is associated with elevated amniotic glucose concentrations. Perhaps abnormal solute movements in the amniotic fluid caused by the elevated levels of glucose are the primary cause of the abnormal volumes of fluid observed in these cases.

▶ [These elegant experiments performed in sheep indicate the importance of constant amniotic fluid solute concentrations, at least in this species. Not surprisingly, fetal urine was the important source of urea and creatinine, but not of sodium or potassium. How little we really know about the dynamics of amniotic fluid production and removal! Although osmolality remained relatively constant in these experiments, amniotic fluid volume did not. The authors suggest that clinical disorders of amniotic fluid volume may reflect water movement initiated to maintain constant solute concentrations.] ◀

1–15 **Effect of Vegetarianism on the Zinc Status of Pregnant Women.** The availability of zinc in a vegetarian diet has been questioned because of the high phytic acid and fiber content of the foods. Zinc requirements are increased in pregnancy, and pregnant vegetarian women may be at a greater risk of poor zinc status. Janet C. King, Terry Stein, and Mary Doyle measured plasma, urine, and hair zinc levels in 12 vegetarian pregnant women, 6 pregnant nonvegetarian women, and 5 nonpregnant vegetarians. All but 1 of the vegetarian women were ovo-lacto vegetarians. None of the women smoked, and none of the nonpregnant subjects was taking oral contraceptives at the time of study. Weight gain was comparable in the two groups of pregnant subjects, and the infants of vegetarians weighed more than those of the nonvegetarians.

All but 2 of the pregnant women had taken some type of vitamin-mineral supplement. Four of the vegetarians used supplements containing zinc, as did 1 in the nonvegetarian group and 1 nonpregnant woman. None of the women in the study followed diets providing recommended amounts of zinc. The plasma zinc levels of nonpregnant women were significantly higher than those of pregnant women. Urinary zinc levels were about twice as high in the pregnant subjects. Hair zinc concentrations were similar in all groups. The use of supplemental zinc did not appear to influence plasma, urine, or hair zinc levels in the pregnant groups.

The plasma zinc level was about one-fifth lower in pregnant than in nonpregnant women, although the pregnant women consumed about twice as much zinc. Zinc status appears to be influenced more by pregnancy than by the ovo-lacto vegetarian dietary habit. Further

---

(1–15) Am. J. Clin. Nutr. 34:1049–1055, June 1981.

study of zinc status in pregnancy is needed to clarify the relationship of plasma, urine, and hair zinc levels to total body zinc levels.

▶ [Zinc nutriture is one of the main theoretical concerns of vegetarianism. In this study, however, dietary, plasma, urinary, and hair zinc levels did not differ in vegetarian and nonvegetarian gravidas. An important caveat is that 11 of the 12 vegetarians were ovo-lacto vegetarians (i.e., eat eggs and milk) and only 1 was a vegan (i.e., eats no animal products of any kind).] ◀

1–16 **Zinc Status of Pregnant Alcoholic Women: Determinant of Fetal Outcome.** Alcohol consumption by pregnant women causes fetal dysmorphogenesis, but the mechanism by which this occurs is unknown. There are relations between zinc deficiency and chronic alcoholism and between low zinc status in pregnancy and fetal malformations. Arthur Flynn, Sue S. Martier, Robert J. Sokol, Sheldon I. Miller, Nancy L. Golden, and Bert C. Del Villano (Cleveland) hypothesized that alcohol-induced fetal dysmorphogenesis may be related to low zinc values. The zinc status of 25 alcoholic and 25 nonalcoholic pregnant women, all of low socioeconomic status, was measured and correlated with fetal outcome.

Both maternal plasma and fetal cord plasma zinc concentrations were significantly lower in the alcoholic than in the nonalcoholic group (table). Eighteen infants in the alcoholic group had a total of 39 birth defects, whereas 14 infants in the nonalcoholic group had 22 defects. The defects of the alcoholic group more closely resembled those of fetal alcohol syndrome. Mean birth weights were 3,090 gm in the alcoholic group and 3,180 gm in the nonalcoholic group. No relation could be found between fetal defects and the alcohol volume index of the mother. There was a strong inverse relation between plasma zinc concentration of the mother and dysmorphological features of the infant; the correlation between fetal cord plasma zinc concentrations and fetal birth defects was less clear.

Alcoholic pregnant women have significantly lower zinc concentrations than comparable nonalcoholic pregnant women. The low zinc values are related to the occurrence of fetal dysmorphogenesis. That maternal zinc deficiency can be corrected with dietary supplementation suggest the possibility of preventing fetal dysmorphogenesis.

ALCOHOL VOLUME INDEX, MATERNAL PLASMA ZINC CONCENTRATION, AND FETAL CORD PLASMA ZINC CONCENTRATION IN ALCOHOLIC AND NONALCOHOLIC PREGNANT WOMEN (MEAN ± SD)

	Alcoholic (n = 25)	Non-alcoholic (n = 25)
Volume index	0·34±0·33	0·11±0·21
Maternal plasma-zinc (μg/ml)	50·7 ±8·5*	72·2 ±7·8
Fetal cord-plasma zinc (μg/ml)	65·5 ±5·0*	81·3 ±6·8

*Group mean was significantly lower than nonalcoholic group mean by Student's *t* test, *P* <.05.

(1–16) Lancet 1:572–575, Mar. 14, 1981.

▶ [At first glance, these observations suggest that zinc deficiency might be involved in production of the fetal alcohol syndrome, because both maternal and cord plasma zinc levels were lower in alcoholics than in controls. However, this may be too simplistic a conclusion for several reasons. In the first place, the observed frequency of "birth defects" was extraordinarily high (18/25 in alcoholics and 14/25 in nonalcoholics). Secondly, a significant correlation with defects was found only for maternal plasma zinc and not for fetal blood zinc concentrations. Finally, it is unfortunate that hair zinc levels, probably a better index of zinc nutriture than that provided by plasma levels, were not studied.] ◀

1–17 **Interrelationships Among Serum Thyroxine, Triiodothyronine, Reverse Triiodothyronine, and Thyroid-Stimulating Hormone in Iodine-Deficient Pregnant Women and Their Offspring: Effects of Iodine Supplementation.** Iodine requirements are expected to increase during pregnancy, and iodine deficiency (ID) is known to cause changes in plasma thyroid hormone concentrations. J. Enrique Silva and Sergio Silva (Santiago, Chile) sought to determine whether moderate or mild ID, which is prevalent in Chile, has effects on serum thyroid hormone and thyrotropin (TSH) concentrations. Blood was sampled at various gestational ages in 250 pregnant women in greater Santiago. They received about 300 μg of iodine daily as potassium iodide solution; one fourth of subjects were not treated.

Significant ID was manifested by excretion of 50 μg of iodine per gm of creatinine or less in 50% of the population. Another fourth of subjects had moderate deficiency, with excretion of 50 to 100 μg of iodine daily. Serum thyroxine (T_4) concentration and urinary iodine excretion correlated linearly in a double reciprocal plot. Serum TSH concentration increased progressively with a decreasing iodine supply. At higher iodine intakes, serum TSH concentration was not influenced by further increases in the iodine supply. Iodine supplementation was associated with significant increases in serum T_4 and reverse triiodothyronine (T_3) concentrations, a decrease in plasma TSH concentration, and no change in plasma T_3 concentration. Serum free T_4 concentrations were reduced in pregnant subjects and increased after potassium iodide treatment to values similar to those in nonpregnant subjects. Serum free T_3 concentrations were normal in the pregnant group and did not change with iodine supplementation. Serum TSH concentrations fell significantly. Infants whose mothers received iodine had higher serum T_4 and reverse T_3 values.

The fall in TSH concentration observed with oral iodine supplementation is due to a rise in serum T_4 concentration. The fetus appears to be relatively protected against ID. The lower plasma T_4 concentration in the fetus may, however, have consequences, since plasma T_4, at least in the rat, is an important source of intracellular T_3 in the brain.

▶ [This article details the biochemical effects of iodine deficiency during pregnancy on mother and infant, a rare complication in developed countries because of the widespread practice of iodization of salt. Iodine deficiency, diagnosed on the basis of urinary iodine excretion, was associated with a fall in T_4 and reverse T_3, a rise in TSH, and unaffected T_3 levels in both maternal and cord blood. Maternal iodine supplementation

---

(1–17) J. Clin. Endocrinol. Metab. 52:671–677, April 1981.

"normalized" the levels. Because the effects were less marked in the fetus than in the mother, it appears that the fetus enjoys some degree of protection against iodine deficiency.] ◄

1–18 **Plasma Antithrombin III Activity in Normal Pregnancy.** The incidence of thromboembolic phenomena increases in pregnancy. Antithrombin III deficiency has been implicated as a possible etiologic factor for the increase of thromboembolic phenomena in women who take exogenous estrogens. Carl P. Weiner and John Brandt (Ohio State Univ.) used a plasma-based assay to measure antithrombin III activity in 73 pregnant women at the 6th to 42nd week of gestation, 17 women in the postpartum period, 112 healthy young women not taking oral contraceptives or other medicines, and 118 women taking a combination oral contraceptive with 50 μg of estrogen or less per pill and 1–1.5 mg of progestogen. No significant difference in antithrombin III activity could be detected within and among the four groups.

A decrease in antithrombin III activity is probably not a cause of increased thromboembolic phenomena during normal pregnancy and oral contraceptive use. The changes noted in other studies may be due to the higher dosage of estrogen than that used in the present study, and to the use of the serum assay technique rather than the plasma-based assay used in the present study. This does not exclude the possibility that a pathologically significant decrease in antithrombin III levels occurs in certain disease states of pregnancy, which would help explain the increased overall incidence of thromboembolic phenomena.

► [Previous studies have suggested that antithrombin III levels are depressed in patients receiving exogenous estrogens and in postpartum patients. It had been postulated that low levels of this inhibitor accounted for the increased tendency for thromboembolism to occur in these circumstances. Back to the drawing board! The present authors, using what they consider to be a superior assay, were unable to demonstrate decreased levels of antithrombin III activity in pregnancy, in the puerperium, or during oral contraceptive use.] ◄

1–19 **Phenytoin Metabolism in Pregnancy.** Changes in phenytoin (DPH) plasma concentrations in epileptics have been suggested as a potential explanation for the increase in frequency of seizures experienced by 45% of epileptic patients during pregnancy. Despite the availability of accurate assays of anticonvulsant plasma levels, there has been essentially no decrease in reported seizure frequency during pregnancy in the past 35 years. To investigate the pharmacokinetics of DPH, Neil K. Kochenour, Maurice G. Emery, and Ronald J. Sawchuck (Univ. of Utah) prospectively measured plasma DPH concentrations and urinary excretion of its major metabolite, 5-(4-hydroxyphenyl)-5-phenylhydantoin (4-OH-DPH), in 5 epileptic patients during pregnancy and in the postpartum period.

A decrease in plasma DPH concentrations was seen in 4 patients, 3 of whom had seizures at a time when DPH levels were low. One patient had 3 seizures. An increase in the dose of DPH caused a corresponding increase in plasma concentration, although the increase

MATERNAL AND UMBILICAL CORD DPH BLOOD LEVELS

Patient no.	Maternal DPH (μg/ml)	Umbilical cord DPH (μg/ml)	Maternal: fetal ratio
1	6.0	6.0	1.0
2	9.0	8.3	1.1
3	3.0	3.0	1.0
4	3.0	3.0	1.0
5	5.0	6.0	0.8

was often of short duration and further increments in dosage were necessary to maintain adequate plasma levels. When plasma levels of DPH approached the therapeutic level, small increments in dosage resulted in a disproportionate increase in plasma concentrations. Those patients who showed a decrease in plasma DPH levels during pregnancy showed a marked increase in DPH levels several weeks after delivery. Although a definite decrease in the percentage of excretion of 4-OH-DPH was observed in patients who remained on a constant dose of DPH during pregnancy, there was no significant change in the renal clearance of unconjugated or conjugated 4-OH-DPH over the course of pregnancy. Maternal plasma and umbilical cord levels of DPH at the time of delivery were quite similar (table).

Since DPH absorption and/or metabolism appears to be altered during pregnancy, periodic measurement of plasma DPH concentration is recommended in managing the pregnant epileptic patient.

▶ [This study confirms the by now well-known tendency of blood anticonvulsant drug levels to fall with gestation. Levels of DPH were lower in pregnancy, in many instances subtherapeutic, than post partum. The level of the principal metabolite (4-OH-DPH) did not rise, suggesting that perhaps an alternative metabolic pathway operates with gestation. In our experience, it is often very difficult to get DPH levels into the "therapeutic range" in pregnant women, even by greatly increasing the dosage. Since, under these circumstances, the patient usually does not experience an increase in seizure frequency, we have tended to rely on her own bioassay.] ◀

1–20 **Organochlorine Pesticide Concentrations in Perinatal Samples From Mothers and Babies.** Organochloride pesticides have been detected in adult human tissues, in the fetus, and in stillborn and newborn infants. There is concern about possible passage of organochlorine pesticides from mother to fetus, transplacentally or otherwise, particularly because of the rapid increase in fat content in the infant's body. F. W. Eckenhausen (Stadskanaal, The Netherlands), D. Bennett, K. I. Beynon, and K. E. Elgar (Sittingbourne, England) obtained samples from Dutch mothers and their infants throughout the perinatal period and analyzed them for a range of organochlorine pesticides by gas-liquid chromatography with electron capture detection.

Confirmation of pp'DDE and HCB in placental tissue and meconium, and of pp'DDE in human milk, was satisfactory, but attempts to confirm these residues in blood and to confirm presence of dieldrin

(1–20) Arch. Environ. Health 36:81–92, Mar.–Apr. 1981.

in any of the samples failed. Organochlorine concentrations were not significantly different in the blood of breast- and bottle-fed infants. Differences in organochlorine levels in blood between mothers who had "slimmed" and those who had not were small, but there were few of the former in the study. From 12 to 21% of the estimated daily intake of dieldrin and 36 to 61% of the intake of DDT by mothers may be eliminated by lactation. The placenta appears to limit the transmission of pesticides to the fetus to some extent. Concentrations of organochlorine in fetal blood were very low.

Breast-feeding appears not to result in higher organochlorine concentrations in infant blood compared to bottle-feeding. The presence of organochlorine pesticides in meconium indicates that these compounds are transferred to the fetus either via the placenta or by ingestion of amniotic fluid, but transfer appears to be limited by the placenta. Concentrations in umbilical cord blood and infants' blood are lower than those in prenatal maternal blood.

▶ [Environmental pollution by pesticides and other chemicals is of great contemporary concern, much of it focused on pregnancy and lactation. This study reports levels of seven organochlorine pesticides, measured with a sensitive analytic technique in maternal and cord blood, placenta, and milk. Comparisons of maternal and cord blood indicate that the fetus enjoys partial protection, with fetal levels 10% to 50% less than those of the mother. Appreciable amounts of some compounds were found in breast milk—in the case of DDT it was estimated that half or more of maternal intake could be eliminated by the breast—but breast-fed babies had no higher blood levels than bottle-fed infants.] ◀

1–21 **High Hemoglobin Levels During Pregnancy and Fetal Risk.** Oddmund Koller, Roar Sandvei, and Norvald Sagen (Univ. of Bergen) investigated the association between unusually high hemoglobin (Hb) levels during pregnancy and fetal disorders in a series of 24 apparently uncomplicated pregnancies with small for dates newborn at or below the tenth percentile. Fifteen of these 24 women had Hb levels 2 SD above the mean value of normal distribution in late pregnancy. Among these, there was only 1 case of intrauterine death of unknown cause.

Two additional series with late abortion or premature delivery were collected from 1975 to 1979, one with 15 cases of intrauterine fetal death of unknown cause prior to labor and one with 16 cases in which the fetus had been alive until labor started. The mothers had not been treated with diuretics, but iron supplementation was routinely given to all pregnant women in the area; however, there is no certainty that these tablets were actually taken. In the series of 15 cases of intrauterine death of unknown cause, before start of labor 10 patients had Hb levels 2 SD above the mean, while in the series of 16 cases of late abortion where the fetus was alive until labor started, only 1 had a Hb level 2 SD above the mean. In 3 cases with serial Hb estimations, the levels were 2 SD above the mean 1 week or more before intrauterine fetal death. Two of these patients also had been observed during a successful pregnancy in which Hb levels were within normal limits, lower by 2.9 gm/100 ml in 1 patient and by 3.2 gm/100 ml in the second.

(1–21) Int. J. Gynaecol. Obstet. 18:53–56, July–Aug. 1980.

A statistical correlation exists between increase of the Hb level and frequency of fetal growth retardation in pregnancies complicated with cyanotic congenital heart disease. In such cases, the raised Hb level is a compensatory phenomenon indicating the degree of hypoxia. Raised Hb levels frequently are found in severe preeclampsia, probably because of reduced plasma volume. The study suggests that high Hb levels per se during the second and third trimester may indicate fetal growth retardation and impending intrauterine fetal death. In one third of cases in which weight of the newborn was at or below the tenth percentile, the Hb concentrations were within normal limits. The reason for this inconsistency might be a different pathogenetic mechanism responsible for the fetal growth retardation.

Decreased viscosity of the blood might be an advantage of the physiologic hemodilution during pregnancy, of importance for maintenance of the uteroplacental circulation. If this is so, a goal of prenatal care should be to prevent unnecessary increase of the Hb level and the hematocrit reading caused, for instance, by exhausting work and by uncritical use of diuretic drugs. The common practice of giving iron in pharmacologic doses to nonanemic pregnant women should be reevaluated because of the risk of inducing an unphysiologically high Hb level. This should not lead to the neglect of the diagnosis of iron-deficiency anemia. Considering the wide physiologic variation of hemodilution among individuals, estimation of the biochemical and morphological characteristics of the erythrocytes would probably provide a better approach to the diagnosis of pathologic anemia than any fixed set of limitations on Hb concentration. Unfortunately, we still lack practical methods of sufficient specificity.

▶ [Given the frequency of maternal anemia as a pregnancy complication, it is generally assumed with hemoglobin levels that the higher, the better. This report, however, notes an apparent association between high hemoglobin concentrations and growth retardation and death of the fetus. The authors seem to believe that the high hemoglobin level is primary and causal, citing such considerations as increased blood viscosity and interference with placental circulation. But couldn't this finding simply identify the patient whose plasma volume fails to expand normally? Low plasma volumes are known to accompany preeclampsia, and some investigators have even suggested that hypovolemia is a causal factor in toxemia; if so, this could explain the adverse fetal effects of a high hemoglobin level.] ◀

1–22 **Effects of Maternal Acetonuria and Low Pregnancy Weight Gain on Children's Psychomotor Development.** Using data from the study of the Collaborative Perinatal Project of the National Institute of Neurological and Communicative Disorders and Stroke, which prospectively followed 53,518 pregnancies, Richard L. Naeye and Ronald A. Chez (Pennsylvania State Univ., Hershey) analyzed the effects of maternal acetonuria, weight loss, and low weight gain during pregnancy on children's psychomotor development. Singleton infants born alive after 20 or more weeks of gestation were studied. Those with major congenital malformations, Down's syndrome, inborn errors of metabolism, head trauma during or after birth, and lead intoxication were excluded. Infants also were excluded if either parent was mentally retarded or the mother had hypothyroidism, convulsive disorder, diabetes mellitus, or alcoholism.

(1–22) Am. J. Obstet. Gynecol. 139:189–193, Jan. 15, 1981.

Gestational acetonuria, weight loss, or low weight gain showed no association with any consistent evidence of mental or motor impairment in offspring during the first year of life. When compared to children whose mothers had weight gains of 22–32 lb, 2 of the 7 tests at 4 years of age were failed more often by children whose mothers lost weight during pregnancy. Combining acetonuria with low weight gain or weight loss produced no consistent evidence of mental or motor impairment at any age. As independent variables, acetonuria, low weight gain, and pregnancy weight loss were not associated with abnormal intelligence quotient (IQ) values at 4 years of age.

The data were extracted from the same population used in the original study that claimed lowered IQ values in offspring resulted from maternal acetonuria. The present findings differ from those in the original study because a number of nonnutritional factors were controlled for that influence psychomotor development and IQ. After an overnight fast, maternal ketone body concentrations are about threefold greater in pregnant than in nonpregnant women; ketonuria often occurs in pregnant women. Expectant mothers have an increased dependence on fat stores for fuel during the second half of pregnancy, with enhanced ketogenesis. Ketones, which are transferred across the placenta, probably represent a normal fuel for the human fetal brain, particularly during late gestations.

▶ [This important study challenges current obstetric teaching. While previous reports indicated that maternal acetonuria during pregnancy was associated with impaired mental performance by the offspring, the present study doesn't demonstrate an adverse effect. Futhermore, weight loss or low maternal weight gains during pregnancy were not associated with lower IQ values of the offspring at age 4 years. The interpretation of these results is hampered by the fact that the studied pregnancies occurred 20 years ago. At the time, low maternal weight gain during pregnancy was encouraged. It may not be right to extrapolate weight gain from an earlier time when weight gain was restricted to today, when the emphasis is just the opposite. Just how *necessary* an "adequate" maternal weight gain by today's standards is remains unresolved.] ◀

2. Medical Complications of Pregnancy

2–1 **Pregnancy and Diabetes: A Survey.** In the diabetes center for pregnant women at Rigshospital, Copenhagen, the principles of management have been aimed at the unspecific but intensive treatment of the diabetic metabolism of pregnancy, its complications, and complications in the newborn. These principles include centralization of management; collaboration among diabetologists, obstetricians, and neonatologists; classification of pregnancy; compensation of the diabetic metabolism; and prophylaxis and treatment of complications. Lars Mølsted-Pedersen presents the results of a survey of some problems of pregnancy complicated by diabetes.

Among 1,885 infants born to diabetic mothers between 1946 and 1978, the perinatal mortality rate fell from 22.1% in 1946 to 1955 to 4.4% in 1976 to 1978. This decline was not attributable to a change in the distribution of the White classifications. When analyzed by White classification and the presence or absence of prognostically bad signs in pregnancy (PBSP), a marked increase in mortality was observed with increasing severity of maternal factors and complications (White classes), irrespective of the PBSP classification. A significantly higher rate of mortality was also observed when PBSP were present in White's classes A, B, C, and D. Congenital malformations accounted for at least 50% of the perinatal deaths.

The frequency of congenital malformations was 3 times as high among diabetic patients compared with control patients. Fetal malformation rate was significantly higher when maternal vascular complications were present. It was found that infants of mothers whose diabetes outside pregnancy was managed at hospitals specializing in the treatment and ambulatory control of diabetes had a markedly lower rate of major congenital malformations than those whose mothers were managed elsewhere (5.6% and 12.2%, respectively). This suggests that poor diabetic control of nonpregnant patients may be teratogenic in the event of pregnancy.

▶ [This paper is interesting because it summarizes the changing concepts of diabetic pregnancy and the resultant improvements in outcome over the professional lifetime of the author. It corresponds almost exactly with the historic review prepared by Steven Gabbe as a special article in the 1980 YEAR BOOK. Perinatal mortality has fallen from 20% or more to 4%. Outcome is improved by attention to the principles of rigid metabolic control. The major remaining problem is malformation, accounting for half of perinatal losses, and there is the suggestion—at this point little more than a suggestion—that tight control periconceptionally may reduce this high incidence.] ◀

2–2 **Elevated Maternal Hemoglobin A_{1c} in Early Pregnancy And Major Congenital Anomalies in Infants of Diabetic Mothers.** Major congenital anomalies are the most important cause of death in

---

(2–1) Acta Endocrinol. [Suppl. 238] (Copenh.) 94:13–19,1980.
(2–2) N. Engl. J. Med. 304:1331–1334, May 28, 1981.

infants of diabetic mothers. These anomalies develop during the first 8 weeks of gestations. Until recently, there has been no objective method to assess retrospectively the control of diabetes during this phase of embryogenesis. Measurement of hemoglobin A_{1c} (HbA_{1c}) has been shown to provide an integrated, retrospective index of glucose control, which reflects the mean blood glucose concentrations during the 4- to 8-week period prior to its measurement. Edith Miller, John W. Hare, John P. Cloherty, Peter J. Dunn, Ray E. Gleason, J. Stuart Soeldner, and John L. Kitzmiller (Brigham and Women's Hosp., Boston) retrospectively studied the relation of the control of diabetes in early pregnancy to the incidence of major congenital anomalies in 116 pregnancies. All 116 women were insulin-dependent diabetics and all had initial HbA_{1c} measurements performed before week 14 of gestation.

Fifteen (13%) of the women were delivered of infants with major congenital anomalies. These included 8 infants with congenital heart defects, 3 of whom died, and 4 infants with malformations of the brain, 3 of whom died. The mean initial HbA_{1c} level was significantly ($P < .01$) higher in those women whose infants had major anomalies than in those giving birth to infants without anomalies (HbA_{1c}, 9.5% $\pm$ 1.0% and 8.4% $\pm$ 1.6%, respectively). Maternal age and sex of the infants did not influence the incidence of anomalies. The gestational age at which the initial HbA_{1c} measurement was made was later in those infants who had major anomalies, but this difference did not bias the HbA_{1c} comparisons. Mothers who had initial HbA_{1c} values less than or equal to 8.5% had a significantly ($P < .01$) lower incidence of infants with major congenital anomalies than those mothers whose initial HbA_{1c} values were greater than 8.5% (table). In the 58 women with an initial HbA_{1c} value greater than 8.5%, the presence of microangiopathy was not associated with a significantly higher incidence of major anomalies in their offspring when compared with the incidence on women without microangiopathy.

The results show that poorly controlled diabetes mellitus in early

DISTRIBUTION OF INITIAL MATERNAL HEMOGLOBIN A_{1c} (HbA_{1c}) VALUES IN RELATION TO INCIDENCE OF MAJOR CONGENITAL ANOMALIES

Group	HbA_{1c} Before 14 Weeks of Gestation	No. with No Anomalies	No. with Major Congenital Anomalies *		Total No. of Subjects
	%				
1	≤6.9	19	0 (0)	} 3.4	19
2	7.0–8.5	37	2 (5.1)		39
3	8.6–9.9	27	8 (22.9)	} 22.4	35
4	≥10.0	18	5 (21.7)		23
All subjects	—	101	15		116

*Chi-square = 8.91 and $P <.01$ for the comparison of groups 1 and 2 versus groups 3 and 4. Figures in parentheses and to the right of brackets denote percentages.

pregnancy is associated with an increased risk of major structural malformations in the offspring.

▶ [With the decrease in perinatal mortality and other complications of diabetes mellitus-associated pregnancy, ascribed in part to rigid blood glucose control, congenital anomalies in infants of diabetic mothers have assumed a greater relative importance. The suggestion has been made previously that the increased tendency for mothers with diabetes to deliver babies with anomalies may be related to abnormal blood glucose levels in early gestation. If so, then rigid periconceptional blood glucose control in diabetic women attempting pregnancy would be indicated. Although this suggestion requires prospective investigation, the present retrospective study of HbA_{1c} levels in early pregnancy (which would generally reflect glucose control during the period of organogenesis) is consistent with this view. When given the chance, we should probably pay the sort of attention to blood sugar levels and insulin dosages in the diabetic patient attempting pregnancy that we would if she presented to us for care during pregnancy.] ◀

2–3 **Pregnancy and Diabetic Retinopathy.** Diabetic retinopathy can be expected in women aged 20–30 years who developed diabetes when they were aged 5–15 years. Glen Paul Johnston (Washington Univ.) retrospectively studied 30 pregnant diabetic patients (35 pregnancies) with juvenile-onset diabetes and a similar group of 30 nonpregnant patients. Xenon photocoagulation was performed under retrobulbar anesthesia in most cases, and Argon laser coagulation was performed as supplementary therapy in a few cases. Treatment was as frequent and extensive as the eye condition warranted. Two patients in each group had pituitary ablation as initial therapy.

The nonpregnant women had retinopathy similar to that in the pregnant group, suggesting duration of diabetes is more important in determining severity of ocular problems than presence or absence of pregnancy. There were no adverse effects on pregnancies in patients treated with photocoagulation; 21 patients gave birth to live infants. Most eyes not treated with photocoagulation before pregnancy deteriorated in visual acuity and grade of classification and were treated during pregnancy. Some eyes treated before pregnancy also deteriorated, but generally to a lesser degree.

Six of 8 patients with background retinopathy in both eyes experienced deterioration to proliferative changes during pregnancy. In patients with background retinopathy in one eye, 15 of 21 eyes progressed to proliferative retinopathy during pregnancy; of the 6 that did not, 5 had been treated previously with photocoagulation. The data indicate an extremely poor prognosis for background retinopathy during pregnancy, but cannot be used to assess the frequency of conversion from background to proliferative retinopathy during pregnancy since all cases were selected for referral.

Of 24 eyes that had photocoagulation for proliferative retinopathy before pregnancy, 7 (29%) deteriorated during pregnancy. Of 30 not treated before pregnancy, 26 (87%) deteriorated. Of the 49 eyes with proliferative retinopathy, 33 (67%) deteriorated during pregnancy; of 26 treated with photocoagulation (7 were considered too far advanced for treatment), 22 (85%) were considered successes on the basis of elimination of neovascular tissue and stabilization of vision.

(2–3) Am. J. Ophthalmol. 90:519–524, October 1980.

Of the 27 patients with proliferative retinopathy, only 3 became blind during or immediately after pregnancy most patients have useful visual acuities. The final visual outcome was essentially the same in women who had interrupted pregnancies as in those who went to full term. In the nonpregnant group, of 8 patients with background retinopathy in both eyes initially, 4 developed proliferative retinopathy in both eyes within 3 years and required photocoagulation. In 3 patients with background retinopathy in one eye and proliferative retinopathy in the other, the background retinopathy deteriorated to proliferative retinopathy within 18 months. Twenty-five patients (47 eyes) had proliferative retinopathy when first examined. All but 2 (who had pituitary ablation surgery) were treated with photocoagulation; 24 patients (80%) retained visual acuities of 6/12 (20/40) or better.

A woman with juvenile-onset diabetes who wishes to become pregnant should do so as early as possible. Evaluation for diabetic retinopathy is necessary; if present, it should be treated before pregnancy. If proliferative retinopathy develops during pregnancy, it should be treated with photocoagulation. Proliferative retinopathy is not an absolute indication for therapeutic abortion. However, it is a serious threat to the mother and a probable cause of morbidity to mother and child and can be considered strong grounds for therapeutic abortion if the prospective mother does not have an intense desire for a child.

▶ [This retrospective analysis of a relatively large number of patients with diabetic retinopathy in pregnancy attests to the value of photocoagulation therapy. Pregnancy per se did not clearly have an adverse effect, although the selection biases inherent in the referral of these patients for care make it difficult to draw firm conclusions. Diabetic retinopathy is not a good thing, as it generally means longstanding diabetes and diffuse vascular disease; however, its presence does not constitute an absolute indication for therapeutic abortion.] ◀

2–4 **Detection of Gestational Diabetes by Means of Ultrasonic Diagnosis of Excessive Fetal Growth.** Hélène Grandjean, Marie-France Sarramon, Jacques de Mouzon, Jean-Michel Reme, and Georges Pontonnier (Toulouse, France) performed an oral glucose tolerance test after the 32d week of pregnancy in 113 women without known diabetes. Of these, 92 met one or more criteria for potential diabetes (diabetes in the close family, obesity, previous child with birth weight over 4,500 gm or unexplained stillbirth, fasting glycosuria, or hydramnios) and 21 had no indications of potential diabetes but had an ultrasonic study showing fetal abdominal transverse diameter to be greater than the 95th percentile.

Abnormal glucose tolerance test results were found in 13 (14%) of the 92 potentially diabetic women and in 8 (38%) of the 21 women with large for date fetuses. An abnormal test was found in 11% of women with a fetal abdominal transverse diameter below the 95th percentile and in 36% of women with this diameter above the 95th percentile. Of the 21 women with abnormal glucose tolerance, 57% had fetal abdominal transverse diameters above the 95th percentile,

(2–4) Am. J. Obstet. Gynecol. 138:790–792, Dec. 1, 1980.

while only 28.5% had fetal biparietal diameters above the 95th percentile.

All infants but 1 were healthy at birth and during the first 6 days. One fetus died 2 days before birth; the mother was obese and had hypertension and normal glucose tolerance. Among the 21 infants of mothers with gestational diabetes, 3 had a birth weight above the 90th percentile and only 1 of these was above the 95th. Mean birth weight of these infants was 3,460 gm and mean duration of gestation was 38.2 weeks (all gestational diabetics had been on restricted diets).

Excessive abdominal transverse fetal diameter is a sensitive indicator of patients with gestational diabetes.

▶ [Several recent reports have called attention to ultrasound measurement of the fetal abdomen in early detection of macrosomia in fetuses of diabetics. This study represents the other side of the coin—detection of diabetes as a result of identifying excessive fetal abdominal growth. Among 21 women with fetuses of 32 weeks or more with abdominal diameters above the 95th percentile, 8 (38%) had diabetic glucose tolerance tests. This yield was significantly higher than that of 14% among 92 women screened because of conventional criteria (family history, obesity, previous macrosomic infant, stillbirth, glucosuria, or hydramnios).] ◀

2–5 **Increased Erythropoiesis and Elevated Erythropoietin in Infants Born to Diabetic Mothers and in Hyperinsulinemic Rhesus Fetuses.** The pathogenesis of the increased erythrocytosis and extramedullary erythropoiesis observed in infants of diabetic mothers (IDMs) has been obscure. In these studies, John A. Widness, John B. Susa, Joseph F. Garcia, Don B. Singer, Prabhat Sehgal, William Oh, Robert Schwartz, and Herbert C. Schwartz found IDM to have elevated umbilical plasma erythropoietin (Ep) concentrations by radioimmunoassay; 22 of 61 nonasphyxiated IDMs (36%) had levels (> 69 mU/ml) above the range of 28 nonasphyxiated, appropriately grown normal infants.

The 3 IDMs with the highest Ep values (6,200–30,000 mU/ml) were not only from the maternal groups with the most severe diabetes; there was no relationship observed between plasma Ep levels and maternal insulin therapy or vascular disease. In 16 control subjects and 20 IDMs, plasma Ep levels correlated directly with plasma insulin levels ($P < .001$, $r = 0.73$). In 31 IDMs who had umbilical blood gases measured at delivery, positive correlations were observed for Ep concentration and ΔP_{O_2} ($P_{uv}O_2 - P_{ua}O_2$) and ΔP_{CO_2}. However, no relationship between umbilical arterial P_{O_2} and Ep level was observed. There was no correlation between plasma Ep and total erythrocyte, nucleated erythrocyte, or reticulocyte counts. The IDMs with elevated Ep values had significantly higher birth weight-to-placental weight ratios than IDMs with normal Ep levels.

A rhesus monkey model with continuous fetal hyperinsulinemia for 21 days in utero in the last third of pregnancy was studied; all mothers were nondiabetic. In 5 experimental fetuses, plasma insulin levels averaged 4,210 µU/ml at delivery (in controls 29–64 µU/ml); plasma Ep levels in hyperinsulinemic fetuses were above the range of 6 con-

(2–5) J. Clin. Invest. 67:637–642, March 1981.

trol monkeys. Arterial plasma glucose levels were lower in the hyperinsulinemic group, but simultaneously obtained umbilical venous glucose values did not differ between groups. Plasma glucagon levels in the hyperinsulinemic group were lower than in control monkeys. The experimental fetuses had elevated reticulocyte counts in umbilical cord blood, but the erythrocyte count was no different between groups. There was no difference in umbilical arterial or venous blood gases (Po_2, Pco_2, or pH) between groups.

The data are most consistent with a secondary effect of fetal hyperinsulinemia on both Ep levels and erythropoiesis. This effect may be related to an increase in cellular proliferation and metabolism resulting in increased oxygen consumption. The fetus, being in a relatively hypoxic state compared with the adult, may be more sensitive to changes in its internal environment.

▶ [Infants of diabetic mothers tend to be polycythemic, an effect previously thought to result from chronic intrauterine hypoxia. This study indicates that it more likely reflects direct stimulation of erythropoietin by insulin. In human studies, cord blood erythropoietin levels were higher in diabetics than in normal subjects (both with normal Apgar scores) and, moreover, correlated positively with insulin levels. In an experiment hyperinsulinemic monkey fetus model developed by this investigative group, erythropoietin levels greatly exceeded those in control fetuses. Thus, it appears that another effect can be added to the long list of consequences of fetal hyperinsulinism.] ◀

2–6 **Follow-up of Children of Diabetic Mothers.** Mary Cummins and Mary Norrish present results of a follow-up study of infants of 51 diabetic mothers who attended the combined antenatal and diabetic clinic at Hammersmith Hospital, London, and delivered 73 infants (one set of twins) of more than 24 weeks' gestation between 1964 and 1972. There were no intrauterine deaths. In 58 pregnancies the mothers required insulin; 1 mother required chlorpropamide. In the other 13 pregnancies, mothers controlled their diabetes with diet alone. Complications of pregnancy included retinopathy (8 patients), renal involvement (1), and severe neuropathy (1). There were 5 deaths from hyaline membrane disease and 2 deaths caused by lethal congenital abnormalities. Sixty-six children survived the neonatal period; there were 3 later deaths. Of the 63 surviving children, 51 were traced in 1977. A medical and developmental history was obtained from the parents. Psychologic assessment (Wechsler Intelligence Scale for children for those aged 6 years or older and the Wechsler Preschool and Primary School Scale of Intelligence for those younger than age 6) was carried out, together with general and neurologic examination, urinalysis, and growth measurements.

Full-scale IQ scores were distributed normally. All but 2 children attend schools for normal children. One child with an IQ below 70 at age $4\frac{1}{2}$ years had delayed speech, poor concentration, and hyperactivity. There was no significant difference between the IQ of children hypoglycemic at birth and those who were not hypoglycemic. The major abnormalities noted at follow-up were severe deafness in 1 child, myopia (1 child), low IQ and hyperactivity (1 child), and epilepsy and

(2–6) Arch. Dis. Child. 55:259–264, April 1980.

urinary infection (1 child). These 4 children had normal neonatal periods without hypoglycemia or other complications. The distribution of height and head circumference centiles was near normal, but one fifth of the children had skinfolds greater than the 90th centile, with very few less than the 10th centile. Obesity correlated well with maternal obesity but not with birth weight.

Lethal congenital malformations remain a serious problem for the infant of the diabetic mother. Congenital malformations were responsible for 20% of the neonatal deaths in this series and 1 of 3 postneonatal deaths. Although there is a greater tendency toward the development of diabetes in children of diabetic mothers, no children in this series have become overtly diabetic, nor have any siblings. The handicaps found at follow-up apparently did not relate to maternal diabetes.

▶ [This report provides long-term follow-up data on children aged 5–13 years born to diabetic women. Generally, the outcome of surviving children does not seem to have been affected by maternal diabetes. Of particular interest is neuropsychological development; mean IQ was 97.5 and school performance appears similar to that of the general population. Previous studies have related intellectual impairment to maternal acetonuria and neonatal hypoglycemia, neither of which was particularly common in this series. There was a suggestion of an increased tendency to childhood obesity in this series, which could be due to influences during diabetic pregnancy but more likely reflects growing up in a household with an overweight mother. For a further consideration of the obesity question, read on.] ◀

2–7 **Somatic Growth of Children of Diabetic Mothers With Reference to Birth Size.** It has been hypothesized that maternal hyperglycemia may cause fetal hyperglycemia and hyperinsulinism, resulting in increased birth size and subsequent macrosomia. Betty R. Vohr, Lewis P. Lipsitt, and William Oh studied the effects of maternal diabetes on the growth of offspring in 52 diabetic women who were enrolled prenatally in the Providence, Rhode Island, cohort of the Perinatal Collaborative Study. There were 12 perinatal deaths, and 6 mothers were lost to follow-up. Of the other 34 diabetic mothers, 6 were insulin dependent, 6 had chemical diabetes, 13 had gestational diabetes, and 9 were classified as suspect. Sequential follow-up evaluations were carried out at 4 months, 1 year, 4 years, and 7 years.

In both diabetic and control subjects a positive correlation was observed between weight before pregnancy, weight gain during pregnancy, and the neonatal weight-height index. At the 7-year follow-up evaluation, 8 of 19 children whose mothers were diabetic and whose size was large for gestation at birth were obese, whereas only 1 of 14 infants whose size was appropriate for gestation at birth were obese.

The results suggest that macrosomia in the neonates of diabetic mothers may predispose toward obesity later in life.

▶ [These findings that infants large for gestational age born to diabetic women are at risk for childhood obesity can be interpreted as indicating that formation of excessive numbers of fat cells during fetal life "programmed" the individual to later fatness. On the other hand, factors in the social environment might be involved in that fat parents tend to overfeed their children. The relative weight of biologic and social influences in the causation of obesity are unknown.] ◀

(2–7) J. Pediatr. 97:196–199, August 1980.

2–8 Successful Outcome of Pregnancy in Women With Hypothyroidism. Pregnancy in women with hypothyroidism is rare, and the literature contains little clear-cut data about the effects of hypothyroidism on fertility, pregnancy, and the offspring. Martin Montoro, Joseph V. Collea, S. Douglas Frasier, and Jorge H. Mestman (Univ. of Southern California) cared for 9 hypothyroid women during 11 pregnancies in 1975–1979.

The women were aged 22–41 years (mean, 29) at conception. Initial evaluation occurred at 8–10 weeks' gestation in 4 pregnancies and at 24–30 weeks in the other 7. The causes of hypothyroidism were thyroidectomy in 3 women, post-^{131}I therapy in 1, Hashimoto's thyroiditis in 2, and idiopathic primary thyroidism in 3. Three patients were asymptomatic, 3 had some symptoms, and 3 had most of the classic symptoms of hypothyroidism. Two cases were first diagnosed during pregnancy. In the others, the diagnosis was known previously but the patients had failed to take their thyroid replacement medication for at least 6 to 8 months before conception. Three patients received no treatment during pregnancy and the others were given 0.15–0.30 mg of L-thyroxine daily. At the initial evaluation, mean serum thyroxine value was 2.3 µg/dl, triiodothyronin was 82 ng/dl, resin triiodothyronine uptake ratio was 0.64, and thyroid-stimulating hormone was 105 mU/ml.

Two deliveries were by cesarean section. There was 1 stillborn infant in the only patient with preeclampsia. Another infant, born to a woman aged 41 years had Down's syndrome and an ostium primum defect. All placentas were normal. All infants were clinically euthyroid at birth, and thyroid function was normal in the 5 infants in whom it was studied. None had goiter. The 7 infants who were followed for up to 2.7 years showed normal thyroid function and somatic development.

Although these 9 women had a prevalence of symptoms and signs of hypothyroidism that was similar to that reported for nonpregnant hypothyroid patients, all were able to conceive and sustain their pregnancies despite hypothyroidism, and the pregnancy outcome was good (90% live born, only 1 infant with anomalies). Thus, conception, embryogenesis, and early fetal development occurred in the absence of significant amounts of maternal thyroid hormone. This agrees with studies showing that the fetal hypothalamic-pituitary-thyroid axis develops and functions independent of maternal thyroid status, and that the fetus does not need maternal thyroid hormone for support. Untreated hypothyroid women should not be discouraged from carrying their pregnancies to term solely because of hypothyroidism.

▶ [Although questions concerning the effects of maternal hypothyroidism on the fetus frequently arise, solid information from the literature is sparse in this area. The present report is generally reassuring, although longer follow-up of the children (e.g., school performance) would be helpful. The early development of the fetal thyroid gland and the lack of significant transplacental passage of thyroid hormone apparently account for the normal outcome despite maternal thyroid insufficiency. A different situation may pertain in regions of severe endemic goiter (see the 1980 YEAR BOOK, pp. 30–31).] ◀

(2–8) Ann. Intern. Med. 94:31–34, January 1981.

2–9 **Neonatal Thyroid Function After Propylthiouracil Therapy for Maternal Graves' Disease.** Propylthiouracil (PTU) is a mainstay of medical treatment for hyperthyroidism during pregnancy. The drug inhibits thyroid-hormone synthesis, extrathyroidal conversion of thyroxine (T_4) to 3,5,3'-triiodothyronine (T_3), and deiodinative degradation of the hormonally inactive T_4 metabolite 3,3',5'-triiodothyronine (reverse T_3, rT_3). Propylthiouracil crosses the placenta, but doses of 300 mg or less daily are thought to control maternal hyperthyroidism without causing clinical neonatal thyroid dysfunction. Neonatal goiters occur with maternal PTU doses of 100–200 mg daily. An infant with fetal goiter and hypothyroidism whose mother was receiving 400 mg of PTU daily prompted Robert G. Cheron, Michael M. Kaplan, P. Reed Larsen, Herbert A. Selenkow, and John F. Crigler, Jr. (Harvard Med. School) to undertake a prospective study of thyroid function at birth, at 1 day of life, and at 3 days of life in infants of 11 hyperthyroid mothers treated with low doses of PTU (100–200 mg daily at term); 7 women also received thyroid-hormone supplementation as liotrix (Euthyroid).

Woman, 20, treated with 400 mg PTU daily for Graves' disease throughout pregnancy, underwent cesarean delivery at 38 weeks' gestation for cephalopelvic disproportion and polyhydramnios. The 2,730-gm male infant was apneic with a pulse of 80 and required assisted ventilation for 20 minutes. The thyroid was enlarged (each lobe, 3.5 by 2 cm). Generalized muscular hypotonia was present, but deep tendon reflexes, skeletal maturation, epiphyseal architecture, and serum bilirubin level were normal. Respiratory distress developed. Tests showed that the mother was euthyroid at delivery, but the infant had a markedly low serum T_4 level and an elevated level of thyroid-stimulating hormone (TSH). These abnormalities resolved in 5 days, and the goiter disappeared within 2 weeks without thyroid hormone therapy.

Serum T_4, TSH, and rT_3 levels, as well as mean free-T_4 index, were normal for those pregnant women studied prospectively. Weights of the babies were normal; they were clinically well except for 1 with choanal atresia and 1 with transient jaundice. None had a goiter. The mean cord serum T_4 value and free-T_4 index were lower than in controls. The serum T_4 concentration in the PTU group rose slightly after 1 day and was further increased at 3 days, but was significantly lower than the control mean at 1 and 3 days. The mean cord serum concentration of TSH in infants of mothers taking PTU was not different from normal values, but there was a pronounced rise at 1 day to 2.5 times the normal mean. The mean serum TSH value at 3 days was normal. The serum T_3 concentration in the PTU group did not differ from control values. There was no definite abnormality in the 3-day serum rT_3 value in the PTU group, but there was a decrease, rather than the normal increase, at 1 day. There was no significant correlation between maternal and cord serum free T_4 indexes, or between PTU dose and cord serum free T_4 index. There was no apparent difference in measurements between neonates whose mothers received liotrix and those whose mothers did not.

These infants, though clinically euthyroid, had biochemical evi-

---

(2–9) N. Engl. J. Med. 304:525–528, Feb. 26, 1981.

dence of mild, transient hypothyroidism, presumably due to maternal PTU therapy. The results emphasize the importance of using the smallest possible PTU dose to treat hyperthyroidism in pregnancy, and of evaluating the neonate for hyperthyroidism and hypothyroidism. Supplementation with liotrix in pregnant women appears not to prevent neonatal hypothyroxinemia.

▶ [Although the baby may appear to be perfectly normal, this study indicates that the neonate delivered of a mother treated with PTU is transiently, mildly hypothyroxinemic. This was true whether or not the mother had concomitantly received thyroid hormone. The authors reemphasize the point that the lowest possible dose of PTU should be used in treating hyperthyroid pregnant women.] ◀

2–10 Pregnancy Complicated by Maternal Heart Disease at the National Maternity Hospital, Dublin, Ireland, 1969 to 1978. Heart disease is the leading cause of indirect maternal death in Ireland, Great Britain, and parts of the United States. Declan Sugrue, Sean Blake, and Dermot MacDonald reviewed data on 387 pregnancies (295 patients) that were complicated by maternal heart disease.

The incidence was 0.5%; 323 (83.5%) were of rheumatic origin (distribution of dominant valve defects, Table 1) 52 (13.4%) were congenital (Table 2), and 12 (3.1%) were a miscellaneous group including cor pulmonale and coronary artery disease. Complications that could be attributed to heart disease occurred in 50 pregnancies: heart failure, 38 (11.8%, Table 3); paroxysmal supraventricular tachycardia, 2 (0.6%); pulmonary embolism, 2 (0.6%); and atrial fibrillation developing during pregnancy, 7 (2.2%). Four patients had chorea during pregnancy that persisted until after delivery despite treatment with phenobarbital, penicillin, and bed rest. The New York Heart Association (NYHA) grading was grade 1 in 39% of patients before onset of failure. Mitral valvotomy was performed at 20 to 21 weeks in 3 patients; ensuing pregnancies were uncomplicated. Three patients with prosthetic valves were treated with oral anticoagulant therapy until the 37th week. Heparin was then given intravenously by continuous infusion pump to keep whole blood clotting time 2 to 3 times normal. The infusion was stopped at onset of labor, and oral anticoagulant therapy was resumed 24 hours post partum. Two offspring were normal; weight of the third infant was less than the fifth percentile for gestational age.

One of the offspring in a patient with congenital heart disease had congenital heart disease. Five pregnancies (3 patients) were complicated by uncorrected cyanotic congenital heart disease. One of 2 maternal deaths was in such a patient on the ninth day post partum (autopsy revealed pulmonary hypertension and a 1.5-cm defect in the membranous portion of the ventricular septum, with no immediate cause of death found); another was from postpartum suicide, unrelated to mild rheumatic heart disease. Perinatal mortality was 3.3%; 3 neonatal deaths were caused by congenital heart disease. Prophylactic antibiotics were not used and infective endocarditis did not occur. Therapeutic abortion was not practiced and a conservative approach was adopted in obstetric intervention and drug therapy.

(2–10) Am. J. Obstet. Gynecol. 139:1–6, Jan. 1, 1981.

TABLE 1.—RHEUMATIC HEART DISEASE: DISTRIBUTION OF DOMINANT VALVE DEFECTS

	Patients		Pregnancies	
Dominant valve defect	No.	%	No.	%
Mitral stenosis:				
Pure	39	16.1	43	13.5
With mitral incompetence	78	32.2	106	33.1
Mitral incompetence	90	37.3	122	38.1
Aortic regurgitation	17	7.0	25	7.8
Aortic stenosis	18	7.4	24	7.5
Total	242	100	320	100

TABLE 2.—HEART FAILURE IN 38 PREGNANCIES COMPLICATED BY RHEUMATIC HEART DISEASE*

		Dominant valve lesion				Time of onset — Trimester				NYHA Class before the onset of failure			
Type of failure	No. of patients	MS	MI	AS	AI	First	Second	Third	Puerperium	U	II	III	IV
Pulmonary congestion	20	7	10	2	1	1	4	15	0	9	8	0	3
Acute pulmonary edema	9	4	3	2	2	1	0	3	5	5	3	0	1
Congestive failure	9	3	5	2	0	1	0	6	2	1	4	2	2

*MS indicates mitral stenosis; MI, mitral incompetence; AS, aortic stenosis; AI, aortic incompetence.

TABLE 3.—TYPE OF CONGENITAL HEART DISEASE COMPLICATING 52 PREGNANCIES (47 PATIENTS)

	Patients		Pregnancies		No. of pregnancies in patients with uncorrected defect
Heart lesion	No.	%	No.	%	
Atrial septal defect	18	38.2	14	26.9	4
Ventricular septal defect	6	12.9	8	15.4	7
Tetralogy of Fallot	6	12.8	7	13.5	0
Coarctation of the aorta	3	6.4	5	9.7	1
Pulmonary stenosis	3	6.4	4	7.6	4
Aortic stenosis	4	8.6	4	7.6	3
Patent ductus arteriosus	2	4.2	3	5.8	1
Eisenmenger complex	2	4.2	3	5.8	3
Total anomalous Pulmonary venous drainage and atrial septal defect	1	2.1	2	3.9	2
Congenital heart block	1	2.1	1	1.9	1
Dextrocardia and aortic stenosis	1	2.1	1	1.9	1

Most pregnancies complicated by heart disease are uneventful, with a favorable outcome for mother and fetus. Adequate daily rest and intense treatment of anemia and infection are essential. Cardiac failure is the most common cause of death. It can occur at any time during pregnancy or the puerperium. Sudden unpredictable changes in NYHA classes I to IV occur. The Eisenmenger syndrome is associated with a particularly high maternal mortality. Preeclamptic toxemia, present antenatally in the Eisenmenger-related death in this series, is associated with a sudden fall in systemic vascular resistance soon after delivery. Immediate replacement of blood loss, bed rest for symptomatic patients, and trial of supplemental oxygen are of value. In general, families should be completed with minimum delay following valvotomy. The teratogenicity of the coumarins is independent of timing of their administration. There is no evidence that long-established antibiotic regimens affect the frequency of endocarditis after high-risk procedures; routine antibiotic prophylaxis carries risks of drug toxicity and antibiotic-resistant endocarditis.

▶ [This is a thoroughly excellent review of cardiac disease in pregnancy. The outcome was excellent—only 1 pregnancy-related maternal death (in a patient with Eisenmenger's syndrome) and a perinatal loss rate of 3.3%. Heart failure was most likely to have its onset during the third trimester but could appear earlier in gestation or during the puerperium. We are somewhat surprised that during this time period (1969–1978) in Dublin most cases (83.5%) were of rheumatic origin. Our experience has been that congenital heart disease has become more common than rheumatic, at least among obstetric patients.] ◀

2–11 **Successful Pregnancies in Women Treated by Dialysis and Kidney Transplantation.** The Registration Committee of the European Dialysis and Transplant Association (St. Thomas' Hosp., London) analyzed findings from successful pregnancies in women undergoing dialysis or renal transplantation. The data were gathered from 67 centers in 19 countries. Table 1 presents findings in 124 children born in Europe and 2 born in Israel to dialysis and transplant patients. The 97 transplant recipients gave birth to 110 babies, including 4 pairs of twins and 1 set of triplets, 5 patients with 2 children, and 1 patient with 3 children. Pregnancy was reported more commonly among recipients of living-donor than cadaveric renal grafts. The mean time between date of transplantation and birth of the first child was 3.3 years (range, 6 months to 10 years). One patient was pregnant at the time of transplantation. Four of the 16 babies born to women undergoing dialysis were conceived before that treatment was started. The remaining 12 pregnancies were completed after a mean of 2.2 years of dialysis.

No abnormalities were noted in offspring of mothers having dialysis; however, abnormalities were recorded in 7 of the children born to mothers with transplants, including 1 pair of twins (Table 2). The transplant patients who gave birth to the children described in Table 2 were taking a significantly higher daily dose of azathioprine than those who had normal children, but there was no significant difference in the daily dose of prednisone between the two groups. About 25% of the mothers took hypotensive drugs, and management of hypertension appears to have been especially difficult in those undergoing dialysis. Additional hematinics and supportive blood transfusions were often required for the dialysis patients. Urinary tract

TABLE 1.—CHILDREN BORN TO DIALYSIS AND TRANSPLANT PATIENTS

Mode of treatment	No. of normal children	No. of abnormal children	Birth weight (kg)		Male:female ratio	Duration of pregnancy (weeks)	
			Mean	Range		Mean	Range
Transplantation	103	7	2·5	0·9–3·9	44:53	35·6	24–43
Dialysis	16	0	1·9	0·8–2·5	5:3	33·2	25–42

(2–11) Br. J. Obstet. Gynaecol. 87:839–845, October 1980.

TABLE 2.—ABNORMALITIES NOTED AT BIRTH IN
CHILDREN OF TRANSPLANT RECIPIENTS

Congenital abnormality

1	Plagiocephaly with neurological damage
2	Congenital heart disease (mild mitral regurgitation)
3	Bilateral pes equinovarus
4 ⎫ twins	Cerebral palsy (frontal haemangioma)
5 ⎭	Cerebral haemorrhage (died 2 days post partum)
6	Hypospadias
7	Congentital cytomegalovirus infection

infections occurred in 17% of patients with transplants, and 4% had pyelitis of pregnancy. Four mothers had complications of pregnancy attributable to immunosuppression: 2 had cholestatic jaundice, a third had thrombocytopenia, and the fourth had a burst abdomen after cesarean section. There was a high incidence of cesarean section in both groups. Dialysis time generally was increased as pregnancy progressed (18 hours per week, mean).

Changes in transplant function occurred. An increased glomerular filtration rate was documented in 3 patients, but in others this was not measured. Eight patients had a slight decline in renal function that did not progress after delivery, but 2 patients experienced a progressive, inexorable decline in renal function. In 1 patient, frank nephrotic syndrome developed and in another, hemolytic uremic syndrome leading to transplant nephrectomy. Two patients experienced acute rejection episodes after delivery.

Management of pregnancies in women with transplants required attention to blood pressure control, anemia, bone disease, and urinary tract infections. The data suggest that the risk of modest doses of azathioprine taken by patients with stable renal function may not be excessive for the fetus. The size of babies born to mothers with transplants and mothers undergoing dialysis was below average, and mean duration of pregnancy was shortened substantially. Of great concern are the changes in transplant function that occurred: 21 patients had evidence of damage to their transplants.

▶ [This review of pregnancies associated with renal dialysis or transplantation, based on 126 live births from 19 western European countries, is an excellent "state of the art" summary. It covers all the important issues of clinical outcome—maternal complications such as hypertension, anemia, altered calcium homeostasis, and urinary tract infection (all increased), congenital malformation (probably not affected), course of renal function (some tendency to deterioration in 20%), manner of delivery (50–50, vaginal vs. cesarean). Our feeling has been—and still is—that pregnancy generally is contraindicated in a patient with end-stage renal disease. Perhaps this may be an overly conservative attitude for, as indicated by this review, a substantial portion of transplant patients seem to get through pregnancy without permanent damage to themselves and with a living normal infant. Not addressed, however, is the issue of long-term prognosis for the woman.] ◀

2–12 Plasma Infusion for Thrombotic Thrombocytopenic Purpura During Pregnancy. Brian K. Walker, Samir K. Ballas, and Jose Martinez describe the development of thrombotic thrombocytopenic purpura (TTP) in a woman aged 26 in the 28th week of pregnancy. Plasma infusions allowed adequate fetal gestation and subsequent survival of both mother and fetus. Symptoms which began 1 week prior to admission, included occipital headaches, transient paresthesias of the arms and legs, and episodes of diplopia. There were petechiae and purpura of the legs, abdomen, and breasts. The patient displayed the classic features of TTP: thrombocytopenia, microangiopathic hemolytic anemia, neurologic signs, and renal dysfunction.

A number of therapeutic approaches were required before resolution of the disease was achieved. Initial treatment with corticosteroids and antiplatelet agents produced no apparent benefit. Exchange transfusion achieved a transient remission, but subsequent relapse responded poorly to a repetition of this procedure. A partial response was attained with long-term administration of plasma infusions, allowing the fetus to reach maturity. Full resolution of the disorder finally was accomplished with simultaneous splenectomy and cesarean section.

The cause of TTP is unknown; however, the variable response to diverse therapeutic measures suggests a multifactorial pathogenesis for this disorder. There may be an immunologic basis for TTP, or it may involve primary defective platelet aggregation leading directly to the development of thrombotic lesions. Several therapeutic modalities have achieved moderate success in selected patients. The success of exchange transfusion and plasmapheresis suggests that removal of a toxic agent or factor might be crucial in the pathogenesis of TTP. The effectiveness of simple plasma infusion indicates the possible deficiency of a necessary plasma factor in these patients. In the patient described, TTP was refractory to prednisone, aspirin, dipyridamole, and sulfinpyrazone; at 25 days of hospitalization the platelet count was only 18,000/μl; the reticulocyte count was 15.2%, and the patient had persistent petechiae and mucosal bleeding. A transfusion regimen of 2 units of fresh frozen plasma every other day was initiated on the 26th hospital day, and the platelet count increased to 50,000/μl. The count was maintained until the 41st hospital day, when the patient underwent cesarean section and splenectomy. Postoperatively, the patient's platelet count was 78,000/μl; antiplatelet drugs were discontinued, and the prednisone dosage was tapered. By the 50th hospital day, the platelet count was 295,000/μl, and the hemoglobin level was 12.0 gm/dl. The patient remains in complete remission 16 months after discharge. The newborn infant had a normal platelet count. These findings suggest that failure of one or several therapeutic approaches in TTP should not discourage attempts at alternative treatment modalities.

▶ [We, too, have seen plasma infusion ameliorate this unusual, but very serious, condition. In our case, the mother survived but the fetus did not. Following delivery, the patient went into a complete remission.] ◀

(2–12) Arch. Intern. Med. 140:981–983, July 1980.

2–13 **Automated Erythrocytopheresis for Sickle Cell Anemia During Pregnancy.** Prophylactic partial exchange transfusion in pregnant women with sickle hemoglobinopathies improves maternal and fetal outcomes, but manual exchange of whole blood phlebotomized from the patient with packed, washed erythrocytes is time-consuming, tedious, technically cumbersome, and requires hospitalization of at least 48 hours. Thomas C. Key, Edgar O. Horger III, Ernest M. Walker, Jr., and Ernestine N. Mitchum (Med. Univ. of South Carolina) used automated erythrocytopheresis in the prophylactic exchange transfusion in 8 pregnant women with sickle hemoglobinopathies.

Automated erythrocytopheresis can be performed on outpatients in as little as $1^{1}/_{2}$ hours. It allows for selective removal of erythrocytes from whole blood by means of extracorporeal centrifugation and separation. Remaining cellular and liquid fractions are returned to the patient, along with donor erythrocytes. Supertransfusion with use of plasmapheresis and simultaneous direct transfusion of erythrocytes increases the hematocrit while maintaining stable intravascular volume.

Of the 8 women treated, 7 were homozygous for hemoglobin (Hb) S and 1 was heterozygous for both Hb S and Hb C. Initial erythrocytopheresis was performed at 17 to 30 weeks of gestation, which was soon after prenatal care began. Two patients initially treated at 17 and 18 weeks' gestation required additional exchanges 7 and 13 weeks later because the hematocrit or Hb A concentration fell below 25%.

Hematocrit was increased significantly by 7 of the 10 procedures, and all patients experienced significant increases in Hb A concentrations to at least 50%. There were no adverse reactions during the procedure. Delivery has occurred in 5 of the 8 pregnancies, all of which went to term uninterrupted for maternal or fetal indications. The infants weighed 3,015 to 3,171 gm, had 5-minute Apgar scores of 7 to 10, enjoyed normal hospital courses, and were discharged with their mothers. One pregnancy was associated with light meconium staining during spontaneous labor at 41 weeks' gestation, and 1 patient had mild puerperal endometritis after vaginal delivery.

Automated erythrocytopheresis is useful in the management of gravid patients with sickle hemoglobinopathies.

▶ [This is an interesting new adjunct to exchange transfusion as used in pregnant women with sickle cell anemia. The technique involves the separation (by centrifugation) of erythrocytes from withdrawn blood so they may be discarded. The patient's plasma, leukocytes, and platelets are returned to her, along with donor erythrocytes containing hemoglobin A.] ◀

2–14 **Iron Studies in Pregnant and Nonpregnant Women with Hemoglobin SS or SC Disease.** O. A. Oluboyede (Univ. Hosp., Ibadan, Nigeria) studied the iron status of 40 women with sickle cell disease in clinical steady state. Of the 22 pregnant women (most in the second trimester), 10 had hemoglobin SS and 12 had hemoglobin SC. Of

(2–13) Am. J. Obstet. Gynecol. 138:731–737, Dec. 1, 1980.
(2–14) Br. J. Obstet. Gynaecol. 87:989, November 1980.

the 18 nonpregnant women, 12 had hemoglobin SS and 6 had hemoglobin SC. All women were taking 5 mg of folic acid and 100 mg of paludrine daily. None had had blood transfusion, none was taking oral iron, and none had evidence of infective, aplastic, or hemolytic crisis.

Mean packed cell volume and hemoglobin level were lower in hemoglobin SS than in hemoglobin SC patients in both the pregnant and nonpregnant groups. Transferrin saturation was lower in pregnant than in nonpregnant women. Serum ferritin values in hemoglobin SS and SC pregnant women were not significantly different. There was a strong correlation between serum ferritin levels and transferrin saturation in the pregnant group. Bone marrow showed scanty or no iron in 14 (63%) of the 22 pregnant women and in 9 (50%) of the 18 nonpregnant women; serum ferritin levels increased progressively with greater amount of hemosiderin in bone marrow.

Thus, evidence of iron deficiency was found in both pregnant and nonpregnant women with hemoglobinopathies. It may be necessary to give oral iron as well as folate and antimalarial drugs to women with sickle cell hemoglobins.

▶ [Because of the hemolysis that occurs in patients with sickle cell anemia, some have suggested that these patients should not be supplemented routinely with iron during pregnancy. Iron deficiency was common in these Nigerian women with sickle hemoglobinopathies, however. Of note, the pregnant patients had not received blood transfusions or iron therapy previously.

Whether or not to prescribe iron for pregnant patients with this problem should be considered on an individual basis. The transfusion history and serum ferritin levels and transferrin saturation will be of help in the decision-making process.] ◀

2-15 **Incidence and Severity of Viral Hepatitis in Pregnancy.** Mohammad Sultan Khuroo, Mohammed Ramzan Teli, Susan Skidmore, Mohammad Amin Soft, and Mohammad Ismail Khuroo carried out a prospective field study during an epidemic of non-A, non-B hepatitis in the Kashmir valley in India (1978) of pregnant women, non-pregnant women of childbearing age, and men 15–45 years old.

In 36 (17.3%) of 208 pregnant women, viral hepatitis developed, as compared with 71 (2.1%) of 3,350 nonpregnant women and 107 (2.8%) of 3,822 men; this was a significantly higher incidence in pregnant women. The incidence in all trimesters (table) was higher than in nonpregnant women. The significantly increased incidence of fulminant hepatitis in pregnancy (8 pregnant women, 22.2%) was indicative of a greater severity of hepatitis during pregnancy. Increased susceptibility to fulminant hepatitis was observed exclusively in the last trimester (fulminant rate, 44.4%). Nonfulminant viral hepatitis did not influence the course of pregnancy or fetal well-being. Fulminant hepatitis resulted in 3 premature deliveries, with 1 neonatal death; 5 patients died during the illness, with the fetus undelivered.

In this common source, water-borne type of epidemic, all groups were exposed equally to the same viral agent, and the higher incidence of hepatitis in pregnant women could only be related to host factors rather than those of the virus. Recent studies have shown that hepatitis viruses (especially hepatitis B) do not behave as cytopathic

(2–15) Am. J. Med. 70:252–255, February 1981.

INCIDENCE OF FULMINANT RATES OF ICTERIC VIRAL
HEPATITIS IN PREGNANT WOMEN, NONPREGNANT
WOMEN, AND MEN

	No.	Viral Hepatitis (no.)	
		Total	Fulminant
Men (15–45 yr old)	3,822	107 (2.8)	3 (2.8)*
Nonpregnant women (15–45 yr old)	2,350	71 (2.1)	0
Pregnant women			
1st trimester	34	3 (8.8)	0
2nd trimester	77	15 (19.4)	0
3rd trimester	97	18 (18.6)	9 (44.4)†

Note: Figures in parentheses are percentages.
*Three fatal cases of hepatitis.
†Six fatal cases of hepatitis.

agents in man. Liver disease is mainly a result of the immunologic response of the host to the virus. It is believed that this holds true for non-B infection, and the increased severity of viral hepatitis in pregnant women could possibly be the result of enhanced immune response to the virus. There was no evidence of malnutrition in pregnant women, as assessed by caloric and protein intake and serum albumin levels. It is believed that hormonal changes may have a role in the course of viral hepatitis in pregnancy. Conclusions on higher incidence of viral and fulminant hepatitis in pregnant women must be restricted to India, Africa, Iran, and the Middle East, where this has been reported. Reports from Europe and the United States have shown that the course of viral hepatitis in pregnancy is not different from that in nonpregnant women. Implications of this study are that during viral hepatitis epidemics, pregnant women in the second and third trimesters should receive appropriate prophylactic preparations of immunoglobulins from human sources; as viral hepatitis in the third trimester is associated with high maternal and fetal mortality, these patients need intensive inpatient care.

▶ [The effect of pregnancy on the course of viral hepatitis is unclear. Many reports from developing countries have indicated an adverse effect (see 1978 YEAR BOOK, pp. 52–53), whereas most reports from Europe and the United States have suggested that pregnancy doesn't influence the course of the disease. Potential bias related to the identification of cases has been a problem in most studies. The comprehensive field study of an epidemic of non-A, non-B hepatitis reported above is valuable, as *every* house in the area was visited several times. Despite adequate diets, pregnant women had higher incidences of both hepatitis and fulminant hepatitis than did men or nonpregnant women.] ◀

2–16 **Transmission of Hepatitis B Antigens From Symptom-Free Carrier Mothers to the Fetus and the Infant.** Hepatitis B surface antigen (HBsAg) is the outer lipoprotein coat of the hepatitis B virus and is known to be a marker of infection. Recently, it has been reported that the presence of hepatitis B-associated e antigen (HBeAg) in serum and the titer of HBsAg in the mother are related to the transmission of HBsAg to the newborn. Vivian C. W. Wong, A. K. Y.

(2–16) Br. J. Obstet. Gynaecol. 87:958–965, November 1980.

Lee, and Henrietta M. H. Ip (Univ. of Hong Kong) prospectively studied maternofetal transmission of hepatitis B virus in 97 symptom free carriers of HBsAg.

Of the 97 carriers, 47 had HBeAg present. Hepatitis B surface antigen was detected in about 25% of the amniotic fluid and 33% of the cord blood samples. In contrast, 96% of the vaginal fluid samples and 90% of the gastric aspirates from the neonates contained HBsAg. Ten infants acquired HBsAg during the first month of life, another 38 by the third month, and 12 more by the fifth month. At the end of the first year, 7 more infants had acquired HBsAg, while 19 remained HBsAg negative. The longer the duration of labor, the greater the prevalence of HBsAg in cord blood. There was a positive correlation between the presence of HBsAg in cord blood and maternal HBsAg titers greater than 1:2,560. An even stronger association was observed between maternal HBeAg and HBsAg in cord blood. The presence of HBeAg in maternal blood was strongly associated with the acquisition of HBsAg by the infants at 3 and 5 months (table). Amniocentesis did not influence the incidence of HBsAg in cord blood or in 1-month-old infants. Considering only those with HBsAg in maternal blood, the presence of HBsAg in amniotic fluid was associated with the acquisition of HBsAg in 1-month-old infants. Hepatitis B surface antigen in the gastric aspirate of infants was associated with the acquisition of HBsAg at 3 months of age but not at 1 month.

It is believed that the 10 infants positive for HBsAg at age 1 month represented cases of intrauterine infection, while as many as 40% of the infants may have acquired HBsAg during labor or by swallowing infective fluid during delivery. It is recommended that in women with HBeAg cesarean section delivery be performed and amniocentesis and breast-feeding be discouraged.

▶ [Vertical transmission of hepatitis B from a chronic carrier mother to her offspring is more common in the Chinese than in other ethnic groups (1979 YEAR BOOK, pp. 195–196). In this study from Hong Kong, the presence of HBeAg was again associated with infectivity. The authors' opinion is that infection can be transmitted antepartum, intrapartum (most frequently), or post partum. Intrapartum transmission was related to the length of labor. Because 90% of neonatal gastric aspirates were positive for HBsAg, the authors conclude that the swallowing of infected fluid during delivery may be the mechanism.

RELATION BETWEEN HBeAg IN MATERNAL SERUM AND HBsAg IN SERUM OF BABIES
AT AGES 3 AND 5 MONTHS

	Maternal blood HBeAg		
	Present	Not present	Total
Babies at three months			
HBsAg present	39	9	48
HBsAg not present	7	35	42
Total	46	44	90 (p <0·0001)
Babies at five months			
HBsAg present	37	10	47
HBsAg not present	1	29	30
Total	38	39	77 (p <0·0001)

The practical application of this clinical investigation is problematic, especially in non-Oriental populations. More knowledge is required before screening for HBsAg is accepted as an obstetric routine in the United States. Perinatal management in the face of acute hepatitis B infection during pregnancy (as opposed to the asymptomatic chronic carrier state considered above) focuses on determination of the HBsAg status of the newborn. If the newborn is antigen negative, hepatitis B immune globulin is indicated.] ◄

2–17   **Acute Liver Disease With Encephalopathy and Renal Failure in Late Pregnancy and the Early Puerperium: A Study of Fourteen Patients.** Although rare, severe acute hepatocellular dysfunction during the third trimester of pregnancy may have fatal results for both mother and fetus. M. H. Davies, S. P. Wilkinson, M. A. Hanid, B. Portmann, J. M. Brudenell, J. R. Newton, and R. Williams (King's College Hosp., London) describe the findings in 14 patients, aged 18 to 38 years, who presented in the third trimester of pregnancy or immediately post partum with severe acute hepatic dysfunction. All but 1 patient also had renal failure.

The patients were divided into four subgroups on the basis of hepatic dysfunction diagnosis: acute fatty liver, presumed viral hepatitis, preeclampsia, and gram-negative septicemia (table). There was one set of twins. Three of 14 mothers (21%) and 5 of 15 infants (33%) died. In the patients with acute fatty liver, the predominant presenting symptoms were anorexia and malaise with abdominal pain and vomiting. Jaundice became apparent 1 to 3 weeks after the onset of illness, followed by encephalopathy and renal failure. Two of these patients subsequently had successful pregnancies without evidence of hepatic dysfunction. Of the 5 patients with presumed viral hepatitis, 4 had a prodrome of anorexia, malaise, and vomiting, 3 had pruritus, and 2 had epigastric pain. Three of these patients showed deterioration with increasing jaundice and development of progressive encephalopathy after delivery. Thrombocytopenia associated with other hematologic disorders consistent with diffuse intravascular coagulation was present in 5 patients. The 2 patients with liver damage associated with preeclampsia also had had preeclampsia in their previous pregnancies. Laboratory findings confirmed severe acute hepatocellular damage with markedly increased serum aspartate aminotransferase levels. One of these patients developed grade IV encephalopathy in the postpartum period and required dialysis for associated renal failure.

Abdominal pain with recurrent vomiting was the most common symptom in all etiologic groups. The occurrence of renal failure in all but 1 patient with acute fatty liver or acute hepatitis (11 patients) is a markedly higher frequency than that seen in nonpregnant patients with fulminant hepatic failure. The extent of renal failure and the rapid improvement in encephalopathy following dialysis in some patients suggests that uremia was a factor in the development of encephalopathy. It is recommended that if there is no evidence of impaired placental function and if the general condition of the affected mother is reasonable, labor should be induced. However, cesarean

(2–17) Br. J. Obstet. Gynaecol. 87:1005–1014, November 1980.

MATERNAL AND FETAL MORTALITIES

Diagnosis	No. of patients	Maternal deaths	Fetal deaths
Acute fatty liver	6	1	4*
Presumed viral hepatitis	5	1	1
Pre-eclampsia	2	1	1
Gram-negative septicaemia	1	0	0
Total	14	3 (21%)	5/15 (33%)

*One set of twins.

section is recommended if there are signs of fetal distress of a failure to progress, with or without a deterioration in the condition of the mother.

▶ [The poor maternal and perinatal outcomes associated with severe hepatic dysfunction in late pregnancy are underscored in this report. It may not be easy clinically to distinguish acute fatty liver of pregnancy from preeclampsia. Hypoglycemia suggests the former. Although firm evidence is lacking, in our view prompt delivery usually is indicated in the ill woman with acute liver failure in late pregnancy.

As has been reported previously, survivors of acute fatty liver of pregnancy may sail through a subsequent gestation without difficulty. Anxiety levels must be high, though, for both patient and obstetrician.] ◀

2–18 **Pregnancy in Inflammatory Bowel Disease: Effect of Sulfasalazine and Corticosteroids on Fetal Outcome.** Michael Mogadam, William O. Dobbins III, Burton I. Korelitz, and Susan W. Ahmed mailed 440-item questionnaires to 2,040 gastroenterologists in the United States to collect data regarding the effect of inflammatory bowel disease on pregnancy and the effect of drugs used to treat the disease on pregnancy. The 976 questionnaires returned provided adequate data on 531 pregnancies in women with inflammatory bowel disease. During pregnancy, 287 women (172 with ulcerative colitis and 115 with Crohn's disease) were treated with steroids of sulfasalazine, or both, and 244 women (137 with ulcerative colitis and 107 with Crohn's disease) did not receive either drug.

The 244 untreated women gave birth to 245 infants. In no instance was birth weight under 2,500 gm. There was 1 premature infant, 2 spontaneous abortions, 1 stillbirth, and 1 infant with a developmental defect. The 287 treated women gave birth to 288 infants. In this group there were only 3 infants of low birth weight, 4 premature infants, 6 spontaneous abortions, 3 stillbirths, and 3 infants with developmental defects. Thus, the frequency of fetal complications was significantly lower in both treated and untreated patients than in the general pregnant population.

Results in ulcerative colitis patients receiving either or both drugs did not differ significantly from those in the entire untreated group. Women with severe Crohn's disease who were treated with steroids or both drugs experienced more complications than untreated pa-

(2–18) Gastroenterology 80:72–76, January 1981.

tients, whereas those receiving sulfasalazine had no more complications than untreated patients.

Inflammatory bowel disease, except for severe active Crohn's disease, does not seem to affect the outcome of concurrent pregnancy adversely. The use of corticosteroids and sulfasalazine during a pregnancy associated with ulcerative colitis is unlikely to increase fetal morbidity or mortality. Women with severe Crohn's disease requiring corticosteroids or both drugs have more complications than patients with untreated disease, but still fewer than the prevailing rates in the general pregnant population. The higher complication rate may be associated more with disease-related than with drug-related factors. In the management of inflammatory bowel disease associated with pregnancy, either or both drugs may be used, just as in nonpregnant patients.

▶ [Although this questionnaire study involving gastroenterologists has obvious limitations, the reported findings generally are reassuring. In inflammatory bowel disease, as in so many other conditions, the right treatment for the nonpregnant patient is the right one for the pregnant patient as well.

In contrast to earlier impressions, sulfasalazine is absorbed to a significant extent and appreciable levels are found in cord serum (1981 YEAR BOOK, pp. 187–188).] ◀

2–19   **Cystic Fibrosis and Pregnancy: National Survey** of 119 cystic fibrosis (CF) centers in the United States and Canada was made by Lawrence F. Cohen, Paul A. di Sant'Agnese, and Jacquelyn Friedlander (Natl. Inst. of Health). The survey identified 129 pregnancies in 100 women with CF. Mean age at pregnancy was 20.7 years (range, 17–32), which is similar to that of normal women. Mean age at diagnosis of CF was 11 years, compared with a mean age of $3^{1}/_{2}$ years for all CF patients.

Of the 129 pregnancies, 97 (75%) were completed, 6 (5%) ended in spontaneous abortion, and 25 (19%) ended in therapeutic abortion. Death within 24 months of delivery occurred in 18% of the women, a mortality rate not exceeding that for all CF women of the same age. The women who died soon after delivery had moderate to severe pulmonary disease before pregnancy, with exacerbation of it during pregnancy. Perinatal death and shortened gestation were also significantly associated with maternal death within 2 years of delivery.

Congestive heart failure complicated 13% of the pregnancies. Maternal weight gain was less than 4.5 kg in 41% of the women; this greatly exceeds the expected rate of 7%. Antibiotics were required to manage pulmonary disease in 65% of the women, and aminoglycosides were given to half of these. Of the 97 completed pregnancies, 86 (89%) resulted in viable infants, a rate that differs significantly from the expected rate of 97.8%. Of the 86 viable infants, only 1 (0.8%) had CF, which confirms the recessive nature of the transmission of CF. None had congenital anomalies. The pregnancies lasted less than 37 weeks in 26.8% of the women, compared with an expected rate of about 6.5%. The 11.3% perinatal death rate was significantly greater than the 3% rate reported in unselected pregnancies. Of the 11 perinatal deaths, 10 were in pregnancies that lasted less than 37 weeks.

(2–19) Lancet 2:842–844, Oct. 18, 1980.

Cyanosis and dyspnea were each associated with increased maternal and perinatal mortality. There were no significant correlations between age at diagnosis of CF or interval between diagnosis and pregnancy, and maternal or perinatal outcome.

Pregnancy normally causes increased respiratory and cardiac work and hypervolemia, and these may be a serious threat to women with CF if they already have significant pulmonary disease. Thus, pregnancy should be avoided if the Schwachman or Taussig clinical score is below 80, indicating serious pulmonary disease. If this advice is not followed, antibiotics may be necessary; if so, penicillin or its derivatives are less toxic than aminoglycosides. The mother should consider the impact of her shortened life span on her child, the fact that reduced exercise tolerance with progressive disease may prevent her from caring for her child, and the fact that her risk of having a child with CF is 1 in 40, compared with 1 in 1,500–2,000 in the general population.

▶ [This review highlights the adverse effects of cystic fibrosis on pregnancy and of pregnancy on cystic fibrosis. Mortality rates, both perinatal and maternal, were high. Forty-one percent of patients gained less than 10 lb during gestation. Serious pulmonary disease prior to conception predicted poor outcome. We recently cared for a gravida with cystic fibrosis; pregnancy was completed and a living infant resulted, but the mother died 3 months post partum.

This problem is becoming more frequent as more cystic fibrosis patients survive into adulthood. At present, it seems that pregnancy is relatively contraindicated.] ◀

2–20 **Herpes Gestationis and Bullous Pemphigoid: A Disease Spectrum.** Herpes gestationis (HG) is a bullous disease of pregnancy and the puerperium that usually resolves itself within a few months after delivery. Direct immunofluorescence of involved skin has shown complement deposition at the basement membrane zone (BMZ) in most patients, with HG and IgG deposition in 50% of the patients. Several investigators have demonstrated a circulating anti-BMZ IgG in some patients with HG. R. Holmes, M. M. Black, D. M. Williamson, and R. W. B. Scutt report the clinical and immunologic features of a case of clinically active HG persisting in a woman for 8 years post partum and evolving into bullous pemphigoid. The patient also had Graves' disease, alopecia totalis, and ulcerative colitis.

Woman, 31, had presented in the last 3 weeks of her only pregnancy at age 23 with an intensely pruritic rash on the extensor surfaces of the arms and legs. Initially, urticated erythematous lesions similar to erythema multiforme were observed, followed by the development of widespread large bullae that were most prominent on the extremities (Fig 2–1). Despite treatment with prednisolone (50 mg/day), widespread bullae continued to develop, and cushingoid changes eventually resulted from steroid therapy. After 3 years, palmoplantar vesicles and lichenification became the predominant lesions, with only occasional bullae on the trunk. The clinical overlap of HG and bullous pemphigoid was paralleled by an immunologic overlap. Initially, both direct and indirect immunofluorescence failed to demonstrate IgG, although this was before C3 staining techniques were available. Direct immunofluorescence of samples obtained 5 years after the onset of the disease demonstrated IgG and C3 at the BMZ, and indirect immunofluorescence was positive at the BMZ for C3 (1:16) and IgG (1:640). Thus, the initial immunoflu-

(2–20) Br. J. Dermatol. 103:535–541, November 1980.

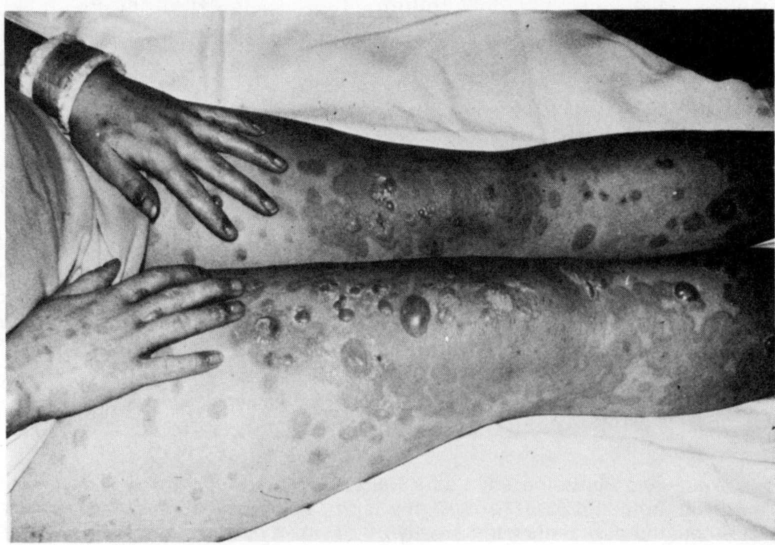

Fig 2−1.—Large blisters with urticated erythema on the legs and hands. (Courtesy of Holmes, R., et al.: Br. J. Dermatol. 103:535−541, November 1980.)

orescence findings were compatible with HG, while the later findings were suggestive of a transformation to bullous pemphigoid.

The findings suggest an autoimmune association of HG and bullous pemphigoid in this patient, which is underscored by the presence of Graves' disease, alopecia totalis, and ulcerative colitis.

▶ [Herpes gestationis, an autoimmune bullous disease of pregnancy and the puerperium, is apparently related to or a variant of bullous pemphigoid. This patient had evidence of multiple autoimmune disorders, including Graves' disease. Other patients with herpes gestationis who have subsequently developed hyperthyroidism have been described (*J. Am. Acad. Dermatol.* 3:474, 1980). Because of the autoimmune basis, plasma exchange may be of value, as indicated in the following article.] ◀

2−21 **Plasma Exchange in Herpes Gestationis.** Herpes gestationis (HG) is a vesiculobullous skin disease that occurs during 1/4,000 pregnancies and puerperium periods. It causes severe itching, usually starts during the second trimester, becomes exacerbated shortly after parturition, and may relapse when menstruation returns or oral contraceptive ingestion begins. Diagnosis is facilitated by finding deposits of C3 along the basement membrane of affected skin and by finding a specific HG factor in the serum (IgG) that can bind complement in the dermoepidermal transition area of normal skin. A. van de Wiel, H. Ch. Hart, J. Flinterman, J. A. M. Kerckhaert, J. A. du Boeuff, and J. W. Imhof (Amersfoort, The Netherlands) treated a patient who had severe HG by using plasma exchange, a treatment suggested by Carruthers and Ewins in 1978.

Woman, 40, had development of HG and severe pruritus in the 20th week of her fifth pregnancy. Her previous pregnancies were normal. The lesions, which included some large bullae, were mostly on the legs and abdomen.

Hypertension was also present. Immunofluorescent examination of biopsy specimens taken from peribullous areas showed C3c and IgG deposits along the basement membrane. Symptomatic treatment with antihistamines and pyridoxine was ineffective. Systemic treatment with corticosteroids was inadvisable in view of the hypertension. In three plasma exchanges carried out during the 26th week of pregnancy, a total of 8 L plasma was replaced with human albumin solution and Haemaccel. Within 24 hours of the first exchange the pruritus subsided significantly. No new lesions developed. After three exchanges the lesions had virtually disappeared, and C3c and IgG were no longer present in a skin biopsy specimen. Pruritus recurred and new skin lesions developed during the 37th week of pregnancy, when a healthy boy, without skin lesions and weighing 2,880 gm, was born. A very severe exacerbation occurred within the next 48 hours. Herpes gestationis factor was again found in maternal serum and in venous umbilical cord blood. After another plasma exchange, the pruritus, skin lesions, and HG factor rapidly disappeared. Four exchanges were made within a week and 12 L of plasma was replaced. A flare-up 3 weeks post partum necessitated two more exchanges.

▶ [Plasma exchange is being used with increasing frequency in certain conditions associated with autoantibodies. Although a report of a single case cannot prove anything, the repeated association temporally of plasma exchange and the amelioration of symptoms is certainly suggestive. This modality should be considered if the more traditional corticosteroid therapy is either contraindicated or ineffective. The appreciable perinatal risks associated with herpes gestationis were considered in the 1979 YEAR BOOK (pp. 72–73).] ◀

2–22 **Decidual Vasculopathy of Placenta in Lupus Erythematosus.** Carlos R. Abramowsky, Maria E. Vegas, Gary Swinehart, and Michael T. Gyves (Case Western Reserve Univ.) reviewed clinical histories and performed histologic and immunofluorescence studies of placentas from 10 patients with systemic lupus erythematosus (SLE) and 1 with discoid lupus (DLE). Four women were primigravidas and 7 were multigravidas. All 4 primigravidas remained clinically stable and delivered live babies; only 1 of the index pregnancies among multigravid women resulted in a live birth. Hypertension, nephritis, and preeclampsia appeared to be more frequent in the multigravid group. The degree of activity of SLE did not correlate with outcome.

On gross examination, 2 placentas had extensive infarcts, whereas others revealed only focal hemorrhages or areas of discoloration. Decidual vessels of 5 multigravida patients who lost fetuses during the index pregnancies showed lesions with fibrinoid necrosis with an associated mononuclear or polymorphonuclear inflammatory component. Vascular architectural disruption ranged from subintimal edema to marked necrotic dissolution of the wall. Infiltration of the vascular wall by cells with clear or foamy cytoplasm (atherosis) was noted (Fig 2–2). Other placental changes noted were infarction, premature aging of villi, and fetal obliterative vascular changes, interpreted as secondary to ischemic injury or fetal death.

Immunofluorescence studies in the 5 patients with decidual vasculopathy showed massive vascular deposits of IgM and a smaller amount of C3 in 2 of them, extensive decidual necrosis in 2 others,

(2–22) N. Engl. J. Med. 303:668–672, Sept. 18, 1980.

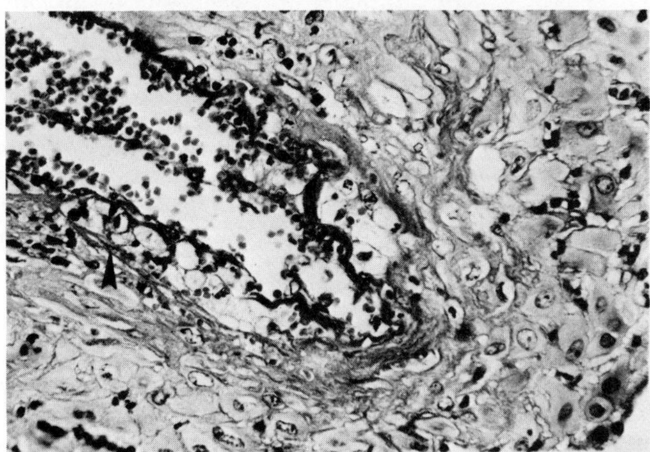

Fig 2–2.—Photomicrograph of placenta showing decidual vessel with early necrosis and infiltration by cells with foamy cytoplasm *(arrowhead)* as example of atherosis. Note darkly stained strands of fibrinoid material and separation of endothelial layers. Hematoxylin-eosin; original magnification ×320. (Courtesy of Abramowsky, C. R., et al.: N. Engl. J. Med. 303:668–672, Sept. 18, 1980.)

and vasculitis in the fifth patient. Four others had findings considered similar to those described in normal placentas.

The histologic lesions described in 5 patients are identical to those described in preeclampsia, severe diabetes, and maternal hypertension. Vascular lesions were associated with all of the fetal deaths in the series beyond the first trimester, and the lesions were not seen in any of the primigravidas. The onset of decidual vasculopathy is triggered by unknown factors that may be related to changes in the physical and chemical characteristics of the complexes, to alterations of the vascular substrate which becomes receptive to the putative complexes, or to a switch to IgM antibody production, with the heavier macroglobulin being more readily deposited in vessels. The consequent decidual vascular injury results in variable placental ischemia, leading to impaired placental development and function with either subsequent impairment of fetal growth or death. Although methods of tissue sampling may be implicated, the absence of lesions in some patients with reproductive failure suggests that alternative mechanisms of fetal damage may exist.

▶ [Relatively little has been written about placental pathology with SLE, which is surprising since SLE is an autoimmune disease and recent studies have noted antigen-antibody deposition in the fetus. This report notes that 5 of 10 placentas from SLE patients demonstrated changes in decidual vessels consisting of fibrinoid necrosis, vessel wall disruption, and "atherosis," illustrated in Figure 2–2. All 5 cases with this decidual vasculopathy had experienced pregnancy wastage (4 stillborns and 1 abortion), which surely suggests a correlation but whether it is cause-effect (and, if so, which is cause and which effect) or mere association is unclear. Immunofluorescence studies were less revealing; although some IgG, IgA, and IgM, along with C3 deposits were identified, their presence did not seem to correlate with the clinical course or outcome.] ◀

2-23 **Effect of Pregnancy on Idiopathic Scoliosis.** Walter P. Blount

(2–23)   J. Bone Joint Surg. [Am.] 62-A:1083–1087, October 1980.

and David D. Mellencamp (Med. College of Wisconsin, Milwaukee) followed 10 patients with idiopathic scoliosis through 19 pregnancies. There were 1 lumbar, 7 thoracic, and 2 double thoracic curves. All patients were treated with a Milwaukee brace. At the start of treatment the curves measured 33 to 74 degrees. A full standing anteroposterior roentgenogram of the spine was obtained prior to conception, soon after delivery, and 1 year later.

Three patients lost 2, 6, and 18 degrees of correction during their initial pregnancies, but the curves remained the same or improved with later pregnancies. The curves of the other 7 women, which had stabilized before conception, did not progress. Scoliosis stability was not related to patient age. Stable scoliotic curves did not progress with pregnancy in teenagers, whereas unstable scolioses progressed in patients older than age 20 years. The amount that the curve increased was not related to the initial size of the curve.

▶ [This study indicates that scoliosis does not progress during pregnancy if it has stabilized prior to conception, information that will be of value in counseling patients with the condition. Two additional aspects of scoliosis that may be of importance obstetrically are (1) the possibility of abnormalities of the pelvis, and (2) cardiac disease secondary to impaired pulmonary function with prolonged and severe kyphoscoliosis.] ◀

2–24 **Heparin-Induced Osteopenia in Pregnancy.** It has been suggested that heparin might be given throughout pregnancy as a therapeutic and prophylactic measure in patients at high risk for thromboembolism. P. H. Wise and A. J. Hall (Charing Cross Hosp., London) report a case of heparin-induced osteopenia in a woman who had taken the drug during pregnancy.

Woman, 38, who was 3 weeks post partum, presented with severe low back pain that had developed suddenly during the eighth month of pregnancy. She had been taking 10,000 units of heparin subcutaneously twice daily by self-administration throughout the pregnancy as a prophylaxis against thromboembolism. Radiologic studies revealed gross thoracolumbar osteoporosis with multiple vertebral compression fractures. The pain rapidly disappeared after heparin was discontinued. The patient was discharged on a regimen of supplemental calcium and physiotherapy.

This phenomenon may occur more often than is recognized clinically, and careful reevaluation of the indications for and the mode of administration of anticoagulants during pregnancy is warranted.

▶ [This case report demonstrates a hazard of long-term heparin anticoagulation during pregnancy noted in the 1980 YEAR BOOK (p. 72). There is no "ideal" regimen available for anticoagulation of the pregnant woman.] ◀

2–25 **Female Reproductive Potential After Treatment for Hodgkin's Disease.** Advances in the treatment of Hodgkin's disease have led to an expectation of long-term survival in more than 70% of cases. Sandra J. Horning, Richard T. Hoppe, Henry S. Kaplan, and Saul A. Rosenberg (Stanford Univ. Med. Center) assessed menstrual status and pregnancies in 103 women who were treated intensively for Hodgkin's disease by total lymphoid irradiation or combination chemotherapy, or both. The median age at the time of treatment was 23

(2–24) Br. Med. J. 281:110–111, July 12, 1980.
(2–25) N. Engl. J. Med. 304:1377–1382, June 4, 1981.

years, and the median interval after completion of treatment was 64 months. Nineteen women had received total lymphoid irradiation, 34 had received chemotherapy, and 50 had received both treatments. Pelvic irradiation was preceded by midline oophoropexy at staging laparotomy.

Nearly one third of the women were amenorrheic after treatment. The only factor significantly predictive of regular menses after treatment was age. Twenty patients conceived after the completion of treatment, while 26 had tried to conceive. However, many sexually active women had not used birth control methods because they assumed that they were sterile. Age at treatment and the presence of menses without menopausal symptoms were significantly related to pregnancies. The median time from treatment to conception was 42 months. The 28 pregnancies resulted in 21 normal live births, including 1 set of twins, 2 premature infants, and 1 infant of low birth weight. There were 5 elective therapeutic abortions. There were no birth defects or developmental abnormalities.

Changes in menstrual pattern and menopausal symptoms following the successful treatment of Hodgkin's disease are related directly to gonadal exposure and age at the time of treatment. Reproductive potential is reduced in women given both pelvic irradiation and combination chemotherapy compared with those given either treatment alone. Young women may retain or recover ovarian function and become pregnant after pelvic irradiation with oophoropexy or combination chemotherapy for Hodgkin's disease.

► [A report abstracted in the 1979 YEAR BOOK (p. 75) suggested that women who had been treated with both radiation therapy and chemotherapy for Hodgkin's disease were predisposed to have babies with congenital malformations. The findings in the current study don't support that view. Both series are small, and more information is needed to permit adequate counseling of such patients. One thing that is clear, however, is that amenorrhea and menopausal symptoms after such therapy, although they indicate ovarian "failure," don't necessarily mean that ovarian function is *permanently* lost. These patients subsequently may menstruate and conceive. Patients should understand this so that they can make informed decisions concerning contraception.] ◄

2–26 ***Chlamydia trachomatis* Infection in Mothers and Infants: Prospective Study.** *Chlamydia trachomatis* infection in males and females is now recognized as a prevalent venereally acquired disease, and genital infection in pregnant women can be expected to confer a risk of transmission of infection to infants at parturition. Alfred D. Heggie, Generosa G. Lumicao, Laurie A. Stuart, and Michael T. Gyves (Case Western Reserve Univ.) examined the occurrence of cervical *C. trachomatis* infection in pregnant women at a large urban hospital and the effect of maternal infection on the outcome of pregnancy. The population included 1,327 women at 8 to 12 or 35 to 37 weeks' gestation. Cervical cultures were obtained at both stages from 131 women.

Cervical infection with *C. trachomatis* was detected in 240 women (18%). Isolations were comparably frequent in the first and third trimesters. Genital gonococcal infection was nearly twice as frequent in *Chlamydia*-infected women as in matched controls. There were no

---

(2–26) Am. J. Dis. Child. 135:507–511, June 1981.

significant differences between these groups in premature births, stillbirths, neonatal deaths, spontaneous abortions, or congenital malformations. Mean birth weights and Apgar scores were similar in the two groups. Infection of the conjunctivas or nasopharynx was detected in 28% of the 95 infants followed after vaginal birth to mothers with chlamydial infection of the cervix. Other respiratory illness occurred in 27% of infected and 16% of uninfected infants.

Cervical infection by *C. trachomatis* was detected in 18% of this population of pregnant women, and transmission of infection to the infant was observed in 28% of cases. Nearly all infected infants will have conjunctivitis if not treated, and a smaller number will have chlamydial pneumonia. Three infected infants in this study had the latter. The effects of such infection on infants with other conditions such as cardiopulmonary disease are unclear.

▶ [A number of recent reports have indicated that chlamydial infections are a common, perhaps the most common, form of venereal disease. This represents a large study of the problem in pregnancy. *Chlamydia trachomatis* was isolated from cervical cultures of 18% of pregnant women, with no difference between early and late gestation. Transmission to the infants was demonstrated in 28% of cases of maternal infection, with most early isolations from the conjunctiva and most later ones from the nasopharynx. Conjunctivitis was the most common clinical problem, in 74% of infected infants, but was relatively benign. There was no apparent association with survival, birth weight, Apgar scores, or other index of pregnancy outcome.] ◀

2–27 **Development of Adverse Sequelae in Children Born With Subclinical Congenital *Toxoplasma* Infection.** Christopher B. Wilson, Jack S. Remington, Sergio Stagno, and David W. Reynolds followed 24 children born with subclinical congenital *Toxoplasma* infection. In 13 children (group 1) the diagnosis was made prospectively, 8 cases being detected as a result of routine screening of cord serum for IgM antibodies specific for *Toxoplasma* and 5 detected as a result of testing for IgG and IgM *Toxoplasma* antibodies. These 13 children were all less than 6 months of age at diagnosis (mean, 2 weeks) and in all, the infection would not have been detected without screening. In the other 11 children (group 2), the diagnosis was considered only after ophthalmologic or neurologic signs of congenital *Toxoplasma* infection developed. These 11 children were aged 17 to 52 weeks at diagnosis (mean, 34 weeks).

The 24 children were last examined at age 1 to 17 years (mean, 8½ years). All children in group 2 and 85% of those in group 1 had chorioretinitis. In group 1, unilateral blindness was present in 3 children (23%); in group 2, unilateral blindness was present in 3 (27%), bilateral blindness in 5 (45%). Severe, permanent neurologic sequelae developed in 1 child (8%) in group 1 and in 2 (18%) in group 2 after they initially presented with eye disease. Two children in each group were retarded (IQ range, 36–62). The 6 children in group 1 who were tested serially had lower IQ scores (mean change from 97 to 74) on repeated testing an average of 5½ years later. Less severe neurologic, intellectual, and audiologic deficits were seen in other children in each group. Only 2 children, both in group 1 and aged 8 to 10 years

(2–27) Pediatrics 66:767–774, November 1980.

at last examination, did not have untoward sequelae of their congenital infection.

Of the 24 children, 11 were never treated, 4 were treated only after adverse sequelae developed or were treated for less than 2 weeks, and 9 were treated for at least 3 weeks before the age of 1 year and before the development of neurologic or intellectual deficits. Treatment in all cases consisted of pyrimethamine and sulfadiazine or pyrimethamine and trisulfapyrimidines. Treated children tended to have fewer or less severe adverse sequelae. Of the 2 children without sequelae, 1 was treated and 1 was not.

Adverse sequelae develop in nearly all children with subclinical congenital *Toxoplasma* infection. The incidence of congenital *Toxoplasma* infection is reportedly 1 per 1,000 live births. Treatment is recommended when the diagnosis is established or, if certain indications are present, before it is established.

▶ [Congenital *Toxoplasma* infections are usually not clinically evident at birth but, as indicated by this long-term follow-up study, nearly always cause sequelae that become evident over the first 5 or 10 years of life. Ophthalmologic complications are most frequent, with chorioretinitis in about 90%. Neurologic sequelae occur in some 40%, but only about a fourth are major. Intelligence seems to be modestly depressed on the average, with significant retardation in 10% to 20%. The data suggest that treatment (pyrimethamine and sulfa) may have some beneficial effect on outcome.] ◀

2–28 **Obesity in Pregnancy: Risks and Outcome.** Obesity has been associated in the literature with other pregnancy risks such as hyper-

---

TABLE 1.—COMPARISONS OF OBESE AND NONOBESE PATIENTS FOR
LABOR ABNORMALITY AND INTRAPARTUM MANAGEMENT
(FREQUENCIES IN %)*

	Obese (N = 249)	Nonobese (N = 2371)
Labor abnormality		
Nulliparas	35.8	37.2
Multiparas	31.2	29.9
Dysfunctional labor patterns		
Prolonged latent phase	1.2	2.8
Protracted active phase dilatation	26.9	26.5
Secondary arrest of dilatation	4.4	5.3
Prolonged deceleration phase	0.8	1.3
Protracted descent	4.4	5.0
Arrest of descent	3.6	3.4
Labor durations		
Labor > 20 hours	4.4	5.9
Precipitous labor (< 3 hours)	7.2	8.1
Second stage > 2.5 hours	1.6	1.5
Labor and delivery management		
Oxytocin augmentation	20.3	20.8
Low forceps	8.0	10.0
Midforceps	1.7	1.5
Primary cesarean section	12.0	9.6

*There were no significant differences for any of these factors.

(2–28)   Obstet. Gynecol. 56:446–450, October 1980.

tension and diabetes mellitus, but disagreement persists about the expected course and complications of labor. Moreover, the effects of obesity on intrauterine growth and gestational duration have not been well defined. Thomas Gross, Robert J. Sokol, and Katherine C. King (Cleveland Metropolitan Genl. Hosp.) studied 2,746 consecutive deliveries using a computer-based uniform perinatal record to compare 300 pregnancy risk and outcome factors for obese and nonobese patients. The 279 obese women (i.e., those weighing over 90 kg at some time during pregnancy) were older and of higher parity than the 2,467 nonobese women. The obese patients were at increased antepartum risk and had increased frequencies of chronic hypertension, inadequate pregnancy weight gain, twin gestation, and diabetes mellitus.

Upon admission for delivery, obese patients were more likely to require medical induction of labor and to have been delivered previously by cesarean section. Comparisons of labor abnormalities among women who were not delivered by repeat cesarean section (Table 1) showed that dysfunctional labor patterns occurred with similar frequency in the two study groups; the need for oxytocin augmentation and incidence of primary cesarean section did not differ in the two groups. Maternal and fetal-infant complications in obese and nonobese groups are shown in Table 2. Trauma to the infant, Apgar scores, and perinatal mortality were similar in the two groups, but there were fewer infants of low birth weight (under 2,500 gm) and

TABLE 2.—MATERNAL AND FETAL-INFANT COMPLICATIONS
AND OUTCOME FOR THE OBESE AND NONOBESE GROUPS
(FREQUENCIES IN %*)

	Obese (N = 279 mothers and 284 infants)	Nonobese (N = 2467 mothers and 2481 infants)	P
Maternal complications			
Vaginal laceration, fourth degree	1.1	4.2	< .025
Postpartum hemorrhage	13.6	10.9	NS
Fetal–infant problems			
Meconium staining	21.8	17.8	NS
Breech presentation	3.0	3.3	NS
Intrapartum trauma	0.3	0.1	NS
Shoulder dystocia	1.1	1.0	NS
Low Apgar score (< 7)			
1 minute	19.6	16.5	NS
5 minutes	2.1	2.3	NS
Perinatal mortality	7.0	16.5	NS

NS = not significant.
*Except perinatal mortality, given as rate per 1,000 births.

more macrosomic babies (over 4,000 gm) born to the obese patients. The increase in birth weight was accounted for not only by an increase in the birth weight percentile, but also by a significant lengthening of the period of gestation.

The increased incidences of oxytocin induction of labor and repeat cesarean section may be related to the increased number of antepartum medical problems found in obese women on entering labor. A lack of increase in perinatal mortality in the obese group may be related to a lower incidence of preterm delivery and intrauterine growth retardation. The obese patient was half as likely to be delivered preterm, and 3.5 times more likely to be delivered post term, than the nonobese mother. The obese mother was half as likely to be delivered of an infant small for gestational age and 2.5 times more likely to be delivered of an infant large for gestational age. It appears that the obese patient is at less risk for labor complications than previously was believed. With careful antepartum and intrapartum management, these patients can be delivered vaginally of larger infants, who are less likely to be preterm or small for gestational age.

► [Obese patients fared as well in labor as did control patients in this study. Although dysfunctional labor patterns occurred with similar frequency in both groups, nulliparity was less common in obese patients. It would have been interesting to characterize the individual labor progress abnormalities by parity in comparing the two groups. We're not surprised that neonatal macrosomia was more common in the obese group, but we would have expected this to be reflected in more frequent shoulder dystocia. This was not the case.] ◄

3. Obstetric Complications

THE MANAGEMENT OF PROLONGED PREGNANCY

ALLAN B. WEINGOLD, M.D.

*Professor and Chairman, Department of Obstetrics and
Gynecology, George Washington University School of
Medicine and Health Sciences*

Introduction

The management of prolonged, or postdate, pregnancy remains an enigma, despite a focus of attention on this clinical situation for more than three decades. While it generally is agreed that it may be hazardous for the fetus to remain in utero beyond the time when maximal benefit from the placenta has been achieved, many authorities have disclaimed additional perinatal risk associated with otherwise uncomplicated prolonged pregnancy. The true postmature fetus in a prolonged pregnancy has reduced resistance for withstanding the stresses of labor or trauma during the birth process. The likelihood of fetal jeopardy is increased greatly by maternal complications that compromise uteroplacental blood flow. Criteria for defining the postmature fetus are relatively well established in the neonatal period. Identification of such affected infants before birth is more complicated. This paper will present a plan of management for prolonged pregnancy based on an assumption of enhanced fetal risk in a minority of such pregnancies while minimizing intervention for the majority of normal fetuses. The protocol is in operation at the George Washington University Hospital.

Definition of Terms

Pregnancy is considered prolonged when it exceeds 294 days calculated from the first day of the last menstrual period. The term "postdatism" is used interchangeably, but implies less certainty about the accuracy of the expected date of delivery. The chance that birth occurs on the expected date is 5%, within ±3 days of the due date it is 29%, within 2 weeks it is 80%. Prematurity occurs in 10% of pregnancies and prolonged pregnancy occurs in 10%. Thus, postdatism is a relatively common clinical problem. The true prolonged pregnancy is less frequent, and within this cohort is an even smaller group wherein the fetus is affected by postmaturity or dysmaturity.

Clifford[1] has described the classic features of postmaturity. They include failure of growth; dehydration; development of dry, cracked, wrinkled, and parchment-like skin (reduction of subcutaneous fat deposits); and thin arms and legs. The fingernails are long and there is advanced hardness of the skull. The skin evidences absence of vernix and lanugo hair with associated full scalp hair. Often there is skin maceration, particularly noted in the flexion folds and the external genital area. In the absence of vernix, the fetal skin loses its protection and the normal red skin color disappears. The skin may be stained brownish green or yellow, with similar discoloration of the umbilical cord and membranes. In postmature infants, the body length is increased in relation to weight; such newborn infants are alert and look almost apprehensive.

Some authors suggest that, despite this classic picture, there is minimal increased risk of perinatal loss and that the dangers of aggressive diagnosis and intervention exceed the observed benefits. Nevertheless, increased perinatal mortality rates have been reported in association with prolonged pregnancy since Clifford's description. Browne,[2] in review of more than 15,000 deliveries, observed that the perinatal mortality rate doubled by the 43d week and more than tripled at 44 weeks. The survey showed that the proportion of both antepartum and intrapartum stillborns increased steadily with lengthened gestation. His study and others stressed the importance of discriminating between the small, growth-retarded postterm fetus and the large, not-at-risk postterm fetus.

The distribution of perinatal mortality is approximately 30% before the onset of labor, 55% during labor, and 15% after birth. These figures attest to the fragility of affected fetuses and confirm the need for accurate identification and cautious labor management. Neonatal death generally is ascribed to respiratory distress secondary to meconium aspiration and to preexisting brain, heart, liver, and adrenal damage. In addition, significant postnatal morbidity occurs in some 20% to 25% of infants.

Demographic Data

The incidence of pregnancy extending beyond 42 weeks has been reported to be between 7.5% and 10%. Between 2% and 4% extend beyond 43 weeks. Many abnormally long gestations are due to delayed ovulation and subsequent fertilization. This is particularly true after recent use of the oral contraceptives with prolongation in the proliferative phase of the cycle. Stewart[3] has shown, utilizing basal temperature graphs, that nearly 70% of postterm pregnancies are a function of delayed ovulation. Unfortunately, the preceding spontaneous menstrual pattern is not associated statistically with prolonged pregnancy[4] even when cycle length is chronically increased (Table 1).

There is a slight tendency toward an increase in male fetuses carried significantly beyond term and a higher perinatal mortality rate in these fetuses (Table 2). The higher death rate of postterm male

TABLE 1.—MENSTRUAL HISTORY IN
PROLONGED PREGNANCY*

	CYCLE	LENGTH
	<25 da	>30 da
Control	9.2%	15.7%
Prolonged pregnancy	10.3%	13.2%

*Adapted from Beischer and Browne[4]

TABLE 2.—SEX-RELATED MORTALITY IN
PROLONGED PREGNANCY*

	MALE	FEMALE
Term	3.4	2.9
Prolonged pregnancy	4.8	3.2

*Adapted from Karn and Penrose.[5]

fetuses may be explained by their more rapid growth, through which they attain maximal placental capacity faster than female fetuses.[5]

There is an increased frequency of prolonged pregnancy and severity of fetal effects in primigravidas versus multigravidas (Table 3). This is particularly apparent from the 43d week of pregnancy onward with a doubling of risk at the 44th week.[6] There is also an increased frequency of dysmaturity with advancing maternal age (Table 4). This is true in both the primigravida and multigravida, but more so

TABLE 3.—GESTATIONAL AGE AND
PARITY IN PROLONGED PREGNANCY*

| | PNM% | |
WEEKS	PRIMIGR.	MULTIP.
39–41	1.4	1.6
42	1.5	1.5
43	2.5	1.6
44	3.5	2.0
45	6.5	3.5

*Adapted from McClure-Browne.[6]

TABLE 4.—MATERNAL AGE
AND PARITY IN PROLONGED
PREGNANCY*

| | PNM% | |
AGE	PRIMIGR.	MULTIP.
<25	1.7	1.4
25–29	2.1	1.4
30–34	2.8	1.9
>35	4.3	2.9

*Adapted from McClure-Browne[6]

in the former, thereby defining the elderly primigravida as a patient of significantly increased risk.

The congenital anomaly rate is increased twofold after the 43d week. The classic example of the anencephalic pregnancy in the absence of hydramnios extending to 300 days or more has been well documented. Even excluding the anticipated repetition of neural tube anomalies, recurrent postterm pregnancies are not uncommon. It is estimated that a woman who carries one pregnancy beyond term has a 50% chance for another postterm pregnancy.

Functional and Biochemical Expressions of Prolonged Pregnancy

Under normal circumstances, the peak of placental function is reached at 36 weeks' gestation, after which diminished rates of placental transfer of labeled sodium are indicative of a decrease in placental efficiency with aging. Accordingly, near term, placental transport processes gradually decline and placental and fetal growth rates are reduced while amniotic fluid volume decreases (Fig 3–1). Yet, various facets of the postmaturity syndrome are observed in no more than 25% of prolonged pregnancies. In the absence of placental insufficiency, 75% of fetuses carried beyond term do well and, in fact, large infants (4,000 gm or more) in good condition are born two to three times more often than in term pregnancies. The postterm fetal death rate is lowest in the average weight group of fetuses carried significantly beyond term. Fetuses who are exceptionally large (with the placenta relatively too small) or very small (small placenta per se) have the highest mortality rate. Placental insufficiency leading to the

Fig 3–1.—Fetal weight (gm), placental weight (gm), and amniotic fluid volume (cu cm) in late pregnancy and post term.

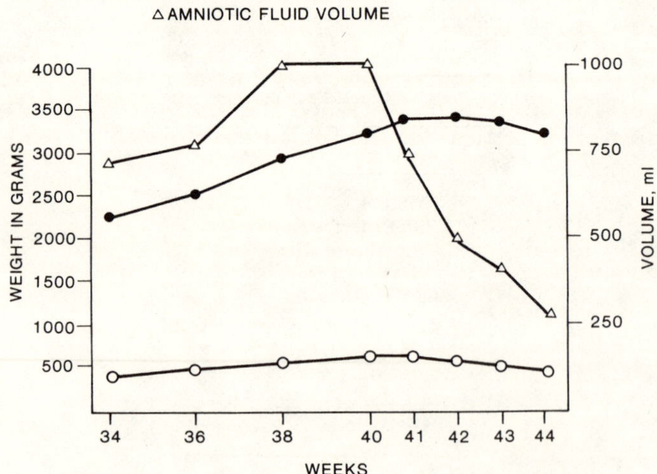

TABLE 5.—PLACENTAL INFARCTS (%) IN
PROLONGED PREGNANCY*

	TOTAL	RED	WHITE
Term	12	9	3
Dysmature postdate	66	20	46

*Adapted from Siegel and Rabanus.[7]

postmaturity syndrome has to be considered as an imbalance between placental capacity and fetal nutritive and respiratory demands.

The morphology of the postterm human placenta is also extremely variable. In the classic advanced case associated with dysmaturity, there is a decrease in placental thickness, a pronounced increase in white infarcts, fibrin deposition, and calcification (Table 5). The inter-villous space is noted to have a decrease in volume due to intervillous thrombosis and fibrin deposition.[7] The villae show absence of regener-ative efforts, stomal edema, hypovascularity, syncytial edema, in-creased syncytial knot formation, and arterial thrombosis with vas-cular hyalinization and degeneration.

The biochemistry of fetal postmaturity is as variable as the appear-ance of the neonates at birth: ranging from large, unaffected infants to those showing the full-blown syndrome and compromise, including fetal death. The minimal fetal oxygen needs are a saturation of 40% (Po_2 of 18 mm/Hg) in the umbilical vein. When the saturation drops below 40%, placental oxygen diffusion must increase to provide com-pensation. This is accomplished by an increase in fetal hemoglobin and an increase in oxygen transport to the fetal tissues. The latter can be measured by a sharp reduction in the oxygen content of the umbilical artery, indicating maximal extraction of oxygen within the fetus.[8] Uterine blood flow may be reduced by 50% (250 ml/minute), and fetal placental blood flow also may be reduced by 50% to 150 ml/ minute, each reduction being individually incompatible with normal fetal growth. Uterine contractions superimpose stress on this already compromised state. Predominantly in older postterm primigravidas and postterm multigravidas with previous complicated pregnancies, fetal hypoxia is likely to occur. When the concentration in the umbil-ical vein becomes critical for the fetus (less than 10%), exhaustion of

TABLE 6.—DURATION OF LABOR
AND PARITY (HOURS) IN
PROLONGED PREGNANCY*

	PRIMIGR.	MULTIP.
Term	18	12
Prolonged pregnancy	28	22

*Adapted from Schubling and Rad-zuweit[10]

the placental reserve capacity occurs and the fetus can no longer survive in utero.

Clinically, there is a paradox in that, despite these placental changes that normally would be associated with decreased placental function specifically including reduced progesterone production, the myometrium is noted for its persistent quiescence. There appears to be a maintenance of the so-called progesterone block beyond term. Postterm gravidas present with an unripe cervix in about 70% of the cases.[9] Not only is there a failure to prepare for labor adequately, resulting in a high rate of failure of induction, there is a tendency during labor toward a sluggish performance.[10] The duration of labor tends to be prolonged in postterm primagravidas and multigravidas (Table 6). The net effect is that the cesarean section rate for the postterm gravida is, in general, increased twofold to threefold over that of the patient at term.

Etiology

Why does postmaturity occur? Why does the uterus not empty itself? If the placenta is undergoing anatomical and, most probably, physiologic senescence, should not the progesterone effect on the myometrium be released? The answer to these questions remains somewhat unclear. For example, it is not only the decrease in progesterone production that releases the myometrium for increased activity, it is an alteration in the estrogen-progesterone ratio that normally requires an estrogen surge near term. If fetoplacental estrogen production is reduced in some postterm gravidas, this trigger may be absent. The markedly reduced intrauterine volume secondary to oligohydramnios and a decrease in fetal and placental weight limits the degree of myometrial stretching, another factor in triggering the onset of labor.

The increasing awareness of the fetal role in the initiation of labor suggests that other etiologic possibilities must be considered, at least theoretically. Nwosu et al.[11] measured neonatal cortisol levels in postterm infants delivered vaginally and by cesarean section with or without "stress" in the antecedent labor period. Term infants born after normal labor had mean cortisol levels of 12.4 μg/dl. Term infants born after stressful labors showed significant reductions in cortisol levels with mean values (8.1 and 4.9 μg/dl, respectively) well below that of the term infant in the absence of stress. This study implied a deficiency in adrenal cortisol production by the fetus and its inability to respond effectively to stress. The decreased fetal adrenal function also may remove the cortisol surge that is a part of the steroidal trigger for the onset of labor. In a subsequent study,[12] Nwosu and co-workers provided further support for the etiologic importance of adrenocortical deficiency in prolonged pregnancy by successfully inducing labor in 8 of 10 postterm patients by intra-amniotic installation of cortisol. None of these possible etiologic factors accounts for the appearance of many postterm infants of large size and good condition. Perhaps these are the infants who are not truly postterm despite clinical evidence to the contrary. In any case, it can be stated that prolongation of pregnancy, placental insufficiency, and fetal postmaturity are closely related to uterine quiescence postterm, uterine dystocia during labor and an increase in operative deliveries.

Diagnosis

In order to select the fetus at risk from among the cohort of postdate pregnancies, we must identify the true prolonged pregnancy. Unfortunately, attempting to do this in the gravida who has proceeded beyond 40 weeks is a difficult, if not impossible, task. The optimal time to establish the accuracy of the expected date of delivery is during the first half of pregnancy, when clinical and laboratory evaluations are most accurate (Table 7). A large portion of potential postterm pregnancies can be eliminated by attention to details of the menstrual, contraceptive, and infertility history and a well-documented early pelvic examination. Noting the first appearance of an audible fetal heart by Doppler instrumentation and the first appearance of an audible fetal heart by auscultation with the fetoscope is critical; these are heard in most patients at 12 and 20 weeks, respectively. Weekly examinations with the fetoscope beginning at the 18th week of pregnancy are necessary to establish the precise timing of initial audibility. Maternal perception of fetal movements has been studied prospectively by Rawlings and Moore.[13]

The first fetal movement was felt at 19 weeks in primigravidas and at 18 weeks in multigravidas. In their study population, 9% of all patients had prolonged pregnancies (beyond 42 weeks) as calculated from the last menstrual period. However, in 61% of these patients, the documented onset of quickening corrected gestational age to less than 42 weeks. Those pregnancies were allowed to continue until spontaneous labor ensued, and no fetal loss occurred. When serial measurement of fundal height is added to these clinical parameters, there is a 95% accuracy in establishing an expected date of delivery. If clinical information is not internally consistent or is discrepant with the last menstrual period, sonography should be utilized early in pregnancy to establish accurate dates. Chilcote and Asoka[14] described the characteristics of the first trimester focusing on the appearance of the gestational sac, discrete fetal structures, crown-rump length measurements, and fetal movements to validate gestational age. Beyond the first trimester, a biparietal diameter obtained be-

---

TABLE 7.—DEFINING GESTATIONAL AGE*

Menstrual history	Doppler FH
Contraceptive history	Audible FH
Infertility history	Uterine size
Early pelvic exam	Fetal movements

IF NOT AVAILABLE OR DISCREPANT: SONOGRAPHY

*FH, fetal heart.

tween 16 and 26 weeks provides a 95% confidence limit for gestational age at ± 10 days. By contrast, as reported by Sabbagha et al.[15] the predictive value of a single biparietal diameter measurement falls precipitously when obtained during the third trimester. In up to 20% of such pregnancies studied, the range of possible age was greater than 3 weeks.

Assessing the Fetus at Risk

Once a true prolonged pregnancy has been identified, a number of techniques may be useful in assessing the degree of risk, if any, for the small cohort of fetuses that will develop true postterm dysmaturity (Table 8).

Postterm placental insufficiency is correlated with diminished production of estriol and human placental lactogen. Plasma and urinary estriol concentrations rise progressively up to the 38th to 40th week of gestation and thereafter level off. From the 42d week on, mean values fall slightly and steadily. This indicates a functional decline of the fetoplacental unit post term. A relationship exists between the incidence of fetal distress and the estriol levels in postterm gravidas: 33% when the estriol level is less than 12 mg/day and 10% when it is in the normal range. As pointed out by Goebelsmann et al.,[16] clinically low estriol levels are useful in corroborating the clinical impression of intrauterine growth retardation. Acute fetal distress, on the other hand, can only be assessed by frequent, perhaps daily, sampling, which is clinically not practical or cost-effective in the management of the 10% of patients whose pregnancies carry beyond 42 weeks of gestation.

Hobbins and co-workers[17] have suggested that decreased serial human chorionic somatomammotropin (hPL) levels correlate well with the presence or absence of the postmaturity syndrome. The overlap, however, between normal and abnormal pregnancies was too high for application of this technique without supporting electronic fetal monitoring information. For this reason, and because of the necessity to obtain frequent serial tests, the cost-effectiveness ratio utilizing hPL determinations does not seem appropriate.

The assessment of fetal activity also has been used as a means of evaluating fetal health during prolonged pregnancy. Sadovsky and Polishuk[18] have stressed that active fetal movements are an expression of fetal well-being. Fetal movements increase steadily from 20 to

---

TABLE 8.—FETAL SURVEILLANCE IN PROLONGED
PREGNANCY*

Estriol	Ultrasound
HPL (hcs)	Amniocentesis
Fetal movement	Nonstress and CST monitoring
Score	

*HPL, human placental lactogen (human chorionic somatomammotropin); CST, contraction stress test.

30 weeks and reach a plateau until the 38th week of pregnancy. Thereafter, probably in association with diminution in amniotic fluid volume, there is a steady decrease that accelerates significantly in the postmature period. The range of fetal movements is broad when self-assessed on an hourly basis by the patient. Nearly 85% of all tocographically monitored movements are perceived by the patient. Each fetus appears to have its own rhythm of movement that must be preestablished in order for this simple clinical tool to be useful. A sudden decrease in fetal movement frequency (movement alarm signal) may precede fetal demise and is associated with a 50% incidence of meconium in the amniotic fluid. This simple and inexpensive form of fetal surveillance has a high false positive rate, but it is an effective screening test when combined with more sophisticated procedures.

Ultrasound is useful in screening the postterm pregnancy by diagnosing two anatomical changes noted in this syndrome: advanced placental senescence and decrease in the size of the uterine contents. After 36 weeks' gestation, the placenta has a distinct echographic appearance that is characterized by rounded transsonic areas measuring 2 to 4 cm in diameter, best noted by real-time scanning at high gain. Anatomical and pathologic study of placentas with these sonographic patterns reveals no characteristic abnormalities. These sonolucent areas represent cotyledonary septa into the intervillous space engorged with blood. As pregnancy progresses into the postterm period, placental mass decreases and the volume of the sonolucent areas increases, producing an ultrasonographic picture characteristic of advanced senescence.[19]

The decrease in reproductive contents when dysmaturity complicates the postterm pregnancy can be measured best by assessing the total intrauterine volume.[20] This technique, utilizing anteroposterior, longitudinal, and transverse measurements of the uterus, obtained in longitudinal and coronal scans, is a useful, although somewhat complex, procedure. As indicated in Figure 3–1, the major decrease in uterine contents occurring during the postterm period is a reduction in amniotic fluid volume, generally to less than 250 ml. This marked oligohydramnios is a significant indicator of dysmaturity. Real-time sonographic scanning can be utilized to provide a simple measurement of amniotic fluid volume, identifying the size of amniotic fluid pockets that are visualized. When such pockets of fluid are less than 1 cm in diameter, or where no amniotic fluid can be obtained on sonographically directed amniocentesis, two of three infants will have significant placental insufficiency. As noted below, oligohydramnios also is associated with an increased frequency in the appearance of noncontraction-related decelerations in the fetal heart rate that may be audible or may be assessed during cardiotachometry.

The amniotic fluid in the postterm patient is characterized by extremely high lecithin-sphingomyelin (L/S) ratios, fat cell contents of 50% or more as determined by Nile blue sulfate staining, and the presence of meconium in a significant percent of patients. For this reason, some authors have suggested that management of the postterm pregnancy may be influenced by the presence of meconium. However, in a retrospective analysis of 392 transabdominal amniocentesis specimens obtained from prolonged pregnancies, Green and Paul[21] found that the presence or absence of meconium could not be correlated with fetal outcome. Ten perinatal deaths occurred within 7 days of obtaining clear fluid, while all cases in which meconium was found eventually received neonatal 5-minute Apgar scores greater than 7. Miller et al.[22] confirm the relative unimportance of meconium in the amniotic fluid. They concluded that the presence of meconium, without signs of fetal asphyxia as determined by fetal heart rate assessment, is not a sign of fetal distress and is not an indication for intervention. It also should be noted that amniocentesis in the postterm patient with significant oligohydramnios or a macrosomic fetus carries a measurable risk of fetal injury. Fetal mortality in association with the procedure has been documented.

The release of meconium into the amniotic fluid is still a valid, although rather insensitive, indicator of placental insufficiency and hypoxia. Meconium passage occurs when oxygen saturation in the umbilical vein drops to half its normal value. Meconium passage is due to hypoxia of the smooth musculature of the gastrointestinal tract resulting in hyperperistalsis and relaxation of the anal sphincter. In our patients at risk for postmaturity in whom the amniotic fluid was clear before labor, there was a less than 5% incidence of low 5-minute Apgar score. However, when meconium was detected before labor and the patient delivered vaginally, there was a 25% incidence of low Apgar score and a 75/100 perinatal mortality rate.

Recently, Yaffe and co-workers[23] attempted to improve the accuracy of diagnosing prolonged pregnancy by measuring the thromboplastic activity of amniotic fluid (TAAF). The TAAF increases with gestational age. Based on this phenomenon, the TAAF of 45 women in the 41st to 43d week of gestation was established, using their amniotic fluid as a source of thromboplastin. It was found that in all cases in which the TAAF value was less than 42 seconds, implying a very high level of thromboplastic activity, the newborns exhibited clinical evidence of postmaturity.

While all of the above tests have been useful in assessing the postdate pregnancy, we have relied increasingly on antepartum fetal heart rate monitoring to screen this relatively common group of patients. Nonstress testing has been utilized on our service as the primary means of screening for fetal status during prolonged pregnancy. The contraction stress test is used to further define fetal status when nonreactivity is evident. With the advent of the nonstress test as a simple, safe, and noninvasive procedure, indications for antepartum assessment of the fetus broadened. For the past year (Table 9), postdate pregnancy has been the most common indication for such evaluation. The false negative rate for the nonstress rate is 0.7%, which compares favorably with the 1.1% false negative rate noted in our earlier contraction stress test series.[24] The false positive rate of the nonstress test is high, producing a poor correlation between a nonreactive nonstress test and the contraction stress test. A reactive non-

TABLE 9.—Nonstress Test Indications

Prolonged pregnancy	263
Vascular disease	149
Diabetes	112
IUGR*	79
Other	56
Total	659

*IUGR, intrauterine growth retardation.

stress test correlates extremely well with a negative contraction stress test.

Considerable debate centers on the issue of which procedure is an earlier detector of fetal distress. We believe that serial nonstress tests demonstrating a progressive decrease in variability and frequency of accelerations is the earliest indicator of distress and has preceded positive contraction stress testing, particularly in cases of fetal dysmaturity (Fig 3–2). For this reason, when a postdate fetus has a fixed baseline, nonreactive nonstress test, we will terminate the pregnancy without delay. This is especially true when atypical variable decelerations or periods of bradycardia occurring spontaneously or associated with contractions are noted on the record. This is a strong indicator of profound oligohydramnios, significant fetal risk, and the need for

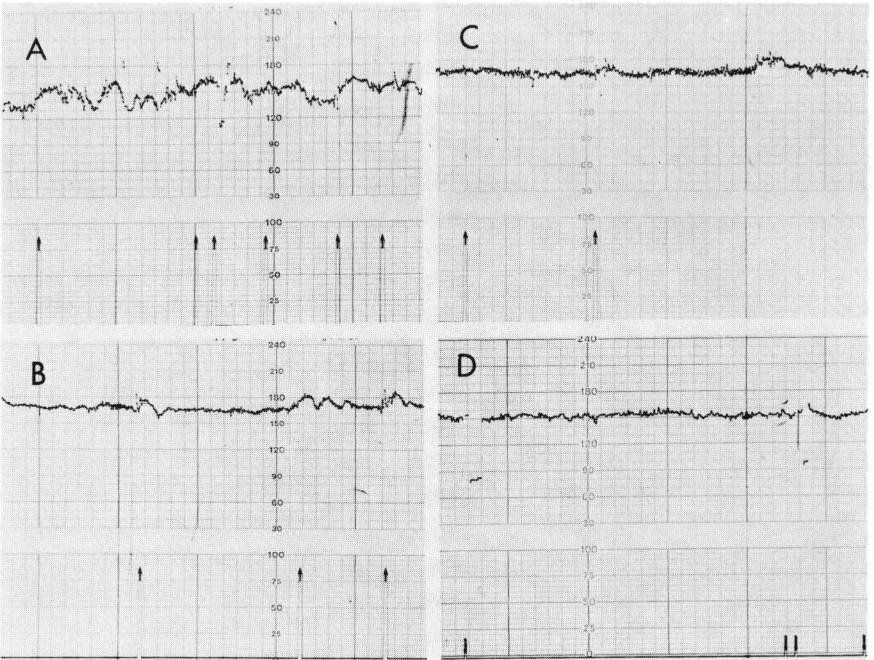

Fig 3–2.—Progressive loss of fetal heart rate reactivity during twice-weekly nonstress test (sequence: **A, B, C, D**).

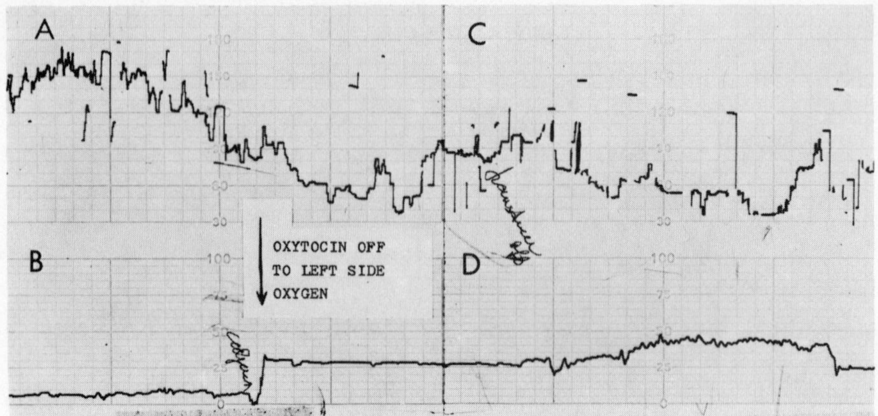

Fig 3–3.—Pronounced bradycardia during oxytocin contraction test with no measurable uterine contractions. Patient had profound oligohydramnios.

delivery (Fig 3–3). The fetus with both a nonreactive nonstress test and a positive contraction stress test does not tolerate induction or stimulation of labor and has a poor prognosis for uncomplicated vaginal delivery. Unless amniotomy can be performed readily with application of an internal monitoring system, patients with prolonged pregnancy evidencing these abnormal tracings should be delivered by cesarean section.[25]

If one elects to allow a pregnancy to continue beyond 42 weeks in order to avoid a long, difficult, and possibly unsuccessful induction of labor, intensive antepartum surveillance will, with a high degree of accuracy, ensure against the possibility of unsuspected fetal compromise.

Perinatal Risks

When postterm dysmaturity occurs, the pattern of fetal compromise occurs in two forms: a chronic phase and a more acute form. The chronic phase is marked by (1) urinary estriol values on the lower limits of normal, (2) meconium release in the amniotic fluid, generally slight, (3) wasting of subcutaneous tissues and dehydration, (4) oligohydramnios, and (5) uncommon changes in the fetal heart rate pattern and rare intrauterine death.

A more acute form extending over a few days immediately before the onset of labor or during labor is noted by (1) subsequent decrease in urinary estriol to critical levels; (2) meconium release and staining of fetal skin and membranes; (3) aspiration of amniotic fluid; (4) necrosis or hemorrhage, or both, into the adrenal glands, secondary to hypoxia; (5) parenchymal damage of the brain, myocardium, and liver secondary to hypoxia; (6) pathologic fetal heart rate patterns, particularly noted by late decelerations or atypical variable deceleration patterns; (7) intrauterine fetal death; and (8) neonatal death.

The major perinatal risks to the fetus are summarized in Table 10. The antepartum stillbirth rate at 43 weeks is threefold that of fetuses between 39 and 41 weeks. Fetal distress before or during labor is well documented by fetal heart rate monitoring, which may show classic late decelerations in response to minimal uterine contractions, marked cord compression patterns in association with contractions or fetal movement, and loss of baseline variability. With fetal distress and meconium passage, aspiration of meconium is a major complication that should be prevented by aggressive management at birth (see below). The fragility of these infants during labor leads to frequent development of acidosis and asphyxia that, when accompanied by meconium aspiration, results in an increased frequency of neonatal mortality from respiratory distress despite clearly mature L/S ratios. In fact, respiratory distress is the most frequent cause of death in liveborn postmature neonates. It is speculated that lack of plasminogen activator in the lung results in the failure to resolve intra-alveolar fibrin deposits caused by aspiration of meconium-filled amniotic fluid. This is compounded by hypoperfusion secondary to vasoconstriction in the lungs produced by acidosis. The incidence of neonatal distress syndrome is further increased when postterm insufficiency of the placenta is complicated by an already existing preterm placental insufficiency.

After birth, the neonate with postterm dysmaturity is subject to temperature instability, hypoglycemia, and polycythemia. The last has been associated with an increased incidence of renal vein thrombosis.

An unresolved question relates to the possible long-term sequelae of postterm dysmaturity. Zwerdling[26] noted a specific risk in postterm infants who were small for gestational age. In this sense, these infants did not differ from preterm infants with intrauterine growth retardation who subsequently show an increased frequency of delayed motor and behavioral milestones during the first 5 years of life. In the larger postterm infant, followed for 5 years, there was no growth or intellectual retardation. Similar evidence of neurologic sequelae has been noted by Lovell.[27]

In a 1-year follow-up of 40 stage I (Clifford) postmature infants matched by sex, race, maternal age, and education with control infants, Field et al.[28] noted lower Denver developmental scores at age 4 months and an increased maternal reporting of "difficult" babies (Table 11). At age 8 months, the Bayley motor scores were equal, but mental scores were lower in the postmature infants who were also prone to an increased incidence of illness, and feeding and sleep disturbances.

TABLE 10.—PERINATAL RISKS IN PROLONGED
PREGNANCY

Stillbirth	Temperature instability
Anomaly	Hypoglycemia
Fetal distress	Polycythemia
Meconium aspiration	Long-term sequelae

TABLE 11.—INFANT FOLLOW-UP IN PROLONGED PREGNANCY

BIRTH	TERM	PROLONGED	VALUE
Gestational age	274	296	.001
Birth weight	3295	3589	.02
Head circumference (cm)	33.9	35.1	.001
AGE 4 MONTHS			
Denver Development			
Rating*	1.37	1.98	.01
Carey Distractability Score*	1.10	1.97	.001
AGE 8 MONTHS			
Hospitalization*	0.60	1.32	.01
Feeding/sleep disturbances*	1.28	1.90	.01
Bayley Mental Scale	102.3	93.5	.05

*Lower score is optimal.
Adapted from Field et al.[28]

Management of Prolonged Pregnancy

With all of the preceding information in mind, we have developed a protocol for the management of prolonged pregnancy that is moderately activist, but readily applicable to a large-volume clinical service. It is predicated on the assumption that there *is* an increased perinatal mortality associated with prolonged pregnancy, although only a minority of fetuses are involved. Because prolonged gestation occurs frequently (7.5% to 10% of pregnancies) and our ability to diagnose antepartum dysmaturity is limited, a standardized clinical approach clearly is indicated and helpful in avoiding both unnecessary intervention and perinatal loss.

The recent literature summarizing similar attempts at prospective management plans is somewhat confusing. Hauth et al.[29] reviewed the mortality and morbidity of 185 postterm pregnancies managed by weekly trial inductions starting at 42 weeks' gestation compared to those of 119 postterm pregnancies with spontaneous labor before a trial of induction was accomplished. One stillbirth occurred in the spontaneous group and none in the induced group. There was no statistical difference in the maternal or fetal morbidity in terms of bradycardia in labor, meconium-stained amniotic fluid, meconium aspiration, 1-minute Apgar scores less than 4, macrosomia (more than 4,000 gm), neonatal pneumonia, and the incidence of cesarean section. The retrospective analysis suggested that standard clinical management is sufficient to ensure optimal perinatal outcome in postterm pregnancies.

In this study, the oxytocin challenge test did not identify clearly the compromised fetuses or reduce perinatal morbidity. Further, the oxytocin challenge test did not predict meconium staining of the amniotic fluid, nor was the presence of a negative oxytocin challenge test associated with decreased perinatal morbidity.

As noted above, Green and Paul[21] reviewed 192 amniocentesis samples performed beyond 41 weeks' gestation. Meconium-stained fluid at amniocentesis was found to be associated with an increased incidence of macrosomia, cesarean deliveries, and low 1-minute Apgar scores. However, 10 perinatal deaths occurred after amniocentesis with clear fluid in prolonged pregnancy, with 4 of these occurring within 7 days of amniocentesis. While no fetal mortality was attributable to amniocentesis, in view of the significant amount of false positive and false negative results, its use solely to demonstrate the presence or absence of meconium staining appeared to be of questionable value in the management of prolonged pregnancy. The authors concluded that other indices of fetal well-being could be utilized to identify affected pregnancies requiring intervention.

Knox and co-workers[30] conducted a prospective randomized study evaluating 180 patients without other complications during prolonged pregnancy. These patients randomly were assigned to be followed serially either by amniocentesis or by contraction stress tests. Labor was induced in each group based on the finding of meconium or the presence of a positive oxytocin challenge test. The incidence of meconium subsequently was shown to be similar in both management groups (22%). Although meconium was associated significantly with abnormal labor progression, intrapartum fetal distress, and low 1- and 5-minute Apgar scores, induction of labor after discovery of meconium, when compared with nonintervention, did not improve perinatal outcome.

Our protocol for the management of prolonged pregnancy is designed to (1) identify the affected fetus, (2) reduce fetal risk by induction when this procedure does not add to maternal risk, and (3) avoid dysmaturity by delivering at term those women at high risk for placental insufficiency.

As noted above, when postterm dysmaturity is superimposed on preterm placental insufficiency, fetal risk is enhanced significantly. Therefore, pregnancy should not be allowed to extend beyond term in women with obstetric complications, such as habitual abortion, previous stillbirth, diabetes mellitus, pregnancy-induced hypertension, intrauterine growth retardation, and erythroblastosis fetalis. The development of placental insufficiency with postmaturity is associated with a high fetal morbidity and mortality in these patients.

Because 70% to 80% of postterm fetuses are delivered in good health, active management of the uncomplicated gravida with prolonged pregnancy should be based on signs of fetal distress or the appearance of additional maternal complicating factors. In the absence of signs of fetal compromise, continuation of pregnancy is indicated when the estimated fetal weight is low, when there is uncertainty about the duration of gestation, and when there is an unfavorable cervix. Conversely, when dates are certain and the cervix is favorable, induction at 42 weeks is logical. Little maternal risk is encumbered and the occasional, but tragic, false negative fetal surveillance score can be avoided. Before induction of labor, assessments of the state of the cervix, the maternal pelvis, and fetal size and position are essential. Higher birth weights of postterm fetuses that may lead to mechanical birth problems and dystocia have been regarded as causes of increased fetal death rate in prolonged pregnancy.

This plan of management for the uncomplicated prolonged pregnancy is predicated on the fact that most patients (70%), as noted by Beischer and Brown,[31] will deliver before the 43d week of pregnancy and 90% will deliver by the 44th week of pregnancy with the onset of spontaneous labor.

When antepartum signs of fetal distress are apparent and the cervix is favorable, an attempt at vaginal delivery is appropriate. Early amniotomy, continuous internal electronic fetal monitoring, and fetal scalp sampling, where appropriate, are mandatory. The high intrapartum mortality in affected fetuses testifies to the fragility of their condition and the need for continuous assessment. When vaginal delivery is attempted for the identified postmature fetus, labor should be conducted in the lateral position with oxygen breathing. Avoidance or limitation of sedatives, narcotics, and conduction anesthesia is important. Delivery by low forceps to shorten the second stage is recommended.

When antepartum fetal compromise is evident and the cervix is unfavorable, cesarean section should be performed. This is particularly true in the elderly primigravida, because of the enhanced risk of perinatal mortality. Anesthesia is best provided by short-acting barbiturates and succinylcholine for intubation, followed by nitrous oxide-oxygen and fentanyl anesthesia after delivery. In our experience, this balanced form of anesthesia is associated with the most favorable neonatal outcome. All general anesthesia in these patients should be preceded by 100% oxygen breathing to raise the arterial oxygen content to the level of 200 torr.

Neonatal attendance is critical because of the high frequency of meconium aspiration and neonatal depression. If meconium is present at the time of delivery of the infant's head, the nasopharynx should be aspirated with a DeLee catheter. Immediately after delivery, the infant should be placed in a position so that the vocal cords can be inspected by direct laryngoscopy. If meconium is found at the level of the cords, intubation and tracheal suction are performed immediately. This pattern of care has been associated with a significant reduction in the incidence of aspiration pneumonia.

In the absence of meconium, the newborn must be observed closely for signs of dehydration, hypoglycemia, hypovolemia, acidosis, cerebral hypoxia, pulmonary complications, and adrenal cortical hypofunction.

Summary

Postdate pregnancies are common clinical events, occurring in 7.5% to 10% of pregnancies. Generally, this is a benign condition from the perinatal perspective, although it is associated with significant anxiety on the part of the prospective parents. True fetal dysmaturity occurs to some degree in 20% of these patients. Perinatal mortality increases after the 42d week in association with fetal dysmaturity. This fetal compromise during prolonged pregnancy can be diagnosed with reasonable accuracy by clinical, endocrine and, particularly, biophysical testing. Because the dysmature fetus is biochemically unstable, its greatest risk period occurs during labor. For this reason, continuous electronic fetal heart rate surveillance during labor is mandatory. An increased cesarean section rate in these patients is anticipated because of fetal distress, failed induction, and a significant incidence of macrosomic babies.

The major logistic problem facing the obstetrician is the application of extensive and expensive antepartum testing procedures for a relatively low incidence but high-risk complication. Accurate establishment of the true expected date of delivery and antepartum fetal heart rate monitoring as outlined above are cost-effective in both medical and human terms.

References

1. Clifford, S.: Postmaturity—with placental dysfunction. *J. Pediatr.*44:1, 1954.
2. Browne, J.C.: Postmaturity. *JAMA* 186:1047, 1963.
3. Stewart, H.L.: Duration of pregnancy and postmaturity. *JAMA* 148:1079, 1952.
4. Beischer, N.A., Brown, J.B.: Postmature pregnancy. *Obstet. Gynecol. Surv.* 27:303, 1972.
5. Karn, M.N., Penrose, L.S.: Newborn sex and perinatal loss. *Ann. Eugenics* 16:147, 1952.
6. McClure-Browne, J.C.: Postmaturity. *Am. J. Obstet. Gynecol.* 85:573, 1963.
7. Siegel, P., Rabanus, W.: The placenta in postmaturity. *Zentralbl. Gynaekol.* 88:345, 1966.
8. Sjostedt, S., et al.: Fetal oxygenation in the dysmature state. *Acta Obstet. Gynecol. Scand.* 39:34, 1960.
9. Walker, J.: Management of postterm pregnancy. *Am. J. Obstet. Gynecol.* 1976:1231, 1958.
10. Schüssling, G., Radzuweit, H.: Zur Ubertragung in der Schwangerschaft. *Zentralbl. Gynaekol.* 90:1705, 1968.
11. Nwosu, U.C., et al.: Possible adrenal cortical insufficiency in postmature neonates. *Am. J. Obstet. Gynecol.* 122:969, 1975.
12. Nwosu, U.C., Wallach, E.E., Bolognese, R.J.: Initiation of labor by intraamniotic cortisol installation in prolonged human pregnancy. *Obstet. Gynecol.* 47:137, 1976.
13. Rawlings, E.E., Moore, B.A.: The accuracy of methods of calculating the expected date of delivery in the diagnosis of postmaturity. *Am. J. Obstet. Gynecol.* 106:676, 1970.
14. Chilcote, W.S., and Asoka, N.: Evaluation of first-trimester pregnancy by ultrasound. *Clin. Obstet. Gynecol.* 20:253, 1977.
15. Sabbagha, R.E., et al.: Sonor BPD and fetal age. *Obstet. Gynecol.* 43:7, 1974.
16. Goebelsmann, U., et al.: Estriol in pregnancy. *Am. J. Obstet. Gynecol.* 115:795, 1973.
17. Hobbins, J. C., Goldstein, L., Hofschild, J. : Value of HCS determinations in management of prolonged pregnancy. *Obstet. Gynecol.* 44:802, 1974.
18. Sadovsky, E., Polishuk, W. Z.: Fetal movements in utero. *Obstet. Gynecol.* 50:49, 1977.
19. Hobbins, J. C., Winsberg, F.: *Ultrasonography in Obstetrics and Gynecology.* Baltimore, Williams & Wilkins Co., 1977.

20. Gohari, P., Berkowitz, R.L., Hobbins, J.C.: Prediction of intrauterine growth retardation by determination of total intrauterine volume. *Am. J. Obstet. Gynecol.* 127:255, 1977.
21. Green, J.N., Paul, R.H.: The value of amniocentesis in prolonged pregnancy. *Obstet. Gynecol.* 51:293, 1978.
22. Miller, E.C., et al.: Significance of meconium during labor. *Am. J. Obstet. Gynecol.* 122:573, 1975.
23. Yaffe, H., Hayam, E., Sadovsky, E.: Thromboplastic activity of amniotic fluid in term and postterm gestation. *Obstet. Gynecol.* 57:490, 1981.
24. Weingold, A.B., DeJesus, T.P.S., O'Kieffe, J.: Oxytocin challenge test. *Am. J. Obstet. Gynecol.* 123:466, 1975.
25. Weingold, A.B., Yonekura, M.L., O'Kieffe, J.: Nonstress testing. *Am. J. Obstet. Gynecol.* 138:195, 1980.
26. Zwerdling, M.A.: Factors pertaining to prolonged pregnancy and its outcome. *Pediatrics* 40:202, 1967.
27. Lovell, K.E.: The effect of postmaturity on the developing child. *Med. J. Aust.* 1:13, 1973.
28. Field, T.M., et al.: Developmental effects of prolonged pregnancy. *J. Pediatr.* 90:836, 1977.
29. Hauth, J.C., et al.: Postterm pregnancy. *Obstet. Gynecol.* 56:467, 1980.
30. Knox, G.E., Huddleston, J.F., Flowers, C.E.: Management of prolonged pregnancy: Results of a prospective randomized trial. *Am. J. Obstet. Gynecol.* 134:376, 1979.
31. Beischer, N.A., Brown, J.B.: Current status of estrogen assays in obstetrics and gynecology. *Obstet. Gynecol. Surv.* 27:303, 1972.

3–1 Prepregnant Blood Pressure, Hypertension During Pregnancy, and Later Blood Pressure of Mothers and Offspring. Mild preeclampsia is relatively common in pregnancy, but little is known of its possible progress to severe proteinuric hypertension in pregnancy. Herbert G. Langford and Robert L. Watson (Univ. of Mississippi) examined the possibility that prepregnancy blood pressure is a major predictor of preeclampsia. High school girls were evaluated and then followed through pregnancy into their postpartum course, and many of their offspring were studied. Subjects were selected in a community-based prospective study of black women in grades 9 through 12.

Prepregnant blood pressures of subjects destined to have the diagnosis of preeclampsia were significantly higher than those of other subjects. The preeclamptics also had significantly higher prepregnant weights. There were no differences in maternal age at delivery, weight gain during pregnancy, recorded edema, Apgar scores, or infant birth weights. No difference in recorded proteinuria was observed between preeclamptic and other subjects. The mean peak blood pressure in the preeclamptics during labor was 157/108 mm Hg, compared with 141/93 mm Hg for the other subjects. In both groups, systolic and diastolic pressures rose steadily through pregnancy. Subsequently the preeclamptic subjects tended to have higher blood pressures than the nonpreeclamptic mothers. Female children of the preeclamptic mothers had higher systolic and diastolic pressures than

(3–1) Hypertension 2(Suppl. I):I130–I133, July–Aug. 1980.

female children of the other mothers. No such difference was found in male children.

Pregnancy-associated hypertension may be an example of a sex-limited variety of essential hypertension, the expression of which is brought about or increased by estrogens. Alternatively, the inheritance of hypertension may be more manifest after puberty has begun in either sex. Further follow-up is needed to determine whether blood pressure differences between girls and boys of mothers with pregnancy-related hypertension persist throughout life.

▶ [This is a provocative study and one with profound clinical implications. It represents a longitudinal study of blood pressure in black women first assessed as schoolgirls and followed through pregnancy and afterward. Blood pressures of patients destined to have the diagnosis of preeclampsia were significantly higher at each point of measurement than those of patients destined to have normal pregnancies. Moreover, female (but not male) offspring of preeclamptics had higher blood pressures than those of normal women. The authors suggest that what is diagnosed as "mild preeclampsia" (i.e., hypertension without proteinuria) is actually a form of essential hypertension unmasked by estrogen. Thus, by implication, mild and severe preeclampsia are two entirely different conditions rather than stages of a similar disease process. In the discussion section of this article, it is stated, "Our data are being further analyzed, but, to date, we cannot ascertain any fetal or maternal damage from 'mild eclampsia' (sic). Also, there is no clear evidence that the mild preeclampsia of our diagnoses leads to eclampsia." This is astounding, even if "mild preeclampsia" is what is meant by "mild eclampsia." It has been said that "clinical experience" is one of the world's three greatest lies; nevertheless, our clinical experience includes a number of instances in which mother or fetus or both have come to harm because of mild preeclampsia and in which the mild form clearly has progressed to the severe variant.] ◀

3–2 **Antihypertensive Effect of Plasma Volume Expansion in Pregnancy-Associated Hypertension.** Gallery et al. in 1979 reported that plasma volume is low in both chronic hypertension in pregnancy and pregnancy-associated hypertension. However, the role of plasma volume expanders in the therapy of hypertension in pregnancy is controversial. E. D. M. Gallery, W. Delprado, and A. Z. Györy (Univ. of Sydney) investigated the clinical effect of intravenous infusion of 500 ml of stable plasma protein substitute (SPPS) given over 15–20 minutes on plasma and total extracellular fluid (ECF) volume in 6 normal nonpregnant women and 6 normotensive and 11 hypertensive women in the third trimester of pregnancy. All but 1 of the hypertensive subjects had pure pregnancy-associated hypertension, and 5 of these also had proteinuria. All subjects were aged 25–37 years.

Plasma and total ECF volume expansion was confirmed in the normotensive women in the third trimester of pregnancy. Twenty-four hours after rapid intravenous infusion of SPPS, the women with pregnancy-associated hypertension showed a significant decrease in both systolic ($P < .01$) and diastolic ($P < .001$) blood pressure, a significant increase in plasma volume ($P < .01$), a significant decrease in interstitial fluid volume ($P < .05$), and a decrease in total ECF and body weight, both of which did not achieve statistical significance (table). In these women, the fall in blood pressure was quite rapid and was sustained for 48 hours after infusion.

(3–2) Aust. N.Z. J. Med. 11:20–24, February 1981.

Plasma Volume (PV), Extracellular Fluid Volume (ECF), and Interstitial Fluid Volume (ISF) in Normal Pregnant Women Before and After Infusion of Stable Plasma Protein Substitute (SPPS)

	PV (ml/cm)	ECF (ml/cm)	ISF (ml/cm)	BP (mmHg)	Wt (kg)
Normal pregnancy	26·9 (11·7)	93·7±5·6	66·8±4·8	$\frac{104}{66}\pm\frac{3\cdot1}{2\cdot1}$	71·6±2·9
Hypertensive pregnancy					
Pre SPPS	24·5 (3·2)	99·1±8·2	74·8±8·7	$\frac{143}{101}\pm\frac{3\cdot3}{2\cdot4}$	72·0±3·5
Post SPPS	‡28·2 (5·9)	87·2±5·3	*59·1±5·0	$\frac{\dagger126}{\ddagger86}\pm\frac{2\cdot4}{2\cdot1}$	70·6±4·0

(**Mean** ± **SE**; *P <0.05; †P <0.01; ‡P <0.001.)

The results suggest that the plasma volume contraction in women with pregnancy-associated hypertension is the result of abnormal vascular permeability, since interstitial fluid volume was abnormally high, while plasma volume was abnormally low. It is concluded that plasma volume expanders are a potentially useful adjunct to traditional antihypertensive regimens, especially in acute management of severe pregnancy-associated hypertension. Further work is in progress to assess the effect of a second daily infusion of SPPS.

▶ [Though it is generally agreed that plasma volume is diminished in hypertensive disorders of pregnancy, particularly acute preeclampsia, whether the plasma volume alteration is primary or secondary is far from clear. If plasma volume contraction is primary, volume expansion would seem to be a logical therapeutic choice. The results of this investigation are certainly consistent with such a view, for rapid infusion (500 ml over 15–20 minutes) of a plasma protein substitute caused a decline in blood pressure and a fluid shift from the interstitial to the intravascular space. These findings are interesting and valuable for the light they may shed on pathophysiology, but we would be cautious about any direct therapeutic implications in view of (1) the potential for cardiac failure (which is, after all, one of the two most common causes of death in toxemia) and (2) concern that any therapeutic maneuver will delay the only known definitive treatment—delivery.] ◀

3–3 **Reassessment of Intravenous MgSO$_4$ Therapy in Preeclampsia-Eclampsia.** The occurrence of seizures in preeclamptic and eclamptic women is considered to be unlikely during treatment with the standard dose of continuous intravenous (IV) administration of magnesium sulfate (MgSO$_4$). There is disagreement as to the recommended dosage and therapeutic levels of MgSO$_4$, but all agree that the dosage should be adjusted according to patellar reflexes, hourly urine output, and respiratory rate. During 21 months, B. M. Sibai, J. Lipshitz, G. D. Anderson, and P. V. Dilts, Jr. (Univ. of Tennessee) encountered, among 1,158 preeclamptic patients, 13 in whom seizures developed while they were receiving IV MgSO$_4$ treatment (table). The type, severity, and duration of seizures did not differ from those observed in patients not receiving MgSO$_4$. One patient was intubated because of respiratory arrest. Serum magnesium levels at the time of seizure were below therapeutic range in 11 patients. All responded to

(3–3) Obstet. Gynecol. 57:199–202, February 1981.

SUMMARY OF PATIENTS IN WHOM SEIZURES DEVELOPED DURING TREATMENT WITH MgSO$_4$

Patient, gravidity, and age	Time of onset of seizure	Mg level (mg/dl)	Hours on maintenance dose before seizure	Maintenance dose (g/hr)	Admitting diagnosis
LS, G1, 23	Ante partum	3.8	5	1	Eclampsia
JM, G1, 19	Ante partum	3.1	3	1	Eclampsia
MT, G1, 19	Intra partum	2.8	24	1	Moderate preeclampsia
HJ, G1, 17	Intra partum	3.4	5	1	Severe preeclampsia
JC, G1, 13	Intra partum	4.2	2	2	Severe preeclampsia
LA, G1, 17	Intra partum	3.4	2	1	Eclampsia
WJ, G2, 25	Intra partum	3.9	4	2	Eclampsia
HA, G1, 17	Intra partum	4.8	9	1	Severe preeclampsia
RH, G2, 23	Post partum	2.6	16	1	Severe preeclampsia
BK, G1, 21	Post partum	3.1	13	1	Severe preeclampsia
BC, G1, 14	Post partum	4.5	22	2	Moderate preeclampsia
NC, G1, 19	Post partum	3.9	11	1	Severe preeclampsia
VR, G1, 18	Post partum	5.1	48	2	Severe preeclampsia

higher maintenance doses of MgSO$_4$ and none had seizures while receiving the higher dose. No perinatal morbidity or mortality occurred in this group. None of these patients had any neurologic deficit. These findings prompted a study of serum magnesium levels in 120 patients who were given IV MgSO$_4$ therapy for preeclampsia-eclampsia. Random serum magnesium samples were obtained 2–48 hours after a loading dose of 4 gm infused over 15 minutes and while patients were taking a maintenance dose of either 1, 2, or 3 gm/hour. The infusion was continued through labor and for 24–96 hours after delivery.

When a maintenance dose of 1 or 2 gm/hour was used, 98% and 50% of the respective serum magnesium values were below levels considered to be therapeutic (4.8–8.4 mg/dl) by several authors. Therapeutic levels were achieved in all patients receiving a maintenance dose of 3 gm/hour. The mean serum magnesium level increased as the maintenance dose increased from 1 to 3 gm/hour. With each of the maintenance doses used, a maximum serum magnesium level was reached at which the levels plateaued irrespective of the duration of infusion. Maximum serum levels were obtained at 18, 8, and 2 hours when maintenance doses of 1, 2, and 3 gm/hour were used, respectively. A poor correlation appeared between the description of patellar reflexes and serum magnesium concentrations; although absence of reflexes seemed to indicate adequate magnesium levels, it was also the first sign of impending magnesium toxicity. Neither symptomatic hypermagnesemia nor hypocalcemia was observed in patients or their newborns.

Magnesium sulfate is the drug of choice in treatment of patients with preeclampsia-eclampsia, but the recommended maintenance dose of 1 gm/hour was insufficient to prevent seizures in some patients. The therapeutic level of serum magnesium remains speculative. Adjusting the dosage of IV-administered MgSO$_4$ according to the response of each patient remains the best approach.

▶ [Our own studies (Cruikshank et al.: *Am. J. Obstet. Gynecol.* 134:243, 1979) are consistent with the findings of this report that current regimens of intravenous magnesium sulfate therapy (4 gm loading dose followed by 1 or 2 gm/hour) give blood levels somewhat lower than the "therapeutic range" of 4–7 mEq/L established with intramuscular administration. However, it certainly has not been our experience that patients treated in this way are at risk of convulsions. In fact, we can recall seeing only 2 patients ever who convulsed after magnesium therapy was well established, and 1 of these patients proved to be hypercalcemic (presumably because of hyperparathyroidism) and the other had an intracranial hemorrhage. This paper describes 13 of 1,158 magnesium-treated preeclamptics or eclamptics who convulsed during therapy at blood levels ranging from 2.2 to 4.3 mEq/L. Perhaps the magnesium sulfate solutions used in Memphis should be analyzed!] ◄

3–4 **Effects of Magnesium Sulfate Treatment on Perinatal Calcium Metabolism: II. Neonatal Responses.** Parenteral magnesium sulfate has been used extensively in the treatment of preeclampsia. Although deleterious effects of hypermagnesemia in the newborn are thought to be rare, there have been reports of neonatal respiratory depression, lethargy, flaccidity, and hyporeflexia that may persist for several days. Gail A. McGuinness, Mary M. Weinstein, Dwight P. Cruikshank, and Roy M. Pitkin (Univ. of Iowa) investigated the effects of maternal magnesium sulfate treatment on neonatal magnesium and calcium homeostasis. Twenty-three pregnant women with preeclampsia were treated at term with intravenous magnesium sulfate, while 14 normotensive gravidas at term served as controls. Serum levels of magnesium, total and ionized calcium, total protein, albumin, and phosphorus were measured in maternal and umbilical cord blood. Each of these parameters, except for ionized calcium, was measured in samples obtained from neonates at 2, 12, 24, 48, and 72 hours after birth.

Treatment with magnesium sulfate produced a 232% increase over maternal baseline serum magnesium levels and a 9% and 11% decline in total and ionized calcium levels, respectively. Although fetuses exposed to maternal magnesium sulfate treatment developed hypermagnesemia, the proportionate increase was not as great as that in maternal serum. At 2, 12, and 24 hours after birth, neonatal serum levels of magnesium were significantly higher in infants exposed to maternal magnesium sulfate than in controls (Fig 3–4). However, at 48 hours and beyond, there were no significant differences between treated and control neonates. Mean serum levels of calcium, total protein, albumin, and phosphorus in umbilical blood and in all subsequent neonatal blood samples were not significantly different between treated and control infants. Among treated mothers, a highly significant correlation between maternal magnesium levels at delivery and magnesium levels in umbilical cord and all neonatal blood samples up to 72 hours after delivery was observed. However, no correlation between maternal serum magnesium levels at delivery and serum calcium levels in umbilical or neonatal blood samples was observed at any time. Birth weights, gestational ages, and Apgar scores were similar in treated and control infants.

Maternal magnesium sulfate treatment for preeclampsia appar-

(3–4) Obstet. Gynecol. 56:595–600, November 1980.

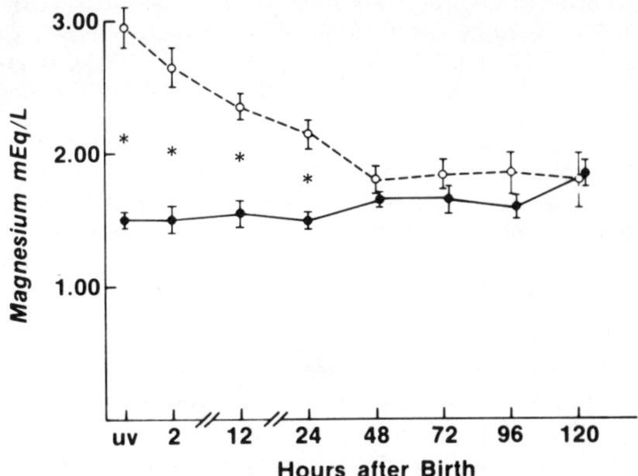

Fig 3–4.—Serial serum magnesium levels in treated versus control neonates. *Open circle,* treated; *solid circle,* control; *asterisk, P* <.001; *uv,* umbilical venous sample. Values are mean ± SEM. (Courtesy of McGuinness, G. A., et al.: Obstet. Gynecol. 56:595–600, November 1980.)

ently does not cause neonatal hypocalcemia, and the neonatal hypermagnesemia induced by treatment resolves by 48 hours after birth.

▶ [This study demonstrates that the elevated serum magnesium levels in the infant following maternal MgSO$_4$ treatment clear quite rapidly and reach normal by 48 hours of age. Moreover, calcium metabolism in the newborn is unaffected by maternal MgSO$_4$. It should be emphasized, however, that the subjects were all term (37 weeks or more) unasphyxiated infants with weight appropriate for gestational age. Magnesium sulfate might not be so safe in conditions accompanied by fetal compromise.] ◀

3–5 **Reduced Umbilical and Placental Vascular Prostacyclin in Severe Preeclampsia.** It is believed that uteroplacental ischemia plays an important role in preeclampsia and that prostaglandin synthesis by vascular walls may modulate uteroplacental blood flow. Recently, it has been reported that fetal blood vessels readily synthesize prostacyclin (PGI$_2$), suggesting that this substance may be involved in the regulation of fetal circulation. G. Remuzzi, D. Marchesi, C. Zoja, D. Muratore, G. Mecca, R. Misiani, E. Rossi, M. Barbato, P. Capetta, M. B. Donati, and G. de Gaetano (Univ. of Milan) investigated this possibility using a bioassay for PGI$_2$ activity in specimens of umbilical and placental vascular tissue obtained from 5 patients with severe preeclampsia and 9 patients with normal pregnancies immediately after expulsion of the fetus. There was 1 case of perinatal death.

Prostacyclin activity was significantly lower ($P < .01$) in the fetal umbilical arteries and placental veins obtained from patients with severe preeclampsia than in those from patients with uncomplicated pregnancies. The amount of PGI$_2$ activity generated by fetal umbilical arteries from women with normal pregnancies was significantly greater ($P < .01$) than that found in vascular tissue from nonpregnant women, while the amount of PGI$_2$ activity in placental veins and control veins was similar.

The results suggest that a deficiency of PGI$_2$ activity in the umbil-

(3–5) Prostaglandins 20:105–110, July 1980.

ical arteries and placental veins could cause a reduction in fetal blood flow resulting in impaired fetal nutrition. The authors advise caution in the use of drugs such as aspirin that may inhibit PGI_2 synthesis during pregnancy.

▶ [Dianna E. Van Orden, of the University of Iowa, reviewed this article at our request and commented as follows:

"The authors showed in a previous publication that human umbilical arteries and placental veins synthesize more prostacyclin (PGI_2) than vessels from adults. Since this prostaglandin-like substance is a potent vasodilator, they postulated that PGI_2 plays an important role in maintenance of the low peripheral vascular resistance in the face of high cardiac output and elevated renin in fetal circulation. In the present study, they compare the PGI_2 production of umbilical arteries from preeclamptic pregnancies to that of vessels from normal pregnancies. Bioassayable PGI_2 activity released upon in vitro incubation was significantly lower in vessels from preeclamptics than controls (preeclamptic umbilical arteries, 65.4 ng/mg tissue versus 191.9 ng/mg tissue in controls, $P < .01$; preeclamptic placental veins, 19.9 ng/mg tissue versus 33.2 ng/mg tissue in controls, $P < .01$). Umbilical arteries generated more PGI_2 than visceral arteries from nonpregnant adults (191.9 ng/mg umbilical artery versus 43.2 ng/mg visceral artery, $P < .01$.)

"The active PGI_2 generation of fetal-placental vessels may be part of a renin-prostaglandin vascular control system. Exposure of endothelium to angiotensin II in vitro causes production of the vasodilator prostaglandin E (PGI_2 not studied), whereas infusions of PGI_2 cause elevation of renin without elevation of blood pressure in human beings. The authors logically suggest that inhibition of prostaglandin and prostacyclin production by aspirin ingestion in pregnancy might be detrimental to placental circulation."] ◄

3–6 **Conservative Management of Premature Rupture of Membranes.** Some have recommended immediate delivery in cases of premature rupture of the membranes because of the risk of infections, but others suggest prolonged observation. Michael W. Varner and Rudolph P. Galask (Univ. of Iowa) reviewed the results of conservative management of 116 pregnancies complicated by premature rupture of the membranes at 28–36 weeks' gestation. Mean maternal age was 25 years. Duration of premature rupture time from rupture to delivery ranged from 6 hours to 45 days.

Labor began spontaneously in 84.5% of patients, and 93% of 127 infants were delivered vaginally. Relationship of gestational age to perinatal survival is shown in Table 1. Respiratory distress syndrome developed in 25% of infants. Incidence appeared to be lower when the membranes were ruptured for longer than 48 hours. Clinical amnionitis developed in 5.2% of patients before labor (Table 2). Endocervical cultures were positive in only three cases. Four patients developed amnionitis during labor. Eight had endometritis after delivery; 4 of the 8 had positive endocervical cultures. Risk of endometritis was not related to the duration of premature rupture of the membranes. Nine infants (7.1%) had culture-proved sepsis. Group B β-hemolytic streptococcus was isolated from 5 infants, including the 1 stillborn infant in the series.

Perinatal survival was 96.9% in these cases of premature membrane rupture managed expectantly. In a predominantly middle-class, well-nourished population, conservative management of premature rupture of the membranes can be used with minimal risk of

(3–6) Am. J. Obstet. Gynecol. 140:39–45, May 1, 1981.

TABLE 1.—PERINATAL SURVIVAL RATES BY GESTATIONAL AGE DURING STUDY PERIOD

Weeks' gestation	*All infants newborn (%)*	*PROM <48 hr (%)*	*PROM ≥48 hr (%)*
28-29	46.5	100	100
30-31	76.7	77.8	90
32-33	96.1	100	100
34-35	97.1	100	96.8
36	99.5	100	100
Total	89.6 (692/772)	96.3 (53/55)	97.3 (70/72)

TABLE 2.—RELATION BETWEEN DURATION OF RUPTURE OF MEMBRANES AND INCIDENCE OF CLINICAL AMNIONITIS PRIOR TO LABOR

Duration (hr)	*% Amnionitis*
<24	0.0 (0/21)
24-48	6.6 (2/30)
48-72	4.2 (1/24)
>72	7.3 (3/41)
Total	5.2 (6/116)

infection of the mother and fetus. Whether the risk of infection is increased with internal fetal monitoring remains unclear. The major cause of neonatal morbidity and mortality in the present series was respiratory distress syndrome. Both this complication and patent ductus arteriosus were less frequent following membrane rupture of more than 24 hours' duration.

▶ [This retrospective analysis makes a compelling argument for a conservative approach to management of premature rupture of the membranes prior to 36 weeks. Treatment was expectant in that labor was not induced unless indicated (e.g., amnionitis, preeclampsia, etc.), and no corticosteroids were given. Survival in these cases was 96.9%, which was actually better than that of all infants of the same gestational age range (89.6%).] ◀

3–7 **C-Reactive Protein as Predictor of Infectious Morbidity With Premature Rupture of Membranes.** In women with premature rupture of membranes (PROM), early delivery increases the risk of prematurity but pregnancy prolongation increases the risk of infection. Although the ability to detect early infection would allow further maturation of the fetus while minimizing the sequelae of infection, early infection is not reliably predicted or detected by standard laboratory parameters. Mark I. Evans, Samir N. Hajj, Lawrence D. Devoe, Neil S. Angerman, and Atef H. Moawad (Univ. of Chicago) assessed the value of measurements of serum C-reactive protein (CRP) in predicting development of infectious morbidity in 109 women; 36 had PROM, 27 had spontaneous rupture of membranes at

(3–7) Am. J. Obstet. Gynecol. 138:648–652, Nov. 15, 1980.

term, 6 had preterm labor with intact membranes, and 40 had term labor with intact membranes. Serum CRP levels were assayed (using a nephelometric method with monospecific antiserums against CRP) along with white blood cell count, differential, and temperature course.

Infectious morbidity developed in 41 of the 109 women. Of the 68 nonmorbid patients, 63 had no detectable levels of CRP and 5 had levels less than 2 mg/dl. All 30 women with CRP levels at or above 2 mg/dl had evidence of morbidity. With 2 mg/dl as a demarcation point, CRP divided morbid from nonmorbid patients with great accuracy. There were no false positive results. There were 11 false nagative results that were also not detected by the other laboratory parameters. The mean CRP level was 4.1 mg/dl in patients with and 0.1 mg/dl in those without morbidity. White blood cell and band counts on differential were also higher when morbidity was present, but less consistently so than CRP.

In the women with PROM who were followed sequentially, the marked elevation of CRP in those with morbidity was again present, along with increased white blood cell and band counts. Of the 36 women with PROM, 31 were correctly categorized by CRP. In 14 of 20 patients with PROM in whom morbidity occurred, CRP tests became positive at least 12 hours before any other parameter. For the other 6 patients, CRP levels became elevated concurrently with at least 1 other parameter.

The serum CRP level is apparently a reliable early predictor of infectious morbidity and thus may be useful in the selective management of women with PROM. In those with gestations of at least 34 weeks or fetuses estimated to weigh at least 2,000 gm, the hazards of infection usually outweigh those of prematurity. The group that presents the greatest dilemma consists of fetuses of 26–33 weeks' gestation or those weighing 750–1,500 gm. Prolongation of such pregnancies is of obvious benefit when infection can be ruled out or predicted very early in its course. Use of CRP measurements may aid in reducing the number of infants delivered unnecessarily because of PROM and allow prompt intervention for those patients in whom chorioamnionitis is developing.

▶ [If it were possible to predict which patients with premature rupture of membranes are apt to become infected, the management of this condition would be on a more rational basis than it is at present. These observations suggest that serial C-reactive protein measurement may provide a clue. From the data presented, it appears that C-reactive protein levels tended to increase some hours prior to indices such as fever and leukocytosis. Another approach to this problem—serum complement activity—is the subject of the following article.] ◀

3–8 **Maternal and Cord Blood Complement Activity: Relationship to Premature Rupture of the Membranes.** Human complement levels are known to reflect presence of clinical infection, with low levels indicative of increased utilization in the body's immune response. Premature rupture of the membranes (PRM) is associated with increased fetal-maternal infectious morbidity, yet histopathologic and

(3–8) Am. J. Obstet. Gynecol. 139:38–40, Jan. 1, 1981.

bacteriologic factors often do not reflect this. In this prospective study by Donald L. Levy and Pierre C. Arquembourg (Ochsner Med. Inst., New Orleans), maternal and cord serum total hemolytic complement activity (CH_{50}) was measured in 102 patients without evidence of infection, with and without PRM.

Maternal serum CH_{50}, regardless of length of gestation, was similar to that of the nonpregnant adult population, except in cases of PRM greater than 12 hours, in which it was significantly lower. Only 2 patients (from the PRM group) had postpartum endometritis, and CH_{50} levels before delivery were both below the mean for the group. Since complement does not cross the placenta, cord serum reflects newborn CH_{50} exclusively. The CH_{50} in term newborns was significantly lower than that of matched maternal samples and dropped with decreasing gestational age. Term newborns of mothers with PRM, when compared to those without PRM, demonstrated an apparent decrease in mean CH_{50}, but the difference was not significant.

The CH_{50} decrease in patients with PRM greater than 12 hours may result from release of fluid containing antigens heterologous to the mother, triggering an antigen-antibody reaction with consumption of complement, and/or from presence of infective agents that initiate the complement reaction as a protective mechanism. The relative state of complement deficiency in term and preterm newborn infants raises the possibility of impaired complement-dependent immunologic function.

▶ [This study notes that maternal serum total complement activity was significantly lower in patients in whom membranes had ruptured more than 12 hours earlier than in those without PRM, implying that complement was consumed in an early response to threat of infection. The results in cord blood are more puzzling; while there was a positive correlation with gestational age, there was no apparent relationship with membrane rupture. Is this a reflection of immunologic immaturity of the fetus?] ◀

3–9   **Studies on Group B β-Hemolytic *Streptococcus:* I. Isolation and Partial Characterization of an Extracellular Toxin.** Group B β-hemolytic *Streptococcus* has become a major pathogen in newborn nurseries in the United States. Early onset disease is characterized by a mortality sometimes above 50% and features resembling those of gram-negative endotoxin shock, suggesting the presence of bacterial products with endotoxin-like properties. Carl G. Hellerqvist, Jorge Rojas, Robert S. Green, Sara Sell, Hakan Sundell, and Mildred T. Stahlman (Vanderbilt Univ.) performed extensive fractionation studies on a group B β-hemolytic *Streptococcus* type III isolated from an infant who died of septicemic shock. Fractions were infused intravenously into unanesthetized adult sheep.

The medium fraction but not the bacteria contained a component with a molecular weight of 2×10^6, composed of 84% carbohydrate and 16% protein, with physiologic activity in the sheep model. Infusion of 2-mg amounts led to a doubling of pulmonary artery pressure, a 20% fall in P_{O_2}, and chills and fever. The active component was degradable by hot phenol-water extraction into a pure polysaccharide with a molecular weight of 200,000, which retained the same physiologic prop-

(3–9) Pediatr. Res. 15:892–898, June 1981.

erties. The degraded component precipitated with group B-specific antiserum.

In sheep, a pure polysaccharide is the physiologically active portion of a high molecular weight toxin synthesized by group B β-hemolytic *Streptococcus* type III. This component has a different carbohydrate composition from that of group B capsular antigen. The means by which the polysaccharide exerts virulence is unknown, but presumably it does so through interaction with a target tissue to cause host-mediated physiologic changes, analogous to the antitumor activity exhibited by polysaccharides in vivo. Alveolar macrophages have receptors for mannose residues, which may be related to release of lysosomal enzymes and resultant tissue destruction.

▶ [This paper is the most exciting work on the *Streptococcus* group B problem we have seen. Many of the clinical features (fulminant onset and course, disparity between carriage and attack rates, etc.) are consistent with the cause being a toxin. If it is indeed a toxin, then the toxin could be isolated and characterized, which could lead to production of an antitoxin for treatment and, better yet, a toxoid for prophylaxis.] ◀

3–10 **Selective Maternal Culturing to Identify Group B Streptococcal Infection.** Group B β-hemolytic streptococci are a major cause of serious early-onset neonatal infection. Attempts at chemoprophylaxis of maternal carriers prior to or during labor and antibiotic therapy of neonates at the time of birth have been criticized because of their huge cost, widespread antibiotic usage, and lack of proven efficacy. An increased rate of infection has been shown among infants with a history of premature onset of labor and prolonged rupture of membranes. Marykay Pasnick, Philip B. Mead, and Alistair G. S. Philip (Univ. of Vermont) obtained vaginal cultures from all women admitted during 1974 to 1979 with onset of labor before 37 weeks' gestation or rupture of membranes without onset of labor. Results with these women and their infants were analyzed to determine if this method of selective culturing would identify infants at risk of serious infection.

With these indications, 1,213 women, representing 12.7% of all parturients, were cultured, and 124 cultures (10.2%) were positive for group B β-hemolytic streptococci. There was no significant difference in ABO blood types between colonized and noncolonized women, in contrast to previous reports. A greater proportion of Rh negativity was seen among colonized than noncolonized mothers (24% vs. 15%), and a greater percentage of Rh-negative women were colonized when compared with Rh-positive women (16% vs. 9%). Maternal age was not associated with streptococcal carriage.

Of the 125 infants born to the 124 women with positive vaginal cultures, 82 (66%) were asymptomatic and were not cultured. Of the remaining 43 infants from whom 1 or more cultures were obtained, 19 (44%) had positive cultures at one or more sites. A total of 10 infants had documented invasive disease (sepsis or meningitis) during the study period; 5 died. All 10 were born to mothers who satisfied the criteria for obtaining vaginal cultures prior to delivery. Eight of these mothers were cultured, and 7 cultures were positive. Early-

(3–10) Am. J. Obstet. Gynecol. 138:480–484, Nov. 1, 1980.

onset disease actually developed in about 1 of every 20 infants designated at high risk.

Selective maternal culturing identifies most infants at high risk for early-onset group B streptococcal disease while subjecting only 12.7% of the parturient population to the culturing procedure. This results in significant cost reduction over previously recommended protocols. By means of new culture techniques, most high-risk infants can be identified at birth or shortly thereafter. The selective maternal culturing protocol decreased the ratio of infants at risk to infants infected to 20:1 (from a previously reported ratio of 100:1), thereby achieving substantial savings in effort and expense without sacrificing screening test sensitivity.

▶ [This suggested approach to the group B streptococcal infection problem is based on culturing selected groups of patients whose neonates are at increased risk for invasive group B streptococcal disease (namely, patients with premature labor or premature rupture of the membranes). In our experience, invasive group B streptococcal disease has not been limited to these two risk groups. Prospective studies are needed to establish whether this sort of approach will provide information soon enough to affect the course of infected neonates.] ◀

3–11 **Group B Streptococcal Disease: Its Diagnosis with Use of Antigen Detection, Gram's Stain, and Presence of Apnea, Hypotension.** Clinically, early onset group B streptococcal (GBS) pneumonia and respiratory distress syndrome are not easily distinguished in neonates. David L. Ingram, Elizabeth L. Pendergrass, Patricia I. Bromberger, James D. Thullen, Charles D. Yoder, and Albert M. Collier evaluated the usefulness of GBS antigen detection, the presence of gram-positive cocci in the gastric aspirate, and the presence of apnea or hypotension, or both, as indicators of GBS infections in neonates. The sensitivities of a latex agglutination (LA) test and a countercurrent immunoelectrophoresis (CIE) test for GBS antigens also were evaluated.

Detection of GBS antigen was found to be a rapid and useful technique. The LA test appeared to be more sensitive than the CIE test, with LA detecting GBS antigens in 100% of 18 neonates able to provide enough urine for concentration. There were no false positive results. Gram-positive cocci were present in the gastric aspirates of 10 (77%) of 13 neonates with early onset GBS pneumonia, but in only 3 (10%) of 30 neonates with RDS. The infection rate in clinically similar neonates without gram-positive cocci in their aspirates was only 4%. Apnea and hypotension were commonly found in both early onset GBS pneumonia and RDS.

The results demonstrate the usefulness of LA in the detection of GBS antigen early in the course of early- and late-onset GBS infections.

▶ [The proper perinatal approach to the problem of early-onset group B streptococcal (GBS) infection has not yet been defined. According to this study, a latex agglutination test done on concentrated urine rapidly and reliably identified GBS antigen, indicating invasive GBS disease. Our pediatric colleagues recommend this test, as a means of making an early diagnosis, for all neonates who present with respiratory distress or with other signs that potentially indicate sepsis.] ◀

(3–11) Am. J. Dis. Child. 134:754–758, August 1980.

3-12 Increased Risk of Group B Streptococcal Disease in Twins.
Morven S. Edwards, Claudia V. Jackson, and Carol J. Baker (Baylor College of Medicine) treated 14 sets of twins or triplets over 5 years, among which 18 infants had proved early- or late-onset group B streptococcal infections. Data were adequate for analysis on 12 of the 14 sets of infants (11 sets of twins and 1 of triplets).

Six sets of infants each had early and late onset of infection. Among 3 of the 12 sets, invasive group B streptococcal infection was diagnosed in the second twin concomitantly or within several days after diagnosis of the index case. Each set of infants with early-onset infection was born prematurely (mean gestational age, 33.3 weeks), and for 3 of the sets symptoms suggesting bacterial infection were evident at birth. The other 3 index patients had symptoms of sepsis within 36 hours of birth. Birth order did not apparently influence the development of early infection. Three of 6 sets of infants with late infection were born at or near term. Type III, group B streptococci were recovered from each patient with late-onset and from 3 of the 6 sets with early-onset infection for whom serotyping of isolates was performed.

Where 1 twin has proved, invasive, early- or late-onset group B streptococcal infection, the other twin is apparently at exceptionally high risk of development of a similar infection for several reasons. Presence of disease in 1 twin reflects a high probability of nonprotective levels of antibody in the other twin. In a prospective study, twins were shown to be at particular risk of early-onset group B streptococcal disease. The similar genetic heritage of twins may place the apparently unaffected infant at increased risk because of as yet unidentified deficient host defense mechanisms. Invasive infection in one twin may denote exposure of the other to a particularly virulent strain of group B streptococci.

To prevent infection in the twin of an affected infant, cultures of blood and cerebrospinal fluid (CSF) should be obtained whether or not symptoms are present. If no CSF abnormalities are found, 150,000 to 200,000 units of penicillin G potassium per kg per day are given intravenously. If cultures of CSF and blood are negative at 72 hours, therapy is discontinued and the patient discharged.

▶ [These observations suggest that an apparently unaffected twin whose twin has group B streptococcal infection is at high risk for the disease. This is not surprising. It could reflect common maternal infection, lack of antibody, or impaired response. The authors propose that twin siblings of affected infants have cultures taken and be treated immediately until culture results are known.] ◀

3-13 Direct Intravascular Fetal Blood Transfusion by Fetoscopy in Severe Rhesus Isoimmunization. C. H. Rodeck, C. A. Holman, J. Karnicki, J. R. Kemp, D. N. Whitmore, and M. A. Austin administered two intravascular blood transfusions (IVTs) between 23 and 25 weeks by fetoscopy to each of 2 fetuses with severe anemia due to rhesus incompatibility.

TECHNIQUE.—Fetoscopy was done under sedation and local anesthesia; point of introduction was selected by real-time ultrasound scanning. Partic-

---

(3–12)   J.A.M.A. 245:2044–2046, May 22/29, 1981.
(3–13)   Lancet 1:625–627, Mar. 21, 1981.

ular care was taken to avoid damaging the thick edematous placenta. Blood was given directly into an umbilical vessel, either at the umbilicus or at the placental cord insertion. Fetal blood samples were taken before and after transfusion to assess hematologic status. A special needle, with an inner diameter of 0.25 mm, a reinforced 20-gauge shaft, and a 3-mm long 26-gauge tip, was threaded through a rubber cap covering the operating channel. A three-way tap and syringe was connected to the hub of the needle and to fresh-packed group-O rhesus-negative blood compatible with the mother. An assistant drew blood into the syringe and infused it into the umbilical vessel, the needle being held in the original puncture by the operator. Studies showed that the infusion rate of 1 ml/minute did not cause significant hemolysis. Fetal heart rate was continually monitored. On completion of infusion, frusemide, 2–5 mg was injected.

One grossly hydropic fetus survived; since chances of survival were low, fetal IVT may have been beneficial. The fetus can receive IVT at an earlier stage than intraperitoneal transfusion (IPT); optimum time for fetoscopy is 18–20 weeks. Absorption of intraperitoneal blood is poor in hydrops fetalis; IVT is more likely to be effective. With IVT, diuretics or albumin can be infused. Perforation of the fetal trunk by a 16-gauge needle is avoided. The second patient's fetus died after IPT. Though necropsy did not clarify cause of death, growth retardation may have been an additional factor. Intravascular blood transfusion conveys diagnostic and prognostic information that amniotic-fluid analysis cannot. Intravascular blood transfusion and IPT have complementary roles; by 26 weeks' gestation, the uterus may be too large, amniotic fluid too cloudy, and quantity of blood for transfusion too great for fetoscopy. Intraperitoneal blood transfusion, with real-time ultrasound to guide the needle, may then be the method of choice. Some 34% of fetuses that have had IPTs survive; of those with hydrops fetalis, the figure may be as low as 7%. When initial IPT is done before 25 weeks' gestation, only 3% of fetuses survive—a reflection both of severity of disease and risk of IPT in a small fetus. Fetal mortality from diagnostic fetoscopy can be about 3%, but risks of IVT are not yet known.

▶ [Whether or not direct intravascular fetal transfusion via fetoscopy is better than early (≤24 weeks' gestation) intraperitoneal fetal transfusion aided by sophisticated ultrasound equipment is problematic. The technical achievement reported here, however, is impressive.] ◀

3–14 **Nonimmunologic Hydrops Fetalis: Review of 19 Cases.** Robert C. Spahr, John J. Botti, Hugh M. MacDonald, and Ian R. Holzman (Univ. of Pittsburgh) reviewed 19 cases of nonimmunologic hydrops fetalis (NHF) occurring over 9 years. The pregnancies were complicated by hydramnios (78%) and preterm delivery (84%). Toxemia was found only twice, and severe maternal anemia did not occur. Delivery was accomplished vaginally in all but 4 patients. Various major fetal anomalies were present in 11 cases; in the other 8 (42%), no major abnormalities could be found except NHF. None of the placentas examined revealed thrombosed vessels or chorioangiomas. Nearly all 13 live-born infants were severely asphyxiated; only 32% survived beyond the neonatal period.

(3–14)   Int. J. Gynaecol. Obstet. 18:303–307, 1980.

Hydramnios appears to be the most useful indicator of the pregnancy at risk and should prompt ultrasonographic investigation for hydrops. A previously affected pregnancy should raise suspicion. Ultrasonographic criteria for diagnosis of hydrops include central displacement of viscera, hepatosplenomegaly, scalp edema, coarse fetal outline, and increased placental thickness. If ultrasonography does not find a cause for NHF, further diagnostic tests are done, such as amniocentesis, serologic tests, fetal cardiac monitoring, Kleihauer-Betke test for fetomaternal bleeding, radiography, hemoglobin electrophoresis, and glucose tolerance testing. It would appear that conditions associated with fetal congestive heart failure, hypoproteinemia, infection, neoplasia, and anemia may be linked with NHF. A specific cause of the hydrops may not be detectable.

Amniocentesis for evaluation of pulmonary maturity may be required when premature delivery is inevitable. Enhancement of pulmonary maturity with corticosteroids may be appropriate. After NHF is diagnosed, fetal heart rate tracings should be performed for evidence of fetal asphyxia; if it is found, delivery should be accomplished urgently in a center with a neonatal intensive care facility. A liberal approach to cesarean delivery is favored because of frequent birth asphyxia. Symptomatic treatment for the neonate includes fluid restriction (fluid requirements estimated with the use of "ideal weight"), maintenance of blood sugar, support of ventilation, and attention to anemia and complications of asphyxia. Genetic counseling is important to provide parents with an understanding of the risk of recurrence.

▶ [This is a nice review of an unusual condition. Nonimmunologic hydrops occurred once in 4,000 pregnancies. Over half of the infants had some type of abnormality and less than one-third survived the perinatal period. The most useful diagnostic method is ultrasound.

In a related study, Perlin and associates (*Obstet. Gynecol.* 57:584, 1981) reported 8 cases of nonimmunologic hydrops seen over 3½ years. Causes or associated conditions included fetomaternal hemorrhage (2 cases), tachyarrhythmia, diaphragmatic hernia, sacral teratoma, neuroblastoma, and heart disease; in 1 case there was no apparent cause. Six of the 8 infants died during the perinatal period.] ◀

3–15 **Antenatal Diagnosis of Chorioangioma of the Placenta.** Large, externally visible chorioangiomas, though uncommon, may cause both maternal and fetal complications, including hydrops, hyponatremia, hypoproteinemia, low birth weight, anemia, cardiomegaly, and congestive heart failure. To date, only 1 case of a placental tumor diagnosed antenatally by sonography has been reported. Beverly A. Spirt, Lawrence Gordon, William N. Cohen, and Thelma Yambao (SUNY, Upstate Med. Center, Syracuse, N.Y.) report a case of a large chorioangioma in a viable pregnancy, which was diagnosed by and followed with sonography.

Woman, 16, presented with a discrepancy between uterine growth and gestational age in the 30th week of pregnancy. Sequential longitudinal and transverse scans at 32 weeks revealed a single fetus in cephalic presentation with a discrete subchorionic lesion, 5 cm in diameter, in the middle of the placenta, consistent with a chorioangioma (Fig 3–5). Follow-up sonograms at

---

(3–15) AJR 135:1273–1275, December 1980.

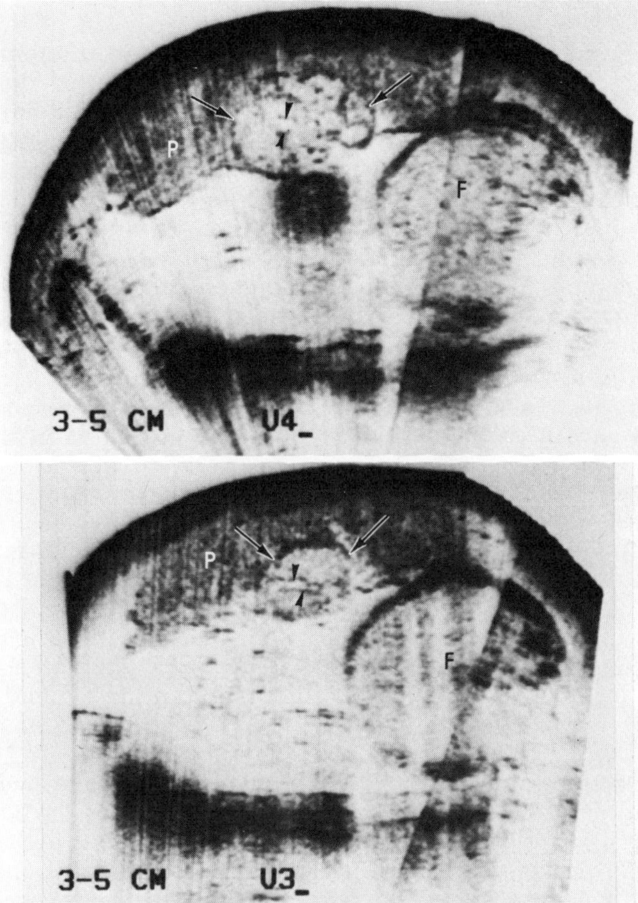

Fig 3–5.—Transverse sonograms in female patient, aged 16, at 34 weeks' gestation, 1 cm apart. Arrowheads show vascular channels within solid subchorionic mass *(arrows)*. *P*, placenta; *F*, fetus. (Courtesy of Spirt, B. A., et al.: AJR 135:1273–1275, December 1980.)

34, 36, and 39 weeks showed a progressive increase in the size of the lesion to 7 cm in diameter. There was no evidence of hydrops, cardiomegaly, or polyhydramnios. At 40 weeks, labor began spontaneously and a normal female infant, larger than average size, was delivered without complication. The neonatal period was uneventful. Pathologic examination of the placenta confirmed that the tumor (6.5 × 9 cm) was a chorioangioma.

Since hemangiomas larger than 5 cm in diameter are often associated with maternal and fetal complications, the absence of complications in this case is unusual. It is speculated that the large tumor infarct protected the fetus by reducing the amount of shunting that usually occurs in a tumor of this size.

▶ [This case report demonstrates that it is possible to make the presumptive diagnosis of chorioangioma of the placenta with ultrasound. Although not present in this patient, chorioangiomas can be associated with hydramnios and fetal hydrops. In the evaluation of a patient with hydramnios, ultrasound routinely is used to rule out twins, anencephaly, and other fetal anomalies, if possible. The reported case indicates that careful scrutiny of the placenta may be rewarding as well.] ◄

3-16 **Triplet and Quadruplet Pregnancies and Management.** The rate of triplet and quadruplet pregnancies has increased significantly since the introduction of ovulation induction agents. Raphael Ron-El, Eliahu Caspi, Peter Schreyer, Zvi Weinraub, Shlomo Arieli, and Michael D. Goldberg (Tel Aviv Univ.) managed 19 triplet and 6 quadruplet births between 1970 and 1978, incidences of 1:1696 and 1:5370, respectively, among all deliveries at the authors' institution.

Of the 25 multiple pregnancies, 18 (72%) followed use of ovulation induction agents (clomiphene in 2 and gonadotropin in 16 cases). Of the 7 spontaneous pregnancies, 4 were not diagnosed as multiple until the third trimester. Of the 18 induced pregnancies, 17 were diagnosed in the first trimester and 1 in the second. Management, initiated upon diagnosis, included bed rest, high-protein diet, β-mimetic agents, progestins, dexamethasone late in the second trimester, and selective cerclage.

Pregnancy lasted an average of 2 weeks longer in parous than in nulliparous women. Weight gain was similar in women carrying triplets and quadruplets (mean, 11 kg; range, 6 to 29). The presentation combination of vertex-vertex-vertex was the most frequent in triplets (Table 1). Mean gestational ages were 34 weeks for triplets and 35 weeks for quadruplets. Cesarean section was used for 44% of the deliveries. Mean infant birth weights were 1,807 gm for triplets and 1,950 gm for quadruplets. The 81 infants had a male-female ratio of 1.7:1. Mean overall Apgar score was 8.16. The perinatal mortality rate was 185/1,000, corrected (more than 28 weeks) to 137/1,000. The prematurity rate was 68% (17 of 25). The main neonatal complications resulted from prematurity; respiratory distress syndrome occurred in 13.7% of the infants. Maternal complications included postpartum hemorrhage necessitating hysterectomy in 2 patients. Apgar scores and perinatal mortality rates were similar after cesarean section and vaginal delivery (Table 2).

For multiple pregnancies, early bed rest and use of β-mimetics and gestagens are probably useful. The value of cerclage is unclear. Although fetal outcomes are similar after vaginal and cesarean deliveries, the latter may be useful in cases of malpresentation of the first fetus regardless of gestational age, prolonged premature rupture of the membranes, dysfunctional labor, and all other medical and obstetric complications as in singletons. As term approaches, there is a place for elective cesarean section for optimum management of neonatal problems.

► [Although this series of triplet and quadruplet pregnancies is relatively large, no one service can accumulate enough patients to answer clearly questions concerning the various techniques used in attempts to prevent premature delivery or the proper mode of delivery. The mean gestation length attained here (34–35 weeks) seems pretty good.] ◄

3-17 **Postterm Pregnancy: I.** John C. Hauth, Michael T. Goodman, Larry C. Gilstrap III, and Jo Ellen R. Gilstrap (Wilford Hall USAF

(3–16) Obstet. Gynecol. 57:458–463, April 1981.
(3–17) Obstet. Gynecol. 56:467–470, October 1980.

TABLE 1.—FETAL PRESENTATION* IN MULTIPLE PREGNANCIES

	1st fetus		2nd fetus		3rd fetus		4th fetus		Total	
Presentation	No.	Percent	No.	Percent	No.	Percent	No.	Percent	No.	Percent
Vertex	17	85	14	70	11	50	2	50	44	67
Breech	2	10	5	25	5	23	1	25	13	20
Transverse	1	5	1	5	6	27	1	25	9	13
Total	20		20		22		4		66	100

*In 4 deliveries, presentation of all fetuses was uncertain.

TABLE 2.—FETAL OUTCOME IN RELATION TO GESTATIONAL AGE AND MODE OF DELIVERY*

	Vaginal delivery					Cesarean section			
Gestational week	No. of cases	No. of cases	Infants	Apgar score (mean)	Perinatal mortality (%)	No. of cases	Infants	Apgar score (mean)	Perinatal mortality (%)
27–32	9	6	19	6.4	53.0	3	10	5.5	50.0
33–36	9	6	18	8.6	5.3	2*	6	8.7	0
≥ 37	7	2*	6	9.0	0	4	15	9.3	0

*One case in each group was not included because of combined vaginal and cesarean section deliveries.

Med. Center, Texas) retrospectively reviewed the perinatal mortality and morbidity of 185 postterm pregnancies managed by weekly trial inductions starting at 42 weeks' gestation. The outcome was compared with that of 119 postterm pregnancies with spontaneous labor before a trial induction was accomplished. The majority of patients (75%) met three or more criteria used in the determination of gestational age, and all patients met at least two. Labor was induced by a standard intravenous infusion of oxytocin. Inductions were conducted over a 6- to 8-hour period and in the absence of abnormal fetal heart rate patterns. Unsuccessful trial inductions were repeated weekly. In patients who had a persistently abnormal fetal heart rate pattern in the absence of hyperstimulation (a positive oxytocin challenge test [OCT]), oxytocin was discontinued. Amniotomy was then performed, and fetal heart rate and uterine pressures were monitored internally. The induction was continued after a period of observation.

Of 185 patients, 115 (62.1%) had labor successfully induced, and 70 (37.9%) entered spontaneous labor or had spontaneous rupture of membranes between inductions. One stillbirth occurred in the group that had no inductions, at 42 weeks, 3 days. This fetus had no congenital abnormalities and no meconium stain. There was no statistically significant difference in perinatal morbidity between the two groups in terms of bradycardia in labor, meconium-stained amniotic fluid, meconium aspiration, 1-minute Apgar scores less than 4, macrosomia (more than 4,000 gm), neonatal pneumonia, and incidence of cesarean section. There were 16 positive OCTs in the induced group. Positive OCT predicted fetal bradycardia in labor that was severe enough to warrant cesarean section in 5 (31%) of these 16 cases; a negative OCT predicted absence of severe bradycardia in 167 (99%) of 169 patients. The perinatal morbidity was not significantly different between patients with negative OCT and those entering spontaneous labor without trial induction or OCT.

The analysis suggests that routine induction of labor may be of no benefit in the management of postterm pregnancies. In this study the OCT did not clearly identify the compromised fetus or reduce perinatal morbidity, as 69% of patients with positive OCT did not show severe bradycardia in labor or depression of the infant at birth. Furthermore, the OCT did not predict meconium staining of amniotic fluid, nor was a negative OCT associated with decreased perinatal morbidity.

▶ [The management of postdatism remains controversial. This retrospective study suggests that a practice of trial inductions on a weekly basis did not offer advantages over expectant management. Because assignment to the treatment groups was not random (pregnancies ≥43 weeks' gestation were twice as frequent in the "trial induction" group), this study doesn't provide us with final answers. The authors promise a randomized, prospective study (presumably comparing trial inductions with expectant management without fetal well-being testing). Such a study would provide very valuable information. Stay tuned.

For a "state of the art" summary of the problem of postdate pregnancy, see the special article by Dr. Weingold at the beginning of this chapter.] ◀

3–18 **Intrauterine Meconium Aspiration** has been reported, but some

---

(3–18) Obstet. Gynecol. 57:26–29, January 1981.

perinatologists regard the phenomenon with skepticism. In an attempt to document its occurrence, Barry L. Brown and Norbert Gleicher (City Univ. of New York) reviewed the autopsy reports and histologic material of 200 successive fetuses that weighed more than 500 gm and were regarded as stillbirths. The cases represent a random sampling of fetal deaths that occurred before the era of fetal electronic surveillance.

Of the 200 fetuses, 25 (12.5%) showed aspiration of amniotic fluid within the alveolar system and 8 of these (4% of the total) had evidence of meconium contamination as shown by special stains for neutral mucopolysaccharides. All cases in which meconium was found within the lung were at 36 weeks' gestation or beyond, and 2 were clearly postmature. In 4 cases significant intrauterine pneumonitis also occurred.

Aspiration of amniotic fluid with or without meconium may thus occur in utero. Meconium aspiration must be regarded as a pathologic state. In many cases it is an acute preterminal event; in others it may develop in a more chronic form, allowing time for actual intrauterine pneumonitis to develop. Although most cases of meconium aspiration are neonatal and therefore largely preventable, others undoubtedly occur at unpredictable moments consequent to unpredictable events during intrauterine life. Recognition that the meconium aspiration syndrome is not necessarily a neonatal event is important, not only for the medical management of these cases but also for its medicolegal implications.

▶ [This study does not in any way minimize the importance of proper management of the airway at the time of birth in cases of meconium staining, but does illustrate that meconium aspiration can occur in utero.] ◀

4. Antepartum Fetal Surveillance

4–1 A Comparison of the Three Methods for External Fetal Cardiography. Techniques for external fetal heart rate monitoring during the antenatal period consist of phonocardiography, abdominal ECG, and ultrasound cardiography. Thore Solum (Univ. Hosp., Lund, Sweden) compared the quality of graphs obtained by these methods in 163 antepartum recordings of 137 patients who were between the 34th and 40th week of pregnancy.

Although an acceptable graph was obtained in 92.6% of the recordings with one or more of the techniques, in only 14% of the recordings did all three methods give equally good results for the same subject. Good or very good recordings (less than 15% failure or artifacts) were found in 23.4% of the phonocardiograms, 55.2% of the abdominal ECGs, and 85.9% of the ultrasound cardiograms. Phonocardiographic quality was significantly lower when the placenta was anteriorly located. The quality of phonocardiograms and abdominal ECGs was slightly, but not significantly, diminished by obesity. Abdominal ECG quality was best when the subjects were 37 weeks or more pregnant.

The results suggest that phonocardiography is of questionable value as standard equipment in cardiotocographs.

▶ [This study compares the three available methods of monitoring the fetal heart externally. Phonocardiography was clearly the least satisfactory, with less than one fourth of tracings rated as good or very good quality, which is consistent with our own experience. New to us is the correlation of placental location and phonocardiographic quality—better with a posterior than with an anterior placenta. Abdominal wall ECG gave good or very good tracings in 70% after 37 weeks' gestation but only in 40% to 45% in the 34- to 37-week interval. Best of all was ultrasound, with 75 to 90% good or very good quality regardless of duration of pregnancy. Unfortunately, ultrasound is known to be least reliable with respect to beat-to-beat variability, so the best technically is the least meaningful clinically. Alas, such is life!] ◀

4–2 Nonstress Testing. Allan B. Weingold, M. Lynne Yonekura, and Jane O'Kieffe (George Washington Univ.) review physiologic considerations on regulation of the fetal heart rate (FHR) and classify and illustrate the types of FHR acceleration. Their study focuses on 509 patients who underwent 1,281 nonstress tests (NST) in 1977 to 1978. Indications for NST included the major high-risk factors. The FHR pattern was assessed for baseline, variability, and occurrence of periodic acceleration or deceleration. The patient was observed for at least 40 minutes, with maternal vital signs recorded every 10 minutes. Palpation and sound stimulation were used to enhance fetal movement when this was not apparent. The NST was defined to include four categories. It was classified as reactive when accelerations of 15 beats per minute or more above baseline occurred and lasted 15

(4–1) Acta Obstet. Gynecol. Scand. 59:123–126, 1980.
(4–2) Am. J. Obstet. Gynecol. 138:195–202, Sept. 15, 1980.

seconds or more, with 5 fetal movements in 20 minutes. The test was nonreactive if no accelerations with fetal movements or fewer than 5 accelerations in 20 minutes occurred in a 40-minute test period. The NST was sinusoidal if oscillations occurred with a frequency of 2–5 cycles per minute, with an amplitude of 5–15 beats per minute. An inadequate NST indicated unreadable FHR data or no fetal movements recorded.

Of the 509 patients, 444 had repetitively reactive tests; 44 patients had 64 nonreactive tests, and there were 178 inadequate tests (13.8%). Use of sound stimulation and other modifications have reduced the number of inadequate procedures in the second year of study. Eight poor outcomes were identified in the reactive NST group; 5 of these had complications of labor clearly unrelated to the previously reactive NSTs, and 3 had false negative results (0.7%). In 21 patients (4.1%) who had persistently inadequate NSTs, there were 3 poor perinatal outcomes, including 1 neonatal death and 1 frequent occurrence of late decelerations during early labor. There were 64 nonreactive tests in 44 patients. There were 2 stillbirths associated with nonreactive NSTs and negative contraction stress tests (CST) within 1 week of delivery. When a nonreactive NST was followed by a positive CST, late decelerations were found during labor, a very poor prognosis for vaginal delivery. In the 39 patients remaining in whom the nonreactive NST appeared to be false positive (87%), 2 patterns evolved: in 22 patients, repeat NST became reactive; in the remaining 17, in whom NST remained nonreactive, fetal monitoring tracings in labor disclosed appearance of late deceleration in only 5.

Apparently a nonreactive NST correlates poorly with the CST, whereas a reactive NST correlates very well with a negative CST. A reactive NST is at least equally predictive of good perinatal outcome to a negative CST. The NST is technically easier to perform than the oxytocin challenge test and has no inherent risk for patient or fetus. The NST can be used as the primary screening tool. Its high false positive incidence requires confirmation by the CST or other indices of fetal distress. However, when an infant with mature lungs has a fixed-baseline nonreactive NST, verified within 12–24 hours, pregnancy should be terminated.

▶ [This study again demonstrates the low false negative rate of reactive NSTs (0.7% perinatal deaths and low 5-minute Apgar scores). The rate of false positive nonreactive tests (i.e., the absence of death or low 5-minute Apgar score) was high (87%). Most of these fetuses showed reactivity on subsequent NST testing and presumably had negative CSTs. The combination of a nonreactive NST and positive CST was ominous, as was a nonreactive NST in which the absence of accelerations was associated with a fixed, flattened baseline. This latter finding seen in conjunction with intrauterine growth retardation was "bad news" even if the CST was negative.] ◀

4–3 **Effects of External Physical Stimulation on Fetuses Near Term.** Bryan Richardson, Karen Campbell, Lesley Carmichael, and John Patrick (Univ. of Western Ontario, London) made measurements in 17 healthy pregnant women between 36 and 42 weeks' gestation 90 minutes before and after a standard physical stimulus was

(4–3) Am. J. Obstet. Gynecol. 139:344–352, Feb. 1, 1981.

applied; this consisted of 10 vigorous shaking movements of the uterine fundus followed by 10 rocking movements of the fetal head suprapubically. A mixed maternal and fetal electrocardiogram was obtained from electrodes placed subcutaneously in the anterior maternal abdominal wall. Fetal QRS complexes were recognized by an abdominal electrocardiogram processor. Fetal breathing movements and gross body movements were measured with a real-time ultrasonic scanner.

The mean fetal heart rate (14 fetuses) was 138 ± 0.4 beats per minute. Mean fetal heart rates at 5, 15, 30, and 90 minutes before external physical stimulation were compared to those noted at the same intervals after stimulation. The median value for the 5-minute standard deviation of successive heartbeat intervals was 30.3 msec, and the percentage of time spent making gross fetal body movements was about 11.1%. These measurements did not change significantly after stimulation. Three fetuses stimulated every 15 minutes over 3 hours also showed no significant changes in such measurements after stimulation. Fetal breathing movements which occurred episodically, were separated by periods of apnea during the control period and after stimulation. Fetal breathing movements diminished significantly over the 180-minute observation period, from 23.4% ± 4.5% during the control period to 10.1% ± 3.8% during the experimental period. However, the decrease in breathing movements began prior to stimulation and did not appear to be changed by it. Periodic increases separated by periodic decreases in fetal heart rate, heart rate variability, gross body movements, and breathing movements seemed unrelated to external fetal stimulation. Fetal outcome confirmed age and good health of the fetuses.

Periodic changes in measurements may have been related to underlying patterns of fetal behavior. It is possible that the acute fetal heart rate response to external physical stimulation may be too short-lived to reach significance when 5-minute time intervals are measured. The decreased fetal breathing activity noted may reflect a normal pattern in fasting women at term. It will be important to account for rest-activity patterns when fetal health is monitored and to recognize that, even in healthy fetuses, external physical stimulation does not reliably produce fetal activity.

▶ [External physical stimulation of the fetus was not associated with consistent changes in fetal heart rate patterns or gross fetal body movements in this study. Although we customarily stimulate the fetus during the performance of antepartum fetal heart rate testing if the mother reports no movements during a 20-minute period, perhaps we simply should "treat" the fetus expectantly. Tincture of time rather than our manipulations may explain any observed increase in fetal activity.] ◀

4–4 **Blind Oxytocin Challenge Test and Perinatal Outcome.** The oxytocin challenge test (OCT) was devised on the assumption that oxytocin-induced uterine contractions might identify the hypoxic and compromised fetus before the onset of labor in high-risk pregnancies. K. J. Staisch, J. R. Westlake, and R. A. Bashore (Univ. of California, Los Angeles) investigated the prognostic value of OCT in 217 patients

(4–4) Am. J. Obstet. Gynecol. 138:399–403, Oct. 15, 1980.

considered to have high-risk pregnancies. A total of 435 OCTs were performed; in no case were the results of the tests known to the attending physician. Management strategy during pregnancy was based on a thorough evaluation of maternal and fetal conditions, which included the use of serial estriol and ultrasound studies and the lecithin-sphingomyelin ratio. The single most ominous OCT result was used as the basis for the grouping of patients. Fetal heart rate was recorded continuously with external and/or internal techniques. The OCT results were correlated with fetal heart rate during labor, 5-minute Apgar scores, a neonatal morbidity score, and perinatal mortality.

The OCT results were positive in 35 patients, suspicious in 52, and negative in 131. Late deceleration of fetal heart rate was observed in 10 of 30 patients with positive OCT results, in 12 of 50 with suspicious results, and in 21 of 123 with negative results (Table 1). No single event alone showed a significant prevalence within the OCT groups. Primary cesarean section delivery was performed in 10 of 34 patients in the positive group, in 11 of 50 in the suspicious group, and in 25 of 123 in the negative group (Table 2). In the positive group, 2 fetuses died in utero and 2 infants died after delivery, for a perinatal mortality of 114:1,000. There were also 4 deaths in the negative group, but none in the suspicious group. Overall, 67% of the OCT

TABLE 1.—FETAL AND NEONATAL PERFORMANCE ASSOCIATED WITH OCT RESULT*

OCT result	Late decelerations in labor		Apgar score ≤6 at 5 minutes		Neonatal morbidity score ≤4	
	No.	%	No.	%	No.	%
Positive (N = 35) (16%)	10 (30*)	33	7 (33)	21	6 (31)	19
Negative (N = 130) (60%)	21 (123)	17	8 (129)	6	9 (127)	7
Suspicious (N = 52) (24%)	12 (50)	24	2 (52)	4	1 (52)	2

*Numbers in parentheses are the numbers of patients evaluated for that particular parameter.

TABLE 2.—CESAREAN SECTION DELIVERIES ACCORDING TO OCT RESULTS

OCT result	No. of patients	Primary cesarean sections		Indicated by late decelerations	
		No.	%	No.	%
Positive	34	10	29	8	80
Negative	123	25	20	5	20
Suspicious	50	11	22	6	55

tests were false positive and 17% were false negative for the parameters studied.

Oxytocin challenge is not a reliable way of identifying fetuses at risk. Clinical judgment remains important in the high-risk pregnancy. Induction of labor in high-risk pregnancies should be performed in a hospital setting where intensive neonatal care is available.

▶ [This is an impeccable study from the point of view of experimental design. Since the results were not made available to those caring for these patients with an assortment of high-risk conditions, it is possible to ask what the OCT might add to clinical information, estriols, ultrasound, and amniotic fluid analysis, which were all available and utilized in management. The "bottom line" seems to be that the OCT provides information of value, but its discriminatory ability is far from perfect. The correlation with the various outcome indices (late decelerations in labor, low 5-minute Apgars, and low neonatal morbidity score) was highest in patients with positive OCTs, intermediate in those with suspicious OCTs, and lowest in those with negative OCTs. However, perhaps the most important finding is that two thirds of those who had at least one positive OCT exhibited none of these "bad" outcomes.] ◀

4–5 **Oxytocin Challenge Test and Intrauterine Growth Retardation.** Intrauterine growth retardation (IUGR) accounts for high rates of perinatal morbidity and mortality and yields the greatest number of positive oxytocin challenge tests (OCTs). Chin-Chu Lin, Lawrence D. Devoe, Philip River, and Atef H. Moawad (Univ. of Chicago) analyzed the nonstressed fetal heart rate test (NST) and the OCT results in 85 fetuses with IUGR. Overall incidence of nonreactive NSTs during the study period was 19.3% in a general high-risk population; rate of positive OCTs was 12.8%. Risk of a nonreactive NST was doubled in cases of IUGR and that of a positive OCT was tripled.

The association between hypertension and a positive OCT in IUGR cases was 50%, significantly greater than that between hypertension and IUGR with a negative reactive fetal heart rate (FHR) pattern. Although the association between abnormal estriol levels and IUGR was very high, no statistically significant differences were found among various FHR response groups. Intrapartum fetal distress correlated well with FHR test outcome in infants with IUGR. Half the infants with IUGR and positive nonreactive tests had 1-minute Apgar scores of 6 or below. The section rate did not differ significantly among FHR response groups. Rate of significant neonatal morbidity was 21.4%. All 4 perinatal deaths were associated with abnormal FHR test responses, 3 with positive nonreactive tests and 1 with a negative nonreactive pattern.

Predictive value of the NST/OCT for perinatal morbidity in IUGR is shown in the table. Weekly evaluation of the NST/OCT is suggested in pregnancies with IUGR. Plasma estriol determinations should be made twice a week. With a positive OCT and normal estriol values or a negative OCT and abnormal estriol values, delivery is indicated if the L/S ratio is mature. With a positive OCT, especially a nonreactive FHR pattern, and abnormal estriol values, immediate delivery is indicated regardless of the L/S ratio. About two thirds of fetuses with IUGR will tolerate the stress of labor without fetal dis-

(4–5)   Am. J. Obstet. Gynecol. 140:282–288, June 1, 1981.

PREDICTIVE VALUE OF NONSTRESSED FETAL HEART RATE TEST AND
OXYTOCIN CHALLENGE TEST ON PERINATAL MORBIDITY
IN INTRAUTERINE GROWTH RETARDATION

NST		OCT		Perinatal morbidity*
Nonreactive	↗	Positive 13 (65%)	→	12/13 (92%)†
20 (39%)	↘	Negative 7 (35%)	→	2/7 (29%)
Reactive	↗	Positive 5 (16%)	→	2/5 (40%)
32 (61%)	↘	Negative 27 (84%)	→	5/27 (18%)

*Perinatal morbidity: combination of intrapartum fetal distress, low 1-minute Apgar score, neonatal complication, and perinatal death.

†Statistical significance at $P < .001$ between nonreactive positive group and combination of other three groups.

tress. Section delivery probably is indicated in cases of severe IUGR with serious maternal complications or IUGR with a positive OCT and an unfavorable cervix.

▶ [This study confirms previous ones in that abnormal antepartum fetal heart rate testing is disproportionately common in cases of IUGR and that the combination of a nonreactive NST and a positive OCT means trouble. Although it was apparently not a problem here, we have had difficulties in this situation by intervening for fetal distress (usually by cesarean section), only to deliver an anomalous baby who doesn't survive. Improved prenatal diagnosis may minimize this problem, but it sort of goes with the territory.] ◀

4–6 **Postdate Pregnancy: Utilization of Contraction Stress Testing for Primary Fetal Surveillance.** In most studies, prolonged pregnancy has been associated with increased fetal and neonatal mortality and morbidity. Recent approaches have focused on fetal surveillance methods that avoid unnecessary interventions but can detect the postmature fetus early enough to allow intervention before permanent damage has occurred. Roger K. Freeman, Thomas J. Garite, Houchang Modanlou, Wendy Dorchester, Catherine Rommal, and Melinda Devaney (Univ. of California at Irvine) prospectively studied 679 consecutive postdate pregnancies assessed with the contraction stress test (CST), along with 500 consecutive normal-term gestations in the same period. The study patients were at or beyond 42 weeks' gestation. Tests producing negative results were repeated after 1 week. Patients with equivocal results began the induction of monitored labor or were observed with frequent nonstress tests (NSTs). A reactive, positive test result called for amniotomy to induce labor and direct fetal heart rate monitoring. If the test was nonreactive and positive, cesarean section was carried out without a trial of labor.

There were no fetal or neonatal deaths in either the postdate or the control group. The rate of Apgar scores below 7 was 0.88% in the study group. Fetal distress occurred in 37% of adequately monitored postdate cases and in 14% of the control cases. Cesarean section was done for this reason in 3.5% of the postdate group and in 1% of the control group. Meconium aspiration occurred in 5 postdate cases. Shoulder dystocia occurred in 10 postdate and 3 control cases. Abnor-

(4–6) Am. J. Obstet. Gynecol. 140:128–135, May 15, 1981.

mal CST results were obtained in 39% of postdate cases, but delivery was elected for this reason in only 5.4% of cases.

No increase in neonatal mortality or morbidity was found in this series of postdate pregnancies. With the use of the CST for primary fetal surveillance, only 1 in 20 patients past 42 weeks' gestation will require intervention on fetal indications. Further efforts are needed to find easy, cost-effective, reliable methods of fetal surveillance in postdate pregnancies.

▶ [Postdatism is far and away the most common reason for antepartum fetal heart rate testing. Most units (including our own) seem to use the NST as the primary approach, with the CST reserved for those with nonreactive NST. Freeman, however, prefers the CST , which he was first to describe in detail, as the initial line of screening. The results reported here are very good—in fact, almost too good! There were no fetal or neonatal deaths in 679 consecutive postdate pregnancies and only 1% of infants had Apgar scores less than 7 at 5 minutes. Among the 500 patients in the comparison group, there were also no perinatal deaths and no low 5-minute Apgar scores. It looks as though Long Beach, California, is the best place to be born.] ◀

4–7 **Clinical Significance of Perceptible Fetal Motion.** It has been proposed that the monitoring of fetal activity during the last trimester of pregnancy is useful in assessing fetal welfare. William F. Rayburn (Ohio State Univ.) tested maternal perception of fetal activity among 82 patients during the third trimester, using real-time ultrasonography in a 15-minute period of testing in late morning and afternoon. All perceived fetal movements were visualized on the scanner and involved motion of the legs.

The patient's subjective sensation registered 82% of all fetal motions that were viewed sonographically. All combined motions of the fetal trunk and legs were perceived by the patients and were described as strong movements (kicks, stretches, rollovers, balling up). Clusters of independent, isolated motions of fetal limbs were less frequent and perceived less accurately (56% accuracy) by patients as weak or flutter movements. The number of fetal movements perceived during the 15-minute test period was significantly ($P < 1.8$) than in those with intact membranes (4.2 ± 0.6). Maternal obesity, parity, gestational age, and Braxton-Hicks uterine contractions had no effect on the patient's sensation of fetal activity.

Fifty-five patients were delivered of infants within 5 days after the ultrasound test. Mean gestational age at delivery was 37 ± 4 weeks. Only 1 fetus among the 45 that had displayed strong movement had any significant neonatal complication; this infant suffered from severe growth retardation and an encephalocele and died shortly after induced vaginal delivery. Of 10 fetuses without visibly strong movement, 5 were perceived as active later the same day and subsequently were delivered without complication. The other 5 fetuses remained motionless that same day and had unfavorable neonatal outcomes related to hydrocephalus (3), severe Rh isoimmunization (1), and an occult prolapsed umbilical cord (1).

Fetal motion after premature rupture of the amniotic membranes (an antepartum complication recorded in 24 patients) had not been

---

(4–7) Am. J. Obstet. Gynecol. 138:210–212, Sept. 15, 1980.

described previously. The decreased intrauterine space was not found to be restrictive. Fetal activity occurred more than twice as frequently in these 24 cases, and maternal perception of fetal motion was as accurate as that of patients with intact amniotic membranes.

The findings of this study reveal that perceived fetal motion is reliable and is related to the strength of lower limb motion, is increased with ruptured amniotic membranes, and is reassuring if the fetus is considered to be visibly active. A lack of visible motion of fetal trunk with limbs may be explained by a fetal rest period, the patient's supine position, or true fetal distress. If the fetus is described as inactive within that same day, testing of fetal heart rate and repeat real-time ultrasonography are indicated.

▶ [The presence of ruptured membranes was associated with increased fetal activity in this study.] ◀

4–8 **Management of Patients With a Live Fetus and Cessation of Fetal Movements.** R. Homburg, A. Matzkel, M. Birger, and V. Insler (Tel-Aviv) managed 67 patients with a history of no fetal movements for at least 12 hours and a live fetus (gestational age 30 weeks), according to a fixed protocol, during an 18-month period. Amnioscopy was done in all but 6 patients who had a tightly closed cervix. Amniocentesis was used to obtain amniotic fluid from these 6 and from 2 patients in whom amnioscopy gave equivocal results. If green or yellow-brown discoloration of the amniotic fluid was revealed, induction of labor was attempted unless an unstressed cardiotocogram (CTG) showed late decelerations of the fetal heart rate or loss of beat-to-beat variability, in which case a Cesarean section was done immediately.

The 67 patients were divided into two groups. Group 1 consisted of 12 patients who were found to have meconium-stained amniotic fluid or abnormal unstressed or stressed CTGs. Labor was induced in all 12, and all were delivered of a live infant within 24 hours of admission. Half of these patients had cesarean section for fetal distress. The 55 patients of group 2 had no signs of fetal distress on admission. They were hospitalized for 2 days; on each of these days they had unstressed CTG and a 24-hour urinary estriol estimation. No abnormalities were found, and all patients in this group felt fetal movements again while hospitalized. After discharge from the hospital, they were seen every week. Half of these pregnancies were classified as high risk. Forty-nine of the 55 patients were allowed to go into labor spontaneously. In the others, labor was induced for reasons unconnected with fetal movements. Seventeen patients had late decelerations or meconium-stained amniotic fluid during labor, or both, 7 had cesarean sections, and 8 required operative vaginal deliveries. Four of the newborn infants had a 1-minute Apgar score of less than 5; the Apgar score at 5 minutes was invariably 8 or above. Of the 67 pregnancies in the entire series, 33 were classified as high risk. The proportion of high-risk pregnancies was the same in both groups, as were the proportion of primiparas to multiparas (1:2) and the ratio of male to female fetuses (2:1).

(4–8) Br. J. Obstet. Gynaecol. 87:804–807, September 1980.

It is reasonable to assume that most fetuses in group 1 were in jeopardy, and prompt delivery saved these babies. The other 55 patients showed no signs of fetal distress, and the pregnancies were allowed to continue. There was a uniformly good outcome, so that unnecessary intervention had been avoided. Half of these patients were delivered within 1 week. A previous study by the authors has noted a significant reduction in fetal movements in the week before delivery in normal pregnancies.

It is suggested that patients of 30 or more weeks' gestation who report a complete cessation of fetal movements for 12 hours or more and have an audible fetal heartbeat be hospitalized. The color of amniotic fluid should be examined. If there is meconium, delivery should be expedited. If no meconium is present, an unstressed 40-minute CTG should be recorded. If this shows late decelerations or loss of beat-to-beat variability, labor should be induced. If the unstressed CTG is normal, an oxytocin-stressed CTG should be recorded, and if this shows late decelerations, labor should be induced. If all examinations prove negative, a CTG is done daily for 2 days and 24-hour urinary estriol levels are measured. If these tests reveal no abnormality, discharge of the patient and conservative management would seem in order.

▶ [There is much current interest in fetal movement assessments ("kick counts") as a means of fetal surveillance. A major clinical problem is what to do with the patient in whom movement ceases. This study provides an answer. If there is no meconium in the amniotic fluid and fetal heart rate studies (stressed or nonstressed, or both) are normal, there seems to be no cause for concern. If, however, either meconium is present or the heart rate monitoring is abnormal, delivery should be effected; in 12 cases of the latter type, all infants were born alive but half required cesarean section for fetal distress.] ◀

4–9 **Qualitative Real-Time Cross-Sectional Echocardiographic Imaging of Human Fetus During Second Half of Pregnancy.** Lothar W. Lange, David J. Sahn, Hugh D. Allen, Stanley J. Goldberg, Caroline Anderson, and Harlan Giles (Univ. of Arizona) investigated how early the normal fetal cardiac anatomy can be identified by means of modern high-resolution, real-time, cross-sectional scanners and assessed the possibilities for prenatal diagnosis of cardiac anomalies. A total of 94 satisfactory (of 106 attempted) real-time fetal examinations were performed in 67 (of 71) normal pregnancies at 19 to 41 weeks' gestation (mean, $31^{1}/_{2}$ weeks). Estimated weights of these fetuses using an ultrasound algorithm were 500–3,100 gm (mean, 1,580 gm). Scans were also made of 14 fetuses of 13 healthy women with high-risk family or obstetric histories for congenital heart disease, and of 3 fetuses of women with Rh incompatibility. Postnatal images were made of 73 of the infants.

No cardiac anomalies were shown in any of the 84 fetuses studied. The four-chamber and short-axis great artery views were most successful for cardiac evaluation. These views could be obtained in nearly 96% of the fetuses. With these views, cardiac chamber and valve structures, as well as two great arteries, could be imaged in

(4–9) Circulation 62:799–806, October 1980.

detail. The ascending and descending aorta, as well as the aortic arch and vessels to the arms and head, were visualized in 87% of the examinations, and the inferior and superior venae cavae were visualized in 76%. In 2 of the 3 Rh fetuses, changes in cardiac chambers compatible with hydrops fetalis were demonstrated. Examination (clinically or noninvasively) of all infants after birth showed that no cardiac malformations were present.

Although no diagnosis of a cardiac malformation was made or missed, diagnosis of gross anomalies of the great arteries, hypoplasia of the right or left ventricles or their atrioventricular valves, the atrioventricular canal, and single or common ventricle should be detectable by this method. Demonstration of normal anatomy in the fetus can also be helpful. Resolution of the systems does not provide enough detail to study fetal hearts at less than 16 weeks' gestation, but 3 recent studies of fetuses at 16 weeks did show the presence of two atrioventricular valves and two ventricular chambers.

▶ [Real-time ultrasound is effective in the evaluation of fetal cardiac anatomy, according to this report. Although there were no cardiac malformations in the cases studied, the authors think that in utero diagnosis of many structural heart defects will be possible. Fetuses with nonimmunologic hydrops, heart block, or arrhythmias would be candidates for this sort of examination.] ◀

4–10   **Successful Treatment of Fetal Congestive Heart Failure Secondary to Tachycardia.** Among the adverse effects of fetal cardiac arrhythmias is persistence of a supraventricular tachycardia in the neonatal period, with or without subsequent congestive heart failure. John T. Harrigan, John J. Kangos, Anju Sikka, Kenneth R. Spisso, Narayanan Natarajan, David Rosenfeld, Sherwin Leiman, and Donald Korn (New Jersey-Rutgers Med. School, Piscataway, N. J.) report a case of fetal tachycardia in which congestive heart failure developed in utero, and was treated successfully by digoxin administration to the mother.

Woman, 31, reported decreased fetal movement at 26 weeks' gestation, and examination disclosed fetal tachycardia of 260 beats per minute, with fetal scalp edema and ascites noted at ultrasonography. The mother was given oral digoxin in a dose of 0.5 mg, repeated twice in a 14-hour period. The fetal heart rate fell to 125–130 beats per minute 1 hour after the third dose, and increased fetal movements were noted soon afterward. The patient continued to receive 0.25 mg of digoxin daily until term. Fetal ascites and scalp edema had resolved on ultrasonography done 19 days after the start of treatment. A 3,268-gm infant was born vaginally at 38 weeks' gestation, with a 1-minute Apgar score of 8 and a 5-minute score of 9. The heart rate, ECG, and M-mode echocardiogram were normal. The cardiothymic image was enlarged moderately but returned to normal by the third day of life. The infant was normal at age 10 weeks.

Digoxin was used successfully in this case to treat congestive heart failure secondary to fetal tachycardia. Delivery appeared inadvisable when cardiac failure was detected, and there was a risk of fetal death from heart failure before maturity. It is not clear why previous attempts at conversion using digoxin have failed. Early treatment when the heart rate consistently exceeds 200 beats per minute can

---

(4–10)   N. Engl. J. Med. 304:1527–1529, June 18, 1981.

reduce the threat of fetal death and make delivery of an immature infant unnecessary.

▶ [In contrast to previous reports (see 1981 YEAR BOOK, pp. 106–107) and our personal experience, maternal administration of digoxin in this case was associated with the conversion of a fetal tachycardia to a normal fetal heart rate. The presence of fetal scalp edema and ascites on ultrasound examination prior to conversion suggests that the fetal tachycardia had been present for some time. Because of the potential risks of digoxin therapy to the mother, direct intrafetal injection of the drug had a certain theoretic appeal, at least as an initial treatment. The variable results reported with digoxin treatment of fetal tachycardias may well relate to the likelihood that the same rhythm disturbance has not been present in all cases.] ◀

4-11 **Fetal Biophysical Profile Scoring: A Prospective Study in 1,184 High-Risk Patients.** Antepartum detection of the fetus at risk for death or damage in utero remains a major challenge. F. A. Manning, T. F. Baskett, I. Morrison, and I. Lange (Univ. of Manitoba, Winnipeg) have based the management of high-risk pregnancies on a fetal biophysical profile score derived from fetal movement, tone, reactivity, breathing, and qualitative amniotic fluid volume. Perinatal nurses were trained in profile scoring based on real-time ultrasound scanning and Doppler fetal heart rate recording. Each variable was scored 2 if normal and 0 if abnormal. A total of 1,184 consecutively referred high-risk infants at gestational ages of 26 weeks or later were included in the study. A total of 2,238 tests were performed.

In 1,801 tests (80.5%), all variables were normal. In 378 tests (17%), all variables but one were normal. Fetal breathing movements were absent in 14% of all tests, and the nonstress test was nonreactive in 6%. The perinatal mortality was 5 per 1,000. It was 3.5 per 1,000 in 1,137 cases in which the last profile score was 8 or above. Only 1 of these deaths occurred unexpectedly in an apparently normal fetus. Two fetal deaths occurred in 47 cases with the last profile score of 6 or under, for a perinatal mortality of 43 per 1,000. Infants with major anomalies incompatible with life were excluded from the study.

Fetal assessment by biophysical profile scoring can be carried out expertly by perinatal nurses trained in real-time B-mode ultrasonography and Doppler ultrasound study. The average time needed to perform the test is about 18 minutes. The use of combined fetal biophysical variables to estimate fetal risk results in a substantial fall in false positive results. Continued improvement in ultrasound imaging systems probably will result in a wider range of fetal biophysical activities that can be observed and recorded.

▶ [The authors of this report promise to compare prospectively their five-item "fetal biophysical profile score" with conventional antepartum fetal heart rate testing. Two fringe benefits of their ultrasound procedure are the identification of intrauterine growth retardation based on the absence of 1-cm pockets of amniotic fluid (as considered elsewhere in this YEAR BOOK) and the antenatal detection of most of the serious congenital malformations in this series.] ◀

4-12 **Alternative to Antepartum Fetal Heart Rate Testing.** William Rayburn, Frederick Zuspan, Mary Ellen Motley, and Marcia Donald-

(4-11) Am. J. Obstet. Gynecol. 140:289–294, June 1, 1981.
(4-12) Ibid., 138:223–226, Sept. 15, 1980.

son prospectively studied the high-risk pregnancies of 203 patients to test the hypothesis that maternal perception of fetal movement is as useful as antepartum fetal heart rate testing (AFHRT) in assessing fetal welfare. Patients whose antepartum course was complicated were asked to participate after 33 weeks of gestation. They were instructed to record perceived fetal motion for a minimum 1-hour rest period each day. A fetus was considered active if 4 or more movements were perceived during each hour of daily counting, and inactive if there were 2 consecutive days of apparent fetal inactivity and if the fetus was classified in the lower 5% of all cases from all weeks. Initially, nonstress testing was done routinely. Within the week prior to delivery, the results of the most recent AFHRT and the daily fetal movement pattern were compared independently to subsequent fetal outcome during labor and delivery.

Most conditions involved an active fetus and subsequently normal AFHRT results (320 of 330 tests, 97%). Evidence for an inactive fetus frequently was followed initially by a nonreactive nonstress test result (14 of 19 results), requiring repeat nonstress testing or contraction stress testing. Ten abnormal AFHRT results with prior evidence of an active fetus involved nonreactant nonstress tests with a contraindication to contraction stress testing (3), suspicious contraction stress tests (4), and positive contraction stress tests (3). The table presents fetal movement patterns and subsequent AFHRT results. A favorable perinatal outcome was present in 175 (86%) of 203 pregnancies. The favorable outcome was equally predicted by an active fetus (168 of 186 pregnancies, or 90%) and a normal AFHRT result (173 of 190 pregnancies, 91%). An unfavorable perinatal outcome following such reassuring results was not more commonly associated with a particular antepartum complication, but was more related to intrapartum complications. An inactive fetal movement pattern was less sensitive than an abnormal AFHRT result in predicting an unfavorable perinatal outcome (10 of 17 pregnancies, 59%, vs. 11 of 13 pregnancies, 86%), but this difference was not significant. Inactivity in a fetus having an abnormal AFHRT result was very predictive of an unfavorable perinatal outcome in 9 of 10 instances. Conditions associated with an unfavorable outcome involved hydrocephalus (2), severe Rh isoimmunization (2), maternal sepsis and acidosis (2), fetal

FETAL MOVEMENT PATTERN AND SUBSEQUENT ANTEPARTUM
FETAL HEART RATE TESTING RESULT

| | | Subsequent AFHRT result | | | |
| | | Normal | | Abnormal | |
Fetal movement pattern	*No of tests*	*No.*	*%*	*No.*	*%*
Active	330	320	97	10	3
Inactive	19	9	44	10	56
Total	349	329	94	20	6

peritonitis, severe fetal growth retardation in a known drug addict, and a nuchal cord accident.

These results suggest that a record of fetal activity by the compliant patient is a reliable alternative to AFHRT for initial screening of fetal well-being. Rest is emphasized while the patient reclines on her left side for 1 hour or more each day; this position should improve uteroplacental perfusion. False positive or reassuring results with this technique were infrequent (18 of 186 cases, 10%).

▶ [It is interesting that three or fewer movements per hour constituted an inactive pattern in this study. A count of fewer than three fetal movements per hour was regarded as an alarm signal by Neldam in a report abstracted in the 1981 YEAR BOOK (pp. 111–112). The correlation between an active fetal pattern as perceived by the patient and a normal subsequent antepartum fetal heart rate test was excellent.] ◀

4–13 **Fetal Movements and Fetal Outcome: A Prospective Study** was conducted by Leo R. Leader, Peter Baillie, and Dirk J. Van Schalkwyk (Univ. of Cape Town). Two hundred sixty-four patients admitted at 26–40 weeks of gestation because of antenatal complications (usually hypertension) were asked to count the number of fetal movements for four 30-minute periods per day. The observations were continued by the patient if she was discharged from the hospital, and duration varied from 3 days to 10 weeks. The fetal movement count was categorized as abnormal if there was a day with no fetal movements or 2 successive days within the week before delivery on which there were less than 10 fetal movements. Fetal condition at birth was regarded as poor if the infant had a 5-minute Apgar score of 6 or less plus a concordant maternofetal arterial base deficit difference of 5 mEq/L or more.

The 264 women were delivered of 15 stillborn infants and 6 infants in poor condition. There was a significant association between abnormal fetal movements and both stillbirth and poor neonatal condition. This association was particularly applicable to the prediction of stillbirths, none of which occurred when fetal movements were normal, and to fetal condition at birth (Table 1). The sensitivity, predictive value, and specificity of evaluation of fetal movements is shown in Table 2. The Youdens index, in which the false positive and false negative errors are combined and subtracted from 100%, was 77%. The mean weekly count decreased with advanced gestational age, but not predictably so in each patient.

Of the 161 patients whose gestational age was greater than 38 weeks, 138 had normal fetal movement counts and 23 had abnormal counts. Perinatal outcome was significantly poorer in the group with abnormal movements ($P = .0015$).

Fetal movement recording by the mother is applicable to virtually all patients and assesses the condition of the fetus at the time of observation. It is simple, safe, inexpensive, noninvasive, and significantly indicative of neonatal outcome. It can be used to screen a population as well as to indicate when a fetus is at risk. Patients who have low fetal movement counts urgently require further investiga-

(4–13) Obstet. Gynecol. 57:431–436, April 1981.

TABLE 1.—FETAL CONDITION AND INCIDENCE OF STILLBIRTH IN ALL PATIENTS

| | Fetal movements | |
Outcome	Normal	Abnormal
Stillbirth	0	15*
Poor condition	3	3†
Good condition	220	21
Total	223‡	39

*$P \leq .00001$.
†$P = .01336$.
‡Excludes 2 neonatal deaths: (1) a hydrocephalic infant who died 3 days after birth; (2) a 900-gm infant delivered for fulminating preeclampsia.

TABLE 2.—EVALUATION OF FETAL MOVEMENTS IN ASSESSING GOOD AND POOR FETAL OUTCOME*

Sensitivity (TP/TP + FN)		Predictive value (TP/TP + FP)		Specificity (TN/FP + TN)	
No.	Percent	No.	Percent	No.	Percent
18/21	86	18/39	46	220/241	91

*TP = true positive; TN = true negative; FP = false positive; FN = false negative.

tion. The presence of normal fetal activity can reassure the clinician, should it be necessary that the pregnancy continue to obtain greater fetal maturity.

▶ [Another enthusiastic report relating fetal movements (FM) as perceived by the mother to perinatal outcome is presented here. The criterion for "abnormality" was 1 day with no movements or 2 successive days within the week prior to delivery with fewer than 10 movements (these hospitalized patients counted movements 2 hours each day). Obstetric patients with complications who are admitted to the hospital prior to labor often spend boring days (bed rest, heart rate testing, urine collections, etc.). Recording fetal movements for an hour each day is probably good therapy for the mother as well an effective means of fetal surveillance.] ◀

4–14 **Ultrasonic Methods of Predicting the Estimated Date of Confinement** were compared by Mazie M. Kopta, Paul G. Tomich, and James P. Crane (Washington Univ.). The most common way to interpret biparietal diameter (BPD) growth curves is to plot the BPD on a graph by the last normal menstrual period, or on the mean, or both. Sabbagha et al. devised the method of growth-adjusted sonographic age (GASA), based on one BPD measurement in the second trimester and another in the third; the first is plotted on the mean and then readjusted, depending on the percentile into which the second falls. The authors have used mean projected gestational age (MPGA) to predict the estimated date of confinement (EDC). Two BPD readings are obtained at 19 to 30 weeks' gestation at an interval of at least 3

(4–14)   Obstet. Gynecol. 57:657–660, May 1981.

CUMULATIVE RESULTS COMPARING INTERVAL BETWEEN PREDICTED EDC
AND ACTUAL DELIVERY DATE

		Accuracy of EDC			
Group	No. patients	± 7 days	± 10 days	± 14 days	> 14 days
MPGA	60	38 (63%)	48 (80%)	54 (90%)	6 (10%)
GASA	60	34 (56%)	41 (68%)	51 (85%)	9 (15%)
Control	60	31 (51%)	38 (63%)	47 (78%)	13 (22%)

weeks and are fitted to the mean of the standard curve as closely as possible to predict the EDC.

The EDC was predicted blindly in 120 cases, in 60 by the MPGA method and in 60 by the GASA technique. In 60 control cases the EDC was predicted from excellent clinical dates. All subjects had singleton pregnancies and had vaginal delivery after spontaneous labor. All birth weights exceeded 2,500 gm. The results are given in the table. No significant difference was found between the MPGA and GASA techniques.

Both the MPGA and the GASA methods proved to be accurate means of calculating the EDC in this study, in comparison with the use of excellent dates. The MPGA method allows a greater time span for the first BPD measurement and greater flexibility in scheduling the second assessment. An EDC is obtained earlier in gestation than with the GASA method. The MPGA method is far less complex. It requires only adjusting two points on a curve, whereas the GASA method requires that each fetus first be assigned to a specific growth pattern, and that the BPD values then be adjusted to varying degrees, depending on the second BPD measurement, before gestational age can be calculated.

▶ [Both of the two-measurement ultrasonographic means of predicting the EDC were of similar accuracy. The mean projected gestational age is simpler and gives the "answer" earlier in gestation than does the growth-adjusted sonographic age. We assume that, since two measurements are taken 3 or 4 weeks apart, random errors overestimating or underestimating the biparietal diameter tend to cancel each other out. Note that the accuracy of the clinically determined estimated date of confinement in the selected patients of the control group wasn't too shabby, either.] ◀

4–15 **Prediction of Intrauterine Growth Retardation by Sonographic Estimation of Total Intrauterine Volume.** Small for gestational age (SGA) infants are liable to increase perinatal and long-term morbidity and mortality. Antenatal identification of the affected fetus is necessary to effectively treat this condition, but clinical examination is of limited use in identifying abnormal fetal growth. Daryl H. Chinn, Roy A. Filly, and Peter W. Callen (Univ. of California Med. Center, San Francisco) evaluated the total intrauterine volume (TIUV) for predicting growth retardation in a series of 252 singleton pregnancies. Measurements were made after 20 weeks' menstrual age and were compared with previously reported normal values from the same institution.

(4–15) JCU 9:175–179, April 1981.

The prevalence of intrauterine growth retardation (IUGR) was 22%. Using a 10% tolerance limit as the threshold, the accuracy of an abnormal TIUV prediction was 41%, and that of a negative measurement was 89%. Eight of 17 false negative fetuses were profoundly growth retarded. Where estimates of gestational age based on the last menstrual period and biparietal diameter agreed, the sensitivity was 70% and specificity was 79%. The accuracy of a positive prediction remained at 41%, while that of a negative prediction was 93%. Among 13 patients having serial examinations who delivered SGA infants, 6 growth-retarded fetuses remained undetected when the last TIUV measurement in each series was used for prediction.

The TIUV is not a sensitive means of detecting growth retardation. The accuracy of a positive prediction is even more disappointing. The method is least predictive when the biparietal diameter is used as an indicator of gestational age. The weakness of this approach may lie in the assumption that all gravid uteri are prolate ellipses. Ultrasonic estimation of the TIUV is limited as a predictor of IUGR.

▶ [The ultrasonographic determination of total intrauterine volume (TIUV) has been advocated by some as a means of identifying intrauterine growth retardation (IUGR). This report is not very enthusiastic. With the lowest 10th percentile used as the cutoff, 70% of growth-retarded fetuses would be identified. This doesn't sound so bad, but 22% of AGA fetuses would be called growth retarded. This means that only 41% of patients with abnormally low TIUVs would actually have growth-retarded babies. Of equal significance, of the 17 small for gestational age babies with normal TIUV determinations (false negative results) 8 were profoundly growth retarded ($\leq$ 3d percentile).

The TIUV determination normal curve relates given values to "normal" values at each week of gestation. As with other means to predict IUGR, herein lies the rub. Very often the gestational age is not known with any certainty. A test for IUGR *independent* of gestational age would be helpful. The qualitative determination of amniotic fluid volume has been advocated as just such a test. Read on.] ◀

4–16 **Qualitative Amniotic Fluid Volume Determination by Ultrasound: Antepartum Detection of Intrauterine Growth Retardation.** Frank A. Manning, Lyndon M. Hill, and Lawrence D. Platt determined qualitative amniotic fluid volume by a linear array real-time ultrasound method prospectively in 120 patients referred with a diagnosis of intrauterine growth retardation (IUGR), defined as a birth weight of less than the tenth percentile for gestational age and sex. Intrauterine growth retardation has been classified broadly into two categories: that resulting from an early embryonic insult with decreased cell number and that caused by impaired cell growth secondary to reduced placental function. Whereas the former condition is rarely amenable to therapy, the latter may be treated by appropriate delivery of the infant. All patients had a minimum of 4 weeks' discrepancy between clinical size and dates. Oligohydramnios is a clinical hallmark of dysmature IUGR. Qualitative amniotic fluid volume was termed normal if at least one pocket of amniotic fluid measuring 1 cm in broadest diameter was identified.

Thirty-one (25.8%) patients were delivered of an infant with IUGR; the false positive rate by clinical means alone was 74.2% (89 patients) (table); 26 (83.9%) of the 31 IUGR fetuses demonstrated decreased

(4–16) Am. J. Obstet. Gynecol. 139:254–258, Feb. 1, 1981.

INCIDENCE OF INTRAUTERINE GROWTH RETARDATION IN PATIENTS
WITH "SUSPECTED" INTRAUTERINE GROWTH RETARDATION

Method	No. of patients	% IUGR N	%	False positive rate (%)	False negative rate (%)
Clinical estimate only	120	31	25.8	74.2	—
Qualitative AFV					
Normal (>1 cm)	91	5	6.6	—	6.6
Decreased (<1 cm)	29	26	89.6*	10.4	—

*$P < .001$, chi-square test.

qualitative amniotic fluid volumes. Qualitative amniotic fluid volume was normal in 91 patients, 86 (93.4%) of whom were delivered of a normal fetus (statistically significant). Three of the 5 infants with IUGR weighed less than the fifth percentile; however, none had neonatal morbidity. The qualitative amniotic fluid volume was decreased in 29 patients, 26 (89.7%) of whom had fetuses with IUGR. The incidence of IUGR was increased significantly in these patients compared to patients with normal qualitative amniotic fluid volumes. Perinatal morbidity (19 of 25 surviving fetuses, or 76%) was increased tenfold in patients with decreased amniotic fluid volumes, and all 4 perinatal deaths occurred in this group. Except for 1, all deaths were directly attributed to congenital anomalies. The incidence of renal agenesis in patients with oligohydramnios was 13.8%.

It is postulated that a mechanism for oligohydramnios in growth-retarded human fetuses may be decreased production of fetal urine and lung liquid as a result of hypoxemia-induced redistribution of cardiac output. This implies that screening for IUGR by qualitative amniotic fluid volume determination may be largely independent of gestational age of the fetus. The high sensitivity (false negative rate, 6.6%) and specificity (false positive rate, 10.4%) of the method, and the rapidity and ease of its application, make screening of high-risk populations practical.

▶ [Ultrasonic qualitative assessment of amniotic fluid volume apparently offers several advantages over other means of detecting intrauterine growth retardation. The sensitivity and specificity of the method are both good and, of greater importance, precise knowledge of gestational age is not necessary for the interpretation of the findings. It is the frequent lack of the latter that creates difficulties in using other methods to identify intrauterine growth retardation. We look forward to reading of others' experience with this technique.] ◀

4–17 **Comparison of Methods for Determining Crown-Rump Measurement by Real-Time Ultrasound.** Determination of gestational age is difficult when the last menstrual period is not known. Unless fetal biparietal diameter (BPD) is determined at an optimum time during pregnancy, usually 18–26 weeks, the correlation between PBD, as determined by ultrasound, and gestational age is compro-

(4–17) JCU 9:67–70, February 1981.

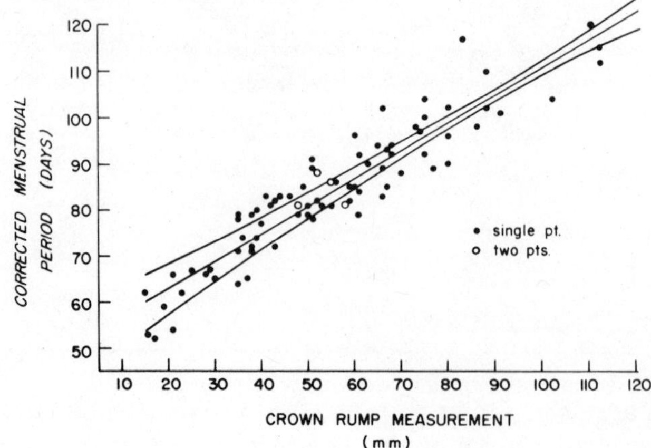

Fig 4–1.—Regression line between the crown-rump measurement (CRM) and gestational age determined by the corrected menstrual cycle. (Courtesy of Nelson, L. H.: JCU 9:67–70, February 1981.)

mised by normal biologic variations in fetal growth rates. Fetal crown-rump measurement (CRM) by B-mode ultrasound in early pregnancy for prediction of gestational age has been described, but has not been evaluated using real-time ultrasound.

Lewis H. Nelson (Bowman Gray School of Medicine) used a linear array real-time ultrasound system for fetal CRM in a group of 83 healthy pregnant women and evaluated currently available tables for determining gestational age from the CRM. The women's menstrual histories, delivery dates, and Dubowitz scores at delivery were known. Three methods were used to determine gestational age by ultrasound, Robinson's "regression analysis" values; Robinson's regression analysis values corrected for random and systematic errors; and Drumm's formula for gestational age.

When the result of each method was compared with the corrected gestational age, a highly significant correlation among all three methods was observed. The correlation coefficients were 0.934 for Drumm's formula, 0.910 for the "corrected" regression analysis, and 0.913 for the "regression analysis." Robinson's "regression analysis" values appeared to be more accurate than the "corrected regression analysis" values. Based on the data for this series, the regression equation between measured CRM and corrected gestational age is as follows: gestation (days) = 51.0008 + 0.6 CRM (in millimeters) with a correlation coefficient of 0.928 (Fig 4–1).

The CRM, as measured by real-time ultrasound, seems to be a practical method of determining gestational age during early pregnancy. It is recommended that CRM should be determined as early as possible. Use of freeze-frame and electronic calipers may help avoid errors of interpolation.

▶ [It has been shown previously that real-time scanning is as effective as conventional scanning in determining the biparietal diameter (1979 YEAR BOOK, pp. 197–198). It is not surprising that the same is true concerning the crown-rump measurement (CRM).

The CRM applicable in the first trimester, is a more accurate predictor of the estimated date of confinement than is the biparietal diameter.] ◄

4–18 Assessment of Gestational Age in Second Trimester by Real-Time Ultrasound Measurement of Femur Length. It has been postulated that ultrasound measurement of fetal femur length can be used to assess gestational age. Using real-time ultrasound, Gregory D. O'Brien, John T. Queenan, and Stuart Campbell (King's College Hosp., London) conducted several studies to determine the reproducibility of femur length measurement, to compare the ultrasound measurements with a radiologic model, and to assess the accuracy of the method in estimating fetal age. Measurements were made until 3 were obtained within a 2-mm range. Linear regression analysis was used to assess the relationship between femur length and gestational age from 12 to 23 weeks, and ultrasound measurements were made between 14 and 23 weeks' gestation in 47 women whose menstrual histories were beyond doubt.

In 30 experiments, the standard deviations of the three measurements of the same femur varied from 0.1 to 1.5 mm, with a mean of 0.8 mm. Increasing femur length was not associated with a clear tendency for the standard deviation to increase. The correlation between femur length as determined by ultrasound and the radiologic model was highly significant ($P < .001$). There was a high degree of positive correlation (r = .987; $P < .001$) between the fetal ages determined by the ultrasound measurement of femur length and those calculated from menstrual age. The regression line for estimating menstrual age was fitted to the data and the 95% confidence limits for the estimate based on ultrasound measurement of femur length was found to be ± 6.7 days (Fig 4–2). In 47 "blind" cases, there was a high degree of correlation between the fetal age estimated from ultrasound measure-

Fig 4–2.—Regression line for estimating gestational age from ultrasound measurement of femur length; confidence limits, 95%. (Courtesy of O'Brien, G. D., et al.: Am. J. Obstet. Gynecol. 139:540–545, Mar. 1, 1981.)

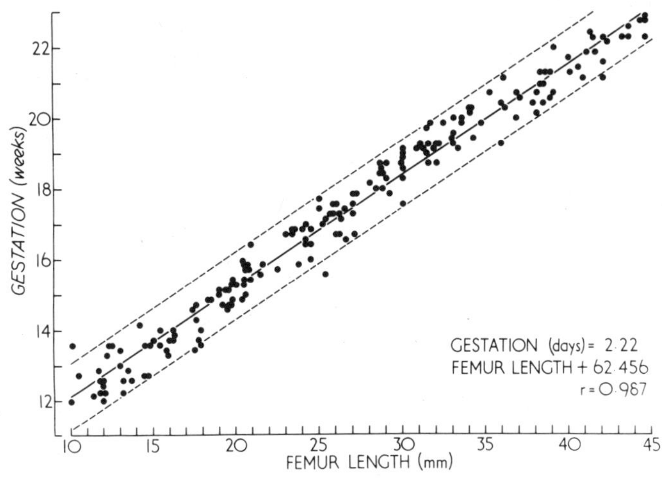

ments of femur length and menstrual age (r = .998; P < .001). The average difference between the estimated and actual ages was 1.5 days, with a maximum of 5 days.

The results demonstrate that ultrasound measurement of femur length is highly reproducible and provides at least as accurate an estimate of fetal age as do estimates based on measurements of the biparietal diameter. Although this method is not intended to replace the parameters currently used to estimate fetal age in the second trimester of pregnancy, it does contribute to the reliability of such estimates.

▶ [These observations indicate that measurement of femur length by real-time ultrasound is a reliable and reproducible means of estimating gestational age during the second trimester. The technique requires some experience, as do all techniques.] ◀

4–19 **Sonograpic Abdominal Circumference: Dynamic Versus Static Imaging.** The ultrasonically derived fetal abdominal circumference (AC) is used to predict birth weight, assess fetal growth, and follow the progress of fetal ascites. Dynamic imaging rapidly identifies the plane showing the liver and ductus venosus/umbilical vein and permits photographing of the AC plane when the fetus is not breathing. However, the outline of the fetal trunk is less sharply outlined than by static imaging, and in some cases the lateral boundaries of the AC cannot be visualized. Carl P. Weiner (Ohio State Univ. Hosp., Columbus), Rudy E. Sabbagha, Ralph K. Tamura, and Sharon DalCompo (Northwestern Univ., Chicago) compared AC values obtained by static and dynamic gray-scale ultrasonic imaging in 39 gravidas at 24–39 weeks' gestational age. A total of 152 echograms of the fetal AC were obtained. The coefficient correlation of the mean AC values derived from dynamic and static imaging was 0.97. Differences, when present, usually were minor; in only 14 studies did the values derived by the two methods differ by 1 cm or more. When the outline of the AC in a fetus near term was larger than the sonic field displayed by dynamic imaging, the partially incomplete boundary could be "filled in" without affecting the accuracy of the result. Extension of borders was necessary in 5 cases.

Values of AC derived by dynamic ultrasound imaging are not significantly different from those derived from static scans. The AC tables generated by static imaging could be used with ACs obtained by a dynamic technique. In dynamic AC scans with an incomplete circumference, the borders can be drawn in without significantly reducing the accuracy of the measurement. Prediction of fetal weight with the use of biparietal diameter-AC tables may be more accurate using AC derived from dynamic ultrasound imaging.

▶ [This study demonstrates a reasonably close correlation between static and dynamic (real-time) techniques in measuring fetal abdominal circumference. This is valuable to know because most standard tables were derived from static imaging, but real-time units rapidly are coming into greater use.] ◀

4–20 **Ultrasonic Evaluation of Fetal Ventricular Growth.** Hydrocephalus may be well established and brain damage present by the

(4–19) Am. J. Obstet. Gynecol. 139:953–955, Apr. 15, 1981.
(4–20) Neuroradiology 21:127–131, April 1981.

time an increased biparietal diameter or head-to-abdomen ratio is observed. The most evident alteration in hydrocephalus is ventricular widening. P. Jeanty, M. Dramaix-Wilmet, D. Delbeke, F. Rodesch, and J. Struyven (Free Univ. of Brussels) studied the evolution of the ratio of lateral ventricular (LV) to hemispheric width (HW) in relation to biparietal diameter and age in a prospective series of 200 pregnancies in white women. All fetuses were clinically normal at term. The LV was measured in a parallel cross section but more cephalad to the plane in which the biparietal diameter was measured. Elevation of the LV/HW ratio was detected much earlier than abnormal biparietal diameter growth.

Real-time ultrasonography permits the rapid and accurate estimation of fetal growth using the LV/HW ratio. Early detection of hydrocephalus is possible using this method. About 30 seconds are added to the examination time. Pulsation of the middle cerebral artery identified the sylvian fissure, which might otherwise be mistaken for the lateral wall of an enlarged ventricle. The ratio decreases rapidly in the first half of pregnancy, and only abnormal subjects in this age group should be closely monitored. The complexity of growth of cerebral tissue explains why raw hyperbolic and parabolic curves have failed to fit the experimental data.

▶ [The increased numbers of ultrasonic scans being performed in pregnancy and the improved resolution of modern ultrasonographic equipment combined with the increased sophistication and knowledge of ultrasonographers have resulted in the more frequent diagnosis of fetal malformations in utero than was possible in the past. Attempts at fetal therapy in cases of hydrocephalus and obstructed bladders have been reported in the lay press. Much remains to be learned about the natural history of these problems diagnosed relatively early in gestation. The present report clearly indicates that dilatation of the ventricles permits the diagnosis of hydrocephalus at a time when the biparietal diameter is still in the normal range. Just what to do in this sort of situation is not yet known.] ◀

4-21 **Effect of Corticosteroids and Fetomaternal Disorders on the L/S Ratio.** Glucocorticoids have been shown to be of benefit in reducing the incidence of fetal respiratory distress syndrome (RDS), but their effect on the lecithin-sphingomyelin (L/S) ratio is less well defined. John C. Morrison, Jack M. Schneider, Walter D. Whybrew, and Edsel T. Bucovaz (Univ. of Tennessee, Memphis) investigated the effect of maternal corticosteroids on the amniotic fluid L/S ratio in 126 women at risk for premature delivery who had immature L/S ratios. Patients received either hydrocortisone or placebo (hydrous lactose) intravenously in a double-blind manner at a dose of 500 mg every 12 hours for four doses. In 70 patients, a second aliquot of amniotic fluid was obtained at or near delivery.

The effect of glucocorticoid therapy on the L/S ratio in previous studies reported in the literature is summarized in the table. Determination of the L/S ratio for a second time between 9 hours and 7 days after treatment in 37 treated patients and 33 controls showed a marked increase in the L/S ratio in those receiving hydrocortisone compared with those receiving the placebo. Treatment also increased the L/S ratio in patients who had fetomaternal disorders that either

(4–21) Obstet. Gynecol. 56:583–590, November 1980.

CHANGE IN LS RATIO AFTER GLUCOCORTICOID THERAPY

Year	Author	Corticosteroid	Route	L:S ratio
1972	Liggins & Howie	Betamethasone	Intramuscular	Unchanged
1973	Spellacy et al	Dexamethasone	Oral	Increased
1973	Caspi et al	Dexamethasone	Intramuscular	Increased
1974	Liggins & Howie	Betamethasone	Intramuscular	Unchanged
1974	Bureau et al	Betamethasone	Intramuscular	Unchanged
1974	Kennedy	Betamethasone	Intramuscular	Unchanged
1974	Fargier et al	Betamethasone	Intravenous	Unchanged
1975	Kling & Kotas	Dexamethasone	Intraamniotic	Unchanged
1975	Schwenzel et al	Betamethasone	Intramuscular	Increased
1976	Caspi et al	Dexamethasone	Intramuscular	Increased
1976	Panter-Brick	Dexamethasone	Intravenous	Increased
1977	Caritis et al	Betamethasone	Intramuscular	Unchanged
1977	Zuspan et al	Hydrocortisone	Intravenous	Increased
1978	Nagy et al	Dexamethasone	Intravenous	Increased
1978	Present study	Hydrocortisone	Intravenous	Increased

accelerated or delayed lecithin production. Fewer neonates of patients treated with hydrocortisone developed RDS than did those in the untreated group. When RDS did occur in treated neonates, the clinical course was milder. None of the 7 diabetic patients from the treatment group developed fetal RDS, which suggests that hydrocortisone may counteract detrimental fetal hyperinsulinemia. The maximal effect of hydrocortisone on changes in the L/S ratio was seen after three intravenous doses.

Hydrocortisone appears to exert an effect on the L/S ratio in women with an immature amniotic L/S ratio.

▶ [Reported studies of the question of whether glucocorticoid administration influences the L/S ratio, listed in the table, are controversial. It is interesting to note that 6 of 7 studies employing betamethasone found no effect, whereas 7 of 8 reports using either dexamethasone or hydrocortisone found an increase. This study, in addition to noting a significant effect of hydrocortisone over placebo, also demonstrated that the effects generally persist when the data are stratified according to the complications in mother and/or fetus.] ◀

4–22 **Amniotic Fluid Phospholipid Profile Determined by Two-Dimensional Thin-Layer Chromatography as Index of Fetal Lung Maturation.** Gluck et al. used two-dimensional thin-layer chromatography to establish the amniotic fluid phospholipid profile, avoid false negative results, and analyze fluids contaminated by blood or meconium. M. J. Whittle, A. I. Wilson, C. R. Whitfield, R. D. Paton, and R. W. Logan (Glasgow) used this method to obtain phospholipid profiles in 188 consecutive patients in which amniotic fluid was sampled within 72 hours before delivery. This method, in addition to the lecithin-sphingomyelin (L/S) ratio, determines the presence or absence of phosphatidylglycerol (PG) and phosphatidylinositol (PI), as well as the less important components phosphatidylethanolamine (PE) and phosphatidylserine (PS).

(4–22) Br. Med. J. 282:428–430, Feb. 7, 1981.

The L/S ratio of amniotic fluid was 2.0 or above in 145 patients, and no respiratory distress syndrome or other respiratory problems developed in this group. A ratio below 2.0 was found in 43 cases. Thirty-one of these samples contained PG. The incidence of respiratory distress syndrome was 27.9%. Seven of 31 infants with immature L/S ratios but PG present had respiratory problems, as did 9 of 12 in whom PG was absent. The amounts of PI and PG in amniotic fluid were not closely related to the development of respiratory distress syndrome; the mere presence or absence of PG was a better predictor. There was no obvious relation between neonatal respiratory function and PI, PE, or PS.

These findings substantiate the remarkable predictive accuracy of an adequate L/S ratio in confirming fetal lung maturation. In practical terms, an amniotic-fluid L/S ratio below 2.0 with no PG present indicates the near certainty of respiratory distress syndrome if delivery cannot be postponed. The identification of PG with an immature L/S ratio should encourage immediate delivery of even a very small preterm fetus judged to be at serious risk in utero. The amniotic-fluid phospholipid profile should be substituted for use of the L/S ratio alone.

▶ [This article reminds us that one must know his or her own laboratory's "normals" and track record in order to interpret amniotic fluid maturity test results wisely. In previous editions of the YEAR BOOK, several reports indicated that phosphatidylglycerol (PG) generally appeared only after a mature L/S ratio (i.e., $\geq$ 2) was achieved, but that, once it did appear, it was the Cadillac (apologies to readers outside the United States)—respiratory distress syndrome did not occur. Different results are reported here. All patients with an L/S ratio $\geq$ 2.0 had PG in their amniotic fluid, as did 72% of patients with immature L/S ratios. Furthermore, respiratory distress syndrome occurred in 10% of cases with PG if the L/S ratio was immature.] ◀

4–23 **Amniotic Fluid Phosphatidylglycerol: A Potentially Useful Predictor of Intrauterine Growth Retardation.** Antenatal diagnosis of intrauterine growth retardation (IUGR) is desirable to plan management so as to minimize perinatal asphyxia. However, recognition of the growth-retarded fetus remains difficult because estimated fetal size is not a reliable predictor of gestational age in the presence of abnormal fetal growth. Thomas L. Gross, Robert J. Sokol, Margaret V. Wilson, Paul M. Kuhnert, and Victor Hirsch (Case Western Reserve Univ., Cleveland) assessed the usefulness of amniotic fluid maturity tests in distinguishing small for gestational age (SGA) infants from appropriate for gestational age (AGA) infants of comparable weight. Review was made of 82 pregnancies resulting in small infants, including 33 SGA and 49 AGA infants, all weighing under 2,700 gm at birth. Birth weights were comparable in the two groups, but estimated gestational age was significantly greater for the SGA group.

The mean percentage of phosphatidylglycerol (PG) and lecithin-sphingomyelin ratio were significantly higher in the SGA group than in the AGA group. No significant difference in phosphatidylinositol, percentage of fat cells, or foam test results were observed. Phospha-

(4–23) Am. J. Obstet. Gynecol. 140:277–281, June 1, 1981.

tidylglycerol was present in 79% of specimens from the SGA group and in 47% of those from the AGA group. A high level of amniotic fluid PG was the most useful predictor of the birth of an SGA infant. The level giving the most accurate prediction was ≥ 7%. Such values were associated with delivery of an SGA infant 60% of the time, and 64% of SGA infants were identified by this criterion. Of the pregnancies with low PG levels, 26% resulted in birth of an SGA infant. Preterm delivery was associated with three fourths of these cases. Birth weights were lower than for SGA infants with high amniotic-fluid PG values.

In this series, a high amniotic fluid PG level was associated with a fourfold increase in SGA births. Estimation of amniotic fluid PG levels late in gestation may improve the differentiation of pregnancies complicated by IUGR from other pregnancies.

▶ [Is a particular patient with a 2,000-gm fetus at 38 weeks' gestation (SGA) or at 34 weeks' gestation (premature AGA)? This is a common clinical question, especially in referral hospitals where patients often are first seen late in pregnancy. Amniotic fluid maturity test results can be helpful in this situation. The authors of this report found that the differences in phosphatidylglycerol concentrations were useful in separating preterm AGA from term SGA fetuses.] ◀

4–24 **Effect of Blood in Amniotic Fluid on Detection of Phosphatidylglycerol.** The amniotic fluid lecithin-sphingomyelin ratio, rapid surfactant (or "shake") test, and phosphatidylglycerol (PG) level are three reliable tests of fetal lung maturity. The first two tests are unreliable however, if blood contaminates the amniotic fluid sample. It has been suggested that PG analysis for assessment of fetal lung maturity may be reliable even in this situation. Howard T. Strassner, Jr., Steven H. Golde, Gladys H. Mosley, and Lawrence D. Platt (Univ. of Southern California) tested this hypothesis.

Samples of amniotic fluid were obtained from women in the second trimester of pregnancy and at term. Phospatidylglycerol standard was added to half of the samples. The samples were then tested for the presence or absence of PG, using two-dimensional thin-layer chromatography, before and after the addition of maternal or fetal serum or red blood cells in concentrations of 1% to 20%. Uncontaminated samples with and without added PG served as controls.

Serum or red blood cell contamination of amniotic fluid without PG did not result in the appearance of a PG spot on the chromatographic plate. Neither serum nor red blood cell contamination interfered with the detection of PG in those fluids in which it was present. Maternal and fetal blood were similar in their failure to affect the detection of PG.

Determination of PG apparently remains a reliable indicator of fetal lung maturity even in the presence of bloody amniotic fluid.

▶ [Previous reports have indicated that the reliability of amniotic fluid phosphatidylglycerol measurement as an index of fetal lung maturity is not affected by the presence of meconium, and this study demonstrates the same with respect to blood contamination.] ◀

(4–24) Am. J. Obstet. Gynecol. 138:697–702, Nov. 15, 1980.

4–25 **Management of Preterm Premature Rupture of Membranes: Assessing Amniotic Fluid in the Vagina for Phosphatidylglycerol.** Management of premature membrane rupture before term remains a challenge. Charles M. Stedman, Scott Crawford, Elise Staten, and Walter B. Cherny (Phoenix, Ariz.) report a prospective study of the usefulness of analyzing amniotic fluid pooled vaginally in patients with premature rupture of the membranes (PROM) before term for evidence of fetal lung maturity. Phosphatidylglycerol (PG) was used because of its reliability as a marker and its virtual absence from body fluids other than lung surfactant. Fifty-five consecutive patients seen at Good Samaritan Hospital in a 6-month period with PROM at 26–36 weeks' gestation were studied. Amniotic fluid was collected by aspiration from the posterior fornix and analyzed for presence of PG. Aspiration was repeated at 24, 48, and 72 hours after PROM. Patients were kept at bed rest and carefully were assessed for infection.

Adequate fluid was obtained in 77 of 99 attempts. Measurable PG was found initially in 6 of 25 patients (24%) at 28–34 weeks' gestation (group A) and in 9 of 22 (41%) at 35 –36 weeks' gestation (group B). Another 47% of group A converted to PG-positive fluid before delivery, as did 31% of group B. Respiratory distress syndrome occurred in 9% of neonates. Its relation to the presence of PG in the amniotic fluid before delivery is shown in the table. Neonatal mortality was 7%; nine patients (16%) had cesarean section. Twelve patients received steroids, and 3 of their infants developed respiratory distress syndrome. Nine mothers (16%) had infectious morbidity. Morbidity rate was 24% when the membranes were ruptured for more than 24 hours. Two infants had infectious morbidity, and 1 of them died of sepsis.

Sampling free amniotic fluid for PG is a reliable noninvasive procedure in the management of preterm PROM. The absence of PG before delivery, however, does not invariably mean that neonatal respiratory distress syndrome will occur. Further studies of fetal lung maturation may reveal an antepartum marker with improved specificity and a sensitivity equal to that of PG. The use of steroids in

---

RELATION OF RESPIRATORY DISTRESS SYNDROME
TO PRESENCE OF PHOSPHATIDYLGLYCEROL
IN AMNIOTIC FLUID PRIOR TO DELIVERY

	Gestation at birth	
PG determination prior to delivery	≤34 wk	>34 wk
Present	0/15	0/13
Absent	4/10	0/9*

*Three infants required > 60 hours of hood oxygen support.

(4–25) Am. J. Obstet. Gynecol. 140:34–38, May 1981.

preterm pregnancies remains controversial, particularly where high-risk factors such as PROM are present.

▶ [This study documents the feasibility of using vaginal-pooled amniotic fluid for fetal lung maturity testing as a guide to management of premature membrane rupture. Phosphatidylglycerol (PG) was measured in preference to other amniotic fluid indices because contamination with other body fluids does not affect levels of this phospholipid. In 80% of cases, sufficient fluid (4 ml) was obtained for testing, and this success rate is at least as good as that expected with transabdominal amniocentesis in patients with ruptured membranes. The presence of PG invariably meant that respiratory distress syndrome would not develop, but only 24% of those without PG developed the syndrome. Thus, as with all other approaches to fetal maturity testing, the false positive rate is low and the false negative rate is high.] ◀

4-26 **Effect of Cervical-Vaginal Secretions on Measurements of Lecithin-Sphingomyelin Ratio and Optical Density of 650 Nm.** Lecithin-sphingomyelin (L/S) ratio analyses of amniotic fluids collected transabdominally is now a well-established procedure for determination of fetal pulmonary maturity. Ratios of L/S above 2.0 generally indicate pulmonary maturity, whereas ratios below 2.0 generally indicate pulmonary immaturity. Amniotic fluid optical density readings at 650 nm equal to or greater than 0.15 correspond to L/S ratios of 2.0 or greater; optical density readings below 0.15 generally correlated with L/S ratios below 2.0. Frequently, in patients with ruptured membranes, a free flow of amniotic fluid into the vagina occurs, which may be the only fluid available for study. A. J. Sbarra, G. Blake, C. L. Cetrulo, R. J. Selvaraj, M. J. Herschel, C. Delise, J. L. Kennedy, and G. W. Mitchell, Jr. (Boston) investigated whether vaginal and cervical secretions interfere with amniotic fluid L/S ratios.

Sterile normal saline (10 ml) was used to wash gently the vagina and cervix of 10 pregnant patients of gestational ages of 10–40 weeks. In another 6 patients, about 10 ml of the patients' transabdominally collected amniotic fluid of known L/S ratio and optical density was gently introduced into the vagina and cervix for lavaging. All fluids were centrifuged at 2,000 × g for 10 minutes, as is done

L/S RATIOS AND OPTICAL DENSITY*

Patient No.	L/S		Optical density at 650 nm	
	Vaginal	Abdominal	Vaginal	Abdominal
1	2.3	2.5	0.27	0.23
2	3.8	3.6	0.70	0.68
3	3.6	3.8	0.41	0.69
4	3.4	3.8	0.60	1.4
5	1.8	1.6	0.05	0.05
6	2.5	2.4	0.92	0.77
7	2.2	2.2	–	–
8	1.3	1.6	–	–

*At 650 nm of amniotic fluid collected transabdominally and subsequently lavaged in vaginal-cervical area.

(4–26) Am. J. Obstet. Gynecol. 139:214–216, Jan. 15, 1981.

when determining amniotic fluid L/S ratios and optical density at 650 nm. Lavaging the vaginal-cervical area with sterile saline and examining the lavage fluid for L/S spots showed no detectable spots in the supernatants (except one sample had faint L/S at a ratio of 1:1) and barely detectable L/S spots in the sediment; all pellets from these centrifuged wash fluids had L/S ratios of 1:1, except two that had ratios of 1.5:1. In all cases, an additional unidentified surfactant was present. Since all fluid samples collected are centrifuged as described before examination, these substances would be removed, with no interference expected. Vaginal-cervical saline-wash fluids did not affect amniotic fluid L/S ratios. Lavaging the vaginal-cervical area with abdominal amniotic fluid did not significantly change the L/S ratio or the optical density of the original amniotic fluid at 650 nm (table).

Free-flowing amniotic fluid collected vaginally can be used reliably to determine fetal pulmonary maturity.

▶ [This study nicely demonstrates that free-flowing amniotic fluid collected vaginally can be used in a reliable way for determination of the L/S ratio or O.D. 650. An important caveat is that the authors routinely centrifuge amniotic fluid specimens at 2,000 × g for 10 minutes prior to testing. The reliability of the vaginal sample may be affected by different centrifugation conditions.] ◀

4–27 **Diagnosis of Fetal Death in Utero With Amniotic Fluid Creatine Kinase.** The standard method for diagnosing the presence or absence of fetal life is real-time ultrasonography, but this procedure is not everywhere available. In 1974, Kerenyi and Sarkozi suggested that the presence of creatine kinase in amniotic fluid indicated fetal death. Laurence E. Stempel and John A. Lott (Ohio State Univ., Columbus) performed real-time ultrasonography and analysis of amniotic fluid for creatine kinase in 108 pregnant women.

In 92 of the women (14 examined in the second trimester and 78 in the third), real-time sonography indicated a live fetus. In 91 of these women, the amniotic fluid creatine kinase activity was 0 to 3 sigma units per milliliter, and in 1 it was 210 units. In the latter case, the fetus was alive but its monochorionic twin in the other sac was dead, with an amniotic fluid creatine kinase activity of 1,070 units.

In 17 women (7 examined in the second trimester and 10 in the third), sonography indicated a dead fetus. These 17 patients had an amniotic fluid creatine kinase activity of 5 to 9,800 sigma units per milliliter. Activity began to rise within 2 days after fetal death, and there was a rough positive relationship between creatine kinase activity and length of time since fetal death (r = 0.39). In all 11 cases of fetal death in which creatine kinase electrophoresis was performed, creatine kinase-MM isoenzyme was the predominant isoenzyme.

Amniotic fluid color was abnormal in 11 of 92 cases in which fetuses were alive and normal in 1 of 17 cases in which fetuses were dead.

Amniotic fluid creatine kinase activity is a sensitive and specific indicator of fetal death. It tends to increase with length of time since fetal death, and it is not affected by a wide variety of maternal and fetal conditions (such as chronic fetal distress and fetal neural tube

(4–27) Am. J. Obstet. Gynecol. 138:1173–1176, Dec. 15, 1980.

defects) or by meconium, blood, and bilirubin pigments in the amniotic fluid. In cases of twins, its presence should be interpreted with caution because the enzyme may have passed from the sac of a dead fetus to that of a living fetus if the dividing membrane was damaged during amniocentesis. Amniotic fluid color is not a reliable indicator of fetal life or death.

► [This study confirms an earlier report indicating the utility of amniotic fluid creatine kinase measurements in diagnosing fetal death. Levels begin to increase within 2 days of fetal death, presumably reflecting seepage from fetal muscle. Various maternal and fetal complications do not seem to interfere with the test.] ◄

4–28 **Potential of Midtrimester Maternal Plasma α-Fetoprotein Measurement in Predicting Infants of Low Birth Weight.** D. J. H. Brock, Lilias Barron, and Gillian M. Raab (Edinburgh) have investigated whether high maternal plasma α-fetoprotein (AFP) levels predicted prematurity, growth retardation, or both. The subjects were 113 women who had been screened for fetal neural tube defects between 15 and 22 weeks of pregnancy and who were subsequently delivered of a live-born singleton infant weighing less than 2.5 kg. Maternal AFP levels were measured at midtrimester. Each subject was matched by taking the next woman screened who was of comparable parity and gestation and who subsequently was delivered of a normal live-born singleton infant weighing more than 2.5 kg.

Median serum AFP levels in the control group increased by 11.7% per week between 15 and 20 weeks of gestation. Plasma AFP levels in pregnancies resulting in a low birth weight infant were significantly higher than in matched controls. Ten subjects and only 3 controls had values above 2.0 times the median. High AFP levels occur in very similar proportions among mothers whose low birth weight infants were born before the 37th week and those who gave birth in the 37th week or later.

Since the median maternal plasma AFP level rises by 11.7% per week between 16 and 22 weeks, an underestimated gestation at the time of screening will lead to a spuriously high AFP concentration and an apparently premature delivery. Also, different policies on induction of labor may lead to different proportions of premature infants. To circumvent these difficulties, the authors selected subjects on the criterion of low birth weight rather than prematurity, and subject and control were from the same antenatal clinic.

Results showed that higher AFP concentrations occur both in pregnancies in which a small premature infant is born and in those in which a small-for-dates baby is born. It is now being explored whether AFP measurements made later in pregnancy will be of more value in predicting low birth weight as a corollary to AFP screening for neural tube defects.

► [Previous reports have indicated an association between elevated maternal blood α-fetoprotein (AFP) levels and the subsequent delivery of low birth weight infants. This report confirms this association, which holds for both preterm birth and intrauterine

(4–28) Br. J. Obstet. Gynaecol. 87:582, July 1980.

growth retardation. Screening for AFP won't serve as a practical or effective predictor of low birth weight infant delivery, however. Only about 9% of low birth weight infants would be identified as a result of elevated second-trimester maternal blood AFP levels.] ◄

4–29 **Origin of Amniocentesis-Induced Rises of α-Fetoprotein Concentrations in Maternal Serum.** Human α-fetoprotein (AFP) exhibits concanavalin A-binding heterogeneity. The relative amounts of AFP present in human amniotic fluid and in fetal serum that do not react with concanavalin A are 15% to 40% and less than 10%, respectively. L. Dallaire, L. Bélanger, Carol J. P. Smith, and P. C. Kelleher obtained serum samples from 65 pregnant women between 15 and 20 weeks of gestation who were undergoing amniocentesis for reasons unrelated to the study. Samples were obtained immediately before and between 15 and 30 minutes after amniocentesis. The concentration of AFP was measured to determine if the pattern of concanavalin A binding of AFP concentration was consistent with fetomaternal hemorrhage (low binding) or transfer of amniotic fluid into the maternal circulation (higher binding). The serums of patients who had a significant increase in AFP concentration after amniocentesis were studied further.

The level of AFP in preamniocentesis serums and amniotic fluids was normal for gestational age in all 65 patients. In 7 patients (11%), serum AFP concentrations were elevated markedly after amniocentesis. On the basis of the percentage of AFP that did not react with concanavalin A, these 7 patients were divided into two groups. In 3 patients, the binding pattern present in serum was similar to that of AFP in fetal serum; in serum in patients 4–7, it was similar to that of AFP present in amniotic fluid. There was no evidence of fetal distress during amniocentesis, and all pregnancies resulted in the birth of a normal infant.

The uniformity with which a significant rise in maternal serum AFP concentration occurs after amniocentesis suggests that in 10% to 15% of cases, there will be an alteration in normal barriers between the fluid compartments of the conceptus and the maternal circulation. The clinical significance of such an event is not known. This study shows that the particular fluid compartment of the conceptus whose relationship with the maternal circulation has been altered can be ascertained by measuring the percentage of maternal serum AFP that does not react with concanavalin A. This enhances the possibility of defining separate groups of patients in whom there may be differences in the risk of complications after amniocentesis. Furthermore, measurements of the percentage of concanavalin A-nonbinding AFP in maternal serum may prove useful in screening programs for the detection of fetuses with neural tube defects and certain other abnormalities.

▶ [A rise in maternal serum α-fetoprotein (AFP) level with amniocentesis occurs in about 10% of instances, and the cause has been assumed to be fetomaternal hemorrhage. This neat little study examines the issue by taking advantage of the different

(4–29) Br. J. Obstet. Gynaecol. 87:856–859, October 1980.

binding characteristics to concanavalin-A exhibited by AFP of amniotic fluid and fetal serum origin. Of the 7 cases in which maternal AFP levels increased with amniocentesis, fetal blood was the apparent source in 3 and amniotic fluid in 4. Thus, the suggestion that maternal AFP levels might be a useful marker of fetomaternal hemorrhage (see 1980 YEAR BOOK, p. 198) is *not* such a good idea.] ◄

5. Labor and Operative Obstetrics

5-1 Appearance of Gap Junctions in the Myometrium of Women During Labor. Studies of uterine tissues from pregnant animals have shown that gap junctions appear between smooth muscle cells with increased frequency during labor and parturition. R. E. Garfield and R. H. Hayashi observed gap junctions between myometrial cells in pregnant women during labor. Myometrial tissues from 29 women having cesarean section at various stages of labor were examined quantitatively by electron microscopy.

Only 4 of 11 women having elective cesarean section or operation because of previous cesarean section had gap junctions in myometrial tissues. All 9 having cesarean section for failure to progress in labor had gap junctions present. These women had greater cervical dilation and contraction frequencies than the elective group. Increased cervical dilation was correlated closely with an increased frequency of contractions and also with the area of smooth muscle membrane occupied by gap junctions. Increased gap junctional area also was correlated with the frequency of uterine contractions.

The formation of gap junctions in myometrial tissue may be stimulated by some physiologic change. The gap junctions may then terminate pregnancy by providing for coordinated, synchronized muscle activity and dilatation of the cervix, followed by expulsion of the fetus. The present study involved women having cesarean section and may not have adequately shown changes that occur in normal vaginal delivery. Studies are under way to define the role of gap junctions in the myometrium with respect to obstetric history, uterine dysfunction, and treatment with excitants and inhibitors of uterine contractility.

▶ [The development of gap junctions in rat myometrium during labor was considered in the 1979 YEAR BOOK (pp. 125–126). The present report indicates that they are present in human labor, both term and preterm, as well. These sites of low resistance to the flow of current are thought to be important in coordinating uterine contractions. Studies of gap junctions may help shed some light on the mechanism of the onset of labor. One technical point: It is understandable that the muscle strips were taken from the lower uterine segment, but can one be sure that the same findings pertain in the upper, contractile portion of the uterus?] ◀

5-2 Morphological and Histochemical Evidence for Occurrence of Collagenolysis and for Role of Neutrophilic Polymorphonuclear Leukocytes During Cervical Dilation. L. C. U. Junqueira, M. Zugaib, G. S. Montes, O. M. S. Toledo, R. M. Krisztán, and K. M. Shigihara (Univ. of São Paulo) present evidence that collagen depolymerization is a widespread phenomenon during cervical dilation.

(5–1)   Am. J. Obstet. Gynecol. 140:254–260, June 1, 1981.
(5–2)   Ibid., 138:273–281, Oct. 1, 1980.

Sixteen biopsy specimens of cervical tissue were obtained from normal patients during parturition, and 10 biopsy specimens were obtained from nonpregnant, sexually active women. The specimens were studied by electron microscopy and by the Picrosirius-polarization method, a specific procedure for the detection of collagen fibers in tissue sections. The method is specific for oriented polymerized collagen molecules.

A and B of Figure 5–1 are photomicrographs of sections of nonpregnant and intrapartum human cervices, respectively. In the nonpregnant cervix, collagen fibers appear continuous and densely packed. Collagen bundles are not birefringent because their orientation is parallel to the direction of polarized light. In intrapartum cervices, collagen fibers appear separated and irregularly fragmented; the amount of collagen fibers per area is reduced drastically. Between regions containing collagen fibers, an amorphous material was seen which stained less intensely with Sirius red. Morphological features suggest that there is local degradation of collagen fibers. Electron microscopy studies supported observations with the optical microscope: the regular arrangement of collagen fibrils was disturbed, and images suggested their corrosion. Deposits of microfibrillar or granular material appeared between the fibrils in intrapartum cervices. Morphometry studies suggest that the diameter of the collagen fibrils in the intrapartum cervices were more variable and smaller than the diameter of fibrils from nonpregnant cervices.

Fig 5–1.—Photomicrographs of sections of **(A)** nonpregnant and **(B)** intrapartum cervices. Picrosirius-polarization method shows collagen fibers as bright birefringent structures against dark background. **A,** collagen appears as bundles of continuous, densely packed fibers. Collagen bundles are not birefringent in apparently empty area *(upper left)* because of their orientation parallel to the direction of the polarized light; original magnification ×100. **B,** collagen fibers appear separated and irregularly fragmented in the intrapartum cervix, and amount of collagen fibers per area is greatly reduced; original magnification ×375. (Courtesy of Junqueira, L. C. U., et al.: Am. J. Obstet. Gynecol. 138:273–281, October 1980.)

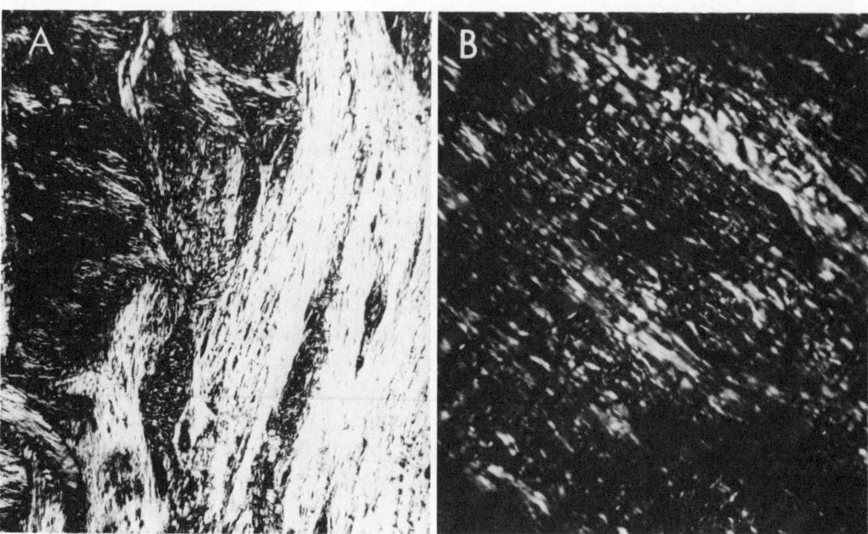

COMPARATIVE BIREFRINGENCY INTENSITY (MEASURED
AS % TRANSMISSION) IN SEVEN SPECIMENS FROM
NONPREGNANT AND INTRAPARTUM CERVICES, WITH USE
OF PICROSIRIUS-POLARIZATION METHOD AND
MICROSPECTROPHOTOMETRY

	Nonpregnant	*Intrapartum*
	38.0	3.5
	40.3	6.6
	42.5	7.3
	49.1	1.4
	31.8	1.4
	65.1	2.8
	56.4	4.0
Average	46.2	3.8

The study of cell populations in cervices of nonpregnant women showed that fibroblasts were the main constituent; in intrapartum material the cellular population increased, and macrophages and mast cells were also present. The most common cell was the neutrophilic polymorphonuclear leukocyte that heavily infiltrated the stroma. In many cases, a positive relationship between the amount of infiltrated cells and the degree of collagenolysis was observed. Using the polarization method in association with microspectrophotometry, comparison of birefringency intensity in nonpregnant and intrapartum cervices (table) corroborates the massive decrease in oriented collagen molecules in cervical dilation.

Results suggest that collagenolysis and infiltration of neutrophils occur throughout pregnancy but are accelerated prior to and during labor. No characteristic changes were seen in the glycosaminoglycans.

▶ [The findings of this morphological and biochemical study suggest that cervical changes with parturition result from lysis of its collagen fibers, perhaps as a result of infiltration with neutrophils containing collagenase. Much of the evidence comes from histochemical studies (illustrated in Figures 5–1 and 5–2) utilizing a technique specific for oriented polymerized collagen molecules.] ◀

5–3 **Premature Labor.**—*I. Prostaglandin precursors in human placental membranes.*—It has been suggested that fetal membranes fulfill a significant metabolic function in human parturition, in which labor is initiated by the release of free arachidonic acid from the phospholipids through the action of fetal membrane of decidual phospholipase A_2, which is probably activated or liberated from the lysosomes by hormonal change. This hypothesis has been derived mainly from data on term pregnancies; little is known about premature labor.

Violeta Curbelo, Raul Bejar, Kurt Benirschke, and Louis Gluck (Univ. of California, San Diego, at La Jolla) studies changes in phospholipids and their fatty acids in amnion and chorion throughout gestation. Membranes from 40 human placentas obtained after spontaneous labor or elective cesarean section after gestations of 26–42

(5–3)   Obstet. Gynecol. 57:473–478, April 1981.

weeks were assayed for phosholipids and fatty acid composition by two-dimensional, thin-layer chromatography and gas-liquid chromatography.

In preterm placental phospholipids, phosphorus concentrations were higher in amnion than in chorion, whereas at term the membranes had similar values due to an increase in phospholipid concentration in the chorion late in gestation. Phosphatidylcholine accounted for 47% of the total phospholipid phosphorus, sphingomyelin for 20%, phosphatidylethanolamine for 15%, phosphatidylserine for 12%, and phosphatidylinositol for 5%. These percentages were similar for amnion and chorion and did not change during gestation. The percentage of arachidonic acid was higher in phosphatidylserine (40% to 65%) than in phosphatidylethanolamine (30% to 53%) and phosphatidylcholine (10% to 13%). The percentage of arachidonic acid was significantly higher in phosphatidylcholine, phosphatidylethanolamine, and phosphatidylserine from the amnion in premature pregnancies than in those of the premature chorion. At term, these amniotic and chorionic phospholipids had similar concentrations of arachidonic acid as a result of a significant increase in this acid in the chorion late in gestation. Amniotic phosphatidylethanolamine obtained after term and preterm elective cesarean section had a significantly higher percentage of arachidonic acid than that obtained after preterm and term labor.

Arachidonic acid is apparently consumed during labor. Amniotic phospholipids, particularly phosphatidylethanolamine, may be its principal source. The amnion seems to be more important for the storage of arachidonic acid than the chorion, particularly in preterm pregnancies in which the concentrations of phospholipids and the percentages of arachidonic acid in phosphatidylcholine, phosphatidylethanolamine, and phosphatidylserine are significantly higher than in the chorion.

5–4 *II. Bacterial sources of phospholipase.*—Human term labor is thought to be initiated by amniotic and chorionic phospholipase A_2, an enzyme that liberates arachidonic acid esters from the phospholipids of these membranes, leading to synthesis of prostaglandins by the placental membranes. The striking association of premature labor with intrauterine infection or contamination, urinary tract infection, and early neonatal sepsis suggested that the microorganisms present in these infections might have phospholipase A_2 activity. To examine this possibility, Bejar, Curbelo, Charles Davis, and Gluck studied the capacity of some 22 bacteria, which occur normally in the vagina and cause perinatal infections, to split fatty acids from the second carbon of the phospholipids.

Activity was found in *Bacteroides fragilis, Peptostreptococcus, Fusobacterium necrophorum, Streptococcus viridans, S. Faecalis, Streptococcus* A and B, *Escherichia coli, Klebsiella, Staphylococcus epidermidis, Pneumococcus, Lactobacillus, and Mycoplasma hominis.* Activities were highest in *B. fragilis, Peptostreptococcus, Fuso-*

(5–4) Obstet. Gynecol. 57:479–482, April 1981.

bacterium, and *S. viridans.* The specific activities of phospholipase A_2 from these organisms were several times higher than that of the membrane phospholipase A_2 of the amnion and chorion.

Premature labor may be initiated by microorganisms with phospholipase A_2 activity from endocervical or intrauterine contamination, infection, or both, producing deacylation of arachidonic acid from amniotic phospholipids, with increased concentrations of free arachidonic acid and increased prostaglandin synthesis, which triggers labor. This hypothesis may also explain why labor starts after rupture of the membranes from any cause, as contamination with anaerobes and streptococci occurs rapidly in either term or preterm pregnancies.

▶ [A current view is that the onset of labor occurs when phospholipase A_2 is activated and hydrolyzes phopholipids producing free arachidonic acid, which is the precursor of prostaglandins E_2 and $F_{2\alpha}$. Phospholipase A_2 is present in membrane lysosomes. These reports indicate that several species of bacteria can produce this enzyme also. This is an important observation, bearing on the still unresolved role of clinically inapparent bacterial infection in triggering parturition.] ◀

5–5   **Coital Activity and Premature Delivery.** Seminal fluid is rich in prostaglandins and conceivably could increase uterine contractility when absorbed from the vaginal mucosa into the maternal circulation. To investigate the relationship of coital activity during pregnancy to premature labor and delivery, William F. Rayburn and Emery A. Wilson (Univ. of Kentucky Med. Center) compared the coital activity of 111 patients who were delivered after spontaneous premature labor with that of a matched group of patients who were delivered at term (table).

The proportion of patients who were sexually active, the mean coital frequency, and the incidence of orgasmic or nonorgasmic coitus within 2 days of delivery were not significantly ($P > .05$) different between the two groups. Only when a predisposing factor for premature delivery could not be identified (18 patients) was coital activity significantly ($P < .05$) greater than in the control group. These sexually active women were delivered in the 33d to 37th week of gestation, a time at which the uterus would be more sensitive to absorbed seminal prostaglandins.

It is concluded that normal coital activity is not an etiologic factor in premature delivery and that it should not be discouraged when there are no obvious preterm complications. However, abstinence may be of some benefit in pregnancies complicated by clinically ar-

COMPARISON IN COITAL ACTIVITY WITHIN ONE WEEK BETWEEN THE
TWO PATIENT POPULATIONS

Coital activity	*Premature group*	*Control group*	*p*
None	66/111	56/111	>0.05
Present	45/111	55/111	>0.05
Recent orgasmic coitus*	8/18	10/17	>0.05
Recent nonorgasmic coitus*	10/18	7/17	>0.05

(5–5)   Am. J. Obstet. Gynecol. 137:972–974, Aug. 15, 1980.

rested premature labor or a previous unexplained premature delivery.

▶ [This report concerns the controversial area of the effects of intercourse and orgasm on premature delivery. Recent studies have reached very different conclusions in this area. Presumably, this relates in large part to the sensitive nature of the behavior being asked about and possibly to guilt-associated recall bias as well. The present study includes an apparently appropriate control group and generally concludes that intercourse doesn't predispose to premature birth. The issue isn't totally settled, however, as those patients who delivered prematurely without underlying cause (e.g., twins, third-trimester bleeding, etc.) had significantly more frequent coitus than did control women. Data concerning orgasm in the absence of coitus aren't provided, but whether or not coitus was orgasmic apparently didn't matter, at least as far as premature delivery was concerned.] ◀

5–6 **Cervical Cerclage Operation for a Dilated Cervix.** Olufemi A. Olatunbosun and Frank Dyck (Univ. of Saskatchewan) treated 12 pregnant women with previously undiagnosed cervical incompetence, who had intact membranes bulging through a cervix dilated at least 4 cm and effaced at least 50%, but with no significant vaginal bleeding. A modification of the McDonald cerclage procedure was used. Average duration of pregnancy at operation was 21.4 weeks. The chief complaint that drew attention to the open cervix was a sensation of lower abdominal pressure, urinary frequency, pink watery discharge, or a vaginal lump.

TECHNIQUE.—An intravenous infusion of isoxsuprine or alcohol is started. During deep general anesthesia with halothane and endotracheal intubation, the woman is placed in a steep Trendelenburg position and supported with strong shoulder braces. The vulva is prepared in the usual manner but the vagina is not cleansed with antiseptic solutions. The cervix is exposed with retractors and 6–10 stay sutures (no. 00 silk) are attached to the edge of the effaced cervix. If traction on the stay sutures does not cause the herniated membranes to fall back into the uterine cavity, a moist swab on sponge-holding forceps or on a finger is used to push them back gently (Fig 5–3). Two purse-string sutures (no. 1 silk), the second 0.5 cm above the first, are placed as high, or proximally, as possible into the exterior aspect of the effaced cervix with deep stitches into the superficial two thirds of the thickness of the cervix while the membranes are held away with a moist swab or finger. Suture placement is normally started anteriorly, and stitches are taken every 60 degrees. The sutures are gently "snugged up" and tied anteriorly. All but 4 stay sutures are removed; the remaining 4 are cross tied over the os. An indwelling Foley catheter is left in place for 24 hours and prophylactic ampicillin is given for 5 days. Intravenous administration of isoxsuprine or alcohol is continued for 24–48 hours or until uterine irritability ceases, and orally administered isoxsuprine is continued 2 weeks more. Normally the woman is allowed to walk about on the 2d day and is discharged on the 5th or 6th day, to be followed up weekly. Sexual intercourse must be avoided for the remainder of the pregnancy. Sutures are removed at 38 weeks' gestation or when labor is established.

The cervix was closed without membrane rupture in all 12 women. Ten pregnancies continued successfully. In two instances, labor could not be arrested with alcohol and isoxsuprine, and sutures had to be removed on the 3d and 7th postoperative days, respectively, resulting in the birth of premature nonviable twins in one instance and of a

(5–6) Obstet. Gynecol. 57:166–170, February 1981.

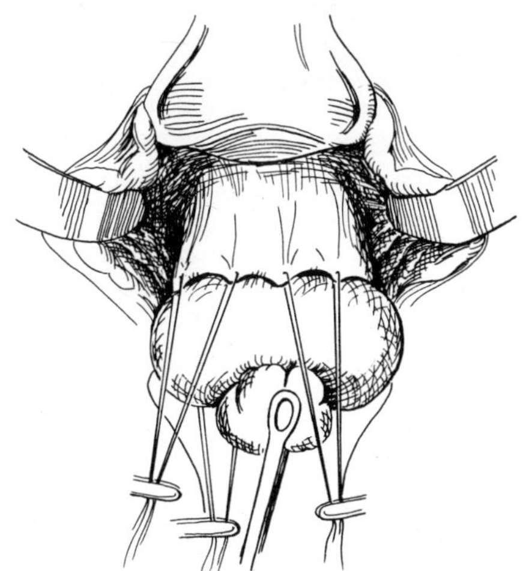

Fig 5–3.—Replacement of membranes into the uterus by gentle traction on stay sutures. (Courtesy of Olatunbosun, O. A., and Dyck, F.: Obstet. Gynecol. 57:166–170, February 1981.)

450-gm fetus in the second. No congenital abnormalities or operative complications were encountered. It was not necessary to repeat the cerclage operation. No patient showed evidence of infection after cervical closure.

Instruments on the cervical edge may accidentally perforate the membranes and must not be used. Ideally, a prophylactic Shirodkar cerclage suture should be placed at 14–16 weeks' gestation for incompetent cervix. Although it is often possible to close an open incompetent cervix, saving the fetus, the operation is contraindicated with ruptured membranes, infection, or labor.

▶ [These results are surprising, for it seems to us that cerclage operations are not often successful when the membranes are hourglassed through the cervix, probably because amnionitis is present. Nonetheless, 10 of 12 patients in this series carried their pregnancies long enough to reach viability. The technique used is a modification of the McDonald method, and the most important point is gentleness, so as to avoid rupturing the membranes. The use of stay sutures in the cervix, illustrated in Figure 5–3, seems to be a helpful adjunct.] ◀

5–7 **Comparison of Success and Morbidity in Cervical Cerclage Procedures.** James H. Harger (Univ. of Pittsburgh) reviewed the charts of the 205 women who underwent 251 cervical cerclage procedures (82 by the Shirodkar technique and 169 by the McDonald method) during 1971 to 1978. The 251 operations were performed by 30 surgeons who usually favored one technique over the other regardless of surgical indication or condition of the cervix.

Fetal survival was 19% before 139 elective McDonald operations and 20% before 63 elective Shirodkar procedures. Fetal survival was 78% after elective McDonald operations and 87% after elective Shirodkar procedures. Fetal survival was 53% after 30 emergency McDonald and 68% after 19 emergency Shirodkar procedures. Grouping of indications for surgery into eight categories showed that improvement in pregnancy outcome was not significant in any category that

(5–7) Obstet. Gynecol. 56:543–548, November 1980.

included cervical dilation as the reason for cerclage. The greatest improvement in pregnancy outcome, an eightfold increase, occurred in operations performed for two or more second-trimester pregnancy losses, i.e., the classic history for cervical insufficiency.

Major postoperative morbidity occurred in 2.0% of the elective cerclage procedures, and acute chorioamnionitis accounted for half the complications (1.2%). Mean blood loss was 30 ml with elective McDonald operations and 44 ml with elective Shirodkar procedures; maximum blood loss of 150 ml occurred in 2 emergency procedures. Cervical laceration at parturition occurred more often with Shirodkar (11%) or McDonald (14%) procedures than with the 55,688 other deliveries (2.2%) that occurred during the study period. Cervical scarring and elective cesarean section increased the cesarean section rate to 16% after McDonald procedures and to 25% after Shirodkar operations.

The finding of cervical dilation to 2–3 cm without effacement does not indicate cervical insufficiency or imminent delivery. Given the uncertainty about the accuracy of diagnosis of cervical insufficiency, and the pregnancy prognosis with and without intervention by a cerclage procedure, it is essential to exclude as causes genetic disorders, müllerian abnormalities, thyroid disorder, collagen-vascular diseases, and perhaps infections by *Ureaplasma urealyticum* or *Mycoplasma hominis* before cerclage is performed. If cerclage is to be carried out, it should be performed after 14 weeks' gestation (to avoid overlapping a spontaneous first-trimester abortion) but before 20 weeks (to avoid any cervical dilation or effacement). Waiting until cervical changes are detected leads to a poorer chance of successful outcome than with elective cerclage (59% vs. 81%, respectively) even though the prior pregnancy success rate was better in the population that had emergency cerclages than in those who had elective cerclages (39% vs. 19%, respectively). The prognosis is much worse if the procedure is delayed until membranes are bulging through the partially dilated cervix; even weekly examination of the cervix will not always forestall this development. Equivalent success and morbidity rates between the two techniques suggests that ease of procedure favors the McDonald operation.

▶ [This is a large and well-analyzed experience with incompetent cervix and its surgical repair. The frequency—1 per 222 deliveries over a 7½-year period—seems high to us, but this may reflect the referral nature of the hospital. Fetal survival was better after elective repair than after emergency procedures, but there was no significant difference between the two types of operations in either elective or emergency categories. This failure to find a difference between McDonald and Shirodkar repairs is interesting, although of uncertain significance because the study is retrospective and there might have been an unrecognized systematic bias in favor or against one procedure (more experienced surgeon, tougher case, etc.). If it is true that there is no real difference in outcome with the two operations, then perhaps the McDonald should be preferred because of its greater simplicity, shorter operating time and smaller blood loss. Our own bias, however, is that the Shirodkar provides a better anatomical repair, at least in the elective case.] ◀

5–8 **Amniocentesis in Evaluation of Premature Labor.** An associa-

---

(5–8) Obstet. Gynecol. 57:483–486, April 1981.

tion between unrecognized amnionitis and prematurity has been suggested, and it has been postulated that diagnostic amniocentesis might aid recognition of early intrauterine infection in patients in premature labor. Roger L. Wallace and C. Neil Herrick (Frankfort Army Regional Med. Center, West Germany) prospectively studied the value of amniocentesis in the management of 25 patients in labor at 26 to 34 weeks' gestation.The patients were receiving tocolytic therapy consisting of terbutaline given intravenously; they later received terbutaline orally for maintenance. Amniocentesis was performed $1^{1}/_{2}$ to 24 hours (mean, $9^{1}/_{2}$) after initiation of tocolytic therapy, at a time when membranes were intact and labor had been successfully arrested in all cases. Amniotic fluid samples were cultured for aerobic and anaerobic organisms.

Three specimens yielded bacterial growth, which in two was considered to be from contaminants. The only patients with significant bacterial growth in the amniotic fluid also had clinical signs and symptoms suggestive of amnionitis. Of the 25 patients, 5 experienced spontaneous rupture of membranes after amniocentesis.

Because amnionitis was not demonstrated in a significant number of otherwise asymptomatic patients in premature labor and because amniocentesis in women with premature labor may be associated with higher risks than have been previously recognized, amniocentesis done only for the possibility of amnionitis seems to be clinically unwarranted. However, it may be useful in the management of patients in premature labor with undefined fever or any signs or symptoms of amnionitis.

▶ [Amnionitis can occur in the presence of intact membranes. This, coupled with the frequent histologic (but not necessarily bacteriologic) evidence of inflammation of the chorioamnion identified in cases of premature delivery, raises the question as to how often threatened premature labor with intact membranes is associated with clinically inapparent intra-amniotic infection. Not very often, according to this study. Others are looking at this problem. It is an important issue with obvious implications concerning the pharmacologic inhibition of threatened premature labor.] ◀

5–9 **Ritodrine in Treatment of Preterm Labor: Clinical Trial to Compare Standard Treatment With Three Regimens Involving Use of Ritodrine** is described by J. Falck Larsen, M. Kern Hansen, H. Hesseldahl, K. Kristoffersen, P. K. Larsen, M. Osler, J. Weber, K. Eldon, and A. Lange (Denmark). Preliminary controlled studies had indicated that this β-sympathomimetic drug inhibits preterm labor. The trial was conducted with 176 otherwise healthy women who presented at 20–36 weeks' gestation with regular contractions or contractions accompanied by effacement or dilation of the cervix, or who were in labor with a fetus thought to weigh less than 2,500 gm. The patients were randomly allocated to one of four treatment groups.

In the "long ritodrine infusion" group, ritodrine was infused intravenously in 5.5% glucose starting at 100 μg/minute and increasing by 50 μg/minute every 5–10 minutes until uterine relaxation or unacceptable side effects occurred (maximum dose, 350 μg/minute). Infusion was continued for 24 hours. Thirty minutes before discontinu-

---

(5–9) Br. J. Obstet. Gynaecol. 87:949–957, November 1980.

ing intravenous infusion, oral ritodrine was begun at a dose of 10 mg four times a day. If uterine irritability occurred, the oral dose was increased to a maximum of 120 mg/day. Oral ritodrine was continued until 37 weeks of gestation or delivery.

In the "short ritodrine infusion" group, initial treatment was as with the long infusion. The infusion was stopped 30 minutes after contractions ceased, at which time oral ritodrine treatment was started at the same dosage scheme as that used for women with long ritodrine infusions.

In the "intramuscular ritodrine treatment" group, ritodrine was given intramuscularly in 10-mg doses every 4 hours for the first 12 hours, and every 6 hours for the next 12 hours. Three hours after the last intramuscular injection, ritodrine was started orally as already described.

In the "standard treatment" group, women were given 5.5% glucose for 24 hours, intravenously, confined to bed, and, in some cases, given injections of diazepam or oral doses of barbiturate, or both. Oral placebo tablets were started 30 minutes after contractions ceased, and 1 such tablet was given four times a day until 37 weeks' gestation or delivery.

All patients were confined to bed for 48 hours. If no contractions occurred after 48 hours, they were kept in the hospital without absolute bed rest for 5 more days. If preterm labor recurred during oral treatment and the patient did not respond to an increased dose of ritodrine or placebo, the initial treatment was repeated.

None of the ritodrine treatments was better in postponing delivery than standard treatment. However, the Bishop scores of patients in the standard treatment group tended to be lower than those of patients treated with ritodrine. Moreover, all cases of congenital malformation and polyhydramnios occurred in patients treated with ritodrine. The incidence of respiratory insufficiency was significantly higher in infants of mothers treated with ritodrine. Mean birth weight was highest in the standard treatment group.

▶ [Although this is a relatively large study, the larger United States multicenter trial did demonstrate a statistically significant, although modest, prolongation of pregnancy with ritodrine (1981 YEAR BOOK, pp. 129–130). Perhaps the absence of infants with congenital malformations and the slightly less favorable cervices in the standard treatment group (the Bishop score was >5 in 7% of the standard group and in 39% of the ritodrine patients) help explain the failure to see an effect.] ◀

5–10 **Suppression of Threatened Premature Labor by Administration of Cortisol and 17α-Hydroxyprogesterone Caproate: Comparison With Ritodrine.** A shift in the progesterone-estradiol balance to estradiol dominance is probably a prerequisite for regular uterine contractions. Antti Kauppila, Anna-Liisa Hartikainen-Sorri, Olli Jänne, Risto Tuimala, and Pentti A. Järvinen (Univ. of Oulu) compared the ability of two methods to antagonize this effect in 48 women admitted at 27 to 36 weeks' gestation with threatened premature labor.

The first 24 women were given a simultaneous intramuscular injec-

---

(5–10) Am. J. Obstet. Gynecol. 138:404–408, Oct. 15, 1980.

tion of 250 mg of 17α-hydroxyprogesterone caproate (17 OHP-C) and an intravenous bolus of 100 mg of cortisol, followed immediately by infusion of 150 mg of cortisol in 500 ml of 5% glucose over 2 hours. The intravenous injection of 100 mg of cortisol was repeated on the second and third days. An intramuscular injection of 250 mg of 17 OHP-C was administered on the third day and then weekly until the 37th week of gestation. The other 24 women were treated with ritodrine, a β-adrenergic agonist widely used for inhibition of premature labor. Ritodrine (50 mg in 500 ml of 5% glucose) was infused at a rate of 50 μg/minute for 10 minutes. The dose was increased by 50 μg/minute at 10-minute intervals until uterine relaxation occurred. The infusion was maintained at the lowest effective dose for at least 48 hours. This intravenous therapy was followed by intramuscular injections of ritodrine, 20 mg 3 times a day for 2 days.

Delivery was postponed by at least 1 week in 21 patients (87.5%) in the steroid group and in 18 (75%) in the ritodrine group. Mean durations of premature labor were 5.1 hours and 2.2 hours, respectively. In singleton pregnancies, gestational age and birth weight of the newborn infants were greater in the steroid group (39.1 weeks and 3,460 gm) than in the ritodrine group (37.7 weeks and 3,106 gm). Steroid treatment suppressed serum estradiol concentrations (maximally by 60%) and, to a lesser extent, testosterone, estradiol, and progesterone levels (maximally by 30%). These hormonal changes were of short duration and did not disturb fetal well-being.

Combined treatment with cortisol and 17 OHP-C is at least as effective in inhibiting premature labor as the widely used therapy with ritodrine.

▶ [Progestational hormones have previously proved disappointing in *treating* premature labor, though there is some suggestion of a beneficial effect in *prophylaxis*. However, the results of this small series suggest there actually may be therapeutic efficacy. Patients with threatened premature labor were given 17α-hydroxyprogesterone caproate intramuscularly and cortisol intravenously (to suppress estradiol), and these results were at least as good as those in patients treated with "standard" tocolytic therapy. It is unfortunate that the numbers are small and the design was not a randomized one. Clearly, more study is needed.] ◀

5–11 **Terbutaline Sulfate in the Prevention of Recurrence of Premature Labor.** Premature labor has been arrested successfully by various tocolytic agents, but the recurrence of premature labor after initial arrest is relatively common. Stanley M. Brown and Nergesh Tejani evaluated the effectiveness of terbutaline sulfate, a β_2-mimetic agent, in the prevention or postponement of recurrent premature labor in a random, double-blind study of 46 patients whose initial episode in the 24th to 36th week of gestation was treated successfully with ethanol infusion. The patients randomly were assigned to the medication group (23 patients) or the placebo group (23 patients). Treatment (5 mg of terbutaline sulfate every 6 hours) was begun 2 hours before the end of ethanol infusion and was continued until the 38th week of gestation or the onset of labor.

Gestational ages were similar between groups, but the Bishop score

(5–11) Obstet. Gynecol. 57:22–25, January 1981.

in the medication group was significantly higher than in the control group, thus placing the medication group at a greater risk of premature delivery (table). Despite this disadvantage, patients treated with terbutaline showed a significant time gain in days until the onset of labor compared with controls. Mean birth weight was significantly greater and the incidence of idiopathic respiratory distress syndrome

SUMMARY OF RESULTS*

Treatment	No. of patients ($N = 46$)	Gestational age at entry (weeks)	Bishop score at entry	Time gained (days)	Birth weight (g)	IRDS
Terbutaline	23	30.9 ± 2.3	4.3 ± 3.2	42.5 ± 22.6	2757 ± 182.3	1/25
Control	23	31.4 ± 3.1	2.8 ± 2.3	29.4 ± 22.2	2386 ± 263.1	6/26
P value		NS	$< .05$	$< .05$	$< .01$	$< .05$

*IRDS, idiopathic respiratory distress syndrome; NS, not significant. All values represented as mean $\pm$ SD.

(IRDS) significantly less in the medication group than in the control group. There were no instances of perinatal mortality in either group. Side effects, primarily mild maternal and fetal tachycardia and elevated maternal blood pressure, were not severe enough to require reduction in dosage or discontinuation of terbutaline.

It is recommended that patients with low birth weight fetuses and premature labor who respond well to tocolytic agents should receive prolonged oral treatment with a β_2-mimetic agent such as terbutaline sulfate to maintain uterine quiescence.

▶ [Although oral β-adrenergic drugs frequently have been used after the successful acute inhibition of threatened premature labor in order to try to prevent or postpone its recurrence, this is the first study we are aware of that demonstrates the efficacy of this prophylactic measure. The study design seems sound, and this sort of oral treatment is probably worthwhile, although we wouldn't continue it for as long as the authors did (until the 38th week).] ◀

5–12 **Metabolic Effects of Intravenous Ritodrine Infusion in Pregnancy.** P. Schreyer, E. Caspi, S. Arieli, J. Maor, and D. Modai (Univ. of Tel-Aviv) examined the effects of intravenous administration of ritodrine, a potent β-adrenergic agent used to suppress uterine contractions in the management of premature labor, on blood glucose, insulin, electrolytes, plasma, red blood cell potassium, and venous pH. The 10 patients studied were considered to be at risk of premature labor because of earlier preterm deliveries with or without cervical incompetence, placenta previa, or premature uterine contractions. Patients with a familial or past history of diabetes were not included in the study. Normal saline infusion was begun via a scalp vein at a rate of 1 ml/minute; blood samples were collected from the collateral antecubital vein at the beginning of the infusion and after 30 and 60 minutes. After 1 hour, ritodrine was administered by an infusion pump at a constant rate of 100 μg/minute. Blood samples were collected at 30, 60, 120, and 180 minutes during the infusion. Urine collected before and after the second and fourth hour of infusion was analyzed for potassium. Pulse rate and blood pressure were measured after each blood sample collection, and ECG was performed in all patients at time zero and during the third hour of infusion.

Blood glucose values were not influenced by saline infusion but rose significantly during ritodrine infusion (mean value 4.12 to 5.91 mmole/L). They had returned to preinfusion values 20 hours therafter. Blood insulin levels significantly were increased 30 and 60 minutes after ritodrine infusion, after which there was an insignificant decrease in insulinemia. Serum potassium levels exhibited a highly significant fall during the first hour of ritodrine administration and a less significant fall thereafter, the difference before and after ritodrine being 1.08 mmole/L. In the first hour of ritodrine infusion, red blood cell potassium showed a highly significant rise; thereafter an insignificant decrease was observed. The correlation coefficient between plasma and red blood cell potassium was highly significant (r = − 0.962). There was a highly significant negative correlation between serum glucose and potassium levels and a positive correlation be-

(5–12) Acta Obstet. Gynecol. Scand. 59:197–201, 1980.

tween insulinemia and red blood cell potassium. Sodium, chloride, calcium, phosphorus, and magnesium were not affected by ritodrine infusion, nor was venous pH or the urinary potassium-creatinine ratio. An increase in heart rate was registered in all patients.

Activation of adenylate cyclase results in an accumulation of intracellular cyclic AMP, which acts on liver enzymes to effect increased output of glucose. Such changes assume importance in the diabetic patient; 3 such women showed a significant increase in insulin requirement. The hypokalemic effect may be secondary to the elevated blood glucose level; this acute effect may be of importance in selected cases, as in patients treated with digitalis or diuretics.

▶ [The package insert for ritodrine, which has only recently become available in the United States, cautions about hypokalemia. This study indicates that the fall in the serum potassium level probably results from migration of potassium ions into the erythrocyte, perhaps reflecting an action of insulin. The mean serum potassium level fell from 3.7 to 2.7 mmole/L over 2 hours of therapy, surely a clinically significant drop. Does this mean that potassium supplements should be given concomitantly?] ◀

5–13 **Cardiovascular Complications Associated With Terbutaline Treatment for Preterm Labor.** Pulmonary edema has been described with the use of terbutaline and other β-adrenergic agents in preterm labors. Michael Katz, Patricia A. Robertson, and Robert K. Creasy (Univ. of California, San Francisco) reviewed experience with 160 patients given terbutaline at 28–36 weeks' gestation in 1978–1980. The drug was given by infusion at increasing rates until uterine contractility was controlled or adverse cardiovascular effects appeared.

Eight patients had severe cardiovascular complications, 7 with clinical and radiologic evidence of pulmonary edema. Three of these 7 patients and 1 other patient had ECG changes indicative of myocardial ischemia. Echocardiography was normal in all 3 patients examined. Pulmonary edema was relieved within 4 to 6 hours by discontinuance of terbutaline infusion and administration of oxygen and intravenous diuretics.

Severe cardiovascular complications occurred in 5% of this series of patients given terbutaline infusion for preterm labor. Four of the 8 patients with complications were among the 13 patients with twin gestations. Maternal blood volume is especially high in such pregnancies. Intravenous fluids are given to most patients in preterm labor, and the risk of volume overload must be kept in mind. Corticosteroids, administered to 5 of the patients who had pulmonary edema, may have mineralocorticoid activity and could thus induce significant electrolyte and fluid balance changes. However, heart failure can occur even in the absence of steroid therapy. The cardiac output may rise markedly during β-adrenergic drug administration, and this might result in damage, leading to cardiogenic pulmonary edema. Complications in the present cases occurred at infusion rates of 10 to 30 µg/ml, in the lower part of the usual dose range. Tachycardia of more than 140 beats per minute for prolonged periods should be avoided. Cardiovascular status should be monitored frequently dur-

(5–13) Am. J. Obstet. Gynecol. 139:605–608, Mar. 1, 1981.

ing tocolytic therapy, and fluid balance should be recorded accurately.

▶ [This report calls attention to a serious complication of tocolytic therapy. Pulmonary edema or myocardial ischemia, or both, occurred in 5% of terbutaline-treated patients. This is not a problem peculiar to terbutaline, but is probably equally likely with all β-agonists. In our own experience, involving terbutaline for several years and ritodrine for the past year, pulmonary edema has been recognized in only two instances, This may reflect the fact that we have virtually never given glucocorticoids to induce lung maturity.] ◀

5–14 **Combined Use of β-Sympathomimetic Drugs and β-Blockers During Labor.** The catecholaminergic labor inhibitors all influence the maternal cardiovascular system as well as the uterus. Cardioselective β-blockers with little effect on β_2-receptors in the blood vessels and bronchi now are available. M. Steyer, W. Poleska, H. P. Diemer, H. Schmidt, and J. Heidenreich used specific cardiac β-blockade to reduce maternal tachycardia without influencing inhibition of labor in women treated with fenoterol. Twelve healthy women with normal singleton pregnancies received a β-blocker in the first stage of labor. All had some degree of uterine hyperactivity. The dose of infused fenoterol ranged from 4 to 5 µg/minute. Five patients received metoprolol in increasing doses up to 2 mg-minute, for a total dose of about 20 mg in 30 minutes. The other patients received a single intravenous injection of 5 mg of atenolol.

Palpitations and tremor resolved after β-blockade. The maternal heart rate declined after administration of both β-blockers. The diastolic blood pressure rose with contractions in fenoterol-treated patients, but not after metoprolol administration. Contractions became sporadic during tocolysis. Amplitudes increased to about 40% of pretreatment levels after metoprolol; the interval between contractions was $1^{1}/_{2}$ times as long as before treatment. Injection of atenolol led to one or two isolated contractions. Fetal heart rate was not influenced significantly by maternal β-blockade. None of the newborn infants showed effects attributable to β-blockade.

Cardioselective β-blockade is effective during tocolysis by fenoterol infusion and does not impair the tocolytic effect significantly. However, the reduction in tachycardia may deprive the mother and child of an important compensatory mechanism, and the general use of this approach cannot be recommended yet.

▶ [This is an interesting approach to minimizing cardiovascular side effects of β-adrenergic tocolytic therapy. Administration of a "cardioselective" β-blocker simultaneously with a β-agonist (fenoterol) lessened maternal and fetal tachycardia. There was a brief increase in uterine activity, though the article states that the β-blockade did not "significantly hamper the tocolytic effects." However, no information is given about outcome in terms of labor suppression. Clearly, more information is needed about this point, as well as about other maternal and fetal side effects.] ◀

5–15 **Comparative Study of Estradiol and Prostaglandin E_2 Vaginal Gel for Ripening the Unfavorable Cervix Before Induction of Labor.** Philip M. Tromans, John M. Beazley, and Peter I. Shenouda (Royal Liverpool Hosp.) compared estradiol, 150 mg, and prostaglandin E_2 (PGE_2), 4 mg suspended in viscous gel, applied intravag-

(5–14) Arch. Gynecol. 203:231–237, May 1981.
(5–15) Br. Med. J. 282:679–681, Feb. 28, 1981.

RESULTS OF COMPARATIVE STUDY GROUPS (NUMBERS OF PATIENTS IN PARENTHESES)

	PGE$_2$ group (n = 30)	Oestradiol group (n = 30)	Significance
Subjective symptoms	90% (27)	17% (5)	p < 0·0005
Uterine activity increased (cardiotocographic findings)	83% (25)	17% (5)	p < 0·0005
Spontaneous onset of labour	7% (2)	0	NS
Decelerative cardiotocographic recording	7% (2)	0	NS
Surgical induction rate after first application	77% (23)	77% (23)	NS
Overall surgical induction rate after second application	87% (26)	90% (27)	NS
Mean cervical score improvement in primigravidae (±1 SD)	3·4 ± 2·0 (20)	2·6 ± 1·3 (18)	NS (NED = 1·85)
Mean cervical score improvement in multiparae (±1 SD)	4·7 ± 2·6 (10)	2·7 ± 0·6 (12)	p < 0·01 (NED = 2·71)
Epidural analgesia	80% (24)	80% (24)	NS
Mean duration of labour in hours (±1 SD)	7·0 ± 3·6 (23)	8·3 ± 4·3 (22)	NS
Patients requiring caesarean section	23% (7)	27% (8)	NS
Mean Apgar score at one minute (±1 SD)	8·5 ± 0·9 (30)	9·0 ± 0·7 (30)	NS

Note: NS indicates not significant (P > .05); NED, normal equivalent deviate.

inally with regard to ripening the unfavorable cervix (assessed at a mean of 12 hours after one application) of patients randomly allocated to two study groups.

Symptoms (backache and lower abdominal pain) occurred within 2 hours of PGE$_2$ gel insertion in 27 patients (table). In primigravidas, no significant difference was observed in efficacy of the two substances. However, some multiparous patients had considerably more uterine sensitivity to PGE$_2$ than to estradiol. Two patients in the PGE$_2$ group quickly had decelerative cardiotocographic tracings after gel insertion, necessitating emergency cesarean section 4 hours after gel insertion in 1 patient.

Findings suggest that estradiol applied vaginally is a safe, comfortable, cheap, and equally effective alternative to PGE$_2$ for ripening the primigravid cervix; in multiparous patients, though both agents were effective for ripening the cervix (PGE$_2$ more than estradiol), PGE$_2$ excited more uterine activity. When PGE$_2$ is employed, cardiotocography is essential.

▶ [Prostaglandin E$_2$ in this study apparently ripened the cervix more effectively than did estradiol (statistically significantly so only in multiparas), but with an associated increase in uterine activity. It is too bad that a placebo group was not included in order to provide another comparison for the estradiol group. Effective cervical ripening in the absence of increased uterine activity is the goal.] ◀

5-16 **Single Application of Prostaglandin E$_2$ in a Viscous Gel for Induction of Labor at Term in Patients With Favorable Cervix.** Prostaglandins given intravenously (IV) or orally do not seem superior to oxytocin to induce labor in patients with favorable inducibility score, and when so given, prostaglandins often cause side effects, es-

(5–16) Acta Obstet. Gynecol. Scand. 60:17–19, 1981.

pecially gastrointestinal disorders. In patients with an unfavorable cervix, prostaglandins given orally or IV seem advantageous compared with oxytocin. With strict intracervical application, prostaglandin E_2 in viscous gel (PGE_2) has been found valuable in induction of labor and/or to ripen the cervix, without side effects. L. Wingerup and U. Ulmsten (Univ. of Lund) introduced a single dose of 0.5 mg of PGE_2 in gel into the cervical canal close to the internal os to induce labor in 150 consecutive patients (79 nulliparas, 71 multiparas) with a favorable cervix. The patient was then requested to stay in bed for 30 minutes; thereafter, she was allowed to walk about. At the time of induction, no patients had spontaneous uterine activity (tocometry) and all had intact membranes. Seven patients had had previous cesarean section, and 5 had had abortion via hysterotomy. Patients with low-implanted placenta were excluded.

All but 5 patients (97%) were delivered within 12 hours. The mean induction delivery time (IDT) was 6.5 hours (range, 2.5–12 hours). Mean IDT was 5.0 in multiparous women and 7.5 hours in nulliparas; the difference resulted from a shorter first stage of labor in multiparas. In only 10 patients (8 nulliparas, 2 multiparas) was the IDT longer than 10 hours. Among those delivered, all were in established labor within 2 hours after gel application except 5 patients whose labor started 3–4 hours after gel application. In the 5 undelivered patients (4 nulliparas, 1 multipara), uterine contractions ceased after approximately 5 hours. In 4 patients (1 nullipara, 3 multiparas) with breech presentations, delivery occurred after 7–11 hours. No adverse maternal or fetal effects were registered. Two nulliparas required cesarean section because of fetal bradycardia in late first stage of labor. Ten patients (8 nulliparas, 2 multiparas) were delivered using ventouse extraction because of abnormal fetal heart rate variations in the second stage of labor. All but 8 neonates had a 1-minute Apgar score >7; after 5 minutes, all infants had an Apgar score >7.

The method enabled induction without primary amniotomy, was easy to perform, safe, and effective, and was well accepted by patients. Labor with intact membranes has advantages over primary amniotomy. In patients with breech presentation, the decreased cervical resistance obtained with PGE_2 may be of particular value.

▶ [These workers previously have described the efficiency of intracervical prostaglandin E_2 in the induction of labor in patients with unfavorable cervices (1981 YEAR BOOK, pp. 137–138), so this report of success in patients with favorable cervices comes as no surprise. Some advantage over amniotomy may pertain in patients in whom the vertex is high; however, in general, amniotomy would be our choice in patients with favorable cervices. We do not share the concerns expressed by others regarding the alleged adverse fetal effects of this standard obstetric intervention.] ◀

5–17 **Induction of Labor by Oxytocin or Prostaglandin E_2.** Katarina Bremme and Marc Bygdeman (Karolinska Hosp., Stockholm) compared the efficacy and safety of the intravenous infusion of oxytocin with the oral administration of prostaglandin E_2 (PGE_2) in the therapeutic induction of labor in a randomized prospective study of 200 women. Amniotomy was performed in both groups at the beginning

---

(5–17) Acta Obstet. Gynecol. Scand. [Suppl.] 92:11–21, 1980.

of therapy or within 2 hours thereafter. Prostaglandin E_2 was administered in an initial dose of 0.5 mg, followed by 1 mg/hour for up to 24 hours, whereas oxytocin was administered in an initial dose of 5 mIU/minute, followed by an incremental increase of 5 mIU/minute every hour up to 20 mIU/minute. Prior to the induction of labor, cervical ripening was assessed and given a Modified Bishop score (Table 1); the number of patients with a Bishop score of 5 or less was significantly higher in the oxytocin treatment group. The outcome of therapy in both groups was compared with that in 1,769 spontaneous deliveries and 249 deliveries induced by oxytocin alone.

Both methods were equally successful in inducing labor. All patients went into labor and delivered within approximately 24 hours. Cesarean section delivery was necessary in 16 patients (8%), and vacuum extraction was required to complete delivery in 52 patients (26%). The frequency of cesarean section was slightly higher in the oxytocin group than in the prostaglandin group, whereas the opposite was the case for the frequency of vacuum extraction. Multiparous patients had a significantly lower incidence of instrumental delivery than primiparous patients. If the patient was multiparous and had a Bishop score of 6 or greater, the combined frequency of cesarean section and instrumental delivery was 2.5% for PGE_2 and 3.1% for oxytocin. The health status of the neonates was similar in both groups.

The mean duration of labor was 1.1 hours longer for those treated

TABLE 1.—MODIFIED BISHOP SCORE IN RANDOMIZED TRIAL

Compound	No. of pat.	Score 0 − 5		Score 6 − 10	
		No.	Per cent	No.	Per cent
PGE_2	104	24*	23	80	77
Oxytocin	96	39*	41	57	59

*P < .05.

TABLE 2.—DURATION OF LABOR IN HOURS FOLLOWING EARLY LOW AMNIOTOMY IN COMBINATION WITH ORAL PGE_2 OR INTRAVENOUS OXYTOCIN INFUSION*

Stage of labor	PGE_2		Oxytocin	
	Primipara	Multipara	Primipara	Multipara
Latency phase	3.1±0.6	1.8±0.3	3.4±1.0	1.5±0.3
Acc. phase	4.8±0.7	2.5±0.4	4.2±0.9	2.0±0.3
Decel. phase	0.8±0.2	0.3±0.1	0.6±0.2	0.3±0.04
Stage I	8.7±1.1	4.6±0.7	8.2±1.6	3.8±0.8
Stage II	0.8±0.2	0.3±0.1	0.8±0.2	0.3±0.1
Stage III	0.1±0.03	0.1±0.03	0.2±0.03	0.1±0.03
Total time	9.7±1.2	5.0±0.7	9.1±1.6	4.3±0.8
Total time	7.2±0.8		6.1±0.9	

*Mean values ± 95% confidence interval. The difference between primiparous and multiparous women was highly statistically significant for the different phases of stage I, for stage II, and for total time for both PGE_2 and oxytocin ($P < .001$). The mean delivery time for all PGE_2 patients was probably significantly longer than that for all oxytocin patients ($P < .05$).

with prostaglandin than those treated with oxytocin (Table 2). This difference was attributed to a prolongation of stage 1 of labor. Multiparous women delivered significantly faster than primiparous women in both groups. The duration of delivery was 2 to 3 hours longer in patients with a Bishop score of 4 or 5 than in patients with a Bishop score of 8 or greater, regardless of parity. Administration of an epidural analgesic significantly prolonged labor, regardless of parity or method. The time to delivery exceeded 22 hours in 7 patients. When oxytocin infusion without amniotomy was done, the mean time to delivery was similar to that for amniotomy with oxytocin or PGE_2 in primiparous patients, but was significantly longer than that for multiparous patients. Most of the women (75% to 81%) bled less than 500 ml at delivery and during the first hours after delivery. Gastrointestinal side effects occurred occasionally. Five primiparous patients showed signs of infection; 3 of these had a time to delivery of 22 hours or more.

Both oxytocin infusion and oral PGE_2 with amniotomy were more effective than intravenous oxytocin alone. Prostaglandin E_2 administered orally is a valuable alternative to intravenous infusion of oxytocin for the induction of labor at or near term.

5–18 **A Comparative Study of Uterine Activity and Fetal Heart Rate Pattern in Labor Induced With Oral Prostaglandin E_2 or Oxytocin.** It is well known that both oxytocin and prostaglandins may cause uterine hyperactivity that could prove dangerous to the fetus and, perhaps, the mother. Katarina Bremme and Marc Bygdeman (Karolinska Hosp., Stockholm) compared the effects of low amniotomy in conjunction with either intravenous infusion of oxytocin or oral administration of prostaglandin E_2 (PGE_2) on uterine contractility in a randomized prospective study of 200 women selected for therapeutic induction of labor. Prostaglandin E_2 was administered in an initial oral dose of 0.5 mg, followed by 1 mg/hour for up to 24 hours, while oxytocin was given as an intravenous pump infusion with an initial dose of 5 mIU/minute, followed by an incremental increase of 5 mIU/minute every hour up to 20 mIU/minute. In 61 women receiving oxytocin and 63 given PGE_2, a cardiotocograph was used to continuously record fetal heart rates and uterine contractility. The uterine contractility recordings of 16 women, 8 from each group, were analyzed in greater detail with regard to the frequency and intensity of contractions.

Labor contractility was established slightly earlier in the oxytocin group than in those receiving PGE_2 (mean, 36 and 94 minutes, respectively). Approximately 2 hours after the induction of labor, the frequency and intensity of uterine contractions were similar in both groups, though the frequency of contractions and increase in intensity of contractions were slightly higher in the oxytocin group. Atypical contractility patterns were significantly more common in the PGE_2 group than the oxytocin group (table). Pairs and triads of contractions were observed in 75% of the PGE_2 group but in only 12.5% of those

(5–18) Acta Obstet. Gynecol. Scand. [Suppl.] 92:23–29, 1980.

FREQUENCY OF ATYPICAL CONTRACTILITY PATTERN IN %
OF ALL 124 RECORDED PATIENTS

Treatment	Frequency of hypertonus	Atypical contractions
L. a.† + oxytocin	0	13*
L. a. + PGE$_2$	4.7	69*

*$P < .001$ (χ^2 analysis).
†Low amniotomy.

treated with oxytocin. When all recordings were examined with regard to both transient episodes of hypertonicity and atypical contractions, the same difference between groups was observed, but at a higher level of significance (table). One patient treated with PGE$_2$ exhibited a period of hypertonus. However, fetal heart rate remained normal and the tonus returned to a normal level without treatment. Both mild and more severe variations in fetal heart rates were observed, but the incidence was similar in both groups. There were no perinatal deaths, and the 5-minute Apgar scores were 8 or higher.

In this study, irregular uterine contractions were more common during oral administration of PGE$_2$ than during the intravenous infusion of oxytocin. However, the association of fetal heart rate abnormalities with atypical uterine contractions and hypertonus was equally rare for both PGE$_2$ and oxytocin.

▶ [This article and the preceding one describe large carefully done studies comparing intravenous oxytocin with oral PGE$_2$ for the induction of labor. Both agents were efficacious. Labor was slightly longer in the PGE$_2$ group even though the distribution of Bishop scores was more favorable in this group. Furthermore, atypical contractions were more common in the prostaglandin group. Oral PGE$_2$ can be used successfully and safely to induce labor, but in this series it apparently offered no advantages over oxytocin for labor induction. The ultimate role of PGE$_2$ in this situation has not been defined.] ◀

5–19 **Factors Affecting Plasma Angiotensin II Concentration in Labor.** E. M. Symonds and Fiona Broughton Pipkin (City Hosp., Nottingham) measured concentrations of plasma angiotensin II (AII) and assessed some factors influencing the levels. Of 134 patients, 115 women (73 primigravid and 42 multigravid) were delivered vaginally, and 19 women (10 primigravid and 9 multigravid) were delivered by elective lower segment cesarean section. In women having vaginal deliveries, blood samples were obtained from the antecubital vein at delivery or during the second stage of labor, within 5–6 minutes of delivery and between contractions. In women undergoing elective cesarean sections, samples were obtained within 1 minute of delivery. All patients were supine. Blood pressure was measured within a minute or so before venipuncture. The data on AII concentrations were analyzed with respect to parity, blood pressure before 20 weeks' gestation and at induction of labor and delivery, maternal body weight,

(5–19) Br. J. Obstet. Gynaecol. 87:869–874, October 1980.

the presence of proteinuria, induction agents used, the length of the second stage of labor, and the method of delivery.

Proteinuria was associated with high AII levels to such an extent that it was necessary to exclude this variable to establish other trends. Therefore, other results relate only to nonproteinuric patients. Concentrations of AII in normotensive primigravidas given epidurals (n = 11) were significantly lower at delivery than in patients not given epidurals (61.3 ± 20.7 and 103.3 ± 15.2 pg/ml, respectively). Concentrations showed an overall positive correlation with the estimated duration of the second stage of labor; when the data were subdivided with respect to parity, the positive relationship persisted in parous women but could not be demonstrated in primigravidas. Patients given oxytocin to augment labor had somewhat lower AII concentrations than patients delivered spontaneously, but in primigravidas also receiving epidurals, AII concentrations were significantly higher following oxytocin. Concentrations of AII showed a statistically significant correlation with the diastolic pressure at delivery in primigravidas, whether normotensive or hypertensive, who had had epidural analgesia. There was also a statistically significant positive relationship between AII concentration and diastolic pressure measured on admission to the labor suite in all the nonproteinuric patients. In nonproteinuric primigravidas not receiving epidural anesthesia, plasma AII showed a significant inverse relationship to body weight and a direct relationship to gestational age. Mean AII concentrations immediately before cesarean section were somewhat lower in both primigravidas and multiparas than levels found before vaginal delivery and were significantly lower (41.8 ± 13.8 versus 83.0 ± 23.5 pg/ml) among normotensive cesarean section patients when compared to patients delivered vaginally. Thus, a number of variables appear to influence AII levels at delivery, but a dominant relationship still emerges among proteinuria, diastolic blood pressure, and AII.

▶ [This study identifies a number of variables which seem to influence maternal angiotensin II levels during labor. The chief finding was that labor itself raised levels of angiotensin II, by an average of about 20%, with a positive correlation between the duration of the second stage of labor and angiotensin II levels. Proteinuric patients had higher levels than nonproteinuric, and epidural anesthesia apparently exerted a lowering effect.] ◀

5–20 **Effect of Supportive Companion on Perinatal Problems, Length of Labor, and Mother-Infant Interaction.** Roberto Sosa, John Kennell, Marshall Klaus, Steven Robertson, and Juan Urrutia (Case Western Reserve Univ.) studied the effects of the presence of a supportive lay woman ("doula") on length of labor and on mother-infant interaction after delivery in healthy Guatemalan primigravid women. All were patients in the Social Security Hospital in Guatemala City. Initial assignment of mothers to the experimental (doula) or control group was random. The control group followed hospital routines that consisted of infrequent vaginal examinations to monitor the course of labor, auscultation of the fetal heart, and assistance to

---

(5–20) N. Engl. J. Med. 303:597–600, Sept. 11, 1980.

the mother during delivery. No electronic monitoring was used. Hospital policies did not permit family members or friends or a continuous nurse caretaker to be present in the labor rooms as a consequence of the large number of deliveries. Mothers in the experimental group received constant support from an untrained lay woman from admission to delivery in addition to routine care. Support consisted of physical contact, conversation, and the presence of a friendly companion whom the mother had not met before.

Controls had higher rates ($P < .001$) of subsequent perinatal problems including evidence of fetal distress requiring intervention during labor or delivery, meconium staining, or other manifestations of neonatal asphyxia. It was necessary to admit 103 mothers to the control group and 33 to the experimental group to obtain 20 in each group with uncomplicated deliveries. In the final sample, the length of time from admission to delivery was shorter in the experimental group (8.7 vs 19.3 hours, $P < .001$). Mothers who had a doula present during labor were awake more after delivery ($P < .02$) and stroked ($P < .001$), smiled at ($P < .009$), and talked to ($P < .002$) their babies more than control mothers did.

The observations suggest that there may be major perinatal benefits of constant human support during labor, and they raise the possibility of an association between acute anxiety and arrests of labor or the development of fetal distress. A possible cause for that association is the increase in levels of catecholamines, which decrease uterine contractility. The combination of crowded hospital conditions, the absence of prenatal preparatory classes, and the unfamiliar hospital environment may have increased maternal anxiety markedly and exaggerated the effect of the supportive companion. Additional studies are needed to determine whether these effects can be correlated with maternal catecholamine levels. The findings suggest that this low-cost intervention may be a simple way to reduce the length of labor and the number of perinatal problems for parturient women and their infants.

▶ [The group of patients exposed to a support person during labor exhibited different maternal behavior in the early postpartum period. These patients stroked, smiled at, and talked to their babies more frequently than did control patients. Support persons are common in most labor units in the United States. Their presence does seem to reduce anxiety. The authors of this study speculate that the longer labors in the control patients may have been due to the inhibition of uterine contractility by elevated catecholamine levels. This may be so, but other differences between the groups in this randomized study are hard to understand. Twenty-four of the originally assigned control patients had meconium staining versus only 3 patients in the experimental group. Since meconium is more apt to be present at the start of labor than to appear during labor when the amniotic fluid is initially clear, it is hard to credit the support person with the striking reduction in meconium staining. Perhaps inadvertent selection artifacts did exist after all.] ◀

5–21 **Antibiotic Prophylaxis Against Infective Endocarditis After Normal Delivery: Is It Necessary?** D. Sugrue, S. Blake, P. Troy, and D. MacDonald (Natl. Maternity Hosp., Dublin) examined the wisdom of the practice of routine antibiotic prophylaxis during normal

(5–21) Br. Heart J. 44:499–502, November 1980.

labor and delivery in women with known heart disease. A survey was made of 2,165 women with rheumatic or congenital heart disease who delivered vaginally between 1959 and 1978 at three large hospitals that did not treat cardiac patients with prophylactic antibiotics routinely at delivery. Two women (0.09%) had puerperal infective endocarditis; neither received antibiotic prophylaxis. Both diagnoses were made clinically, although blood cultures were negative. In each case, manual removal had been performed.

A questionnaire of 19 obstetricians in Ireland showed that 12 (63%) gave antibiotics routinely to cardiac patients during labor and after delivery, 5 (26%) did not, and 2 (11%) used them occasionally.

In 83 women without heart disease, 299 peripheral vein blood samples were drawn serially from 0 to 30 minutes after vaginal delivery to study the incidence of asymptomatic puerperal bacteremia. Of the 299 cultures, 3 (from 3 different women) gave positive results (3.6% of patients, 0.1% of cultures). One of the positive cultures was obtained from a woman who had a manual removal.

These results, together with findings reported in the literature, show that well-documented cases of infective endocarditis and asymptomatic puerperal bacteremia after normal vaginal delivery are uncommon. Indeed, antibiotic prophylaxis may increase the risk of development of antibiotic-resistant endocarditis. Recommended prophylactic regimens carry considerable risk of drug toxicity. These facts, coupled with the lack of direct evidence supporting the efficacy of antibiotic prophylaxis, suggest that routine peripartum antibiotic prophylaxis is not indicated in women with heart disease. The occurrence of both cases of endocarditis and 1 case of asymptomatic bacteremia after manual removal of the placenta suggests that this procedure may increase the risk of endocarditis, making it prudent to give antibiotic prophylaxis in this situation.

▶ [The viewpoint expressed here differs from standard obstetric opinion in the United States. One wonders whether bacterial endocarditis presenting later in the puerperium than the first few days would be identified in this survey. A more pertinent issue concerns the incidence of bacteremia after vaginal delivery. The authors' experience and those reports cited from the literature suggest that the incidence is much smaller than that found after dental or urinary tract manipulations. This merits further study. We will continue to use antibiotic prophylaxis in the laboring patient with known congenital or rheumatic heart disease, but are less certain that it is absolutely necessary.] ◀

5–22 **Is Your Enema Really Necessary?** It has long been established practice in many midwifery units to administer an enema to all patients in labor to facilitate descent of the presenting part, reduce fecal contamination, and stimulate uterine activity. Mona L. Romney and H. Gordon (Harrow, England), having found that shaving the pubic area is not beneficial, evaluated the practice of administering an enema in a series of 274 women admitted for delivery of singleton infants, 149 of whom received an enema. Most medical staff and midwives favored the use of an enema, whereas many patients considered the procedure degrading and uncomfortable but accepted it as necessary for a "clean" delivery. A low-volume enema containing sodium acid phosphate and sodium phosphate was used.

(5–22) Br. Med. J. 282:1269–1271, Apr. 18, 1981.

The two groups of patients showed no significant differences in degree of fecal contamination in the first and second stages of labor or in the incidence of gross contamination. Seven neonates in each group showed evidence of infection. Bowel organisms were isolated from 4 in the no-enema group and 2 in the enema group. The duration of labor was comparable in the two groups. Where contamination occurred, women given an enema were likelier to have fluid contamination, which was particularly difficult to control. One mother, an enema-treated patient with fecal contamination in the second stage, had an extensive episiotomy infection caused by *Escherichia coli*.

During the preparation for normal labor, an enema should be reserved for women who have not had a bowel movement in the past 24 hours and have an obviously full rectum on initial pelvic examination. Similar trials elsewhere are needed to confirm these findings and reinforce the conclusion that an enema is generally not necessary for women in labor.

▶ [We are not surprised at the strong feelings of the staff concerning a practice so ingrained as that of the enema given to laboring patients. We also are not surprised that the length of labor and the incidence of infectious complaints didn't differ in the two groups. The loss either of formed stool in the absence of an enema or of watery stool in the second stage of labor related to an enema is somewhat embarrassing to the patient and is at least esthetically disconcerting to the obstetrician. The authors' suggestion of withholding the enema if the patient recently has moved her bowels and if the rectum is empty on the initial pelvic examination is probably appropriate.] ◀

5–23 **Urinary Bladder Distention: Effect on Labor and Uterine Activity.** John A. Read, Frank C. Miller, Sze-Ya Yeh, and Lawrence D. Platt (Univ. of Southern California) refute the long-held belief that urinary bladder distention inhibits labor. Direct intrauterine pressure recordings and on-line measurements of uterine activity units were used to determine quantitatively the effect on labor and uterine activity of urinary bladder distention of a degree frequently found.

Studies were performed in 68 women, aged 15 to 40 years (mean, $23^1/_2$ years), in the active phase of labor and in whom catheterization was required. There were 38 nulliparas. Range of gravidity was 1–9. In all patients the cervix was at least 4 cm dilated. Membranes were ruptured at the start of the study. Patients were studied in the same lateral position for 30 minutes before and after a catheterization interval, during which time uterine activity units were quantitated on-line and changes were noted in cervical dilation and station and contraction frequency and tonus. Results were analyzed for the entire group, for individual patients, and by urine volumes (10–550 ml) obtained at catheterization.

Total uterine activity units increased in 43 women and decreased in 25 after catheterization. When these measurements were compared with expected increases calculated from the slopes of the precatheterization interval in individual patients, there were 36 increases and 32 decreases. Individual slopes of uterine activity increased in 36 and decreased in 31 cases. There were no differences when the data were analyzed by urine volume, parity, or birth weight except possibly at

(5–23) Obstet. Gynecol. 56:565–570, November 1980.

large volumes. Changes in rates of cervical dilation and descent of the presenting part conformed to the expected normal labor pattern.

Most clinicians have seen patients with the presenting part at a high station but whose labor was arrested seemingly due to mechanical dystocia by the bladder, such as by cystocele or by massive distention, and in whom labor progressed after catheterization. This study, however, suggests the act of emptying the urinary bladder has no effect on uterine activity progress or the course of labor, except possibly with very large volumes. This would seem to confirm anatomical evidence of a passive role of the urinary bladder during labor at urine volumes usually encountered.

▶ [Most clinicians recall the occasional parturient in which an arrested labor, usually at high station, is corrected by emptying a greatly distended bladder. This study indicates, however, that at least moderate degrees of bladder distention generally have little, if any, effect on uterine activity in labor. After removal of 10 to 550 ml of urine some patients did exhibit more than the expected uterine activity, but about an equal proportion exhibited less, and the net changes in either case were modest.] ◀

5–24 **Predictability of Labor Outcome From Comparison of Birth Weight and X-ray Pelvimetry.** The value of x-ray pelvimetry in labor recently has been questioned, but few morphometric data on the fetopelvic relationship have been presented. Naseem Jagani, Harold Schulman, Prasanta Chandra, Rosa Gonzalez and Adiel Fleischer (Albert Einstein College of Medicine, New York) compared maternal pelvic measurements with infant birth weight in 51 women having dysfunctional labor, in whom both x-ray pelvimetry and oxytocin had been used. Twenty-seven babies were delivered by cesarean section, and 24 were delivered vaginally. Multiple regression analysis was used to compare multiple pelvic indices against birth weight in the two groups.

The infants in the cesarean group weighed 228 gm more than those in the vaginal delivery group, but the difference was not significant. The most common indication for pelvimetry was arrest of labor. A random distribution of birth weight and pelvic dimensions was observed, with no significant differences between the cesarean section and vaginal delivery groups. The pelvic measurements did not provide a predictive tool for delivery outcome. The approximately 15% margin of dimensional differences between a successful and a failed outcome is too small to be detected by current diagnostic methods.

The application of current statistical methods to the clear end points of birth weight and pelvic dimensions fails to define an entity of fetopelvic disproportion. X-ray pelvimetry, as currently used during labor, is of no proved value in predicting the outcome of labor in at least 95% of cases. Management should be based on objective evidence that an adequate trial of labor has occurred. O'Driscoll et al. have obtained a very low perinatal morbidity rate and a very low cesarean section rate using a program of monitoring labor by a graphic record of such factors as centimeters dilated plotted against time. Women who deviate significantly from normal progress receive

(5–24) Am. J. Obstet. Gynecol. 139:507–511, Mar. 1, 1981.

oxytocin if there are no significant fetal heart rate abnormalities or meconium in the amniotic fluid.

▶ [Obstetricians seem to be coming increasingly to the point of view that x-ray pelvimetry is of limited or no value in labor management. In this study, pelvimetry findings of patients with labor abnormalities did not seem to correlate at all well with outcome in terms of vaginal delivery versus cesarean section. Further evidence that x-ray pelvimetry is an idea whose time has passed comes from a recent prospective study in our department (to be published in *JAMA*) which a physician ordering the procedure had to state what he or she would do without it. In general, the x-ray findings did not alter management.

Concerns about the value of pelvimetry, in our judgment at least, are limited to vertex presentation. We feel it has a definite place in the assessment of the patient with a breech presentation in whom vaginal delivery is being considered.] ◀

5–25 **Randomized Trial of Ambulation Versus Oxytocin for Labor Enhancement: A Preliminary Report.** Intrapartum assumption of the vertical position has been associated with a shortened duration of labor. In addition to an increase in intensity of contractions, a synergistic effect of gravity has been observed. John A. Read, Frank C. Miller, and Richard H. Paul (Univ. of Southern California) evaluated ambulation in 14 patients who had failed to progress in active-phase labor and who required augmentation for "inadequate" contractions. All had ruptured membranes. Six patients received oxytocin, while 8 remained out of bed walking or standing, and occasionally sitting, for 2 hours. The two groups were similar in age of the mother and gestational age of fetus.

All ambulatory patients made progress in both descent and dilation in the first hour of study, while only 3 of the 6 oxytocin-treated patients made progress. Two patients in the ambulation group withdrew because of fatigue. One was delivered after $1^{1}/_{2}$ hours of ambulation. All 7 other ambulation patients and 4 of 6 oxytocin-treated patients made progress in the second hour of study. The mean change in dilation and mean station change were comparable over the 2-hour study period. Uterine activity was similar in the two groups at most intervals. No significant differences in outcome were apparent. Six ambulation patients required oxytocin after the study. All oxytocin-treated patients reported increased pain, whereas several ambulated patients felt less pain. No significant changes in fetal heart rate variability or pattern were noted with ambulation.

The immediate effect of ambulation and enhanced tolerance to pain would seem to recommend it over oxytocin, but fatigue and motivation are limiting factors. Further study will be needed to assess the relative merits of ambulation and oxytocin administration for enhancing labor.

▶ [Several papers abstracted in recent editions of the YEAR BOOK have addressed the question of whether ambulation benefits the course of labor. The results have been mixed. This report focuses on abnormal labor; patients with arrest in the active phase were assigned randomly to either oxytocin or ambulation. The number of subjects was small and no clear (i.e., statistically significant) differences were found, but the results do suggest some reason to think that ambulation may have been more efficacious. Further study clearly is indicated.] ◀

(5–25) Am. J. Obstet. Gynecol. 139:669–672, Mar. 15, 1981.

INCIDENCE OF FETOMATERNAL BLEEDING AT DELIVERY

Fetal red cells in maternal blood (ml)	No. of patients (%)
0.0	1031 (85.5)
> 0.0–7.5	132 (10.9)
7.5–15.0	31 (2.6)
> 15.0	12 (1.0)
Total	1206

5–26 **Intrapartum Fetomaternal Bleeding in Rh-Negative Women.** The use of Rh-immune globulin has reduced considerably the incidence of pregnancies complicated by Rh immunization, although the failure rate in ABO-compatible pairs is 1% to 2% post partum. L. Kimball Lloyd, Fred Miya, Richard M. Hebertson, Neil K. Kochenour, and James R. Scott (Salt Lake City) prospectively studied the presence of fetal erythrocytes in maternal circulation in a consecutive series of 1,206 Rh-negative women who were delivered of Rh-positive infants.

Fetal erythrocytes were present in the blood of 175 (14.5%) of the mothers during the immediate postpartum period (table). There was evidence that 12 of these patients had at least 15 ml of circulating fetal erythrocytes, which indicates a greater Rh-immune globulin requirement than the standard 300 µg postpartum dose for neutralization. With the exception of manual removal of the fetus, there was no correlation between excessive fetomaternal hemorrhage and obstetric manipulations, complications of delivery, or surgery. The incidence of ABO incompatibility was 15.4% in cases of fetomaternal hemorrhage and 19.5% in those without fetal erythrocytes.

It is recommended that all Rh-negative patients be screened during the postpartum period to determine the adequacy of Rh-immune globulin prophylaxis.

▶ [The most important message from this study is that 1% of Rh-negative women delivering Rh-positive infants had fetomaternal bleeding in amounts greater than 15 ml of erythrocytes, the maximal amount theoretically neutralized by one vial of Rh-immune globulin. On this basis, the authors advocate routine screening of Rh-negative women after birth of an Rh-positive infant to identify those who need more than one vial. The cost-benefit aspects of this recommendation are not addressed. Our friends in the blood bank tell us that this is now considered "standard" care in the United States.] ◀

5–27 **Intrapartum Electronic Fetal Monitoring in Low-Risk Pregnancies.** Magnus Westgren, Eva Ingemarsson, Ingemar Ingemarsson, and Thore Solum (Univ. Hosp. of Lund, Sweden) evaluated the benefits and hazards of intrapartum electronic fetal monitoring (EFM) in 5,037 low-risk pregnancies in 1977 and 1978. Early amniotomy, performed routinely, made possible a high frequency of internal fetal heart rate (FHR) recordings by scalp electrode (90%) and

---

(5–26) Obstet. Gynecol. 56:285–288, September 1980.
(5–27) Ibid., pp. 301–304.

tocography with intrauterine catheter (30%). When ominous FHR changes were recorded, blood samples for pH determinations were taken routinely.

In 85% of all deliveries (4,278 patients), a technically acceptable registration could be obtained during the first stage of labor. The baseline and variability in FHR were normal in 87.5% and 80.3%, respectively. Decelerations occurred in half of the recordings. An irreproachable tracing was recorded in less than half of the cases. The FHR changes demanding scalp pH measurements or operative intervention for fetal distress occurred in about 10% of all deliveries. Instrumental vaginal deliveries were performed in 6.5% of all patients, cesarean sections in 1.5%. In only 30 patients (0.7%) was cesarean section performed for fetal distress. Scalp pH determinations were made in 4.9% of all 1977 deliveries and in 10.4% of all 1978 deliveries. In 1977, the distress diagnosis was in most cases based solely on an abnormal FHR tracing, whereas in 1978, an abnormal scalp pH (below 7.25) usually supported the diagnosis. In deliveries in which late decelerations were recorded, normal fetal acid-base balance (pH above 7.25) was found in 56%, and vaginal delivery was performed in most cases. Ninety of 5,037 newborns had an Apgar score less than 7 at 1 minute; 15 newborns (0.3%) had a score less than 7 at 5 minutes. No intrapartum deaths occurred during the study. The corrected perinatal mortality (antenatal deaths excluded) was 0.14%. Causes of death in the 7 dead infants were lethal malformation (2 infants), sudden infant death syndrome 2–3 days after delivery (3 infants), traumatic instrumental delivery (1 infant), and intrauterine asphyxia (1 infant). Only the last 15 minutes of delivery were monitored in this last case.

The sharp distinction between high- and low-risk pregnancies made in debates of EFM is often difficult to maintain in clinical practice. Moreover, results of this investigation indicate that occurrence of fetal distress demanding cesarean section in a low-risk group is rare. Therefore, the fetal distress diagnosis must be supported by pH measurements. If these demands are not fulfilled, the disadvantages of EFM in overdiagnosis of fetal distress might outweigh the benefits in the low-risk patient.

▶ [Whereas the value of intrapartum fetal heart rate monitoring in high-risk patients is accepted by all but the most strident opponent of the technique, the place of monitoring in low-risk pregnancy is quite open to question. The recent National Institute of Health Consensus Conference concluded that it was of uncertain value in normal patients. This study is certainly not definitive because it lacks controls, but the results support the contention that there is some benefit in normal situations. In a series of over 5,000 low-risk deliveries there were no intrapartum deaths and only 0.14% neonatal mortality. Moreover, the cesarean section rate was only 1.5% overall and 0.6% for fetal distress, due, no doubt, to the availability of fetal blood sampling, so monitoring hardly can be said to lead to large numbers of unnecessary cesarean sections. Unfortunately, no data are given about possible complications of monitoring, such as puerperal morbidity statistics, fetal scalp infection frequency, or other untoward events.] ◀

5–28 **Correlation of Meconium-Stained Amniotic Fluid, Early Intrapartum Fetal pH, and Apgar Scores as Predictors of Perinatal Outcome.** It has been suggested by many investigators that

---

(5–28) Obstet. Gynecol. 56:604–609, November 1980.

the type of meconium passed and its time of passage are the most significant factors affecting fetal outcome. Gregory C. Starks (Case Western Reserve Univ., Cleveland) conducted a prospective study of 278 pregnant women to determine if the passage of meconium during the early intrapartum period, the consistency of the meconium passed, and fetal scalp pH values could be correlated with 1- and 5-minute Apgar scores as predictors of neonatal outcome. One hundred seventy-seven of the women studied were in early labor, had a cervical dilation of 3 cm or less, and had ruptured membranes and meconium-stained amniotic fluid. Thick meconium was found in 101 patients and thin meconium in the other 76.

Patients with thick meconium, compared with nonmeconium controls, had significantly lower 1- and 5-minute Apgar scores, a significantly greater incidence of pH values less than 7.25, and increased risk factors such as abnormal fetal heart rates, prolonged pregnancy, and a fetus small for gestational age. Except for abnormal fetal heart rates and prolonged pregnancy in patients with thin meconium, nonmeconium controls and patients with thin meconium did not appear to have increased associated risks. Thick meconium, in and of itself, seemed to be the most significant factor influencing neonatal outcome. The presence of a fetal heart rate abnormality in association

Fig 5–4.—Etiology and management of meconium-stained amniotic fluid passage using a modern obstetric approach. *GI,* gastrointestinal; *FHR,* fetal heart rate; *NL,* normal; *ABNL,* abnormal; *C-section,* cesarean section. (Courtesy of Starks, G. C.: Obstet. Gynecol. 56:604–609, November 1980.)

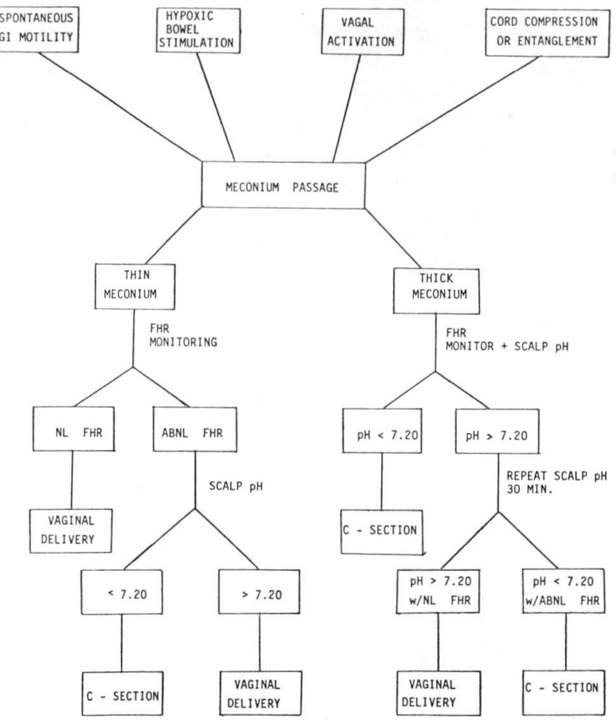

with thick meconium greatly increased perinatal morbidity, as indicated by fetal acidosis and 1- and 5-minute Apgar scores of 6 or less.

The passage of meconium in the early intrapartum period appears to correlate with neonatal outcome and increased perinatal morbidity. The significance of the passage of meconium is discussed and a modern obstetric approach to the management of patients with meconium-stained amniotic fluid is presented schematically (Fig 5–4).

▶ [This is a well-designed and conducted clinical study of a common obstetric dilemma, meconium passage during labor. Its major finding is that there is a marked prognostic difference between thin and thick meconium; whereas the former is not generally indicative of any problems, the latter indicates the likelihood of prior hypoxia, and moreover, presages complications later in labor (heart rate abnormalities, hypoxia in scalp blood, and low Apgar scores). Clearly, meconium passage is a high-risk condition and the plan outlined in Figure 5–4 seems a reasonable approach. Also of great importance is immediate management of the newborn. A different view concerning thin versus thick meconium staining follows. Read on.] ◀

5–29 **Intrapartum Fetal Heart Rate Monitoring: III. Association of Meconium With Abnormal Fetal Heart Rate Patterns.** There is some disagreement as to whether meconium-stained amniotic fluid (MSAF) in labor is an indicator of fetal distress in the absence of abnormal fetal heart rate (FHR) changes. H. B. Krebs, R. E. Petres, L. J. Dunn, H. V. F. Jordaan, and A. Segreti (Med. College of Virginia, Richmond) investigated the significance of meconium associated with normal and abnormal FHR patterns in a retrospective study of the FHR tracings of 284 fetuses with MSAF and 1,672 fetuses without MSAF. One- and 5-minute Apgar scores were used to quantify changes in FHR patterns.

The neonatal death rate was 2.5% in the MSAF group and 0.8% in the non-MSAF group ($P < .05$). Low 1- and 5-minute Apgar scores were associated significantly with MSAF. In the last 30 minutes of

COMPARISON OF INCIDENCE OF VARIOUS FHR PATTERNS IN LAST 30
MINUTES OF MONITORED LABOR OF PREGNANCIES WITH AND
WITHOUT MSAF

	Meconium		No meconium		
FHR patterns in last 30 minutes	N	% of total	N	% of total	P
Tachycardia	18	6.3	90	5.4	>0.5
Bradycardia	65	22.9	293	17.5	<0.05
Oscillatory amplitude ≤ 5 bpm	104	36.6	414	24.8	<0.001
Oscillatory frequency quency ≤ 6 op'n	23	8.1	66	3.9	<0.001
Accelerations ≤ 4/30 min.	141	49.6	639	38.2	<0.005
Early decelerations	56	19.7	266	15.6	>0.1
Variable decelerations	137	48.2	836	50.0	>0.5
Late decelerations	23	8.1	65	3.8	<0.01

Note: Analysis by χ^2 test.

(5–29) Am. J. Obstet. Gynecol. 137:936–943, Aug. 15, 1980.

FHR monitoring during labor, reductions in oscillatory amplitude, oscillatory frequency, and accelerations and increases in bradycardia and late decelerations were significantly more common in the MSAF group than in the non-MSAF group (table). Similar reductions in FHR patterns were observed during the first 30 minutes of monitoring.

It is concluded that MSAF has an unfavorable influence on fetal outcome and that its presence should be regarded as a warning sign of fetal distress, warranting close intrapartum observation.

▶ [Meconium serves as both an indicator of fetal distress and as a potential cause of neonatal distress secondary to meconium aspiration. In contrast to other recent reports, meconium staining was associated with increased incidences of abnormal fetal heart rate patterns, and the nature of the meconium staining ("light" versus "heavy") was not prognostically important in this study.] ◀

5–30 **Neonatal Performance of Selected Term Vaginal Breech Delivery.** Many clinicians perform cesarean section for all intrapartum breech presentations. Martin L. Gimovsky, Roy H. Petrie, and W. Duane Todd (Columbia Univ.) suggest that judiciously selected fetuses at term in breech presentation may be safely delivered vaginally by a selective management protocol that requires cesarean section when mandated criteria are not met.

METHOD.—Gravidas with term breech presentations are allowed a trial of labor if they are prepared immediately for cesarean section, estimated fetal weight is 2,000 to 4,000 gm and gestational age is 36 to 42 weeks, pelvimetry is adequate clinically and radiologically, intensive intrapartum fetal assessment by both biophysical and biochemical techniques is performed, and analysis of labor by a Friedman curve shows progress in cervical dilation of greater than 1 cm/hour in nulliparas and 1.3 cm/hour in multiparas. Cesarean section may be initiated in less than 5 minutes in emergencies and usually is performed under general anesthesia.

If the membranes have been ruptured for more than 18 hours with a term breech presentation, engagement of the fetus, and no labor, low-dose oxytocin is administered by continuous intravenous infusion to initiate labor. Oxytocin is not used to augment dysfunctional active-phase labor with a breech presentation. Nulliparas and multiparas are managed similarly, as are frank, complete, and footling breech presentations. Assisted breech delivery usually is used, including spontaneous delivery of the breech just past the umbilicus, manual rotation of the shoulders for delivery of the arms, and delivery of the after-coming head by manual maneuvers or Piper forceps. Delivery anesthesia is mainly pudendal nerve block supplemented with mask nitrous oxide.

Between 1972 and 1977, 488 infants weighing more than 2,000 gm were in breech presentation. Of these, 208 (43%) were delivered vaginally, 130 by protocol and 78 outside protocol because the mothers were admitted in advanced labor, the pregnancies were electively managed outside protocol, or there were other indications for a protocol bypass. The 130 protocol vaginal breech deliveries were matched with 130 spontaneous vaginal vertex deliveries and 130 elective repeated cesarean sections.

Neonatal morbidity occurred in 3.1% of breech infants delivered

(5–30)   Obstet. Gynecol. 56:687–691, December 1980.

vaginally by protocol, 15.4% of breech infants delivered vaginally outside protocol, 2.3% of vertex infants delivered vaginally, and 1.5% of infants delivered by elective cesarean section. Thus, morbidity in the protocol breech vaginal delivery group was not different from that of controls. Mortality occurred only in the nonprotocol-managed breech vaginal delivery group. There were no significant differences in outcome in the protocol group of vaginal breech deliveries between ward and private patients, between primiparas and multiparas, or among the various breech presentations.

When time is inadequate for full clinical evaluation, cesarean section is recommended for vaginal breech presentations. About 50% of term breech presentations that are properly selected and managed may be safely delivered vaginally.

▶ [This paper is representative of several in the recent literature supporting vaginal delivery of selected cases of breech presentation. Five to 10 years ago the literature contained many references advocating routine or near-routine use of cesarean section, but the pendulum seems to be swinging back toward a middle-ground position. Our criteria for selecting breeches for vaginal delivery—and we believe this is the appropriate way to view it, rather than to list the indications for cesarean section—are virtually identical to the protocol of these authors: fetus not large, pelvis adequate by clinical and radiographic assessments, and entirely normal course of labor terminating in assisted breech delivery. We agree that parity and type of breech do alter the approach. The frequency of cesarean section with breech presentations on our service is 35% to 40% compared with 57% in this report.] ◀

5–31 **Management of Low Birth Weight Breech Delivery: Should Cesarean Section be Routine?** To determine the optimum method of delivery of low birth weight infants in breech presentation, Olavi Kauppila, Matti Grönroos, Paavo Aro, Pirjo Aittoniemi, and Mirja Kuoppala retrospectively studied 217 singleton infants weighing 1,000 to 2,499 gm, presenting in breech positions, and delivered between 1967 and 1976. Findings were compared with those in 217 infants in vertex presentation matched for birth weight. During the second half of the study the cesarean section rate for low birth weight infants in breech presentation increased threefold over that of the first half, whereas the rate for comparable cephalic presentations increased only 1.7-fold.

Infant mortality was significantly higher after breech than after cephalic deliveries; perinatal and neonatal mortality rates were 1.8-fold and 2.9-fold greater, respectively. Despite the much greater increase in cesarean section rate in the second 5-year period for infants in breech than for those in cephalic positions, the perinatal and neonatal mortality rates were no better for breech than for cephalic deliveries in the later period; on the contrary, the perinatal mortality index deteriorated from 1.7 to 2.2 and the neonatal mortality index from 2.5 to 4.0 (table).

The cesarean section rate rose in the second half of the study in infants weighing 1,500 to 2,499 gm but not in those weighing 1,000 to 1,499 gm. Even in the larger infants, the prognosis did not improve with the increased cesarean section rate. Malformations and respiratory distress syndrome were more frequent in infants in breech than

(5–31) Obstet. Gynecol. 57:289–294, March 1981.

EFFECT OF CESAREAN SECTION FREQUENCY ON MORTALITY* IN BREECH
AND CEPHALIC DELIVERIES (INFANT WEIGHT GROUP 1,000 TO 2,499 GM)

	Breech deliveries (%)	Cephalic deliveries (%)	Index (breech/cephalic)	
Cesarean section frequency				
1967–1971	14/109 (12.8)	14/109 (12.8)	1.0	
1972–1976	41/108 (38.0)	24/108 (22.2)	1.7	$P < .01$
	$P < .001$	$P > .05$		
PNM				
1967–1971	38/109 (34.9)	23/109 (21.1)	1.7	$P < .05$
1972–1976	24/108 (22.2)	11/108 (10.2)	2.2	$P < .05$
NNM				
1967–1971	22/93 (23.7)	9/95 (9.5)	2.5	$P < .01$
1972–1976	16/100 (16.0)	4/101 (4.0)	4.0	$P < .01$

*PNM, perinatal mortality; NNM, neonatal mortality.

in cephalic presentations. Conditions associated with the corrected perinatal mortality (cerebral hemorrhage, fetal asphyxia, prolapsed cord) were also more common among breech presentations, but especially in infants weighing less than 1,500 gm. This weight group, for which the cesarean section rate did not rise, thus appears to be a special area of concern.

Vaginal delivery of an infant in breech position is justified after 32 weeks of gestation if estimated fetal weight is 1,500 gm or more, if labor can be monitored, and if prompt operative intervention is available if disturbances occur or if there are signs that delivery may be prolonged. Primary cesarean section should be undertaken in footling breech presentation or in the presence of other obstetric complications (toxemia, hypertension, diabetes mellitus, small for dates infant, complicated obstetric history), but it cannot otherwise be recommended automatically. For infants of less than 32 weeks' gestation, i.e., with a birth weight of less than 1,500 gm, the higher incidence of cerebral hemorrhage with cephalic delivery suggests that primary cesarean section be recommended. The coexistence of respiratory distress syndrome, however, makes conclusiveness on this point difficult.

▶ [This is yet another retrospective study of breech presentation in the low birth weight fetus. As has been found many times previously, perinatal mortality is higher in breech than in comparable weight vertex (1.8 times in this series) presentations, with malformations and respiratory distress syndrome largely responsible. The study, though retrospective, does give some insights into the highly controversial matter of delivery. By dividing their data into two time periods, 1967–1971 and 1972–1976, the authors could compare differing cesarean section rates. Although the frequency of cesarean section for breech increased from 12.8 to 38% over the two periods, the decline in neonatal and perinatal mortality rates was actually less than that observed with vertex, suggesting that universal or near-universal cesarean section is not the answer. However, the cesarean section rate for fetuses of < 32 weeks or < 1,500 gm, or both, did not change, and their outcome remained poor. The authors conclude that a trial labor, with constant monitoring and capacity for prompt operative intervention, is indicated for frank breeches of 32 weeks or longer (1,500 gm or more) without other complications. For younger and smaller infants, they tentatively suggest more liberal use of cesarean section.] ◀

5-32 Cesarean Section for Delivery of the Second Twin. Fetal indications for cesarean section are increasingly responsible for rising primary cesarean section rates. Higher mortality for twin B than for twin A is well documented, and vaginal delivery of twin A is no assurance of safe passage for twin B, particularly if this is the larger infant. John R. Evrard and Edwin M. Gold (Providence, R.I.) report 4 cases of combined vaginal-abdominal delivery of twins and review of 5 other cases from the recent literature. Multiple gestation was clinically confirmed ante partum in 5 of the 9 cases. The interval between the two births was 90 minutes or less in all cases but 1 and was 13 to 24 minutes in all the author's cases. Three second twins presented in transverse or oblique lie, and there was 1 compound presentation. In 3 cases the cervix contracted after delivery of twin A. Two neonatal deaths occurred, both of second twins; 1 was due to intracranial hemorrhage and 1 to severe hypoxia.

Malposition, malpresentation, and cervical contraction were the chief indications for cesarean delivery of the second twin in these cases. Difficult vaginal delivery of the second twin was associated with transverse lie, oblique lie, compound presentation, and contraction of the cervix after delivery of the first twin. When difficulty is encountered in delivery of the second twin, cesarean section should be considered.

▶ [It is certainly worth remembering that cesarean section is a perfectly legitimate way to deliver twin B, even though twin A has been delivered vaginally. This won't be a common occurrence. Our routine practice with twins is to have the anesthesiologist in the delivery room. After delivery of twin A, if twin B is in breech presentation, we either await descent of the breech or induce general anesthesia (halothane) and perform a breech extraction. If twin B is in vertex presentation, the head is guided over the inlet, the membranes are ruptured, and an internal monitor scalp lead is attached. The fetal heart rate pattern, if normal, permits us to ignore the length of the interval between twin A and twin B. Oxytocin often is required. Twin B usually delivers spontaneously or is delivered with low forceps under pudendal block. If twin B is in transverse lie and is small, we attempt to convert it to a vertex. If this cannot be done, general anesthesia is instituted and a version and extraction are performed. If there is difficulty turning the fetus or if the large size of the fetus causes concern, one can back off and perform a cesarean section.] ◀

5-33 Maternal Death After Cesarean Section in Georgia. There are few reliable data on the risk of maternal death from cesarean section. George L. Rubin, Herbert B. Peterson, Roger W. Rochat, Brian J. McCarthy, and Jules S. Terry (Atlanta) attempted to identify more deaths after cesarean section than are reported in vital records alone by linking data from Georgia resident live-birth certificates to those from death certificates of Georgia women aged 10–44 years in 1975–1976. Maternal death was defined as a death resulting from a complication of pregnancy or childbirth within 42 days of delivery of a live-born infant.

Thirty-six percent more total maternal deaths and 45% more deaths after cesarean section were identified by the record linkage procedure than by the death certificate reporting system. There were 9 cesarean-attributed deaths and 7 non-cesarean-attributed deaths.

(5–32) Obstet. Gynecol. 57:581–583, May 1981.
(5–33) Am. J. Obstet. Gynecol. 139:681–685, Mar. 15, 1981.

MATERNAL DEATHS BY TYPE OF DELIVERY, GEORGIA, 1975 AND 1976

Method of delivery	Maternal deaths	No. of live births	Mortality rate*	95% Confidence interval
Vaginal	14	144,045	9.7	5.3-16.3
Cesarean section	16	15,188	105.3	60.2-171.1
Total	30	159,233	18.8	12.7-26.9

*Maternal deaths per 100,000 deliveries of live-born infants by specified method.

Five of the former were detected by the record linkage procedure alone. The cesarean-attributed maternal mortality rate was 59 per 100,000 cesarean section deliveries. Maternal deaths by type of delivery are shown in the table. The total maternal mortality after cesarean section was about 10 times that after vaginal delivery. Three women in the cesarean-attributed death group and 1 in the non-cesarean-attributed death group had had a previous cesarean section. Three patients, 2 in the cesarean-attributed death group, had surgical sterilization at the time of delivery. The leading causes of death were pulmonary embolism and cardiopulmonary arrest.

Maternal mortality from cesarean section delivery appears to be higher in this survey than indicated in other reports based on vital records or hospital records alone. Further studies are needed to determine whether the risk of death from cesarean section delivery in Georgia is representative of that for the general population. Preventive measures aimed at reducing pulmonary embolism and cardiopulmonary arrest during general anesthesia may reduce deaths after cesarean section.

▶ [Cesarean section is certainly one of the safest of major operations. While it carries more risk than vaginal birth, all other factors being equal, the magnitude of the increased risk is uncertain because of the confounding effect of the reason for which the cesarean section is done. In other words, how much is due to the operation itself and how much to the associated condition (previa, abruption, toxemia, etc.) responsible for the operation? This study gives some indication. Among 16 maternal deaths with cesarean section in Georgia during 1975 to 1976 (identified by linking birth and death certificates to circumvent the typical underreporting of maternal mortality statistics), 9 were judged by a panel of obstetricians to be "reasonably attributed" to the cesarean delivery. On this basis, the maternal mortality, as listed in the table, is about 10 times greater with cesarean section as with vaginal delivery, and the cesarean-attributed mortality rate is 59.3 per 100,000 cesarean births.] ◀

5–34 **Maternal, Fetal, and Neonatal Effects of β-Adrenergic Stimulation in Connection With Cesarean Section.** To investigate the combined effects of β-mimetic therapy and general anesthesia on maternal and fetal-neonatal metabolism, R. Jouppila, A. Kauppila, R. Tuimala, A. Pakarinen, and K. Moilanen (Univ. of Oulu, Finland) treated 34 healthy women in the thirty-eighth to forty-third week of normal pregnancy: 14 (controls) with isotonic saline, 11 with intravenous fenoterol (3 μg/minute), and 9 with intravenous isoxsuprine (150 μg/minute) for 30 minutes before elective cesarean section. General anesthesia was induced 10 minutes after cessation of infusion.

Heart rate and diastolic and systolic blood pressures increased dur-

(5–34) Acta Obstet. Gynecol. Scand. 59:489–493, 1980.

ing operation in each group. In the isoxsuprine group, mean heart rate at beginning of surgery was significantly higher than the initial value or the corresponding value in the control group. At delivery, mean heart rate in the isoxsuprine and fenoterol groups was significantly higher than in the control group.

Before anesthesia induction, the lowest mean systolic blood pressure was recorded in the isoxsuprine group. This differed significantly from that in the fenoterol group. At other times there were no statistically significant intergroup differences in systolic blood pressures. In the fenoterol and isoxsuprine groups, systolic blood pressure increased more rapidly during anesthesia and operation than in the control group. The lowest mean initial diastolic pressure was seen in the isoxsuprine group. This differed significantly from that in the control group.

Mean pulse pressure did not change significantly during surgery in any group. At delivery, mean pulse pressure in the isoxsuprine group was significantly lower than in the fenoterol group.

At delivery, the mean maternal base-deficit was significantly higher in fenoterol patients than in control patients, indicating a trend toward metabolic acidosis. Other acid-base balance values in maternal and umbilical blood did not reveal differences between groups. Neonatal glucose at 2 hours after delivery was significantly higher in the fenoterol group than in the control group. Other values recorded during 36 hours revealed no differences between groups. The decrease between 2 and 6 hours in the fenoterol group was significant.

β-Mimetic treatment preceding general anesthesia in the present and in elective cases of normal pregnancy without placental disturbances cesarean sections without uterine contractions did not have unfavorable effects on the mother, fetus, or newborn. Such therapy thus does not seem contraindicated when uterine contractions should be rapidly suppressed in cases of fetal distress before operation. In cases of an acidotic fetus and uterine contractions, findings could be different.

Maternal cardiovascular effects of β-mimetic drugs, evident in a few minutes, are tachycardia and hypotension. In patients with cardiovascular diseases, β-mimetics should be avoided because of risk of cardiac decompensation. The main maternal metabolic changes with β-mimetics are lipolysis and glycogenolysis, which are triggered immediately after the beginning of infusion. Changes in maternal acid-base balance (acute metabolic acidosis) are sequelae of those primary changes. Ideal placental blood flow is the primary factor for fetal well-being. β-Stimulated peripheral vasodilatation together with widened pulse amplitude and increased cardiac output enhance placental perfusion.

▶ [As noted in the 1979 YEAR BOOK (pp. 145–147), tocolytic agents have been used to treat fetal distress. The rationale, of course, is that decreased uterine activity should permit better placental perfusion. Before this sort of therapy is advocated, one must be convinced that β-adrenergic treatment will not result in *decreased* uterine blood flow. This study by Jouppila et al. is a first step in looking at this question. These were *normal* patients and were *not* in labor. β-Agonists infused prior to general anesthesia for cesarean section did not affect umbilical cord blood gas values adversely. So far so good, but we must be careful in extrapolating data from these findings.] ◄

5–35 **Intrauterine Irrigation With Cefamandole Nafate Solution at Cesarean Section: Preliminary Report.** Endometritis occurs after cesarean section in up to 85% of high-risk patients. Prophylactic use of parenteral antibiotics has reduced this rate, but uterine contractions after delivery may prevent access of such antibiotics to the surgical site. William H. Long, Eugene G. Rudd, and Michael B. Dillon (Tripler Army Med. Center, Honolulu) hypothesized that topical use of antibiotics may avoid this and other disadvantages.

A prospective, double-blind trial was carried out in 90 women undergoing cesarean section. After delivery, 30 underwent intrauterine irrigation with 800 ml of normal saline solution containing 2 gm of cefamandole nafate (chosen because it has high tissue affinity, relatively long half-life, and broad-spectrum activity against organisms that commonly cause puerperal endometritis), 30 underwent irrigation with 800 ml of saline, and 30 received no irrigation.

METHOD.—After delivery of the infant, placenta, and membranes, the uterus was delivered through the abdominal incision. Irrigation was performed with a bulb syringe with some force, creating a jetlike effect. Care was taken to ensure that the uterine incision margins received a direct application. The irrigant was suctioned simultaneously. The uterine incision then was repaired. Additional irrigant was applied to the closed incision and bladder flap. The uterus was replaced in the abdomen and, with the patient in reverse Trendelenburg position, the abdominal gutters were irrigated and suctioned. Any solution remaining was used to irrigate the abdominal incision during closure.

Endometritis occurred in none of 30 women in the antibiotic irrigation group, 8 of 30 (26.7%) in the control irrigation group, and 7 of 30 (23.3%) in the nonirrigation group. The treated group had a slightly larger number of women with high-risk conditions (e.g., membranes ruptured over 6 hours, labor present, invasive fetal monitoring used) than the two control groups. There were no long-term complications or late infections in the treated group.

Intrauterine irrigation with cefamandole nafate solution at the time of cesarean section is useful in reducing the incidence of endometritis.

► [The results of this preliminary study indicate that uterine irrigation with an antibiotic solution at cesarean section markedly lowers the incidence of puerperal infection. If these data are confirmed, perhaps this technique might replace systemic antibiotic prophylaxis.] ◄

(5–35) Am. J. Obstet. Gynecol. 138:755–758, Dec. 1, 1980.

6. Obstetric Analgesia and Anesthesia

6-1 **Neonatal Depression After Obstetric Analgesia With Pethidine: Role of Injection-Delivery Time Interval and of Plasma Concentrations of Pethidine and Norpethidine.** P. Belfrage, L. O. Boréus, P. Hartvig, L. Irestedt, and N. Raabe administered a single dose of pethidine (100 mg) intramuscularly to 28 healthy women in labor with uncomplicated pregnancies (gestational age, 37–42 weeks) at 26–180 minutes before delivery. During continuous monitoring of their respiratory and heart rates, 18 randomly selected newborns received, intramuscularly, 60 µg of naloxone, and 10 newborns received an injection of saline and served as controls.

At birth, all newborns were clinically unaffected. The interval before respiration in the newborn became sustained was shorter if pethidine was given less than 1 hour before delivery. The respiratory rate increased after naloxone injection in 40% of the newborns, and heart rate increased in 6 of 18, mostly when intrauterine exposure to pethidine exceeded 1 hour; newborns showing an increase in respiratory or heart rate after naloxone administration did not have higher concentrations of pethidine or norpethidine than other newborns.

The pethidine level fell and the norpethidine level rose in maternal plasma with increasing time between administration and sampling. Data for pethidine seemed to conform to a two-compartment model with a plasma half-life of about 4.5 hours. Maternal plasma pethidine concentrations at delivery ranged from 105 to 535 ng/ml, corresponding to mild or moderate analgesia. At delivery, the pethidine concentration in the maternal vein plasma was always higher than that in the umbilical vein (Fig 6–1). Concentrations in the umbilical vein and artery indicated a continuous net transfer of pethidine from mother to fetus for about 2 hours (Fig 6–2), which correlated with the finding of maximum neonatal depression 2–3 hours after maternal injection. After this period of accumulation in the fetus, a backflow seemed to occur from fetus to mother. Umbilical vein norpethidine concentrations increased with a longer interval between injection and delivery but were probably too low to have any effect on the newborn. In the newborn, plasma pethidine concentration seemed to level off after about 3 hours; norpethidine plasma concentration increased over the entire observation period (almost 4 hours after maternal pethidine administration).

Neonatal depression seems to be related to the amount of unmetabolized pethidine transferred from mother to fetus. It seems reasonably safe to administer pethidine shortly before delivery, provided none has been given earlier during labor. Low concentration and low activ-

<hr>

(6–1) Acta Obstet. Gynecol. Scand. 60:43–49, 1981.

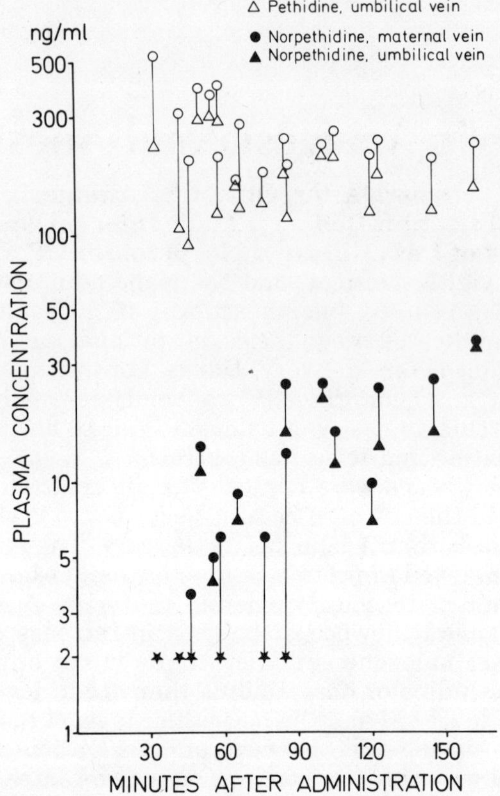

Fig 6–1.—Concentrations of pethidine (n = 18) and norpethidine (n = 16) in maternal vein plasma and in umbilical vein plasma. Samples were taken at time of delivery. Stars denote that the concentration of norpethidine was below the limit of detection (lower than 2 ng/ml). (Courtesy of Belfrage, P., et al.: Acta Obstet. Gynecol. Scand. 60:43–49, 1981.)

Fig 6–2.—Ratios of pethidine concentrations in umbilical artery *(UA)* to umbilical vein *(UV)* in relation to the time interval between administration and delivery (n = 18). (Courtesy of Belfrage, P., et al.: Acta Obstet. Gynecol. Scand. 60:43–49, 1981.)

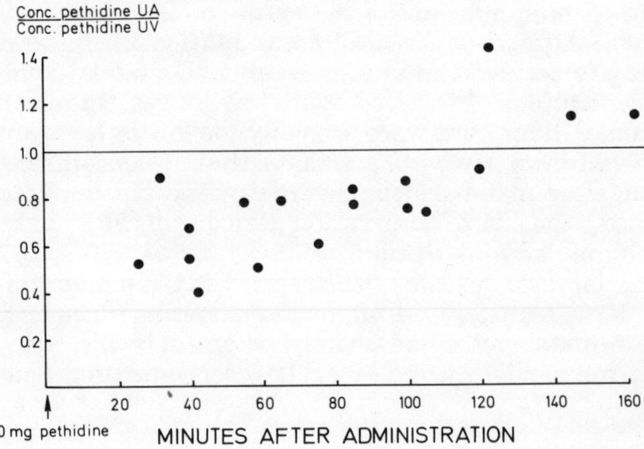

ity of norpethidine strongly speak against its role in respiratory problems in the newborn. However, if pethidine is given as repeated injections, norpethidine, which is excreted more slowly than pethidine, tends to accumulate in the plasma.

▶ [When pethidine (meperidine HC in the United States) is given to a laboring patient shortly before delivery, although there may be anxiety concerning the possibility of neonatal depression due to the drug, there is usually no problem. Clinical narcotic depression of the neonate is observed more frequently if the drug has been given 2 to 3 hours before birth. This study suggests that neonatal meperidine levels are highest at this time, and that the clinical observations therefore have a ready explanation. Although others have suggested that meperidine metabolites play a central role in narcotic neonatal depression (see the 1978 YEAR BOOK, pp. 147–148, and the 1981 YEAR BOOK, pp. 157–158), the authors of this study think that the drug itself is the culprit.] ◀

6–2   **Transcutaneous Nerve Stimulation for Pain Relief During Labor: A Controlled Study.** R. Erkkola, P. Pikkola, and J. Kanto (Univ. Central Hosp., Turku, Finland) applied transcutaneous nerve stimulation (TNS) at T10–L1 and S2–S4 levels on both sides of the spinous processes (two intensities—just below where stimulation led to sensation of fasciculation and about 20–25 V lower) to 100 parturients to attempt to decrease pain during labor. One to 2 hours after delivery, mothers, midwives, and 100 randomly selected control parturients independently submitted questionnaires regarding pain during labor.

The desire for and administration of analgesics was not significantly different between groups. Despite TNS, 23 mothers requested additional analgesia. Significantly more mothers in the TNS group reported labor as moderately or intensely painful compared with the control group during cervical dilatation to 7 cm; thereafter, there were no differences between groups. At no stage did mothers in the TNS group consider their pains to have been less than those in the control group. Of mothers in the TNS group, 31 considered the pain-relieving effect of TNS good and 55 considered it moderate; 32 mothers in the TNS group wanted a more efficient analgesic method for the next labor, 62 considered TNS sufficient, and 6 considered that they needed no analgesia for the next labor.

A drawback that greatly may diminish the role of TNS in management of labor pains is that in most cases fetal electronic monitoring becomes difficult or impossible.

▶ [Transcutaneous nerve stimulation was not effective in providing analgesia during labor in this study. An interesting disadvantage of the technique is that it interfered with both internal and external electronic fetal heart rate monitoring.] ◀

6–3   **Intrathecal Morphine as Sole Analgesic During Labor.** Peter V. Scott, Fiona E. Bowen, P. Cartwright, B. C. Mohan Rao, D. Deeley, H. G. Wotherspoon, and I. M. A. Sumrien (Bromsgrove, England) conducted a pilot study of 12 unselected, consecutive pregnant women to evaluate the efficacy of intrathecal morphine in the management of pain during labor. Prior to labor, the patients received a single subarachnoid injection of 1.5 mg of morphine sulfate, 8 by barbotage. In 4 patients, barbotage was not used.

(6–2)   Ann. Chir. Gynaecol. 69:273–277, 1980.
(6–3)   Br. Med. J. 281: 351–353, Aug. 2, 1980.

None of the patients experienced pain during the first stage of labor; 2 were not even aware they were in labor. During the second stage of labor, pain was abolished in 4 patients and was diminished markedly in 3. Pain at the site of episiotomy was reduced considerably. All the patients experienced itching of the face, particularly of the nose, approximately 30 minutes after injection. Nine patients became nauseated, and 5 vomited. Three patients acquired frontal headache 24 to 48 hours after the delivery. The side effects were mild and easily treated. Those patients who were given injections without barbotage had less severe side effects. There was no apparent association between the rate of forceps delivery (3 cases) and cesarean section (3 cases) and the use of intrathecal morphine. There was 1 case of fetal distress that required immediate cesarean section.

The results demonstrate that intrathecal morphine can abolish the pain of labor while allowing maternal cooperation for the second stage of labor. The results justify controlled studies of intrathecal morphine in the treatment and prevention of pain during labor.

▶ [We have heard of spinal anesthesia with morphine but this is the first report we have seen of its use in obstetric patients. The results are quite encouraging. With a very small dose (1–1.5 mg) given into the subarachnoid space, rapid and complete anesthesia was attained. It is not clear from this article how long the duration of anesthesia was, but it must have been considerable because some of the subjects were induced *after* the block, and the effect continued into the puerperium. There were some side effects—itching around the mouth and nose occurred in all subjects, 9 of 12 patients became nauseated, 4 were unable to void, and 1 experienced transient diplopia. This approach to obstetric anesthesia is intriguing, though, clearly, more study is needed.

Magora and associates (*Am. J. Obstet. Gynecol.* 138:260, 1980) reported the use of morphine (2 mg) injected into the epidural space for analgesia for second-trimester abortion. The effect lasted for several hours in 10 of 16 patients.

Dirksen and Nijhuis (*Acta Anaesthesiol. Scand.* 24:367, 1980) used epidural opiate for gynecologic operations and found a duration of at least 3½ hours. Less satisfactory results with epidural administration of morphine are reported below. Read on.] ◀

6–4 **Maternal and Fetal Concentrations of Morphine After Epidural Administration During Labor.** Gunilla Nybell-Lindahl, Christer Carlsson, Ingemar Ingemarsson, Magnus Westgren, and Lennart Paalzow studied the efficacy of epidural morphine as an analgesic in 20 healthy women in labor. During the first stage of labor, 4 to 6 mg of morphine diluted in 0.9% saline to a total volume of 10 ml was given via epidural catheter inserted at T11–12 or T12–L1.

Four patients experienced some pain relief; 16 reported no effect on pain. One newborn infant whose mother had been given 5 mg of morphine 1 hour and 50 minutes before delivery had possible morphine-induced respiratory depression. The highest morphine concentrations, analyzed in maternal and cord blood at delivery, were found in those mothers and fetuses with the shortest time interval between injection and delivery. This indicates rapid morphine absorption from the epidural space and rapid transport across the placenta and suggests drug redistribution and degradation in mother and fetus. There was close correlation between maternal and fetal drug concentrations.

It would appear that the analgesic effect of 4 to 6 mg of extradu-

---

(6–4) Am. J. Obstet. Gynecol. 139:20–21, Jan. 1, 1981.

rally administered morphine during labor is poor. Rapid morphine transport from the extradural space across the placenta implies a potential risk to the fetus. When there is a short injection-delivery time, when high drug doses are given, and when the fetus is premature, this risk might be clinically important.

6–5 **Prophylactic Single-Dose Oral Antacid Therapy in the Preoperative Period: Comparison of Cimetidine and Maalox.** Cimetidine (Tagamet), a histamine H_2-receptor-blocking agent, is a potent inhibitor of all phases of gastric secretion. Michael D. Detmer, Sujit K. Pandit, and Peter J. Cohen (Univ. of Michigan) evaluated the possible role of cimetidine in the prophylaxis of aspiration pneumonitis in 34 patients undergoing laparoscopic examination or sterilization. Twelve patients received 300 mg of cimetidine orally 2 hours before induction of anesthesia, and another 12 received 30 ml of Maalox orally 1 hour prior to anesthesia; all patients also received 10 mg of diazepam orally. An additional group of 10 patients treated only with diazepam served as controls. No patient was given anticholinergic medication. The treatments were evaluated by measurement of aspirated gastric fluid pH values and volumes.

All gastric fluid samples from patients treated with cimetidine had pH values greater than 2.5, whereas 7 of the controls and 5 of the patients treated with Maalox had pH values less than 2.5. Gastric fluid volumes greater than or equal to 20 ml were obtained from 3 of the patients treated with cimetidine, 10 of those treated with Maalox, and 6 of the controls. Of these patients with elevated, potentially hazardous fluid volume levels, 5 of the controls, 4 of the patients treated with Maalox, and none of those treated with cimetidine also had pH values less than 2.5. Cimetidine had a longer duration of action than Maalox.

The results strongly suggest that cimetidine would be an effective agent in the prophylaxis of aspiration pneumonitis, even in the absence of anticholinergic premedication. Because cimetidine is more palatable, increases gastric pH more consistently, and has a longer duration of action than Maalox, it is recommended that it be given routinely before induction of anesthesia in all surgical cases.

▶ [A potential problem with antacid prophylaxis against aspiration pneumonitis, i.e., the adverse pulmonary effects of the aspirated antacid itself, was considered in the 1981 YEAR BOOK (pp. 162–163). This study indicates that cimetidine (a histamine H_2-receptor antagonist), when given orally 2 hours before the induction of anesthesia in *nonpregnant* patients, was efficacious in increasing the pH of the gastric fluid. The important questions to be answered now concern (1) the efficacy of cimetidine in laboring patients and (2) the effects of the drug on the fetus/neonate. Different results with cimetidine are reported below. Read on.] ◀

6–6 **Prophylaxis for Mendelson's Syndrome Before Elective Cesarean Section: A Comparison of Cimetidine and Magnesium Trisilicate Mixture Regimens.** Acid aspiration pneumonitis (Mendelson's syndrome) is an important cause of maternal death related to general anesthesia. Reducing the acidity of gastric fluids by inhibiting acid secretion may be preferable to alkali neutralization in pa-

---

(6–5) Anesthesiology 51:270–273, September 1979.
(6–6) Br. J. Obstet. Gynaecol. 87:565–570, July 1980.

GASTRIC ASPIRATES FROM PATIENTS TREATED WITH CIMETIDINE AND MAGNESIUM TRISILICATE

	No. of patients	Volume (ml)		pH		pH $<2\cdot5$	
		Mean $\pm$ SD	Range	Median	Range	No.	per cent
Cimetidine	31	$7\cdot6\pm 8\cdot8$	4–25	$4\cdot3$	$1\cdot6$–$7\cdot2$	8	26
Magnesium trisilicate BPC	31	$18\cdot4\pm25\cdot3$	4–85	$7\cdot9$	$3\cdot1$–$8\cdot8$	0	0
		$p <0\cdot05$*		$p <0\cdot001$†		$p = 0\cdot002$‡	

*Student's *t* test.
†Wilcoxon's rank sum test.
‡Fisher's exact test (one tail).

tients undergoing general anesthesia who are at high risk for this syndrome. R. P. Husemeyer and H. T. Davenport compared the effects of 400 mg of oral cimetidine with those of 20 ml of magnesium trisilicate mixture BPC on gastric fluids in 62 patients undergoing elective cesarean section. Cimetidine was given 2 to 6 hours before anesthesia, and magnesium trisilicate BPC was administered within 1 hour of general anesthesia.

Those patients who received the magnesium trisilicate BPC showed a significantly higher volume of gastric fluid, significantly higher gastric fluid pH values, and a significantly lower incidence of pH values less than 2.5 than those who received cimetidine (table). Gastric fluids from all newborn infants were neutral or slightly alkaline and there were no significant differences in gastric fluid volume or pH between the two groups. All the infants were healthy at birth.

The results suggest that 20 ml of magnesium trisilicate BPC is more effective than a single oral dose of 400 mg of cimetidine as a prophylactic for Mendelson's syndrome in patients undergoing elective cesarean section.

▶ [In this study, cimetidine was less effective in raising the pH of the gastric aspirate in patients undergoing elective cesarean section than was the antacid magnesium trisilicate. Although the dosage schedule was slightly different, it is hard to reconcile these results with those of Detmer et al. in the preceding article. The final answers concerning prophylaxis against Mendelson's syndrome in general, and the role of cimetidine in particular, are not yet available.] ◀

6–7 **Fetal Acid-Base State Following Spinal or Epidural Anesthesia for Cesarean Section.** Steve N. Caritis, Ezzat Abouleish, Daniel I. Edelstone, and Eberhard Mueller-Heubach (Univ. of Pittsburgh) prospectively studied fetal acid-base state and maternal blood pressure in 111 unselected healthy women who underwent elective repeat cesarean section. Sixty-four of the women chose spinal and 47 chose epidural anesthesia. All were given 500–1,500 ml of 5% dextrose in Ringer's lactate intravenously during the 30 minutes before injection of the local anesthetic. For epidural anesthesia, 15–22 ml of 0.75% bupivacaine was used without epinephrine. For spinal anesthesia, 50–75 mg of 5% lidocaine in 7.5% dextrose with 0.2 mg epinephrine was injected intrathecally.

In each anesthetic group the mean values for umbilical venous and arterial pH were well above those indicating fetal acidemia. Umbilical venous and arterial pH values, however, were significantly higher and base deficit was significantly lower in fetuses of women who received epidural anesthesia, compared with fetuses whose mothers received spinal anesthesia, despite similar maternal blood gas and acid-base values. Maximum reductions in systolic and mean blood pressure after induction of anesthesia were significantly greater in women who received spinal anesthesia than in those who received epidural anesthesia. The incidence of systolic hypotension of varying degrees and the incidence of vasopressor use were significantly greater in patients who received spinal anesthesia.

With a preanesthetic fluid load of 500–999 ml, fetal umbilical acidemia (umbilical venous pH less than 7.25 or umbilical arterial pH less than 7.20) was more often observed after spinal than with epidural anesthesia (20% vs. 4% of the cases). When 1,000–1,500 ml of fluid was infused prior to anesthesia, the incidence of fetal acidemia after spinal anesthesia was similar to that after epidural anesthesia. The maximum reduction in systolic blood pressure after spinal anesthesia was not related to preanesthetic fluid load. In cases of severe hypotension, however, the hypotensive episode was shorter and easier to treat when the preanesthetic fluid load was above rather than be-

(6–7) Obstet. Gynecol. 56:610–615, November 1980.

low 1,000 ml. Fetal umbilical venous and arterial pH was slightly lower and base deficit was significantly higher in infants whose mothers received the smaller fluid loads. No infant had a low Apgar score at 5 minutes. There was no relationship between umbilical acid-base state and the induction-delivery interval.

Infants delivered electively by cesarean section with epidural anesthesia have higher pH and lower base deficit values in cord blood than infants delivered with spinal anesthesia. These differences are related to the greater degree and higher incidence of hypotension in the latter group. Thus, because spinal anesthesia poses some hazard to the fetus, its use for cesarean section may not be advisable in cases of preexisting fetal acidemia. Spinal anesthesia is well tolerated by a healthy fetus, however, when a fluid load in excess of 1,000 ml precedes the injection of anesthetic. After an episode of post-spinal anesthetic hypotension, rapid delivery is not essential; if maternal blood pressure is rapidly restored, it may be more prudent to allow the fetus to recover from the respiratory acidemia for 4 or 5 minutes than to deliver it immediately.

▶ [These observations suggest that, among infants born by elective repeat cesarean section, there is a slightly greater tendency toward metabolic acidosis with spinal than with epidural anesthesia, a difference apparently reflecting more severe hypotension with spinal than with epidural anesthesia. The difference in hypotension was minimized by preloading the spinal anesthesia patients with at least 1,000 ml of intravenous fluids. Thus, the clinical message is that women having spinal anesthesia for cesarean section should be given an intravenous infusion of at least 1 L before the administration of the anesthetic.] ◀

6–8 **Case for Abandonment of Explosive Anesthetic Agents.** The use of inflammable anesthetics in the United States has been controversial for some time. Harvey V. Fineberg, Laurie A. Pearlman, and Ronald A. Gabel (Harvard Univ.) review the arguments for retaining the use of inflammable anesthetics and present arguments for banning their use.

Although virtually all hospitals in the United States used explosive anesthetics in 1956, their use had been banned by 85% of the hospitals by 1978. Those who favor the continued use of explosive agents cite the educational value to anesthesiology programs, professional prerogative, the pharmacologic advantages and safety of diethyl ether and cyclopropane, and retention of the option to use agents whose effects are well established. Those who favor the elimination of the use of explosive agents argue that they offer no important pharmacologic advantages, that as the familiarity of the anesthesiologist with these agents diminishes, the risk to the patient increases; and that the risk of explosion increases because of the likelihood of relaxed safety precautions. Further, it is conservatively estimated that the use of inflammable anesthetics adds $9.4 million annually to the cost of surgical care. Because the costs are fixed for the most part, a further decline in the use of explosive agents would increase the cost per patient.

Because the use of inflammable anesthetics is likely to continue at

(6–8) N. Engl. J. Med. 303:613–617, Sept. 11, 1980.

a very low and expensive rate without definitive action by policy makers, it is urged that their use be abolished.

▶ [A few years ago when we were planning our new labor and delivery unit, the question arose as to the need for conductive floors. In the future, would we ever use explosive anesthetic agents in the delivery rooms? We equipped them to handle explosive agents "just in case." We probably made a mistake. The authors of this article make a good argument for the total abandonment of explosive anesthetic agents.] ◀

7. Genetics and Teratology

7–1 **Utilization of Prenatal Genetic Diagnosis in Women 35 Years of Age and Older in the United States, 1977 to 1978.** Melissa M. Adams, Sara Finley, Holger Hansen, Rene I. Jahiel, Godfrey P. Oakley, Jr., Warren Sanger, Gwynne Wells, and Wladamir Wertelecki assessed access to and acceptability of prenatal chromosomal diagnosis among older gravidas by determining the ratio of use of prenatal diagnosis by women aged 35 and older in Alabama, California, Manhattan, and Nebraska for the period 1977–1978. The number of amniotic fluid specimens tested for fetal karyotype was divided by the corresponding number of live births.

Utilization ratios are given in the table. The ratios were higher in 1978 than in 1977. Overall ratios were 6%–28%, well below the adjusted rates of 40%–50% found in certain other states and in British localities. Urban women tended to have higher utilization ratios than rural women, and white women had higher ratios than blacks. Ratios for black and rural residents were extremely low. Women aged 40 and older, who were at a fivefold greater risk than those aged 35–36 years, had less than a onefold rise in utilization over the latter group. The great majority of older gravidas began prenatal care early enough to receive prenatal diagnosis. Generally, only 10%–30% of women were initially seen too late to receive prenatal diagnosis.

Program strategies must ensure access to prenatal diagnosis for women aged 40 years and older, blacks, and women who live in rural areas. The best course would be to expand capacities, but resources to achieve this are limited. If providers cannot meet present demands, they might consider preferentially selecting women aged 40 and older for prenatal diagnosis. This will ensure the greatest impact of prenatal diagnosis on disease prevention.

▶ [This study compared utilization of prenatal genetic diagnosis by women aged 35

UTILIZATION RATIOS FOR PRENATAL CHROMOSOMAL
DIAGNOSIS IN WOMEN ≥ 35 YEARS OF AGE IN
ALABAMA, CALIFORNIA, MANHATTAN, AND NEBRASKA,
1977–1978

	Year	
	1977	*1978*
Alabama	7.3%	10.9%
California	14.3%	19.8%
Nebraska	6.4%	6.7%
Manhattan	24.8%	28.9%

(7–1) Am. J. Obstet. Gynecol. 139:673–677, Mar. 15, 1981.

years or older in four geographic areas. There was a considerable difference by geography, with rural populations substantially below urban in utilizing this diagnostic test. In rural areas of Nebraska and Alabama, only 2%–10% of women of 40 years and older were tested, compared with 30% or more in Manhattan and San Francisco. Whether this reflects lack of availability, lack of information, or lack of interest is unclear.] ◄

7-2 **Genetic Disease in the Offspring of Older Fathers.** Geneticists have recognized that the mean age of fathers of offspring with some autosomal dominant diseases due to new mutations is higher than expected, but the magnitude of the risk is unknown. A paternal age effect has been suggested for X-linked recessive disorders as well. J. M. Friedman (Univ. of Texas Health Science Center at Dallas) determined the relative and absolute frequencies of offspring with autosomal dominant diseases due to mutation in the sperm from fathers of various ages. Achondroplasia is the condition for which the best data on paternal age effect are available. As in Down's syndrome, the relative frequency of achondroplasia exhibits a strong direct relation to age of the relevant parent (Fig 7–1).

The estimated risk of a man older than age 40 years having a child with an autosomal dominant disease due to a new mutation is 0.3% to 0.5%. Although this estimate is crude, regardless of the absolute risk, about one third of infants with diseases due to new autosomal dominant mutations are fathered by men aged 40 and older. If men fathered their children before age 40, a significant reduction in the frequency of disease due to new mutation would be expected. Both men and women should complete their families before age 40 years if possible.

Fig 7–1.—Relative frequency of Down's syndrome *(open circles)* and achondroplasia *(solid circles)* in offspring of mothers (Down's syndrome) and fathers (achondroplasia) of various ages. (Courtesy of Friedman, J. M.: Obstet. Gynecol. 57:745–749, June 1981.)

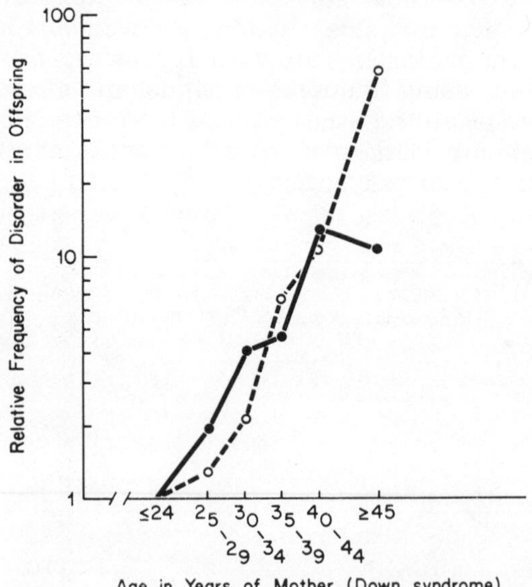

(7–2) Obstet. Gynecol. 57:745–749, June 1981.

▶ [Although the association between advanced maternal age and chromosomally abnormal offspring is appreciated by both the medical profession and the public, Friedman's point in this article is not well understood by either. A genetic disorder with dominant inheritance may appear in an individual with a negative family history, because of a point mutation in the germ cell of one of his parents. These mutations often occur during DNA replication and cell division, and are therefore more common in the sperm than in the egg. The sperm of older men are more apt to harbor such mutations. The message is that, although one can assure the May–December couple that the young bride is not predisposed to a chromosomally abnormal baby, the graying husband's sperm may not be as good as they once were. Ain't it the truth?] ◀

▶ ↓ The following article provides specific data regarding paternal age and the risk of Down's syndrome. ◀

7–3 **Down's Syndrome Associated With Father's Age in Norway.** Recently, there has been renewed interest in the possibility that older fathers might be at a higher risk of producing infants with Down's syndrome. J. David Erickson and Tor Bjerkedal reviewed records of births in Norway in 1967–1978 for evidence of an increased risk of Down's syndrome associated with older paternal age. In some 685,000 total births with known parental ages, 693 cases of Down's syndrome were reported. When fathers were considered young if aged 49 years and less, a significant effect was obtained at the 0.05 level. An increased risk of perhaps 20%–30% appeared to be associated with older fathers, independent of any maternal age effect.

These findings suggest that the risk of Down's syndrome may be modestly increased when fathers are older than age 50 years or so. This is the first indication of such an effect where stringent control of the maternal age effect was exercised. If there is an effect of older paternal age, it is much smaller than the increase in risk associated with advancing maternal age. Since older men contribute a relatively small proportion of total births, their contribution to the total burden of Down's syndrome would be quite small. If the paternal age effect is quite small and the rate of paternal nondisjunction is quite high, it is possible that the maternal age effect has causes other than, or in addition to, an increasing frequency of nondisjunction with increasing age. An example would be an age-related decrease in the effectiveness of the screening mechanism of spontaneous abortion. Younger mothers may abort a higher proportion of affected fetuses than older mothers.

▶ [These observations, based on birth certificate data during a 12-year period in Norway, suggest that risk of Down's syndrome increases with paternal age, presumably reflecting paternal nondisjunction. The increase was modest in comparison with that related to maternal age and was statistically significant only at the over-age-50 vs. under-age-50 breakpoint.] ◀

7–4 **Genetic Amniocentesis in Twin Gestations.** Sherman Elias, Albert B. Gerbie, Joe Leigh Simpson, Henry L. Nadler, Rudy E. Sabbagha, and Arnold Shkolnik describe two genetics programs at Northwestern University, one at Children's Memorial Hospital (CMH) and another at Prentice Women's Hospital and Maternity Center (PWHMC), in Chicago, and discuss results in 1,613 women studied with routine ultrasonography prior to genetic amniocentesis.

(7–3) J. Med. Genet. 18:22–28, February 1981.
(7–4) Am. J. Obstet. Gynecol. 138:169–174, Sept. 15, 1980.

In the CMH program, patients undergo routine ultrasound monitoring (USM) at CMH, after which they travel to PWHMC for amniocentesis. In singleton pregnancies, the amniocentesis is performed without repeating USM studies; in multiple gestations, amniocentesis is performed after further visualization in the USM laboratory at PWHMC. In the PWHMC program, all amniocenteses in singleton and multiple gestations are performed in the ultrasonography laboratory immediately after USM (gray-scale and real-time). In twin gestations, the procedure of amniocentesis is performed no earlier than 17 weeks' gestation, 1 week later than is routine for singleton gestations. Separate amniotic sacs are distinguished by injecting a dye (1–3 ml of 0.8% indigo carmine diluted with sterile water to give a final concentration of 0.08%) into the sac, from which the first sample of fluid (20 ml) is aspirated (Fig 7–2). After ambulation of the patient for 5 minutes, a second amniocentesis is performed in the ultrasonographically determined location of the other fetus. Aspiration of bluish fluid indicates that the first amniotic sac has been reentered.

Among 786 women who underwent amniocentesis prior to the routine use of USM at CMH, there were 2 sets of twins, neither detected at the time of amniocentesis. Among 1,080 women who underwent routine USM, there were 16 (1.4%) with multiple gestations. Only once was a twin gestation not detected; in this case, real-time USM was not used. Amniotic fluid was thus aspirated from only 1 amniotic sac. In the other 15 cases, USM detected multiple gestations. Three of these patients elected not to undergo amniocentesis. Among 533 women who underwent amniocentesis in the PWHMC program, there were 10 (1.9%) with twin gestations. All 10 cases were detected with USM. One patient elected not to undergo amniocentesis and later was delivered of 2 normal infants. In another case, USM at 19 weeks showed a severely growth-retarded fetus with oligohydramnios; the other fetus was of normal size. The couple elected to have 1 amniocentesis directed toward the apparently normal sac. The α-fetoprotein level was 1.79 mg/dl and chromosomal analysis of amniotic fluid fibroblasts revealed a 47 XX, +21 complement. When the pregnancy was terminated, a 47 XX, +21 complement was confirmed in the larger fetus. Eight other women with twins requested amniocentesis on both sacs.

From the two programs, there were 20 sets of twins in which both fetuses were normal and viable and in which the mother requested sampling from both amniotic sacs. With the technique shown in Figure 7–2, fluid was obtained successfully from both sacs in 19 of 20 sets. The remaining patient was subsequently delivered at term of 1 stillborn and 1 liveborn infant. Two attempts to obtain fluid in the second amniotic sac had failed in this patient. Both infants had craniocarpotarsal dysplasia, an autosomal dominant disorder. In the other 19 women, fluid from each amniotic sac was successfully obtained; 2 or 3 insertions of the needle were required per patient. All 19 sets of twins were cytogenetically normal. It is concluded that twin gestations can be detected reliably by routine USM, that both amniotic sacs usually can be sampled, and that the complication rate

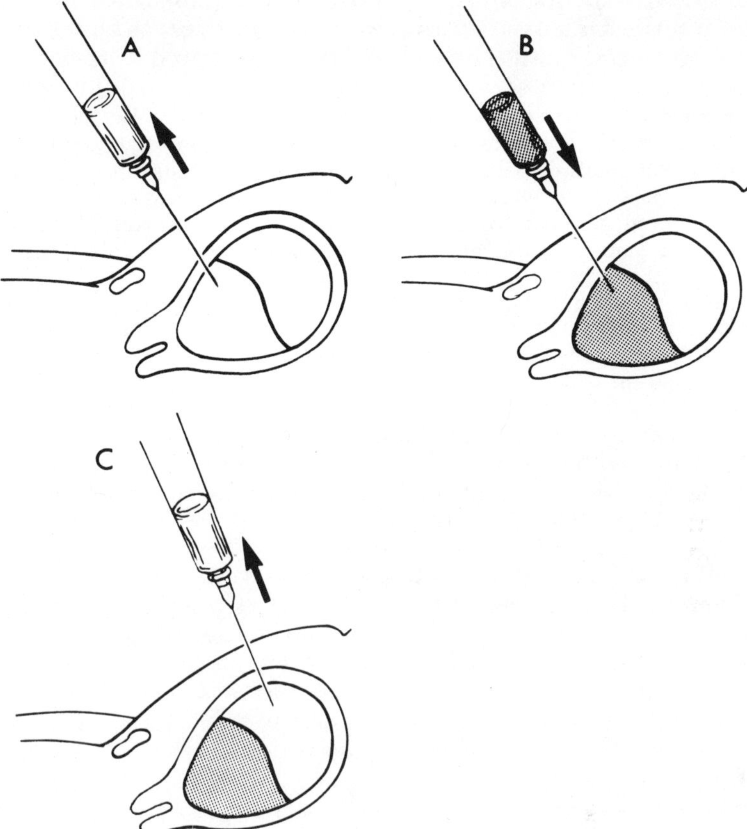

Fig 7–2.—Technique for amniocentesis in twin gestations, performed immediately after ultrasonographic examination. **A,** fluid aspirated from the first amniotic sac. **B,** indigo carmine injected into the first amniotic sac. **C,** second tap in the ultrasonographically determined location of the second fetus. Clear fluid confirms that the second amniotic sac was successfully aspirated. (Courtesy of Elias, S., et al.: Am. J. Obstet. Gynecol. 138:169–174, Sept. 15, 1980.)

appears to be minimal. Findings are important because multiple gestation increases with advancing maternal age. If both amniotic sacs are investigated, it is inevitable that in certain cases the dilemma will arise of having 1 normal and 1 abnormal fetus. In this case, the couple must then be counseled in regard to the prognosis of the abnormal fetus. The final decision of whether to terminate the pregnancy should be made by the couple.

7–5 **Selective Birth in Twin Pregnancy With Discordancy for Down's Syndrome.** At least 5 recent reports have appeared of cases in second trimester in which one twin fetus had a major congenital malformation and the other was normal. Thomas D. Kerenyi and Usha Chitkara (Mt. Sinai School of Medicine, New York) report a case of twin pregnancy with discordancy for trisomy 21 in which an

(7–5) N. Engl. J. Med. 304:1525–1527, June 18, 1981.

aggressive approach was taken to terminate the abnormal fetus selectively by intracardiac puncture and exsanguination at 20 weeks' gestation. The normal fetus subsequently was delivered at term.

Woman, 40, a nullipara previously treated for hypothyroidism, was found at 17 weeks' gestation to have a twin pregnancy. Amniotic fluid analysis indicated two male fetuses, one with a normal male karyotype and one with trisomy 21. The mother wanted to have the normal child but could not face the need to care for an abnormal child. At 20 weeks' gestation, under real-time ultrasound guidance and after diazepam and meperidine administration, 40 ml of amniotic fluid was removed from the sac of the abnormal fetus, and a second attempt at cardiac puncture and exsanguination succeeded. Later chromosomal analysis confirmed that the blood was from the fetus with trisomy 21. The normal fetus retained normal motion and cardiac activity. The mother remained stable throughout the procedure. Prophylactic antibiotics were given for 5 days. Uterine irritability was mild and usually subsided with rest.

Follow-up sonography showed normal growth of the normal twin and decreasing head and body size of the twin with trisomy 21. A normal infant was delivered at 40 weeks, followed by a fetus papyraceus weighing 120 gm. The placental area corresponding to the abnormal fetus was small, fibrosed, and infarcted. The mother and infant were doing well 7 months later.

Cephalometry indicated normal growth of the surviving twin and regression of the affected twin in this case as pregnancy progressed. In the absence of a persisting marker differentiating the two fetuses, it may be difficult to identify the fetus with the abnormality when the chromosomal analysis is reported. The site of implantation of the placenta is an important technical consideration. There may be risk of maternal disseminated intravascular coagulation after the death of one of monozygous twins in utero.

▶ [This experience reported by Gerbie and associates is similar to that on our service. Twins should be diagnosed at the time of ultrasonography and the simple technique described should enable the physician to obtain amniotic fluid from both sacs. Discordant results from the two fetuses create more of a dilemma than does the technical matter of obtaining the fluid samples. The case reported by Kerenyi and Chitkara represents an interesting, albeit controversial, approach to this dilemma.] ◀

7–6 **Prenatal Detection of Neural Tube Defects: VI. Experience With 20,000 Pregnancies.** Elevated amniotic fluid levels of α-fetoprotein (AFP) have been associated with an open, leaking neural tube defect (NTD). By measuring amniotic fluid levels of AFP, prenatal detection of NTDs is possible in approximately 95% of cases. Aubrey Milunsky (Harvard Med. School) reports the findings on amniotic fluid AFP assays performed in 20,000 pregnancies.

Elevated amniotic fluid levels of AFP were present in 334 of the 20,000 pregnancies (1.7%). Of these, there were 143 NTDs, 136 of which were open lesions (40.7%). In addition, there were 90 pregnancies with other fetal defects or conditions associated with elevated AFP levels, and 108 with elevated AFP levels with or without fetal blood admixture. No adequate explanation for elevated AFP could be found in 8 of these. A false negative result (defined as a normal AFP in the presence of a *closed* NTD) was found in 7 of the 143 NTDs

---

(7–6) JAMA 244:2731–2735, Dec. 19, 1980.

(4.9%), while the practical false positive rate for all NTDs was less than 0.06%. Eleven women with elevated AFP levels chose to terminate their pregnancies; all had an apparently normal fetus. However, an explanation for the elevated AFP levels was found in all but 2 of these 11 patients. Based on the data presented, the risk of a woman who has had a previous child with an NTD having another is approximately 1.5% (36/2,389), while the risk of an unexpected NTD is 0.2% (38/16,605).

Couples at risk for bearing children with NTDs should be offered counseling and prenatal diagnosis when indicated. Various points should be kept in mind when evaluating a patient at risk: (1) accurate assessment of gestational age is important for reliable interpretation of the AFP assay, (2) ultrasonography and amniocentesis should be performed at 15 to 16 weeks' gestation, (3) amniotic fluid samples should not be centrifuged, (4) amniotic fluid samples should be tested for the presence of urine, (5) if fetal blood is present in the sample and associated with elevated AFP levels, a second amniocentesis 10 days later is recommended, (6) if the AFP level is elevated, corroborative evidence should be obtained before the patient elects therapeutic abortion, and (7) if a pregnancy is aborted after 2 elevated AFP assays, preparations should be made before the procedure to obtain fetal kidney tissue for electron microscopy.

▶ [Dwight P. Cruikshank, of the University of Iowa, reviewed this article at our request and commented as follows:

"This enormous experience demonstrates that amniotic fluid AFP determinations are effective in detecting open NTD—no case was missed. However, the test is not entirely specific, and 108 of 20,000 patients initially had false positive AFP elevations. Careful follow-up testing reduced the number of true false positives to 2 (0.01%). High amniotic fluid AFP levels must be evaluated with repeat amniocentesis, determination of fetal blood contamination, and sophisticated ultrasound studies, coupled with expert counseling to insure against unnecessary pregnancy terminations. Thus, NTD testing, as all other forms of prenatal genetic diagnosis, requires broad expertise. The 1.5%–2.0% recurrence rate of NTD found in couples with one previously involved child is lower than the 3%–5% risk formerly quoted."

In a related study, Robinson and associates (*Obstet. Gynecol.* 56:705, 1981) reported their experience with ultrasound diagnosis of NTDs. Ultrasound proved to be quite accurate and was regarded as complementary to amniotic fluid AFP measurement.] ◀

7–7 **Relation of Glucose to α-Fetoprotein in Amniotic Fluid.** Low glucose concentrations have been found in amniotic fluid of women who have delivered anencephalic fetuses. A. H. Rule, V. Sliogeris, M. Farber, G. Britton, and J. Vandervoorde studied the relation between glucose and α-fetoprotein concentrations in amniotic fluid samples obtained between the 16th and 22nd weeks of gestation from women who subsequently delivered normal infants. α-Fetoprotein was measured by radioimmunoassay and glucose by the glucose oxidase assay.

A direct relation, significant in each of the 6 gestational weeks tested, was found between amniotic fluid glucose and α-fetoprotein concentrations. The coefficients of correlation varied from .74 to .91. The relation between amniotic fluid α-fetoprotein and urea nitrogen, another metabolite, was not significant ($r = -.34$), suggesting that

---

(7–7) Obstet. Gynecol. 57:310–312, March 1981.

the α-fetoprotein-glucose relation was not spurious. Absence of pregnancy-associated macroglobulins in the samples indicated that they were not contaminated by maternal serum.

The clinical significance of the linear relation between α-fetoprotein and glucose concentrations in amniotic fluid from normal gestations at 16 to 22 weeks is obvious in light of the dichotomy in those values reported with anencephalic fetuses. The relation between neural tube defects and glucose concentrations is unknown. Further studies are needed to analyze the difference between amniotic fluid glucose to α-fetoprotein ratios in normal pregnancies and in those that terminate in delivery of an anencephalic fetus or a fetus with a neural tube defect.

▶ [This report notes a significant positive correlation between glucose and α-fetoprotein concentrations in amniotic fluid between 16 and 22 weeks' gestation. All α-fetoprotein levels were normal. It would be interesting to examine amniotic fluid glucose levels in a group of cases of neural tube defect.] ◀

7–8 **Glial Origin of Rapidly Adhering Amniotic Fluid Cells.** Amniotic fluid from pregnancies complicated by fetal anencephaly or spina bifida contains an excess of cells that adhere rapidly to glass or plastic under tissue culture conditions. The gross morphological appearance of these rapidly adhering cells suggests a CNS origin. Pertti Aula, Harriet von Koskull, Kari Teramo, Olavi Karjalainen, Ismo Virtanen, Veli-Pekka Lehto, and Doris Dahl describe immunofluorescent studies showing the cells to be of glial origin.

Woman, 28, who had been taking phenytoin and carbamazepine as anticonvulsants for several years, was found to have a raised serum α-fetoprotein (AFP) level at 20 weeks' gestation. Ultrasonography at 23 weeks suggested fetal anencephaly. Amniocentesis yielded amniotic fluid with an AFP level of 56.3 mg/L. Amniotic fluid cells were cultured for 24 hours and then examined by phase-contrast microscopy and indirect immunofluorescence microscopy with a glial cell-specific, glial fibrillary acidic protein antiserum. A high proportion of the cells showed glial-specific fluorescence. No such staining was seen in cells from samples of normal amniotic fluid. A stillborn infant with typical anencephaly was delivered at 24 weeks. Autopsy showed a large defect in the cranial end of the neural tube that permitted direct contact between spinal and amniotic cavities.

The rapidly adhering cells in amniotic fluid from pregnancies complicated by fetal anencephaly are apparently glial cells of CNS origin. Rapidly adhering cells of different morphology are also present in amniotic fluid from pregnancies with other fetal abnormalities such as exomphalos and urogenital atresia. Tissue-specific immunofluorescence techniques may be of use in these cases to distinguish among the various types of malformations.

▶ [Several tools can be used to evaluate the fetal condition when an elevated amniotic fluid AFP level is detected. Ultrasonography may indicate anencephaly (or spina bifida in certain expert hands), elevated acetylcholinesterase levels may suggest an open neural tube defect, or the morphology of rapidly adhering amniotic fluid cells in tissue culture may provide clues as to why the AFP level is high. Gosden and Brock (1980 YEAR BOOK, pp. 200–202) have described what look like "neural" cells in cases of open neural tube defects. The present report adds confirmation to this morphological impression. A glial cell-specific antibody coated these rapidly adhering cells from a

(7–8) Br. Med. J. 281:1456–1457, Nov. 29, 1980.

patient with an anencephalic fetus. For suggestions regarding prevention of neural tube defects, see the following two articles.] ◄

7–9 **Diet as a Factor in Etiology of Neural Tube Defects.** Neural tube defects (NTDs) have been more frequent in British mothers from the lower social classes, who more often have an inadequate diet in early pregnancy and sometimes have actual deficiencies of essential dietary constituents such as folic acid. Nansi James, K. M. Laurence, and Mary Miller (Welsh Natl. School of Medicine, Cardiff) undertook a dietary survey of women who had had a child with NTD. A total of 174 women who wished another pregnancy participated in a prospective study of the role of diet in early pregnancy, and 103 women received dietary counseling. Subjects received 2 mg of folic acid or placebo twice daily from the time contraception was discontinued. Sixty women given folic acid and 61 receiving placebo were compared.

The subjects described a poorer diet during affected pregnancies than during those with a normal outcome or during interpregnancy periods. About two thirds of counseled patients improved their diets, whereas diets of the other subjects were unchanged. There were 3 recurrences of NTD in 109 pregnancies of counseled patients and 5 recurrences in 77 pregnancies of noncounseled patients. All 8 recurrences were among women taking a poor diet, as were all but 3 of 18 miscarriages. Only 1 of 45 folic acid-treated women with high serum folate concentrations had a recurrence, and this subject had not used tablets for the first 7 weeks of gestation. Six recurrences of NTD took place among 130 nonsupplemented women.

Neural tube defects are probably of multifactorial origin. Poor diet is one obvious etiologic factor, and one that can be modified by counseling and by supplementation. Women should be taught to take a well-balanced diet, starting in school. This and supplementation with folic acid or other vitamins may reduce the risk of recurrence of NTD.

7–10 **Double-Blind, Randomized, Controlled Trial of Folate Treatment Before Conception to Prevent Recurrence of Neural Tube Defects.** Neural tube defects (NTDs) are the most common serious malformation found at birth in the United Kingdom. Women from the lower social classes are affected more often, and blood concentrations of various essential substances including folic acid are lower in these subjects and lower still in women bearing a child with an NTD. K. M. Laurence, Nansi James, Mary H. Miller, G. B. Tennant, and H. Campbell (Welsh Natl. School of Medicine, Cardiff) examined the role of folic acid supplementation before conception in the prevention of NTDs in a double-blind trial conducted in south Wales. Sixty women who had had 1 child with an NTD were allocated before conception to take 4 mg of folic acid daily, and 44 complied. Fifty-one other women were allocated to placebo.

At 6 to 9 weeks' gestation, compliant women had serum folate concentrations above 10 μg/L. One of the noncompliers, who took no folate in early pregnancy but took a large amount at 7 weeks' gestation, had a spontaneous abortion of an anencephalic fetus. Two noncom-

(7–9) Z. Kinderchir. 31:302–307, December 1980.
(7–10) Br. Med. J. 282:1509–1511, May 9, 1981.

NUMBERS OF WOMEN TAKING GOOD, FAIR, OR INADEQUATE DIETS
CLASSIFIED ACCORDING TO WHETHER THEY RECEIVED FOLATE TREATMENT
AND WHETHER FETUS WAS NORMAL OR HAD NEURAL TUBE DEFECT

| | Received folate | | Did not receive folate | | |
Diet	Normal	Neural-tube defect	Normal	Neural-tube defect	All cases
Good	17	0	26	0	43
Fair	17	0	24	0	41
Inadequate	10	0	11	6	27
All cases	44	0	61	6	111

pliers and 4 placebo-treated women but no compliant patients had a fetus with an NTD. The proportion of women with inadequate diets was similar in the two treatment groups (table). All 6 recurrences of NTD were in women taking an inadequate diet. Compliers in each dietary group had significantly higher red blood cell folate concentrations than placebo patients. Concentrations in noncompliers were similar to those in the placebo group. The mean concentration in women with NTD recurrences was 249 μg/L, lower than the mean in the untreated women but not significantly different from it.

Folic acid supplementation may be an inexpensive, safe, and effective means of primary prevention of NTDs, but a large, multicenter trial is needed to confirm this. If effective, folic acid supplementation would greatly reduce the costs and hazards of screening for α-fetoprotein, amniocentesis, termination of pregnancies, and the medical and custodial care of liveborn infants with NTDs.

▶ [The results of these studies are consistent with those of a report abstracted in the 1981 YEAR BOOK (pp. 179–180). The implication is that recurrent NTDs reflect dietary inadequacy, particularly of folate. However, there are problems in interpretation. In the study by James et al., the retrospective analysis relied on diet history, a crude tool at best, but even more suspect when taken from women who have delivered a defective child; moreover, although recurrence rates were less with improved diet and folate supplementation, in no cases were the differences statistically significant. In this article by Laurence and associates, compliance was defined solely by serum folate levels, and those 16 patients judged noncompliant had a higher recurrence rate than did those patients who received the placebo. As we commented in the 1981 YEAR BOOK, these results seem almost too good.

Just as presently there is attention being focused on periconceptional blood glucose control in the hope of decreasing the prevalence of malformations in infants of diabetic mothers, perhaps more emphasis will soon be placed on the quality of the diet of women attempting pregnancy. As intriguing as these reports are, we don't think the final answer is in.] ◀

7–11   **Methylumbelliferylguanidinobenzoate-reactive Proteases in Human Amniotic Fluid: Promising Marker for the Intrauterine Detection of Cystic Fibrosis.** M. M. J. Walsh and Henry L. Nadler (Northwestern Univ.) have analyzed 1,162 specimens of second-trimester human amniotic fluid for 4-methylumbelliferylguanidinobenzoate (MUGB) reactivity to document possible differences in mean specific activity of control specimens versus that of four specimens of cystic fibrosis (CF) amniotic fluid (3 second-trimester and 1

(7–11)   Am. J. Obstet. Gynecol. 137:978–982, Aug. 15, 1980.

term). As previously reported, MUGB is a sensitive active site titrant of many serine proteases that have certain properties in common with the arginine esterases in plasma that are known to be deficient in CF.

The mean specific activity value, measured in nanomoles of methylumbelliferone (MU) formed per milligram of protein, for the control population (1,037) was 2.37 ± 0.41. The mean specific activity values from a series of specimens of amniotic fluid from abnormal pregnancies (chromosomal and biochemical abnormalities, confirmed neural tube defects, abortions, and stillbirths) were found not to vary significantly from the values in the control population. The mean specific activity value of blood-tinged samples centrifuged to remove red blood cell contaminants prior to freezing at − 20 C did not vary from the value for the control group, in contrast to the value for samples frozen without centrifugation and containing hemolyzed red blood cells (1.76 ± 0.30). The mean specific activity values for all four groups (control, abnormal, centrifuged, and noncentrifuged) were found to be significantly different ($P <$ .001) from the mean specific activity value of 1.24 ± 0.12 for the four CF amniotic fluids. In addition, when the control and CF fluids were focused isoelectrically on polyacrylamide gels at pH 5.0 to 7.0, and were stained subsequently for α-N-benzoyl-L-arginine ethyl ester activity, the controls gave a pattern of five activity bands with a pI of 5.1 to 5.4, whereas the CF fluids consistently gave only four. These data suggest the potential value of the MUGB-reactive protease assay for intrauterine detection of CF.

One theoretical problem that must be evaluated is the ability of the assay to distinguish heterozygotes from affected fetuses. It has not yet been possible to define the value of MUGB in amniotic fluid for heterozygotes. However, on the basis of the results of the study, a number of pregnancies at risk for CF currently are being monitored.

▶ [Cystic fibrosis is a more common disease than many others for which prenatal diagnosis is already available; and, thus, an accurate test is much needed. These preliminary reports indicate that MUGB reactivity is decreased in amniotic fluid from affected pregnancies (the abbreviation is necessary for the 14-syllable name of the chemical used in the determination). The number of cases studied so far is small, and the level of reactivity in fluids from heterozygote fetuses has not yet been established. Therefore, it is too early to be certain that this represents an important breakthrough in prenatal diagnosis. We have had one case on our service in which amniotic fluid MUGB testing indicated a normal fetus but the infant was subsequently diagnosed as having the disease, so there is some risk of false negative results.] ◀

7–12 **Intrauterine Detection of Cystic Fibrosis.** Significant differences were found in the extent of protease-methylumbelliferylguanidinobenzoate (MUGB) reactivity when plasma of patients with cystic fibrosis, obligate heterozygotes, and control subjects were compared. Amniotic fluid contains MUGB-reactive proteases that appear to be physiochemically similar to those found in plasma. Henry L. Nadler and M. M. J. Walsh (Northwestern Univ.) studied MUGB-reactive proteases in 1,898 amniotic fluid samples obtained during routine diagnostic midtrimester amniocenteses and in 13 samples of amniotic fluid from pregnancies at risk for cystic fibrosis. Each of the latter 13

(7–12) *Pediatrics* 66:690–692, November 1980.

cases, the couples were obligate heterozygotes, having previously produced children with cystic fibrosis.

Mean titer value, expressed as nanomoles of methylumbelliferone (MU) formed per milliliter of amniotic fluid, was 11.93 (range, 4.9–27.8) in control samples and 4.32 (range, 3.01–5.52) in 7 samples from women carrying fetuses later proved to have cystic fibrosis. Mean specific activity, expressed as nanomoles of MU formed per milligram of protein, was 2.35 (range, 1.5–3.8) in control samples and 1.20 (range 1.06–1.34) in samples from women with affected fetuses.

The 13 pregnancies at risk for cystic fibrosis were monitored by a combination of quantitative determination of MUGB activity, gel electrophoresis, and gel filtration. These studies indicated 3 affected and 10 normal fetuses. In each case the diagnosis was confirmed after delivery. The likelihood of this occurring by chance is about 1 in 10,000.

Assessment of MUGB-reactive proteases in midtrimester amniotic fluid by three different procedures (quantitative analysis, polyacrylamide isoelectric focusing, and column filtration) may provide a practical and reliable method for the intrauterine detection of cystic fibrosis. Neither the precise origin nor identification of these proteases in amniotic fluid is known, and the relationship of the proteases to the basic defect in cystic fibrosis is highly speculative. It is not known whether the test will detect all cases of cystic fibrosis or only the 85% with pancreatic insufficiency, or whether false positive results occur. No method is available to confirm the diagnosis of cystic fibrosis in midtrimester abortion material.

7–13 **Prenatal Identification of Paternity: HLA Typing After Rape.** The extreme genetic polymorphism of the HLA antigen system offers a highly discriminating system for testing paternity. Marilyn S. Pollack, Irwin A. Schafer, Donald Barford, and Bo DuPont report a case in which HLA typing was used to identify the father of a fetus in a pregnant woman, aged 24 years, who had been raped. Although the woman was delivered of identical twin girls, the presence of twin fetuses was not detected at the time of amniocentesis.

The HLA typing indicated that the amniotic cells had a paternal HLA haplotype that was also present in the woman's husband and their son, aged 2 years. Based on the frequency of this particular paternal halotype (A1, B17) in the white population, it was calculated that the probability of the woman's husband being the father was 25:1 (96%), even though the rapist's HLA type had not been established yet. The rapist was excluded as the father because the fetal cells lacked all the specificities found on his cells and he lacked the specificities found in the fetal cells and absent in the mother. The results were confirmed after delivery.

It is concluded that HLA typing for prenatal determination of paternity can be a clinically important procedure, especially when a possible unnecessary abortion is being considered.

▶ [The HLA typing of the cells obtained at amniocentesis was useful in paternity testing in this case.] ◀

(7–13) JAMA 244:1954–1956, Oct. 24/31, 1980.

7-14 **Congenital Rubella Affecting an Infant Whose Mother had Rubella Antibodies Before Conception.** Virologically confirmed rubella reinfections, with disease in a fetus, are rare. J. W. Partridge, T. H. Flewett, and J. E. M. Whitehead describe an infant with severe congenital rubella, whose mother had high titers of rubella antibody some months before conceiving.

Female infant was the first child of healthy parents. The mother had been told that she had rubella at age 7 but had not been immunized, and she deliberately made contact with a case of suspected rubella before conceiving. A rubella hemagglutination inhibition titer of 400 units was documented, but rubella-specific IgM antibody was not estimated. Pregnancy began $7^{1}/_{2}$ months after the last antibody estimate. Slight malaise occurred at $2^{1}/_{2}$ months' gestation. The infant, with disproportionately small hands and eyes, fed with difficulty. Lens opacities were noted at age $3^{1}/_{2}$ months, and there was increased limb muscle tone. Weight increased slowly; head circumference was 34 cm. Rubella virus was isolated from the nose and throat at age 4 months. Severe thoracic kyphoscoliosis, coxa vara, spastic quadriplegia, and microcephaly subsequently were confirmed. The infant responded only to loud sounds and was visually inattentive. She died at age $3^{1}/_{2}$ years after a series of chest infections. Rubella virus could not be isolated from a cervical swab from the mother 9 months after delivery of the affected infant. The mother had no apparent immunologic abnormality, and she was delivered of a normal infant 2 years after the death of the first infant.

This infant clearly had features of congenital rubella, and the diagnosis was confirmed by isolation of virus, despite a maternal antibody titer usually considered to indicate immunity several months before conception. Rubella reinfection now is known to occur; it usually is subclinical. Reports of presumed reinfection during pregnancy suggest that the fetus may be severely affected. Rubella antibody titers must be interpreted cautiously when deciding whether rubella infection has occurred in pregnancy. High levels preceding conception do not exclude the possibility of congenital rubella in a subsequent gestation. Pregnant women should avoid unnecessary contact with rubella even when they consider themselves immune.

▶ [This must be a rare phenomenon, but, as with other infections, rubella infection with viremia can occur in the face of "protective" antibody levels. The implication here is that pregnant women should avoid unnecessary contact with rubella, even if they show serologic evidence of immunity. Even though they've got it, they shouldn't flaunt it!] ◀

7-15 **Maternal Phenylketonuria and Hyperphenylalaninemia: An International Survey of the Outcome of Untreated and Treated Pregnancies.** Phenylketonuria (PKU) is well recognized as an inborn metabolic error that can cause mental retardation and other signs of brain damage. It is now apparent that nonphenylketonuric offspring of phenylketonuric mothers may develop microcephaly, congenital heart disease, intrauterine growth retardation, and mental retardation. A high incidence of spontaneous abortion among phenylketonuric women also has been reported. To ascertain the effect of maternal PKU and hyperphenylalaninemia on the offspring of phen-

---

(7–14) Br. Med. J. 282:187–188, Jan. 17, 1981.
(7–15) N. Engl. J. Med. 303:1202–1208, Nov. 20, 1980.

ylketonuric women, Roger R. Lenke and Harvey L. Levy (Boston) reviewed the literature on this subject and obtained additional unpublished data through an international survey. Data were obtained on 524 pregnancies, including 101 spontaneous abortions, in 155 women. In 34 pregnancies, a low-phenylalanine diet was begun shortly before or after pregnancy was established.

Among 444 untreated pregnancies, the frequency of spontaneous abortion was 25% at maternal blood phenylalanine concentrations of 16 mg/dl or greater, compared with the expected rate of 15% to 20% in the white population. The incidences of mental retardation, microcephaly, congenital heart disease, and low birth weight in the offspring of untreated pregnancies were considerably higher than in the normal population and correlated with maternal blood levels of phenylalanine (Table 1). Phenylketonuria or some degree of hyperphenylalaninemia was present in 40 offspring of 27 mothers. Ninety-five percent of mothers with phenylalanine levels greater than or equal to 20 mg/dl and 72% of those with concentrations of 16 to 19 mg/dl had one or more mentally retarded children. In the 34 pregnancies in which a low-phenylalanine diet was administered, there was no consistent relation between treatment and the prevention of abnormalities (Table 2). Death from congenital heart disease occurred in 4 of 11 offspring from pregnancies in which treatment began in the first trimester of pregnancy. There did, however, appear to be a trend toward higher IQ and normal head circumference when treatment was initiated early.

Women with PKU are at very high risk of delivering a mentally retarded, microcephalic child and at a somewhat lower, but still increased, risk of having children with congenital heart disease and low

TABLE 1.—FREQUENCY OF SPONTANEOUS ABORTION AND ABNORMALITIES IN OFFSPRING FROM UNTREATED PREGNANCIES OF WOMEN WITH PHENYLKETONURIA OR HYPERPHENYLALANINEMIA*

COMPLICATION	GROUPINGS OF MATERNAL PHENYLALANINE LEVELS				FREQUENCY (%) IN NORMAL POPULATION
	>20 mg/dl	16–19 mg/dl	11–15 mg/dl	3–10 mg/dl	
	percentage affected in each group				
Spontaneous abortions (%)	24 (297)	30 (66)	0 (33)	8 (48)	15–20 (ref. 17)
Mental retardation (%)	92 (172)	73 (37)	22 (23)	21 (29)	5.0 †
Microcephaly (%)	73 (138)	68 (44)	35 (23)	24 (21)	4.8 †
Congenital heart disease (%)	12 (225)	15 (46)	6 (33)	0 (44)	0.8 (ref. 23)
Birth weight ≤2500 g (%)	40 (89)	52 (33)	56 (9)	13 (16)	9.6 †

*Figures in parentheses denote the size of the sample from which the percentages were calculated. Offspring with phenylketonuria or hyperphenylalaninemia are excluded.

†Perinatal Collaborative Study Data were supplied by Joseph S. Drage and colleagues.

TABLE 2.—SUMMARY OF RESULTS IN OFFSPRING, RELATED TO START OF DIETARY THERAPY DURING PREGNANCY

WHEN TREATMENT BEGAN	NUMBER OF PREGNANCIES STUDIED	OFFSPRING				
		IQ OR DQ *	MICROCEPHALY †	CONGENITAL HEART DISEASE †	BIRTH WEIGHT ≤2500 G †	OTHER EFFECTS
Before conception	3	90 (80–100)[2]	0 (0 of 3) ‡	0 (0 of 3)	0 (0 of 3)	—
First trimester	11	103 (74–127)[7]	20 (2 of 10)	36 (4 of 11)	0 (0 of 9)	§
Second trimester	16	84 (53–108)[13]	53 (8 of 15)	13 (2 of 16)	33 (4 of 12)	¶
Third trimester	4	79 (48–100)[3]	67 (2 of 3)	0 (0 of 4)	0 (0 of 2)	—

*First figure in the line is mean, range is in parentheses, and number of offspring measured appears in brackets.
†Figures denote percentages; those in parentheses indicate number of offspring with defect out of total number for which data were reported.
‡One of the 3 had a head circumference of 2 SD below the mean and thus may be considered to have "borderline" microcephaly.
§Esophageal atresia.
¶Stillbirth; cleft palate; skeletal defects.

birth weight. It could not be clearly established whether PKU increases the risk of spontaneous abortion. Treatment of women with PKU with a low-phenylalanine diet before conception merits further evaluation.

▶ [With maternal PKU, in contrast to the infantile variety, the fetus is generally normal genetically but at risk for damage in utero by virtue of exposure to high phenylalanine levels. Since the placenta normally "concentrates" amino acids on the fetal side (i.e., fetal blood levels exceed maternal), hyperphenylalaninemia in the mother will be reflected in even higher levels in the fetus. This large survey documents the devastating effect of maternal PKU: more than 90% of infants born to women with blood phenylalanine levels of 20 mg/dl or higher were mentally retarded, and the frequencies of low birth weight, microcephaly, and congenital heart disease all were increased as well. Theoretically, maternal dietary treatment (i.e., low phenylalanine diet) should be beneficial, but the results reported here on 34 patients treated during gestation do not appear very encouraging. Therapy should begin preconceptionally, but there were only 3 cases where this was done; 2 produced normal infants and 1 resulted in a borderline microcephalic baby with an IQ of 80.

In a related report, Scott and colleagues (*Arch. Dis. Child.* 55:634, 1980) described a woman with PKU recognized at 16 weeks' gestation and treated thereafter with a low phenylalanine diet. Though her blood levels were lowered, the infant was born small for gestational age and had Pierre Robin syndrome.

7–16 **Congenital Malformations and Maternal Occupation in Finland: Multivariate Analysis.** Original analysis of parental occupation in relation to congenital malformations in offspring showed increased odds ratios for certain maternal but not paternal occupational groups. K. Hemminki, P. Mutanen, I. Saloniemi, and K. Luoma (Inst. of Occupational Health, Helsinki) used the Finnish Register of Congenital Malformations in a multivariate analysis to explore the associations between maternal occupation in industrial trades (industry, construction, transport, and communications) and children born with CNS, musculoskeletal, or oral cleft malformations. Possible confounding factors were selected in preliminary screening of risk indicators for malformations. These factors included characteristics of the mother, child, and family; maternal illnesses (first trimester); and maternal medication at time of pregnancy.

Tobacco smoking was a confounding factor for all types of malformations; number of children born to the mother, maternal age, malformations in the family, number of rooms occupied by the family, sex of the child, threatened abortion, and continuous medication of the mother during the first trimester confounded the association for certain types of malformations. After adjusting for confounding factors, maternal occupation in industrial trades significantly correlated with CNS, oral cleft, and musculoskeletal malformations in offspring. Central nervous system malformations appeared to be particularly common among children of industrial and construction workers, while oral cleft and musculoskeletal malformations were common among children of transport and communications workers, although this group was so small that it could not be analyzed separately.

▶ [Questions concerning the possible adverse fetal effects of occupational exposures to various agents are becoming increasingly common; answers based on solid information are hard to give. The 1981 YEAR BOOK (pp. 180–181) contained a report also from Finland suggesting an association between organic solvent exposure in pregnancy and CNS anomalies. This more general study attempts to correct for socioeconomic and behavioral variables. Again, maternal occupation in industry was associated with CNS malformations. It is unlikely that quick and easy answers will soon be forthcoming in this complicated area.] ◀

(7–16) J. Epidemiol. Community Health 35:5–10, March 1981.

7–17 **Is Bendectin a Teratogen?** Bendectin is widely prescribed in the United States for nausea in pregnancy. In 1978, about 3 million prescriptions were written for the drug, which contains doxylamine succinate and pyridoxine hydrochloride. A possible association with limb reductions has been suggested. José F. Cordero, Godfrey P. Oakley, Frank Greenberg, and Levy M. James (Center for Disease Control, Atlanta) examined first-trimester exposure to Bendectin for several major groups of birth defects in infants entered in the Metropolitan Atlanta Congenital Defects Program from 1968 to 1978. More than 280,000 births had been monitored through the program through 1978.

There was a total of 1,493 cases with an interviewable birth defect, and 1,231 interviews were completed. First-trimester exposure to Bendectin was reported by 9.5% of the interviewees. There were no significant differences in exposure to the drug among any of the 12 categories of defects analyzed. Among subgroups of limb defects, the amniotic bands complex exhibited significantly increased exposure to Bendectin. When the data were stratified for two periods of exposure, a significant association was found between encephalocele and exposure to two-component Bendectin. A significant association was found between esophageal atresia and exposure to three-component Bendectin, including dicyclomine hydrochloride. With stratification, no significant association was found for the amniotic bands complex.

The findings do not suggest that exposure to Bendectin is associated causally with birth defects. If any causal association does exist, the actual risks appear to be extremely small. It is not possible to prove any agent safe, and the potential risks from all drugs used during pregnancy must be weighed against their potential benefits.

7–18 **Birth Defects Related to Bendectin Use in Pregnancy: I. Oral Clefts and Cardiac Defects.** Nausea and vomiting in early pregnancy can be very debilitating. Bendectin is the antiemetic agent most widely prescribed in pregnancy in the United States and is the only one specifically approved for use in pregnancy by the Food and Drug Administration. It contains 10 mg each of doxylamine succinate and pyridoxine hydrochloride; dicyclomine has been deleted. Allen A. Mitchell, Lynn Rosenberg, Samuel Shapiro and Dennis Slone evaluated the risks of birth defects in a case-control study of malformed infants whose mothers were interviewed at three regional centers. The 98 infants with isolated cleft palate, 221 with cleft lip with or without cleft palate, and 122 with selected cardiac defects were compared with 970 other malformed infants who served as control subjects.

The relative risk estimates for first-trimester exposure to Bendectin were 0.9 for the cleft palate group, 0.6 for the cleft lip-palate group, and 1.0 for the cardiac defect group. The risk estimates were not altered appreciably by allowance for a large number of potentially confounding factors.

(7–17) JAMA 245:2307–2310, June 12, 1981.
(7–18) Ibid., pp. 2311–2314.

In utero exposure to Bendectin in early pregnancy appears not to increase the risk of oral clefts or selected cardiac defects in the infants materially. The findings do not confirm previous reports of positive associations between antenatal exposure to Bendectin and the development in offspring of oral clefts or selected cardiac defects. The possibility that a particular drug may be a weak teratogen cannot be excluded completely because of the impracticality of entirely eliminating unrecognized confounding or other forms of bias in nonexperimental studies of human populations.

▶ [These two reports are reassuring. The evidence suggests that Bendectin is not a teratogen. Because it is a commonly used preparation that is *prescribed* for patients who are known to be pregnant, rather than a drug taken *inadvertently* by women who do not suspect pregnancy, close scrutiny as to its potential effects is entirely appropriate. The choice of mothers of babies with other congenital anomalies as controls in both of these studies is a good one, as recall bias should be eliminated. If a regimen based on expectancy and frequent small feedings is insufficient for a patient with nausea and vomiting in early pregnancy, our personal practice is to prescribe Bendectin. The preparation combines an antihistaminic and vitamin B_6. It would be interesting to see a blinded study comparing the efficacy of the combination, each agent singly, and a placebo.] ◀

7–19 **Pregnancy Outcome in Women Exposed to Diethylstilbestrol In Utero.** The occurrence of anomalies of the vagina, cervix, and uterus in women exposed to diethylstilbestrol (DES) in utero has aroused interest and concern regarding the reproductive potential of these women. To better evaluate the current knowledge on this matter, Eugene C. Sandberg, Nancy L. Riffle, Jane V. Higdon, and Carolyn E. Getman (Stanford Univ.) retrospectively examined the pregnancy outcomes of 167 women, representing 255 pregnancies, with confirmed intrauterine exposure to DES who were registered in the Stilbestrol Clinic at the Stanford University Medical Center. The findings were combined with the published results of similar investigations at other institutions, and all available data were summarized.

Based on the combined data, 27% of the women exposed to DES and 16% of the unexposed control women had experienced a spontaneous abortion (table). Preterm delivery had been experienced by 20% of the exposed women and 7% of the unexposed control women, while 69% of the exposed women and 93% of the unexposed control women had experienced a term delivery. Overall, 79% of the exposed women and 95% of the unexposed control women had had at least 1 living infant. In exposed women, 1 of every 30 pregnancies was ectopically located.

The evidence suggested that exposed patients with teratologic changes had a higher incidence of pregnancy loss or preterm delivery than those women without such changes. Exposed women with abnormal hysterographic findings had a higher incidence of spontaneous abortion, ectopic pregnancy, and premature delivery than those without abnormal findings. However, there was no evidence that the presence of teratologic changes in exposed patients precluded normal pregnancy and term delivery.

It should be noted that most of the observed differences were not

(7–19) Am. J. Obstet. Gynecol. 140:194–205, May 15, 1981.

NUMBERS AND PERCENTAGES OF WOMEN EXPOSED TO DES AND UNEXPOSED CONTROL WOMEN WHO HAVE EXPERIENCED EACH TYPE OF PREGNANCY OUTCOME (PERCENTAGES RELATE TO EVALUABLE WOMEN—THOSE WITH PREGNANCY OUTCOME OTHER THAN ELECTIVE ABORTION ONLY)

	Herbst et al.		Barnes et al.		Kaufman et al. (exposed)	This study (exposed)	All studies combined	
	Exposed	Unexposed	Exposed	Unexposed			Exposed	Unexposed
Experienced pregnancy	82	112	289	310	93*	167	631	422
Had elective abortion only	15	21	69	86	17	56	157	107
Evaluable women	67	91	220	224	76	111	474	315
Had spontaneous abortion	17	15	57†	36†	25	27	126 (27%)	51 (16%)
Had ectopic pregnancy	4	0	8	3	7	7	26	3
Had preterm delivery	26	10	25‡	13‡	18	26	95 (20%)	23(7%)
Had term delivery	40	79	178†	213†	41	70	329 (69%)	292 (93%)
Had surviving infant	55	85	178§	213§	–‖	83	316 (79%)‖	298 (95%)

*Includes only women "who agreed to undergo" hysterosalpingographic evaluation.
†Only the differences in incidence represented by these numbers are reported to be statistically significant.
‡Numbers for "stillbirth" and "premature birth" in original report are combined here as "preterm deliveries."
§These are minimal figures, as they do not include the unknown number of prematurely born infants who survived.
‖Results from the study of Kaufman et al. do not include information regarding infant survival and are not included in this tabulation.

statistically significant. In the few instances in which a statistically valid difference was observed, a similar significant difference for the same outcome was not obtained by other investigators. Although virtually all studies show a poorer pregnancy outcome in women exposed in utero to DES than in unexposed women, there also has been reassuring data regarding the potential of exposed patients to reproduce successfully.

▶ [This is a thorough review of the literature and tabulation of reported results, along with those from Stanford University, of the effects of intrauterine DES exposure on subsequent reproductive performance. The "bottom line" is that spontaneous abortion is doubled, preterm delivery tripled, and ectopic pregnancy increased fivefold to tenfold.] ◀

7–20 **Genital Abnormalities and Abnormal Semen Analyses in Male Patients Exposed to Diethylstilbestrol In Utero.** E. Douglas Whitehead and Elliot Leiter (Beth Israel Med. Center, New York) report that urologic examination of 48 male patients aged 12–35 years exposed to diethylstilbestrol in utero found genital abnormalities in 29. Fourteen (29%) had a varicocele, 6 (13%) had epididymal cysts, 5 (10%) had hypoplastic testes and 4 (8%) had cryptorchidism. In addition, 2 (4%) had a rudimentary double urethral meatus, 2 (4%) had monorchism, and 1 each had a meatal narrowing, hypoplastic glans, and hypoplastic penis. Nine patients (19%) had more than one abnormality. Semen analyses in 20 men aged 20–35 years disclosed abnormal sperm morphology with <60% normal oval forms in 9 (45%), sperm count $< 20 \times 10^6$/ml in 5 (25%), sperm motility <40% in 4 (20%), and semen volume <1.5 ml in 1. Semen analyses categorized further by the Eliasson scoring system in 18 patients, measuring sperm count/10^6, percentage of motile sperm cells, grade of motility, and percentage of morphologically normal sperm, showed an Eliasson score >10 (severely pathologic) in 6 (33%) patients and a score between 5 and 10 (pathologic) in 3 (17%). Only 6 patients (33%) had scores between 0 and 1 (normal). None of 24 patients had elevations of the α-fetoprotein or β-subunit human chorionic gonadotropin levels. Of the 48 patients, 11 (23%) had a history of penicillin allergy.

The occurrence of varicocele in 29% of patients is 3 times the 9.5% incidence reported in the population at large. The occurrence of epididymal cysts in 13% and hypoplastic testes in 10% is considerably above the 5% and 1% incidences in 161 control patients, respectively. The incidence of cryptorchidism in the population at large is 0.3% to 0.7%. The incidence of monorchism in the population at large has been estimated as 1 in 5,000. Monorchism, rudimentary double urethral meatus, and hypoplastic glans do not appear to have been reported previously in association with diethylstilbestrol exposure in male subjects. Of 6 patients with Eliasson scores >10, 5 had significant genital tract abnormalities. All patients with an Eliasson score between 5 and 10 had genital abnormalities. Only 1 patient with normal semen had no genital abnormalities. It is recommended that all males exposed to diethylstilbestrol undergo urologic examination and semen analyses; a history of diethylstilbestrol exposure should be sought in patients with infertility or pathologic semen analyses of unknown etiology.

▶ [This study confirms earlier ones in demonstrating genital tract abnormalities in the male exposed in utero to diethylstilbestrol. One third of the patients tested had markedly abnormal semen analyses. Another report describing the effects of intrauterine

(7–20) J. Urol. 125:47–50, January 1981.

exposure to diethylstilbestrol on male offspring is included in the chapter on infertility.] ◄

7–21 **Oral Contraception and Congenital Abnormalities.** Pravin N. Kasan and Joan Andrews (St. David's Hosp., Cardiff) retrospectively investigated the relationship between oral contraceptives and congenital abnormalities in offspring of all women living in the city of Cardiff and the towns of Barry and Penarth in Wales who were delivered of a single child between January 1974 and June 1976. Comparison was made between those who used oral contraception in the 3 months before their last menstrual period or in early pregnancy, either by accident or by design (users, 27.3%), and those who had not taken oral contraceptives during this period (nonusers, 72.7%). It is not known how long the effects last after oral contraception has been discontinued. The significance of differences in findings between users and nonusers was tested by chi-square analysis. The 20- to 29-year age group accounted for 80% of all pill users and 62% of nonusers. There were greater numbers of nonusers among women aged 16–19 years and women older than 30 years of age. In the user group there was a preponderance of women in social class III. Users also smoked more than nonusers.

There were 81 (2.83%) infants with abnormalities among users and 225 (2.95%) among nonusers. There was no significant difference in the number of infants with one or more abnormalities born to users compared with those born to nonusers. There was no significant difference in the incidence of abnormality of the gastrointestinal tract, cardiovascular system, urogenital system, bones, muscle and connective tissue, or endocrine and hematologic system, or of microcephaly or cleft palate and harelip. There was no increase in the incidence of chromosomal abnormality among users. There were 18 (0.63%) infants with neural tube defects born to users, compared with 19 (0.25%) among nonusers. This difference is statistically significant.

There was no definite evidence found that the difference in incidence of neural tube defects was due to a third factor such as maternal age, parity, social class, or smoking habit. There is a known association between lower social class and increased incidence of neural tube defect, and this study shows a preponderance of pill users in social class III. Either oral contraception has an effect, or some unidentified factor associated with social class exists. Results suggest that the use of mechanical contraception be recommended for 2 to 3 months after elective cessation of oral contraception. There is an urgent need for coordinated prospective studies of the effect of oral contraception on subsequent offspring.

► [These results are generally reassuring. The "user" group included both patients with recent oral contraceptive use and those with inadvertent exposure in early pregnancy. Although neural tube defects were more common in users, the overall malformation rate was not. Users differed from nonusers in several respects, including smoking habits. It is too bad that the user group was not characterized by time of exposure to oral contraceptives, i.e., that prepregnancy use was not considered separately from that during pregnancy. Most recent studies have not found an association between

(7–21) Br. J. Obstet. Gynaecol. 87:545–551, July 1980.

recent oral contraceptive use and congenital malformations. For further consideration of the issue, read on.] ◄

7-22 **Relationship Between Hormonal Pregnancy Tests and Congenital Anomalies: Prospective Study.** Epidemiologic studies of the possible teratogenic effect of estrogen-progestogen preparations (EPP) given during pregnancy have yielded conflicting results. Claudine P. Torfs, Lucille Milkovich, and Bea J. van den Berg (Univ. of California, Berkeley) examined this possible relationship by reviewing longitudinal data from the Child Health and Development Studies, a prospective study of some 20,000 pregnancies in the San Francisco East Bay area. A total of 227 gravidas were tested for pregnancy with EPP. Controls had been tested with either a serum or a urine procedure. Gestest was used for hormone testing in about two thirds of study pregnancies. This preparation consists of 2.5 mg of norethindrone and 0.05 mg of ethinyl estradiol.

No significant differences were found in rates of severe congenital anomalies between the hormone test subjects and the two control groups. The relative risks and 95% confidence intervals were 1.01 (0.47 to 2.19) for the hormone-serum test comparison and 1.60 (0.60 to 4.18) for the hormone-urine test comparison. No clustering of any particular type of severe anomaly was observed. Among nonsevere anomalies, a higher rate of genitourinary tract defects was observed for male offspring in the hormone test group. The rate was 5.5/100 live births, compared with 3.1 for the serum test group and 1.2 for the urine test group.

This survey does not support the hypothesis that EPP, given for pregnancy testing, are associated with an excess of severe congenital anomalies. However, a small increase in congenital anomalies may have gone undetected. A possible weak association with genitourinary tract defects in male infants was observed. Because nonrisk pregnancy tests are now readily available, any further use of hormone pregnancy tests seems to be unwarranted.

► [Studies seem to be divided about equally on the question of teratogenicity of hormonal pregnancy tests. This one, which comes down on the negative side, is quite convincing because it is large, well designed, and well analyzed. Nevertheless, we do not believe there is currently any place for hormonal pregnancy tests, because other ways of answering the question are readily available and inexpensive. However, when a patient presents who, for one reason or another, has received an estrogen-progestin drug in early pregnancy, data such as these are helpful in counseling her. In such situations, we do not feel that a medical indication for abortion exists although we do tell the patient that there *may* be some slight increased risk of malformation.] ◄

7-23 **Vaginal Spermicides and Congenital Disorders.** Contraceptive methods that use vaginal spermicides have an appreciable failure rate, but little is known of the prevalence of abnormalities in conceptuses of women using spermicides near the time of conception. Hershel Jick, Alexander M. Walker, Kenneth J. Rothman, Judith R. Hunter, Lewis B. Holmes, Richard N. Watkins, Diane C. D'Ewart, Anne Danford, and Sue Madsen used the computerized records of the Group Health Cooperative in Seattle to study the prevalence of cer-

(7–22) Am. J. Epidemiol. 113:563–574, May 1981.
(7–23) JAMA 245:1329–1332, Apr. 3, 1981.

tain major congenital anomalies among 763 liveborn infants of white women who had filled a prescription for a vaginal spermicide (nonoxynol 9 in 20% and octoxynol in 80%) in the 10 months before conception and among 3,902 comparable infants of women who had not used spermicides.

Anomalies occurred in 2.2% of infants of mothers presumed to have used spermicides and in 1.0% of control infants (P = .002). The difference between these groups was due to an excess of limb reduction deformities, neoplasms (nesidioblastosis and medulloblastoma), chromosomal abnormalities (Down's syndrome), and hypospadias in infants whose mothers were presumed to have used vaginal spermicides. Pregnancies in women who had used vaginal spermicides ended in spontaneous abortion requiring hospitalization 1.8 times more commonly than did pregnancies in those who had not.

The data show a positive association between vaginal spermicide use and limb reduction deformities, neoplasms, chromosomal abnormalities, and hypospadias. However, because a well-defined syndrome among babies with congenital disorders whose mothers used spermicides was not present, these results should be considered to be tentative.

▶ [Roger A. Williamson, of the University of Iowa, reviewed this article at our request and commented as follows:

"Vaginal spermicides have an actual failure rate considerably in excess of the theoretical failure rate, which raises some question about usage patterns. Because of the known difficulties of patient recall, no attempt was made in this study to determine if those who had filled a prescription for a spermicide preparation actually used it, either preconceptually or inadvertently after conception. Another difficulty acknowledged by the authors was the absence of a well-defined syndrome suggestive of the degree of specificity common for the known teratogens. Instead, there was an increase in four general categories of congenital disorders and an increased incidence of spontaneous abortion requiring hospitalization. Nonetheless, an association was found and definitive studies are needed."] ◀

7–24 **Pregnancy Outcome Following Cancer Chemotherapy.** Most drugs used against human cancer cause malformations in laboratory animals, but little is known of the teratogenicity and mutagenicity of most drugs in human beings. Julie Blatt, John J. Mulvihill, John L. Ziegler, Robert C. Young, and David G. Poplack (Natl. Inst. of Health) studied the reproductive histories of 448 patients of childbearing age (10–45 years in female patients and at least 10 years in male patients) who are being or who have been treated with cancer chemotherapy.

Of 212 female patients, 23 had 30 pregnancies. Of 236 male patients, wives of 7 had 12 pregnancies. Diagnoses varied, but all patients received moderate to high doses of combination chemotherapy, including adriamycin (7 patients), cytoxan (11), methotrexate (12), vincristin (24), and prednisone (16). Two patients received immunoadjuvants. Only 1 received direct radiation to the abdomen or pelvis.

Of the 23 female patients, 19 (83%) conceived 1 month to 9 years (median, 4 years) after all chemotherapy was stopped, 1 was in the

(7–24) Am. J. Med. 69:828–832, December 1980.

second trimester of pregnancy when leukemia was diagnosed and chemotherapy begun, 1 was in the third trimester when leukemia recurred and therapy was reinstituted, and 2 conceived during treatment, which was continued for the first 2 months of gestation. Of the 7 male patients whose wives conceived, 2 were receiving chemotherapy at the time of conception, and although no formal paternity testing was done, the sperm count of 1 patient was normal just prior to conception.

Complications of pregnancy were toxemia (1 patient) and vaginal bleeding (1). Two spontaneous abortions occurred and 10 elective abortions were performed, all because of the risk of having an abnormal child after chemotherapy. None of the abortuses had obvious malformations.

Of the 42 pregnancies, 2 are continuing, 12 ended in abortion, and 28 ended in term births of single live infants with normal birth weights. At follow-up, the children were aged several days to 12 years (median, $2^{1}/_{2}$ years). Problems included bilateral pilonidal dimples without spina bifida in 1 infant, history of simple febrile convulsions in 1, skull fracture secondary to forceps trauma in 1, congenital hip dysplasia and fractured clavicle at birth in 1, and a capillary nevus in 1. Growth, development, and school performance were normal. There were no major abnormalities.

Chemotherapy administered to women prior to gestation or after the first trimester or to men at or prior to the time of conception does not appear to result in fetal damage.

▶ [The numbers here are too small to be reassuring, but what news there is is good. Four patients received intensive multiagent chemotherapy during pregnancy (two in the first trimester) and had healthy babies of normal size. Previous chemotherapy of either patient or husband wasn't associated with an excessive risk of congenital malformations. There have been case reports of malformations associated with chemotherapy in the first trimester, however, so advising patients in this situation is not easy.] ◀

7–25 **Prenatal Exposure to Synthetic Progestins Increases Potential for Aggression in Human Beings.** In most mammalian species, early androgenic stimulation is necessary for many characteristic male behaviors to develop in adulthood, and aggressive behaviors have been clearly shown to be hormonally mediated. Among human subjects, males exhibit more intraspecific aggressive behavior than do females. Many pregnant women have received progestins and estrogens for threatened abortion, and synthetic progestins may have some androgenic potential when given during pregnancy. June Machover Reinisch (Rutgers Univ.) evaluated 17 girls and 8 boys whose mothers received synthetic progestins for complications of current or previous pregnancies. Each was compared with at least 1 same-sexed sibling who had not been exposed to exogenous hormones. Mean age was about $11^{1}/_{2}$ years. Average total dose of synthetic progestin to which study subjects were exposed was 3,412 mg. Treatment always was begun in the first trimester.

The Leifer-Roberts Response Hierarchy was used to assess the po-

(7–25) Science 211:1171–1173, Mar. 13, 1981.

tential for aggressive behavior by eliciting verbal estimates of responses to a variety of common conflict situations. Exposure to progestins appeared to have a significant effect on the scores of both girls and boys, compared with their unexposed siblings. Twelve of 17 exposed girls and 7 of 8 exposed boys had higher scores than their sisters and brothers, respectively, for physical aggression. No differences in verbal aggression scores were observed. Aggression scores were not related to age or birth order. No IQ differences were found between exposed and unexposed siblings.

Verbal estimates of aggressive response appear to be enhanced in both males and females by prenatal exposure to synthetic progestins with androgenic potential. Whether the probability of choosing physically aggressive behavior in response to hypothetical conflict situations is related to aggressive action in real life situations is uncertain. Differences in frequency of aggressive behavior between males and females and also personal differences may be related to natural variations in hormone concentrations before birth.

▶ [This report notes that children, both male and female, exposed to synthetic progestins in utero exhibited more aggressive tendencies on psychological testing at age 6–18 years than did their unexposed siblings. The implication is that behavior can be "masculinized" by prenatal exposure to hormones with adrogenic action. Similar effects have been demonstrated in several experimental animals, including nonhuman primates.] ◀

7–26 **Danazol May Cause Female Pseudohermaphroditism.** Danazol, the 2,3-*d*-isoxazole derivative of 17α-ethinyltestosterone, is used for treatment of endometriosis in anticipation that the patient may become pregnant. In animals, danazol crosses the placenta and affects the fetus as would a compound with mild androgenic activity. Stephen C. Duck and E. Paul Katayama (Med. College of Wisconsin) evaluated a girl exposed to danazol in utero.

Woman, 27, began receiving danazol, 800 mg daily, on March 1, 1977, and found to be pregnant on May 10. Danazol therapy was stopped on June 9; a total of 81 gm had been ingested during 101 days. The mother had no evidence of virilization. A girl, born on November 10, was in the fifth percentile for height and weight. Mild clitoral enlargement and a urogenital sinus were evident. At age 2 years, height was 83.6 cm (25th percentile) and weight was 10.1 kg (fifth percentile). Physical findings of note were limited to the perineum: some clitoral enlargement; empty, darkened, rugated labia majora; complete urogenital sinus formation; normally positioned anus. Laboratory testing excluded other causes of first-trimester-dependent virilization: chromosomes, 46 XX (Q-banded); serum 17-hydroxyprogesterone level, under 15 ng/dl; androstenedione level, under 5 ng/dl; testosterone, 26 ng/dl; luteinizing hormone, 3.7 mIU/ml; and renin activity, 6.8 ng/ml/hour. Radiography showed a bone age of 21 months; genitogram revealed a large vagina with separate urethral orifice. Well-formed prepuberal cervix, uterus, fallopian tubes, and ovaries (2 × 1 cm) were seen at laparotomy.

Androgenic side effects of danazol are dose related. The "anabolic" to "androgenic" ratio is greater than unity. In human beings, danazol partially inhibits the 3β-hydroxysteroid dehydrogenase-Δ^{4-5}-isomerase complex, 11β-hydroxylase enzymes, and the fetal adrenal 21-hy-

(7–26) Fertil. Steril. 35:230–231, February 1981.

droxylase enzyme; resultant increases in dehydroepiandrosterone and Δ^4-androstenedione levels could contribute to fetal virilization. The human fetus is exquisitely sensitive to androgen excess, particularly during the first trimester. A combination of danazol's direct and indirect androgenic effects probably accounted for the patient's findings. The absence of marked clitoral enlargement reflected absence of an androgenic effect during the last two trimesters of pregnancy. From this case, it is recommended that danazol therapy be initiated on about the fifth day of the normal menstrual cycle. Pregnancy tests should be carried out 6 and 8 weeks after initiation of therapy. If a pregnancy test is positive, danazol therapy should be discontinued immediately.

▶ [Although anovulation is expected with danazol treatment and therefore pregnancy during therapy should be uncommon, this report reminds us that the drug is a weak androgen and that inadvertent exposure of a female fetus in the first trimester may result in virilization of the external genitalia. Pregnancy should be ruled out before treatment with danazol is initiated.] ◀

7–27 **Vascular Pathogenesis of Gastroschisis: Intrauterine Interruption of the Omphalomesenteric Artery.** Gastroschisis is a specific defect of the abdominal wall that allows extrusion of abdominal contents without involving the umbilical cord. It has been postulated that most cases of gastroschisis are the result of an intrauterine vascular accident that involves the omphalomesenteric artery, with subsequent disruption of the umbilical ring and herniation of the abdominal contents. H. Eugene Hoyme, Marilyn C. Higginbottom, and Kenneth L. Jones reviewed patient records from a 10-year period to identify all children with gastroschisis and to determine the incidence and nature of associated structural anomalies that may share the same etiology and pathogenesis as gastroschisis.

Of 26 cases of gastroschisis, 10 were associated with a structural defect. Except for bilateral hydronephrosis in 1 child, all the associated abnormalities involved the absence or disruption of structure. Most of the associated defects showed strong clinical and experimental evidence of having resulted from an in utero vascular accident. Nonduodenal intestinal atresia or stenosis was found in 3 patients, atresia of the appendix in 1, "apple peel" bowel in 2, and porencephaly in 1. Atresia of the gallbladder and absence of one kidney were present in 1 patient each.

It is hypothesized that intrauterine disruption of the omphalomesenteric artery leads to infarction and necrosis of the base of the umbilical cord, herniation of the gut through this area, and healing and resorption of the tissue on the margins of the defect. Paired omphalomesenteric arteries arise in early gestation as a plexus of smaller vessels from the dorsal aorta (Fig 7–3). Through cell death and rearrangement of vascular connections, the left omphalomesenteric artery disappears, while the right artery persists. The proximal portion of the right omphalomesenteric artery becomes the superior mesenteric artery and follows, distally, the omphalomesenteric duct through the umbilical ring. The midgut is normally herniated into

---

(7–27) J. Pediatr. 98:228–231, February 1981.

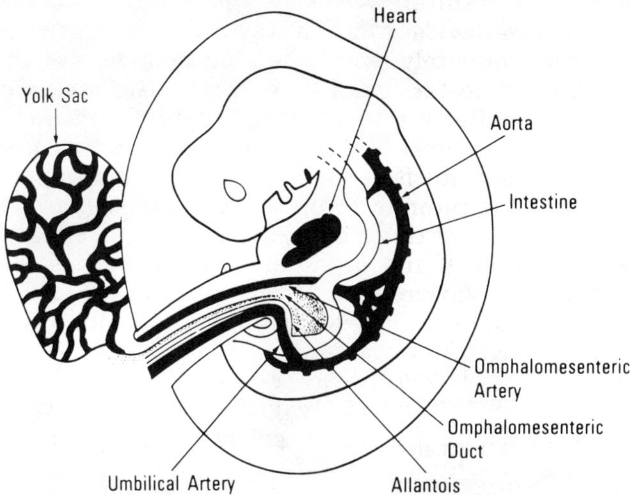

Fig 7–3.—Diagrammatic representation of sagittal view of human embryo (32 days), 5-mm crown-rump length. Arteries are shown in black; the extraembryonic coelom and peritoneal cavity are stippled; veins have been deleted. (Courtesy of Hoyme, H. E., et al.: J. Pediatr. 98:228–231, February 1981.) (Adapted from Cullen, T. S.: *Embryology, Anatomy, and Diseases of the Umbilicus.* Philadelphia, W. B. Saunders Co., 1916.)

the extraembryonic coelom between weeks 6 and 10 of gestation. The extraembryonic coelom, which contains the "herniated" gut and the omphalomesenteric duct and vessels, comprises the right portion of the umbilical ring and is continuous with the peritoneal cavity. By the end of week 10, the intestine returns to the peritoneal cavity. The omphalomesenteric vessels course through the small remnant of extraembryonic coelom that persists at the right of the base of the umbilical cord. Interruption of the superior mesenteric artery leads to gastroschisis and intestinal atresia or stenosis, as well as many other associated defects. Any defect seen in association with gastroschisis, porencephaly, or intestinal atresia should raise the question of a possible vascular pathogenesis.

▶ [This is an interesting speculation. Ten of 26 cases of gastroschisis had associated malformations, most of which were thought to be associated with a vascular accident during development. The authors propose that gastroschisis results from disruption of the omphalomesenteric artery, causing infarction and necrosis of the base of the cord and herniation of the gut through the defect. The more proximal the interruption, the more likely are associated malformations such as intestinal atresia or stenosis.] ◀

7–28 **Compression-Related Defects From Early Amnion Rupture: Evidence for Mechanical Teratogenesis.** Non-band-related limb defects are thought to be caused by intrauterine compression. Marvin E. Miller, John M. Graham, Jr., Marilyn C. Higginbottom, and David W. Smith obtained evidence that the structural defects pleurosomus, a lateral body wall deficiency with an ipsilateral upper limb deficiency, and cyllosomus, a lateral body wall deficiency with an ipsilateral lower limb deficiency, result from intrauterine compression caused by early amnion rupture.

(7–28) J. Pediatr. 98:292–297, February 1981.

Ten new cases of limb-body wall deficiency and 17 reported cases were reviewed. The sex distribution was about equal. In the 21 cases with lateral body wall deficiency, the affected side was the same as that of the major limb deficiency. Severe scoloisis was present in 19 of 26 cases; the convexity usually was toward the same side as the limb and body wall defects. Neural tube defects ranged from a membrane-covered encephalocele or skin-covered meningocele to complete absence of the calvarium and brain. All 8 open cranial defects were associated with major upper limb deficiencies and upper body wall deficiencies. Three of 4 lumbar meningoceles were associated with major lower limb deficiencies and abdominal wall deficiencies. A short umbilical cord was a consistent finding. Amniotic bands or placental adhesions, or both, were found in 41% of cases. Postural deformations, usually of the feet, were common. Prenatal growth deficiency was noted in 15 of 16 evaluable cases. Early death was invariable. In live-born infants, respiratory insufficiency was the chief cause of death. Chromosome studies were negative in all 9 cases evaluated. No maternal exposure to known teratogens was noted, and there was no history of recurrence in any of the families.

Early amnion rupture, acting through compression from the loss of amniotic fluid, appears to be the cause of non-band-related defects in cases of limb-body wall deficiency. The scoliosis and postural deformities result from prolonged intrauterine constraint. Ultrasonographic recognition of limb-body wall deficiency before birth could prevent unnecessary cesarean births.

▶ [Limb malformations including amputations due to entanglement of the fetal limb with an amniotic band have been recognized for several years. The authors of this report make a good case for what they call "the amnion rupture sequence." Limb and lateral abdominal wall defects are thought to result from compression secondary to the early loss of (or failure to produce) sufficient amniotic fluid to cushion the embryo. Amniotic bands, as such, may not be identified. The umbilical cord is very short in these cases. The importance of all of this is that one apparently is dealing with a sporadic event without a genetic basis. Therefore, couples can be reassured that the recurrence risk in such situations is very low.] ◀

7–29 **Follow-up of Methadone-Treated and Untreated Narcotic-Dependent Women and Their Infants: Health, Developmental, and Social Implications.** Programs providing methadone treatment have improved the use of medical and supportive services by narcotic-dependent pregnant women and reduced obstetric risks, but a more severe and prolonged neonatal abstinence syndrome has been described in infants of methadone-treated women. Geraldine S. Wilson, Murdina M. Desmond and Raymond B. Wait (Baylor College of Medicine, Houston), compared the health, neurodevelopmental course, and home evironment in the first postnatal year for infants of methadone-treated women, those of other narcotic-dependent women, and those of drug-free women. The 68 narcotic-dependent women in the study gave birth to 69 live-born infants. Thirty-nine were born to methadone-treated mothers and 30 to untreated heroin-dependent women. Fifty-seven drug-free mothers were delivered of 58 infants.

(7–29) J. Pediatr. 98:716–722, May 1981.

The mean duration of methadone maintenance before delivery was 15 months. The average duration of addiction was 6.2 years.

The rate of prenatal care among methadone-treated women was significantly greater than for untreated drug-dependent women, but the former subjects continued to use a variety of psychoactive drugs, both illicit and prescribed. Prenatal and intrapartum risk scores were comparable in the various groups. Neonatal abstinence syndrome lasted longer in the methadone-treated group. Neonatal infections were more frequent in this group than in drug-free control subjects. Medical problems in the first year of life were comparable in the drug-exposed and drug-free groups. Infants in the methadone group often cried excessively and had trouble sleeping. Psychomotor development was normal in the methadone group but lower than in the untreated group. Fine motor coordination was poorer than in drug-free control subjects. Eighty percent of methadone infants were living with their parents at age 1 year, while 48% of untreated drug-dependent women had relinquished responsibility for their child's care.

The greatest benefit of methadone treatment may be the mother's ongoing involvement in the care of her child. Methadone-treated mothers compare favorably with drug-free women on ratings of family stability, and their children do not appear to be at an increased risk of abuse or deprivation in the first year of life.

▶ [The data from the neonatal period didn't indicate differences between the methadone-treated drug-dependent group and the untreated drug-dependent group. At age 1 year, infants of methadone-treated women were more apt to be living with their parent(s) than were the offspring of untreated mothers. This undoubtedly partly reflects underlying differences between those addicted women who chose methadone programs and those who did not. The most interesting " real world" finding reported here is that 92% of the methadone-treated women used other psychoactive drugs (often illicit ones) during pregnancy. Indeed, two thirds of them used heroin!] ◀

7-30 **Alcohol, Smoking, and Incidence of Spontaneous Abortions in First and Second Trimester.** S. Harlap and P. H. Shiono examined the incidence of spontaneous fetal loss at different stages of pregnancy in 32,019 women who completed a questionnaire on alcohol use at their first antenatal visit. Outcomes of pregnancy were ascertained by surveillance of hospital admissions. Of the women participating, 51.7% reported drinking no alcohol in early pregnancy; 44.7% had less than 1 drink daily; and 2.4%, 0.4%, and 0.1% had averages of 1–2, 3–5, or more than 6 drinks daily, respectively. Because drinkers began antenatal care later than did nondrinkers, results were analyzed with life-table methods. The number of women under observation (at risk) each day was calculated from the number who had started antenatal care prior to that day minus those whose pregnancies had already terminated.

Life-table analysis showed that the age-adjusted relative risks of second-trimester losses (15–27 weeks) were 1.03 (not significant: ns), 1.98 (P <.01), and 3.53 (P <.01), respectively, for women having less than 1, 1–2, and more than 3 drinks daily, compared with nondrinkers. The corresponding relative risks for first trimester losses (5–14

(7–30) Lancet 2:173–176, July 26, 1980.

weeks) were 1.12 (ns), 1.15 (ns), and 1.15, respectively. Smokers had relative risks of 1.01 (ns) and 1.21 (ns) in the first and second trimesters, respectively, compared with nonsmokers. The increased risk of second-trimester miscarriage in drinkers was not explained by age, parity, race, marital status, smoking, or number of previous spontaneous or induced abortions.

Alcohol use tends to be correlated with smoking. An examination of the combined effects of smoking and drinking on second-trimester losses showed that regular drinkers had a higher incidence of miscarriages in all smoking groups. Within categories of drinkers the effect of smoking per se was weak and inconsistent. The independent effects of both drinking and smoking were confirmed in a linear multiple-regression analysis. Based on regression results, about 69 (10%) of 690 second-trimester abortions were attributed to the effects of drinking or smoking.

These results suggest that alcohol may harm human fetuses not only when it is abused, but also when it is taken in moderation. The findings should not be taken to imply with certainty that alcohol has no effect in the first trimester. The women who initiated antenatal care early in pregnancy (and therefore entered the study early) would have been a selected group and perhaps at higher risk for miscarriage. Therefore, findings for early pregnancy may contain biases which could invalidate the conclusions drawn about first-trimester alcohol effects.

7–31 **Drinking During Pregnancy and Spontaneous Abortion.** Jennie Kline, Patrick Shrout, Zena Stein, Mervyn Susser, and Dorothy Warburton (Columbia Univ.) compared the drinking habits before and during pregnancy of 616 women who aborted spontaneously (cases) with those of 632 women who delivered after at least 28 weeks' gestation (controls). The amount and type of alcohol, frequency of drinking, and time of exposure were considered. The cases comprised a consecutive series of women having spontaneous abortions, the data being collected from three Manhattan hospitals between 1974 and 1978. Overall, 17.0% of the cases, compared to 8.1% of controls, reported drinking twice a week or more during pregnancy. The hypothesis that drinking during pregnancy is associated with spontaneous abortion was tested by maximum-likelihood logistic regression analysis. The adjusted-odds ratio for this association was 2.62. It was estimated that more than 25% of pregnant women drinking twice a week or more are likely to abort, compared with about 14% of women who drink less often. Consideration of wine, beer, and spirits separately suggested that the minimum harmful dosage was 1 oz of absolute alcohol. Several potentially confounding variables, including maternal age, gestation, prior spontaneous abortions, smoking habits, and the occurrence of nausea or vomiting were controlled in the analysis. The association between drinking during pregnancy and spontaneous abortion did not vary with consideration of these factors.

(7–31) Lancet 2:176–180, July 26, 1980.

Even moderate consumption of alcohol during pregnancy is a risk factor for, and may be a cause of, spontaneous abortion. Karyotype analyses, recently completed, showed that drinking during pregnancy was associated with the abortion of euploid, and not aneuploid, conceptions. Drinking during pregnancy could bring about spontaneous abortion by acting as a teratogen, abortifacient, or fetotoxin, of which the latter seems most likely. The association between drinking and spontaneous abortion was unrelated to gestation at abortion, and mean gestational age did not vary among cases; therefore, it is unlikely that teratogenesis is the primary mechanism. Because there was no coincidence in timing of spontaneous abortion shortly after episodes of drinking, alcohol is not likely to act as an abortifacient. Rather, the results suggest that alcohol is mainly an acute fetotoxin and that the developing fetus is highly sensitive throughout the first and second trimesters.

▶ [This study and the one discussed in the preceding article (one prospective and one retrospective) suggest that moderate alcohol consumption in pregnancy is associated with an increased risk of spontaneous abortion (limited to the second trimester in the first study). The enormous difficulties in the interpretation of these data are apparent (recall bias, unappreciated covariables, inaccurate reporting of alcohol intake, etc.). Despite these limitations, it would seem prudent to advise women to drink very little, if at all, during pregnancy.] ◀

7–32 **Decreased Birth Weight in Infants of Alcoholic Women Who Abstained During Pregnancy.** Fetal alcohol syndrome is characterized by prenatal and postnatal growth deficiency, mental retardation, and a characteristic pattern of malformation. Ruth E. Little, Ann Pytkowicz Streissguth, Helen M. Barr, and Cynthia S. Herman (Univ. of Washington, Seattle) retrospectively interviewed three groups of women: (1) 50 who had a history of alcoholism prior to conception of the study child who reported abstinence during the entire pregnancy, (2) 50 who had a history of alcoholism prior to conception of the study child and reported heavy drinking during pregnancy; and (3) 50 with no history of alcoholism who were essentially abstinent during pregnancy (mean daily ethanol intake less than 0.1 oz).

The mean birth weight of children born to abstinent alcoholic mothers was 258 gm less than the mean birth weight of children born to controls; in the heavy drinking group, the mean birth weight of the infants was 493 gm below that of the controls. These differences in birth weight were statistically significant after adjusting for maternal smoking, height, age, and parity as well as gestational age and sex of the child. The mean birth weight in the control group was high (3,391 gm) considering that 74% of the mothers were smokers; however, it is comparable to birth weights reported in other series in which alcohol use was minimal. It is possible that mean birth weights in the three groups may reflect differences in maternal characteristics not evident in the group profiles. A self-selection bias and diet are other factors that could account for these differences. However, abstaining alcoholics had a high mean level of education and 90% were of at least lower-middle socioeconomic status; thus, it is not likely that they could not afford an adequate diet.

The reduction in birth weight of children of abstinent alcoholics is important because it suggests that there may be lasting reproductive impairment associated with a history of alcohol abuse. The biologic nature of such impairment can only be hypothesized, but certainly liver function may be involved. There is evidence that cirrhosis tends to develop earlier and with lower doses of alcohol in women than in men. Onset of other diseases also may be accelerated. The decrements in birth weight observed in this study are not explained by differences in demographic variables or tobacco use. The findings suggest that a history of maternal alcoholism as well as heavy drinking may pose a risk to optimal development of the fetus.

► [Abstinent alcoholics, although delivering heavier babies than drinking alcoholics, had lighter babies than control women. It is too bad that data concerning maternal weight at the start of pregnancy and weight gain during pregnancy were not considered here. As we have stated elsewhere, this is a difficult subject to study; solid answers are hard to come by.] ◄

7–33 **Immune Deficiency in Fetal Alcohol Syndrome.** There is increasing awareness of a distinct dysmorphic phenotype termed fetal alcohol syndrome (FAS). A high frequency of acquired overt infectious diseases has been observed among affected children. Sharron Johnson, Richard Knight, Daniel J. Marmer, and Russell W. Steele reviewed 13 documented cases of FAS in subjects aged 1 to $10^{1/2}$ years. All had most of the clinical features characterizing FAS and a history of excessive maternal alcohol consumption. Thirteen age- and sex-matched normal children also were evaluated, and since most FAS patients were small for gestational age (SGA), 13 control SGA patients also were studied. Placental insufficiency was responsible in all instances.

Both an increased incidence of life-threatening bacterial infection and a propensity to minor infections were found in the FAS group (table). Clinical infections could not be correlated with degree of immune deficiency. Absolute lymphocyte counts, E rosettes, and responses to mitogen stimulation were depressed in the FAS group, but

INFECTIOUS DISEASES EXPERIENCED BY 13 INFANTS AND CHILDREN WITH FAS

Infectious process	No. affected
Sepsis	1
Meningitis	2
Soft tissue infection *	3
Pneumonia	5
Other infection †	6
Recurrent otitis media	9
Frequent upper respiratory infection	11

*Cellulitis, abscesses, or impetigo.
†Urinary tract infection, gastroenteritis, or monilial diaper rash.

(7–33) Pediatr. Res. 15:908–911, June 1981.

skin reactivity to recall antigens was not. Decreased numbers of lymphocytes could be attributed to intrauterine growth retardation alone. The absolute number of B lymphocytes was significantly lower in FAS children than in either control group. Nine FAS children had abnormal immunoglobulin concentrations; decreased IgA was most common. Total hemolytic complement was normal in all subjects. Absolute neutrophil counts were similar in the various groups, as was endotoxin-stimulated nitroblue tetrazolium dye reduction, but absolute numbers of eosinophils were increased in the FAS group.

Children with FAS appear to have a greatly increased susceptibility to both life-threatening and minor infections. Numerous immune deficiencies were identified in the present population. If these deficiencies persist into adulthood, other conditions associated with immune defects such as neoplastic and autoimmune processes might be anticipated.

▶ [This study found evidence of immune deficiency on several tests (E rosette-forming lymphocytes, EAC rosette-forming lymphocytes, stimulation response to mitogens, dysgammaglobulinemia, and eosinophilia) in infants and children with the fetal alcohol syndrome. As indicated in the table, the subjects seemed to have histories of unusually frequent infection. It would not be particularly surprising if the fetal alcohol syndrome has functional as well as morphological components.] ◀

7–34 **Influence of Maternal Cigarette Smoking During Pregnancy on Fetal and Childhood Growth.** It has been reported widely that the offspring of cigarette smokers are mildly growth retarded in comparison with the offspring of nonsmokers. Among the possible mechanisms that may be associated with growth retardation are suboptimal maternal food intake during pregnancy, low pregravid body weight, carboxyhemoglobin-induced fetal hypoxia, reduced uteroplacental perfusion, genetic differences between smokers and nonsmokers, and maternal hypotension during pregnancy. Richard L. Naeye (Pennsylvania State Univ.) analyzed the data from a major prospective study of 8,193 pregnancies for clues to the mechanisms responsible for impaired fetal growth associated with maternal cigarette smoking.

The infants of women who smoked during pregnancy had lower body weights than the infants of women who had never smoked (Fig 7–4). Body lengths and head circumferences also were affected. The degree of growth retardation increased with the number of cigarettes smoked and was independent of pregravid weight for height and net pregnancy weight gain. Growth retardation was also evident in intrapair comparisons of siblings whose mothers had smoked in one, but not both, of their pregnancies. In these paired pregnancies, there were no significant differences in the sex ratio of infants, mean neonatal hemoglobin levels, maternal age, maternal hemoglobin levels, intervals between pregnancies, or socioeconomic status. Thus, genetic factors would not appear to explain growth retardation. Although birth weights were somewhat less for infants whose mothers had stopped smoking during pregnancy than for those whose mothers never smoked, growth retardation was not apparent. A small degree

(7–34) Obstet. Gynecol. 57:18–21, January 1981.

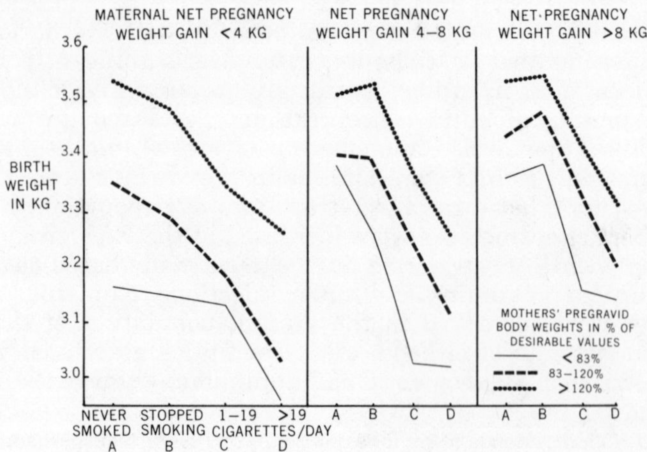

Fig 7–4.—Effects of maternal cigarette smoking on birth weights of full-term white infants. Lines represent mothers' pregravid body weights in percent of desirable values; *solid line,* less than 83%; *broken line,* 83–120%; *dotted line,* more than 120%. (Coutesy of Naeye, R. L.: Obstet. Gynecol. 57:18–21, January 1981.)

of growth retardation was evident at 7 years of age in the offspring of mothers who smoked. Stratification of the data by peak maternal diastolic blood pressures, socioeconomic status, birth order, and maternal age had virtually no effect on fetal and childhood growth retardation associated with smoking.

The results confirm previous reports that infants of women who smoke are smaller at birth than infants of nonsmokers. The results also suggest that growth retardation associated with smoking is independent of maternal undernutrition, genetic factors, and reduced uteroplacental perfusion.

▶ [Based on data from more than 8,000 pregnancies, Figure 7–4 nicely demonstrates again that the adverse effect of maternal smoking on birth weight is apparently independent of dietary intake or nutritional status. Smoking exerted an effect regardless of maternal prepregnancy weight or weight gain during pregnancy. Uterine arterial vasoconstriction secondary to nicotine or impaired oxygen transport secondary to elevated carboxy-hemoglobin levels, or both, probably is involved.] ◀

7-35 **Smoking in Pregnancy: Associations With Skin-fold Thickness, Maternal Weight Gain, and Fetal Size at Birth.** Smoking during pregnancy is associated with a reduction in the baby's birth weight. A fall in maternal weight gain also is noted, suggesting that the adverse effects are due to maternal nutritional deficiency. S. W. D'Souza, Patricia Black, and B. Richards (Manchester, England) examined the effects of smoking during pregnancy on skin-fold thickness, maternal weight gain, and fetal size at birth in a series of 452 women who attended antenatal clinics at St. Mary's Hospital. All had normal singleton pregnancies; age range was 19–35 years. They had no history of stillbirth. The nonsmokers, light to moderate smokers

(7–35) Br. Med. J. 282:1661–1663, May 23, 1981.

(1–14 cigarettes daily), and heavy smokers were comparable in age, height, parity, and duration of pregnancy.

Nonsmokers gained 60 mg a week more than the heavy smokers. Triceps and subscapular skin-fold thicknesses were lower in smokers than in nonsmokers, but the differences were not significant. Infants of nonsmokers were heavier, longer, and had larger head circumferences than those born to heavy smokers. Most values for infants of light to moderate smokers were intermediate. Lower birth weights were noted for heavy smokers in all social class groups.

Smoking in pregnancy appears to be associated with a general retardation in intrauterine growth. However, in this study, skin-fold thickness was not affected in infants of women who smoked. These infants resembled constitutionally small, growth-retarded babies rather than truly undernourished infants. It seems unlikely that smoking restricts fetal growth mainly through undernutrition. The effect might well be due to fetal hypoxia caused by some constituent of tobacco smoke, probably carbon monoxide. In any case, the adverse effects are reduced when mothers give up smoking.

▶ [Several articles in recent years have examined the relationship in cigarette smokers between weight gain in pregnancy and birth weight of the offspring. Most investigators have concluded that the growth retardation associated with smoking is not based on inadequate maternal nutrition. Although the approach here is indirect, the failure to find a difference in skin-fold thickness between infants of smoking mothers and infants of nonsmoking mothers is consistent with the majority opinion.] ◀

7–36 **Effect of Maternal Cigarette Smoking on Apgar Scores.** Many adverse effects of cigarette smoking during pregnancy have emerged in recent years, including restriction of fetal growth and increased frequency of prematurity. Stanley M. Garn, Michael Johnston, Stephen A. Ridella, and Audrey S. Petzold (Univ. of Michigan) obtained data on maternal cigarette smoking in pregnancy and on 1- and 5-minute Apgar scores in 43,492 pregnancies yielding live-born singleton infants in the National Collaborative Perinatal Project.

Successively higher levels of maternal cigarette smoking were associated with increased percentages of "low" or "depressed" Apgar scores in both blacks and whites, and for both the 1- and 5-minute scores. A nearly fourfold rise in low scores was associated with the smoking of two packs or more a day. Results were similar when only gestations of 38 weeks and longer were analyzed.

Maternal cigarette use during pregnancy is strikingly related to the proportion of low or depressed Apgar scores in the newborn infants. Smoking of two to three packs a day is associated with a near-quadrupling of low and depressed Apgar scores, even when premature infants are excluded. The elevated hemoglobin concentrations found in these infants and the finding of elevated carbon monoxide concentrations in cord blood suggest that the depressed Apgar scores may reflect prenatal carbon monoxide poisoning. An increase in intensity of smoking may act to offset any changes in cigarette manufacturing,

---

(7–36) Am. J. Dis. Child. 135:503–506, June 1981.

such as the use of low-tar and low-nicotine tobaccos and more effective filters.

▶ [These data provide further evidence, if any is needed, of the adverse effects of smoking during pregnancy. Using the data base of the Collaborative Perinatal Project, these investigators found a dose-response relationship between maternal smoking and low Apgar scores at both 1 and 5 minutes. It is well known that smoking is associated with decreased birth size and increased placental size. Taken together, these observations point to chronic fetal hypoxia as the mechanism.] ◀

8. The Puerperium

⁸⁻¹ **1980 Update: Recent Trend in Breast-Feeding.** Gilbert A. Martinez and John P. Nalezienski (Ross Labs., Columbus, Ohio) reviewed surveys conducted from 1955 to 1979 to identify trends in breast-feeding compared with the feeding of whole cow's milk (WCM)-evaporated milk (EM) and commercial formulas. Questionnaires were sent to a sample of about 47,000 mothers in 1979, and replies were received from 57%. The incidence of breast-feeding was seen to have risen in 1979 at all infant ages, continuing the trend observed since 1971. Breast-feeding in hospitals more than doubled during this period. The change was most marked in younger groups. Among infants aged 5 to 6 months, the use of WCM-EM declined and that of prepared infant formulas increased, primarily because of the use of iron-fortified formulas. Breast-feeding in hospitals increased in all United States census regions in 1979. The highest rate was in mothers with some college education and higher family incomes, but rapid increases were shown by women with less education.

The trend toward an increase in breast-feeding continued in 1979. The increase has occurred at all infant ages, in all parts of the United States, and in all demographic groups examined. The use of iron-fortified formulas also has increased at all infant ages. The increase in breast-feeding has not been restricted to mothers from higher socioeconomic levels.

▶ [This survey documents the increasing popularity of breast-feeding in the United States. Before we feel too sorry for the nice folks at the formula companies, however, we should note that formula feeding of infants at 5 to 6 months of age is on the increase, at the expense of whole cow's milk and evaporated milk. Both of these trends are probably desirable.] ◀

⁸⁻² **Effect of Nursing on Neurohypophyseal Hormone and Prolactin Secretion in Human Subjects.** Although nursing is known to stimulate oxytocin (OT) secretion, the specificity of the suckling response has not been confirmed by sensitive radioimmunoassay measurements of arginine vasopressin (AVP). Using highly specific radioimmunoassay systems, Richard E. Weitzman, Rosemary D. Leake, Robert T. Rubin, and Delbert A. Fisher (Harbor-UCLA Med. Center, Torrance, Calif.) measured the plasma OT, AVP, and serum prolactin responses to nursing in 6 normal women 2 to 3 days postpartum. Blood samples were obtained for radioimmunoassay 3 and 0 minutes before nursing, at 3-minute intervals during nursing for 15 minutes, and 5 minutes after nursing was completed. Six women who were not nursing during the postpartum period served as controls.

During nursing, plasma OT levels increased from a mean baseline

---

(8–1) Pediatrics 67:260–263, February 1981.
(8–2) J. Clin. Endocrinol. Metab. 51:836–839, October 1980.

value of 1.1 ± 0.2 to 3.6 ± 0.6 μU/ml at 3 minutes, peaked at 6.4 ± 1.5 μU/ml at 6 minutes, remained above baseline values for the remainder of the 15-minute nursing period and then returned to, or close to, baseline values 5 minutes later. There was no evidence of variations in OT concentrations suggestive of pulsatile episodic secretion. No change in plasma AVP concentrations was noted in either the nursing mothers or controls. This was also the case for mean plasma osmolality and plasma sodium concentration. After 15 minutes of nursing, plasma prolactin levels rose from a mean baseline value of 268 ± 24 to 362 ± 31 ng/ml. Apparently, nursing is a specific stimulus for OT and prolactin release but has no effect on the release of AVP.

▶ [These investigators found nursing during the early puerperium to be associated with prompt oxytocin release, more gradual prolactin secretion, and no change in vasopressin levels. These results with respect to oxytocin differ somewhat from those reported by Lucas and associates (*Br. Med. J.* 281:834, 1980), who found that an oxytocin response did not always occur during established lactation. A positive association between oxytocin release and multiparity was found. The following article discusses a therapeutic application of these findings.] ◀

8–3 **A Dose-Response Relation Between Improved Lactation and Metoclopramide.** Many mothers are unable to breast-feed their infants because lactation does not become established or stops too soon. Such women may be deficient in prolactin, the chief hormonal mediator of milk secretion. Antti Kauppila, Seppo Kivinen, and Olavi Ylikorkala (Univ. of Oulu) evaluated metoclopramide, an antidopaminergic prolactin secretion-stimulating agent, in a placebo-controlled crossover study of 37 puerperal women with inadequate breast milk production in the first 2 months after delivery. All had an average yield of breast milk at least 30% less than the estimated normal intake. Metoclopramide was given in a dose of 5, 10, or 15 mg 3 times daily for 2 weeks, and a placebo was given for another 2 weeks.

Significant increases in maternal serum prolactin levels occurred with the higher doses of metoclopramide. These doses also increased the milk yield significantly and reduced the amount of supplementary feeding necessary. The larger dose produced an effect more rapidly. Nine of the 27 women given 30 or 45 mg of metoclopramide daily were able to stop giving supplementary feeds. The response was similar in the first, second, and third to fourth months after delivery. The initial serum prolactin level did not correlate with the lactational response. Nearly half of the mothers wished to continue the preferred medication, which in every instance was metoclopramide. Seven women reported side effects, and an infant of a mother given 45 mg daily had intestinal discomfort. Three women had similar side effects during placebo intake.

Treatment with 30–45 mg of metoclopramide daily improved milk secretion in mothers with lactational insufficiency. A rise in serum prolactin level probably was responsible. Breast milk is considered preferable to formula in the first weeks of life. Metoclopramide may be particularly indicated for mothers with a family history of allergy. The risk of serious side effects appears to be negligible. It is not clear

---

(8–3) Lancet 1:1175–1177, May 30, 1981.

whether the drug is absorbed sufficiently to stimulate prolactin secretion in the infant.

▶ [Metoclopramide stimulates prolactin secretion and, as indicated by this study, can increase milk output substantially. A dose of 10 mg three times daily increased milk yield by 40%, decreased the need for supplemental feeding, and improved infant weight gain. This approach has obvious therapeutic implications for the woman whose milk supply seems inadequate. Before it can be used clinically, however, much more work is needed to establish safety.] ◀

8–4 Prostacyclin, Thromboxane, and Prostaglandin $F_{2\alpha}$ in Maternal Plasma During Breast-Feeding. Animal and human studies have suggested a role for some classic prostaglandins in lactogenesis or milk ejection. O. Ylikorkala and L. Viinikka (Univ. of Oulu), measured levels of the stable metabolites of the prostanoids with smooth muscle cell activity, prostacyclin, thromboxane A_2, and prostaglandin $F_{2\alpha}$ in the plasma of 11 women before, during, and after nursing in the early puerperium. The respective metabolites estimated were 6-keto-prostaglandin $F_{1\alpha}$ (6-keto-PGF$_{1\alpha}$), thromboxane B_2, and 13,14-dihydro-15-keto-PGF$_{2\alpha}$ (M-PGF$_{2\alpha}$). The women, aged 21–32 years, all had vaginal delivery of healthy infants, and lactation had begun normally. Studies were done 4–5 days post partum. The metabolite levels were estimated by radioimmunoassay.

The presence of the infant on the breast without suckling caused no changes in prostanoid levels, but suckling was associated with a decrease in M-PGF$_{2\alpha}$ level from 254 to 204 pg/ml. The level returned to 235 pg/ml 1 hour after the end of nursing. A significant fall in 6-keto-PGF$_{2\alpha}$ level was noted after 15 minutes of nursing, but there were no changes in the thromboxane B_2 level.

The finding of a decrease in the M-PGF$_{2\alpha}$ level in maternal plasma during suckling is in accord with a report that administration of PGF$_{2\alpha}$ inhibits milk ejection in lactating rats. The relatively high amount of PGF$_{2\alpha}$ present before suckling may keep milk in the breast and may inhibit further lactogenesis, which could resume after the PGF$_{2\alpha}$ level has decreased following milk ejection. The production of prostacyclin in the maternal vascular bed may decrease with the increased secretion of oxytocin and prolactin during suckling. Repeated reductions in production of prostacyclin during suckling might contribute to the frequent occurrence of thromboembolic complications in the puerperium.

▶ [From these findings that metabolites of prostaglandin $F_{2\alpha}$ and prostacyclin decrease with suckling, it appears that prostanoids should be added to prolactin and oxytocin as humoral substances involved in lactation.] ◀

8–5 Effect of Modification of Fluid Intake in the Puerperium on Serum Prolactin Levels and Lactation. Lactating women sometimes are advised to take considerable fluids, whereas fluid restriction may be advised to suppress lactation. Impaired lactation has been attributed to excessive water drinking. If such effects exist, they may represent prolactin responses to osmotic stimuli. M. Horowitz, G. D. Higgins, J. J. Graham, Helen Berriman, and P. E. Harding (Adelaide,

(8–4)   Am. J. Obstet. Gynecol. 139:690–692, Mar. 15, 1981.
(8–5)   Med. J. Aust. 2:625–626, Nov. 29, 1980.

Australia) examined the effects of physiologic variations in fluid intake on prolactin secretion and milk yield in the puerperium.

Twenty-one multiparas were assigned to fluid excess and fluid-restricted groups. Ten subjects took 4 L of fluid per 24 hours, while 11 took 800 ml per 24 hours. The groups were similar in age and weight distribution. Studies were done 4–6 days post partum. Urinary osmolalities reflected substantial stimulation of antidiuretic hormone secretion in the fluid-restricted group. The rise of serum prolactin level in response to suckling was similar in the two groups of subjects, but basal serum prolactin levels fell in the fluid-restricted group. Mean levels on day 6 were 44 ng/ml in this group and 88 ng/ml in the fluid-excess group, a difference of doubtful significance. Milk yields were similar in the two groups of subjects.

Physiologic variations in fluid intake in this study, while resulting in a clear stimulus to vasopressin secretion, produced no definite change in serum prolactin levels. Water regulation and prolactin secretion may be interrelated in other species, but there is little evidence for this in human beings, and there is no basis for recommending changes in fluid intake for lactating women.

► [The clinical lesson here is that suggesting increased or decreased fluid intake won't improve milk production or help hasten lactation suppression. Water regulation and prolactin secretion are related in other species, but apparently are not related to a clinically significant degree in human beings.] ◄

8-6 **Dietary Supplementation of Gambian Nursing Mothers and Lactational Performance.** It has been postulated that a more adequate maternal energy and nutrient intake will lead to improved lactational performance. A. M. Prentice, Susan B. Roberts, M. Watkinson, R. G. Whitehead, Alison A. Paul, Ann Prentice, and Anne A. Watkinson (Med. Res. Council Dunn Nutrition Unit, Cambridge, England) assessed the lactational response to a dietary supplement in nursing mothers of a Gambian village over a 1-year period. Presupplementation dietary energy intakes averaged only 40% to 60% of the World Health Organization and Food and Agriculture Organization theoretical requirements. Consumption was carefully supervised and quantified. The supplement provided, on average, an additional 800 to 900 kcal/day, which increased the mean total energy intake to 2,291 kcal/day. New subjects were enrolled in the study at 8 days post partum.

The supplemented diet caused an initial weight gain of 1 to 2 kg, which was maintained over nonsupplemented women, but did not eliminate the weight loss that occurs in all adults of this village during the "hungry season." Subcutaneous fat stores showed a similar pattern. However, there was no consistent improvement in breast milk intake by infants, even when the data for 24-hour test weighings were analyzed, and the increase in milk fat concentrations was not significant (3.94 ± 0.03 vs. 3.86 ± 0.05 gm/dl). This may be due to the possibility that the supplemented diet resulted in a somewhat less

(8–6) Lancet 2:886–887, Oct. 25, 1980.

efficient maternal metabolism or that lactational performance became fixed very early in lactation.

Dietary supplement in this study did not enhance lactational performance. Nutritionists and health planners are cautioned not to oversimplify the physiology of diet-lactation interrelationships nor to draw premature conclusions about the relative merits of maternal, in contrast to infant, diet supplementation.

8–7 **Effect of Protein Intake on Protein and Nitrogen Composition of Breast Milk.** Elisabet Forsum and Bo Lönnerdal (Univ. of Uppsala) investigated the effect of a low- and a high-protein diet (approximately 8% and 20% energy from protein, respectively) on the contents of different nitrogen-containing substances in breast milk. The subjects were 3 healthy Swedish mothers in full lactation. Each experimental diet was fed during a 4-day period; milk samples were collected during the last day. The milk volume was estimated by weighing the child before and after each feeding.

The 24-hour outputs and concentrations of total nitrogen, true protein, and nonprotein nitrogen were significantly higher when the subjects ate the high-protein diet. The higher content of nonprotein nitrogen was due to increased urea levels as well as to increased free amino acid levels. Milk urea levels were closely correlated with plasma urea levels in samples collected after overnight fasting; at this time, the subjects had consumed the experimental diets for 4 days. The 24-hour output of lactoferrin, α-lactalbumin, and serum albumin were greater with the high-protein diet, but the differences were not significant.

These results show that it is possible to change the nitrogen output in breast milk by changing the mother's protein intake. However, the number of subjects was small and the observation period was short. Also, the fact that the order of treatment was the same for all subjects might have affected the results. The difference in average protein output of mothers when fed the 2 diets corresponded to approximately 20% of the daily protein intake of the breast-fed infant. A difference of this magnitude can be important to the nutrition of a suckling baby. The practical significance may be limited, however, since the average percentage of energy derived from protein in the normal diet will rarely be as low as 8% or as high as 20%.

▶ [This article and the preceding one address the question of maternal nutritional status and lactation. The results seem contradictory. In the report of Prentice et al., from Gambia, nutritional supplements providing 800–900 kcal per day to a chronically malnourished population had no effect on milk production or fat content. By contrast, Forsum and Lönnerdal noted a relationship between high- and low-protein intake (20% and 8%, respectively, of energy intake as protein) and milk nitrogen content; the amount of total nitrogen in milk was approximately 30% higher with high- than with low-protein intake, reflecting significant differences in protein, amino acids, and, particularly, nonprotein nitrogen. It should be emphasized that the dietary manipulations used in the Swedish study were indeed extreme (e.g., the usual American diet consists of 12% or 13% of calories as protein), and it is doubtful if levels as low as 8% or as high as 20% occur with any frequency in developed countries.

(8–7) Am. J. Clin. Nutr. 33:1809–1813, August 1980.

The general rule seems to be that quantitative and qualitative aspects of milk production seem to be maintained across a wide range of maternal diets, although perhaps effects may be seen with marked protein deficiency.] ◄

8–8 **Induced Lactation: A Study of Adoptive Nursing by 240 Women.** Adoptive nursing is not a new idea, but it has received little more than speculative attention in the literature. Kathleen G. Auerbach and Jimmie Lynne Avery (Univ. of Nebraska, Omaha) examined adoptive nursing in 240 women. Eighty-three had never been pregnant, while 55 had been pregnant but had never lactated, and 102 had nursed one or more biologic infants before their adoptive nursing experience. The median age was 27 years.

The decision to nurse the adopted infant often hinged on the mother-infant relationship and emotional benefits to the infant. Body contact, nutritional benefits, and nurturing opportunities also ranked high. Most of the adoptive mothers supplemented their diets in some way, usually adding extra fluids and taking brewer's yeast or a B-complex vitamin. Most used two or more methods of nipple stimulation, including infant suckling, nipple exercises, and hand-operated or electric breast pumps. Nipple exercises were the most effective method. Half of the respondents were able to express milk before the infant's arrival. Only 6% of the women used hormones before the infant's arrival. The average infant age at placement was 6 weeks. Most infants had been exclusively bottle-fed before arrival. Within a week, three fourths of the infants were willing to suckle. Nearly all respondents reported having supplemented their own milk supply, often with the Lact-Aid nursing trainer. The infants did not appear to differ from breast-fed biologic infants in the way in which they nursed. Tandem nursing of an adoptive infant and an older biologic infant did not assure an increase in milk production sufficient to meet the adoptive infant's needs.

Three fourths of these women evaluated their experience positively. The women expressed a wish for the infant to know its mother in a way unrelated to biologic kinship. They suggested that every infant is entitled to nurturance at the breast, regardless of parentage or the amount of milk produced.

► [Although these study subjects may not be representative of the entire population of women who attempt induced lactation, the number of participants (240) is impressive. Nipple stimulation, not surprisingly, was the most effective means of inducing lactation. One half of the study subjects had colostrum-like or milky breast secretion prior to the arrival of the infant. Only 4% of the respondents noted amenorrhea after the initiation of breast-feeding. We would have guessed a higher figure (assuming that breast stimulation leads to hyperprolactinemia, which leads to milk production and anovulation).] ◄

► ↓ For data regarding protein levels in milk from mothers nursing by induced lactation, read on. ◄

8–9 **Protein Values of Milk Samples From Mothers Without Biologic Pregnancies.** Milk from mothers giving birth to premature and term infants has been studied in depth, but few data are available for milk produced by women in whom relactation is induced.

(8–8) Am. J. Dis. Child. 135:340–343, April 1981.
(8–9) J. Pediatr. 97:612–615, October 1980.

Ronald Kleinman, Linda Jacobson, Elizabeth Hormann, and W. Allan Walker (Harvard Med. School) studied milk samples donated by 5 women who adopted infants and induced lactation by having the infant suckle. Two women had breast-fed biologic infants in the past and 3 women had no biologic children. No medication was taken to help accomplish lactation. In all cases, lactation was achieved within 11 days of putting the infant to the breast. A total of 10 milk samples was collected during the first 5 days of lactation. Milk samples also were collected serially for up to 245 days from 5 women who breast-fed their own infants.

In biologic mothers, the mean total protein level was about 36 mg/ml in colostrum (first 5 days of lactation), 15 mg/ml in transitional milk (day 6–15), and 9 mg/ml in mature milk (day 16–245). In the initial milk of nonbiologic mothers, the mean total protein level was about 14 mg/ml.

The concentrations of proteins that together constitute total protein did not change uniformly with time. The IgA concentration in biologic milk was about 16.5, 4.0, and 2.5 mg/ml in colostral, transitional, and mature samples, respectively; in nonbiologic milk, the IgA level was about 3 mg/ml. In biologic milk, the level of albumin rose from 2 to 3 to 4 mg/ml in colostral, transitional, and mature samples, respectively; in nonbiologic milk, the level was 3.5 mg/ml. The level of α-lactalbumin in biologic milk rose from 5.5 to 17.5 to 34 mg/ml during the three time periods, respectively; in nonbiologic milk, the concentration was about 27 mg/ml.

Thus, milk collected during the first 5 days of relactation contains protein levels that are similar to those of transitional and mature biologic milk. Nonbiologic milk is lower in IgA and total protein and higher in α-lactalbumin than colostrum. The first milk of nonbiologic mothers does not pass through a colostral phase. Pregnancy and delivery, and their accompanying hormonal changes, apparently are required for colostrum production; suckling alone is not a sufficient stimulus.

▶ [Nursing adopted infants by women who have never been pregnant, or at least not within a period of some time, is an interesting phenomenon. This study indicates that the early milk produced under these circumstances resembles mature milk produced by biologic mothers with respect to protein content. It does not go through the colostral phase (high total protein and IgA; low albumin and α-lactalbumin).] ◀

8–10 **Elevated Levels of LRH in Human Milk.** Luteinizing hormone-releasing hormone (LRH) acts on the anterior pituitary gonadotropes to stimulate synthesis and release of gonadotropins. It has been described in the milk of various animal species. A. K. Sarda and R. M. G. Nair (Charleston, S. C.) found that relatively large amounts of LRH are present in human milk. The amount was estimated by radioimmunoassay of milk samples from 6 healthy women who had normal pregnancies and deliveries. The milk samples contained 5–6 times more LRH than corresponding plasma samples. The mean immunoreactive level of LRH in milk was 107 pg/ml, compared to 17 pg/ml for plasma.

(8–10) J. Clin. Endocrinol. Metab. 52:826–828, April 1981.

This is the first demonstration of correlation between immunoreactive LRH levels in human milk and levels in corresponding plasma samples. If the LRH in milk is of hypothalamic origin, there may be passive diffusion of LRH from the peripheral circulation into milk or, more likely, an active concentrating mechanism may be operative. There also may be an extrahypothalamic source for LRH in the mammary gland. The LRH in milk may be responsible for inducing elevated gonadotropin levels in neonates. Intrauterine exposure to high levels of LRH from the placenta may continue into the neonatal period by the high levels of LRH in breast milk. Milk may prove to be an excellent source for complete characterization of human LRH.

▶ [This finding of relatively high levels of luteining hormone-releasing hormone (LRH) in milk raises, a number of questions. How does it get there? The breast might "concentrate" it from the blood, but the fivefold to sixfold higher levels in milk over those in plasma call for a remarkable concentrating ability. Perhaps the breast synthesizes LRH—after all, the placenta apparently does (see 1981 YEAR BOOK, p. 28). But what is LRH doing there?] ◀

8–11 **High Milk Lipase Activity Associated With Breast Milk Jaundice.** Breast milk jaundice is a syndrome of prolonged neonatal unconjugated hyperbilirubinemia related to ingestion of certain abnormal human milks. These milks inhibit hepatic bilirubin-UDP-glucuronyl transferase (UDPGT) in vitro. Some reports have identified the inhibitor as 3α, 20β-pregnanediol, but others point to free fatty acids as the inhibitor. Ronald L. Poland, Gary E. Schultz, and Gayatri Garg (Wayne State Univ.) measured the levels of nonesterified fatty acids (total and individual fatty acids), total fat and protein, and lipase activities (with and without bile salt stimulation) in milk samples from 9 women whose infants had prolonged unconjugated hyperbilirubinemia and whose milk inhibited the activity of UDPGT and from 130 women with healthy babies.

Inhibitory milk contained more nonesterified fatty acids (total, palmitic, and oleic) than did controls. Fat and protein levels and bile salt-stimulated lipase activities were similar in the two groups. Unstimulated lipase activity was almost twice as high in the inhibitory milks as in control milks. Specific activity of unstimulated lipase was also higher in the inhibitory milks.

The inhibitor of UDPGT activity in breast milks that cause breast milk jaundice appears to be nonesterified fatty acids, which occur in the abnormal milks in excess quantities due to the action of an abnormal lipolytic activity. Whether this defect is genetically determined or is due to some stimulant of lipase activity and how it leads to prolonged unconjugated hyperbilirubinemia are unknown. Fat digestion and absorption may have important effects on the metabolism of bilirubin in newborn infants. Continued study of the influence of the digestive process on the absorption and further metabolism of dietary lipid in neonates may help to illuminate the relation between lipid metabolism and neonatal hyperbilirubinemia.

▶ [Early studies suggested that some breast-fed infants exhibit prolonged unconjugated hyperbilirubinemia because of inhibition of glucuronyl transferase by a pregna-

(8–11) Pediatr. Res. 14:1328–1331, December 1980.

nediol metabolite in milk. More recent reports, however, have indicated that the inhibiting factor may be free fatty acids. This study confirms the role of free fatty acids and indicates further that high levels in inhibitory milks reflect unstimulated lipase activity. Why milk lipase contents should vary from one patient to another is unclear. Breast milk jaundice generally is not regarded as serious in terms of causing complications, but it certainly can lead to prolonged hospitalization and parent anxiety.] ◄

8–12 **Analgesic Drugs in Breast Milk and Plasma.** The possible excretion of drugs in breast milk often raises questions concerning the safety of the infant in continued nursing during periods of maternal drug therapy. John W. A. Findlay, Richard L. DeAngelis, Marlene F. Kearney, Richard M. Welch, and Jean M. Findlay examined the disposition of salicylic acid, phenacetin, caffeine, codeine, and two metabolites, acetaminophen and morphine, in the breast milk and plasma of two lactating mothers after single oral doses of a compound analgesic, Empirin Compound with Codeine No. 3. The compound contains 454 mg of aspirin, 324 mg of phenacetin, 64 mg of caffeine, and 60 mg of codeine phosphate.

Salicylic acid was found to penetrate poorly into breast milk, and it was eliminated more slowly from milk than from plasma. Caffeine and phenacetin kinetics were similar in breast milk and plasma, but milk levels were somewhat lower than plasma levels in both subjects. Levels of acetaminophen were much higher than those of the parent drug, phenacetin, in 1 subject, but the reverse was true for the other subject early after ingestion of the compound. Acetaminophen was eliminated more slowly from milk than from plasma. Codeine levels in milk were 1.5–2.4 times the plasma levels. Levels of metabolically produced morphine in milk were low in both subjects, but exceeded levels in plasma after 1 hour. Calculations based on predicted steady-state milk concentrations indicated maximum milk excretion of 0.7% and 2.7% of the ingested dose of each drug in the 2 subjects. In both cases, caffeine was excreted in milk in the greatest quantity.

These findings are in accordance with the acid-base properties of the various compounds with respect to their distribution in plasma and in the slightly more acidic breast milk. The infant presumably would not be at risk from drug effects during continued nursing by mothers taking recommended doses of the preparation, but this may not be so when excessive doses are taken continuously. Caffeine concentrations in milk should be estimated in mothers who ingest large amounts of caffeine-containing beverages.

► [This is an excellent pharmacokinetic study of analgesic drugs in lactation. All the drugs measured were found in milk but, with the exception of codeine, milk levels were lower than those in plasma. Caffeine was excreted in milk in the greatest amounts, raising the obvious question of the advisability of caffeine ingestion by the nursing mother.] ◄

8–13 **Bromocriptine Mesylate for Prevention of Postpartum Lactation.** Claude Duchesne and Robert Leke (Univ. of Montreal) administered bromocriptine mesylate to 420 normal puerperal women who did not wish to nurse their infants. The usual dosage was 2.5 mg twice daily with meals for 14 days, beginning on the day of vaginal

(8–12) Clin. Pharmacol. Ther. 29:625–633, May 1981.
(8–13) Obstet. Gynecol. 57:464–467, April 1981.

delivery (mean interval between delivery and onset of therapy, 4 hours), or at the start of oral intake in women delivered by cesarean section (mean interval, 28 hours).

Complete inhibition of breast engorgement and milk secretion was obtained in 97% of the women after 5 days of therapy. Of 370 women who completed 14 days of therapy, 74% were completely symptom free and the rest showed only grade I or II breast engorgement and secretion. Side effects such as nausea, vomiting, and dizziness were experienced by 3% of the women, and 7% reported rebound engorgement and secretion after treatment was concluded. Of the women with rebound symptoms, a third became symptom free on another 7-day course of bromocriptine therapy and in the rest, symptoms spontaneously disappeared. No patient had evidence of thromboembolism.

Bromocriptine is safe and effective for prevention of postpartum breast engorgement and milk secretion. Its apparent lack of thromboembolic complications and low incidence of rebound effects suggest possible advantages over other pharmacologic preparations currently used to prevent postpartum lactation, i.e., estrogen-containing drugs. No explanation is apparent for the finding that only 3% of women reported side effects, compared with about 65% of women taking the same drug as treatment for amenorrhea-galactorrhea.

▶ [A few years ago, our service stopped using pharmacologic means to inhibit lactation in non-breast-feeding mothers, but relied only on binders, ice, and simple analgesics for those patients who experienced moderately severe symptoms. We expected an outcry from the nursing staff of our postpartum unit. It never came. The question, it seems to us, is not whether bromocriptine works (it does), but rather whether this or other pharmacologic suppression of lactation is really necessary.] ◀

8–14 **Postpartum Lymphocytic Thyroiditis in American Women: A Spectrum of Thyroid Dysfunction.** The recently described syndrome of postpartum thyroiditis is characterized by transient hypothyroidism, goiter, and antithyroid autoantibodies occurring within 6 months of delivery and remitting by 1 year. Henry G. Fein, Joel M. Goldman, and Bruce D. Weintraub describe 5 women who experienced six episodes of postpartum primary hypothyroidism. Three women were examined when goiter appeared post partum, and 2 were being followed up for prior thyroid disease.

Within 6 months post partum, all women were clinically hypothyroid, with a diffuse goiter 2–3 times normal size, altered thyroid function (average thyroxine level, 2.6 µg/dl; thyroid-stimulating hormone [TSH], 58.2 µU/ml), and elevated levels of antithyroid antibodies (antimicrosomal antibody titers of 1:6,400 or more). After 5 more months, all patients had decreased antibody titer, resolution of symptoms, and increased thyroid hormone levels (average thyroxine level, 7.3 µg/dl), although 2 women had compensated hypothyroidism (average TSH level, 9.3 µU/ml). Four patients had lymphocytic thyroiditis diagnosed by fine-needle aspiration biopsy.

Despite the apparent transience of postpartum hypothyroidism, all 5 patients have chronic thyroid dysfunction. Three have persistent goiters (all less than twice the normal size) and 2 have compensated

---

(8–14) Am. J. Obstet. Gynecol. 138:504–510, Nov. 1, 1980.

hypothyroidism. One patient had previous Graves' hyperthyroidism, and 2 had recurrent transient hypothyroidism (at 21 months post partum in 1 patient and 5 months after another pregnancy in the other). Three women had transient, painless hyperthyroidism (average thyroxine level, 16.1 μg/dl) before becoming hypothyroid: 2 patients within 8 weeks post partum and 1 at 20 months (preceding an episode of recurrent hypothyroidism).

Previous reports of postpartum hypothyroidism have come from scattered locales abroad, and it is unclear whether local environmental factors are pathogenic. Nevertheless, in general, this syndrome may have gone unrecognized and may be a significant cause of illness in postpartum women. Women in whom goiters appear during pregnancy or after delivery and those with a history of thyroid dysfunction before pregnancy must have close follow-up.

▶ [Reports from several parts of the world suggest that postpartum thyroiditis is increasing in frequency, or at least is becoming more frequently recognized. Several weeks to a few months after delivery, patients present with goiter, antithyroid antibodies, and hypothyroidism (often preceded by transient hyperthyroidism). Euthyroidism returns, but goiter or elevated TSH levels may persist. Thyroid dysfunction may recur after a subsequent pregnancy. Just what all this means is unclear, but there are two implications for the obstetrician-gynecologist: We must be careful not to assume that all postpartum fatigue is due to motherhood and we must have close follow-up of pregnant patients with a history of previous thyroid dysfunction, both throughout gestation and for several months thereafter.] ◀

8–15 **Infection With *Mycoplasma hominis* in Postpartum Fever.** Richard Platt, John W. Warren, Kenneth C. Edelin, Juey-Shin L. Lin, Bernard Rosner, and William M. McCormack (Boston) studied the frequency with which *M. hominis* causes fever after vaginal delivery by followup of 535 women who delivered vaginally at Boston City Hospital. Data and specimens were collected from 147 for extended study.

Of the 535 women, 9% had a temperature of 37.7 C or higher on 2 days after delivery and 2% had a temperature of 38 C or higher. The most common cause of both categories of fever was *M. hominis* infection, as defined by a fourfold or greater rise in mucoplasmacidal antibody titer. Among women for whom serum was available, this agent caused 50% (14 of 28) of all fevers and 71% (5 of 7) of high fevers. Absence or low titer (less than 1:8) of antibody against *M. hominis* was the strongest single predictor of otherwise unexplained fever (fever occurred in 16 of 40 women with low antibody titer and in 7 of 50 with high titer). Among women with absent or low antibody titers, both rise in titer of antibody to *M. hominis* and lochial colonization by it were significantly associated with fever. Standard microbiologic and clinical techniques identified probable causes in only 18% (5 of 28) of all fevers and 29% (2 of 7) of high fevers. Women with *M. hominis* postpartum infection remained hospitalized 31% longer than noninfected women (4¹⁄₂ vs. 3¹⁄₂ days). Low antibody to and lochial colonization with *M. hominis* occurred together in 17% of women, who accounted for 71% of all those with high fevers.

(8–15) Lancet 2:1217–1221, Dec. 6, 1980.

Antibody to and lochial colonization with *M. hominis*, risk factors for postpartum fever, can be identified before delivery. Prophylactic measures applied selectively to women with these risk factors may prevent many postpartum fevers and the excess hospital stay associated with them.

▶ [R. P. Galask, of the University of Iowa, reviewed this paper at our request and commented as follows:

"This report concerning the occurrence of fever with an association of *Mycoplasma hominis* colonization and an increase in the mycoplasmocidal antibody titer presents an intriguing concept for the etiology of puerperal infection. Half of all postpartum fevers and 71% of significant fevers were related to *M. hominis.* The authors used a criterion for fever of 37.7 C, rather than the standard criterion of a fever of 38 C or higher on at least 2 of the first 10 postpartum days. Lochial cultures were obtained just within the introitus, and no attempt was made to culture the intrauterine cavity, making it uncertain how the results relate to infections within the endometrium. Also, the authors studied microbiologically only the presence of *Neisseria gonorrhoeae,* β-hemolytic streptococci group B, *Gardnerella vaginalis, Trichomonas vaginalis,* and *Candida albicans* without attempting to isolate other facultative organisms or anaerobic bacteria that commonly have been associated with peripheral sepsis. The isolation of *Ureaplasma urealyticum* from a blood culture does appear to be a significant finding.

"The use of mycoplasmacidal antibody titers is an important aspect of this study. However, it is not apparent from this or previous reports from the same laboratory whether or not specificity for the antibody was determined. It would be important to know if there were any cross reactivity with maternal serum from an infected patient. However, it is interesting that a majority of all of the febrile patients had antibody titers to *M. hominis.*

"Although this report is intriguing, it lacks careful microbiologic evaluation of the site of infection to include those microorganisms that commonly are felt to be etiologic agents of puerperal sepsis. Further studies utilizing the mycoplasma antibody are required to determine its specificity for mycoplasma."] ◀

8–16 Puerperal Infectious Morbidity: Relationship to Route of Delivery and to Antepartum *Chlamydia trachomatis* Infection was studied by Gael P. Wager, David H. Martin, Laura Koutsky, David A. Eschenbach, Janet R. Daling, W. T. Chiang, E. R. Alexander, and King K. Holmes (Univ. of Washington, Seattle). *Chlamydia trachomatis* was recovered from 45 (9.3%) of the 486 women who underwent antepartum cervical culture during 1977 to 1979, including 32 (8.2%) of the 391 women who were followed completely through 6 weeks post partum or until earlier onset of puerperal pelvic infection. Compared with patients who did not have antepartum *C. trachomatis* infection, those with infection were significantly younger, had lower mean gravidity, were more often receiving welfare, were more often nonwhite, and were more often unmarried.

Infectious morbidity occurred in 27 (44%) of 62 women who underwent cesarean section and in 33 (10%) of 329 who had vaginal deliveries. Infectious morbidity after cesarean section was not correlated with *C. trachomatis* infection and was largely limited to early (within 48 hours) postpartum fever not attributable to infections of sites outside the uterus. Among women who had vaginal deliveries, infectious morbidity occurred in 10 (34%) of 29 women with and in 23 (8%) of 300 without *C. trachomatis* infection. Chlamydial infection was associated only with intrapartum fever and late (48 hours to 6 weeks)

(8–16) Am. J. Obstet. Gynecol. 138:1028–1033, Dec. 1, 1980.

postpartum endometritis. Separate matched case-control analyses confirmed that cesarean section was associated with an increased risk of early postpartum fever, whereas among women who had vaginal deliveries, antepartum *C. trachomatis* infection was associated with an increased risk of the development of intrapartum fever or late postpartum endometritis.

▶ [Other articles in this YEAR BOOK deal with the role of *Chlamydia trachomatis* in acute pelvic inflammatory disease. The present study suggests that this organism may play a significant role in obstetric infections as well. Routine antepartum testing showed that 9.3% of the population were colonized. Late postpartum endometritis and intrapartum chorioamnionitis were diagnosed more frequently in patients harboring chlamydiae. The organism lives intracellularly, and sophisticated techniques are required to culture it. Further investigations will, in all likelihood, better define its place in the scheme of things concerning genital tract infections in women.] ◀

8–17 **Erythromycin Ointment for Ocular Prophylaxis of Neonatal Chlamydial Infection.** Most states require some form of prophylaxis against neonatal gonococcal ophthalmia, and 1% silver nitrate generally is used for this purpose. The incidence of neonatal chlamydial ophthalmia is now much greater than that of gonococcal ophthalmia (0.4% vs. 0.04%, respectively), however, and neonatal ocular prophylaxis with silver nitrate reportedly does not prevent chlamydial ophthalmia. Margaret R. Hammerschlag, John W. Chandler, E. Russell Alexander, Marilyn English, Wen-Tsuo Chiang, Laura Koutsky, David A. Eschenbach, and James R. Smith compared the efficacy of erythromycin ophthalmic ointment and silver nitrate drops for the prevention of neonatal conjunctivitis and respiratory tract infection from *Chlamydia trachomatis*.

The organism was isolated from the cervix of 67 (12%) of 572 women in the third trimester of pregnancy. Seventeen mother-infant pairs were excluded, usually because of delivery elsewhere. The remaining 555 women gave birth to 559 infants, 60 of whom were born to *Chlamydia*-positive women. The infants were randomly assigned to receive ocular prophylaxis with either 1% silver nitrate (2 drops into each conjunctival sac) or erythromycin ointment (a 2.5-cm ribbon to each eye).

Chlamydial conjunctivitis occurred in 12 (33%) of the 36 infants who received silver nitrate but in none of the 24 who received erythromycin. Chlamydial nasopharyngeal infection occurred in 10 (28%) of the infants who received silver nitrate (3 of these 10 later had pneumonia) and in 5 (21%) of those who received erythromycin (1 had pneumonia). There were no cases of gonococcal ophthalmia among the 559 infants, although *Neisseria gonorrhoeae* was isolated from the endocervix at some time during pregnancy in 11 (3%) of 389 women. There were no adverse effects to erythromycin prophylaxis.

Erythromycin ointment apparently is effective in preventing chlamydial conjunctivitis, but it may not reduce nasopharyngeal infection or subsequent pneumonia.

▶ [Since the natural history of neonatal chlamydial conjunctivitis has not been defined well, it is hard to gauge the importance of these observations. Perhaps silver nitrate as "the drug" for ophthalmic prophylaxis will be replaced by an agent effective against

(8–17) JAMA 244:2291–2293, Nov. 21, 1980.

both chlamydial and gonococcal infections. Some of our new mothers object to the chemical irritation caused by silver nitrate and worry about adverse effects on bonding. Perhaps erythromycin ointment would be more acceptable to them. Speaking of chemical conjunctivitis due to silver nitrate, do we mistakenly make this diagnosis at times when the real problem is undiagnosed chlamydial infection?] ◄

8-18 **Molecular Epidemiology of Cytomegalovirus Infections in Women and Their Infants.** Normal women immune to cytomegaloviruses (CMV) often shed virus from various sites, including the genital and urinary tracts, pharynx, and breasts. Cytomegalovirus can be transmitted in utero to the fetus and in the postpartum period to the infant, resulting in congenital infection. Because live vaccine is being contemplated for the control of congenital CMV infection, it is important to determine whether recurrent viral shedding and intrauterine transmission in immune women is caused by reactivation of latent virus or reinfection by exogenous strains of CMV. Eng-Shang Huang, Charles A. Alford, David W. Reynolds, Sergio Stagno, and Robert F. Pass investigated the source of recurrent CMV infection by studying the genetic relatedness of 21 strains of CMV from 6 mother-infant pairs, 2 congenitally infected siblings, and repeat isolates from 4 women. The examinations were made by restriction endonuclease analysis of purified viral DNA.

Major genetic differences were found among CMV from unrelated persons. In contrast, strains from 5 of 6 congenitally infected infants were identical or very similar to those from their mothers. Concordance was observed among strains from congenitally infected infants as well as in repeat isolates from 3 of 4 women. In 2 cases, major genetic differences between viruses were detected from the same person or from related persons: in one, a virus recovered from the genital tract of a mother differed from the isolate obtained from her congenitally infected infant 6 years earlier, and the other involved repeat isolates from the genital tract of a woman that were obtained 1 year apart.

Endogenous virus is most frequently the source of recurrent CMV infection in women. It can be transmitted to the fetus years after initial acquisition despite maternal immunity. Reinfection of the genital tract by different genetic variants also occurs, but is not as common.

► [Lightning can strike the same place twice! Although it is uncommon, a mother who has previously given birth to a baby with congenital CMV infection and has circulating anti-CMV antibody can deliver another infected infant. Does this represent reinfection of the mother with a new strain of CMV or does it indicate persistence or reactivation of her previous CMV strain? This DNA "fingerprinting" study suggests that the latter is usually the case.] ◄

(8-18) N. Engl. J. Med. 303:958–962, Oct. 23, 1980.

9. The Newborn

9-1 **Outcome for Infants of Very Low Birth Weight: Survey of World Literature.** To determine if any inferences could be drawn about trends in healthy survival, mortality rate, and handicap rate in infants of very low birth weight (VLBW; equal to or less than 1,500 gm) born in countries with modern medical services, Ann L. Stewart, E. O. R. Reynolds, and A. P. Lipscomb (Univ. College, London) analyzed 22 reports from developed countries worldwide on the outcome of VLBW infants born since 1946. The data were pooled according to the quinquennium of birth.

Generally, the results from each quinquennium were similar. During the first 3 quinquennia (1946–1960), there was no change in the proportion of healthy survivors when compared with the combined proportions of dead and handicapped infants (Fig 9–1), but there were significant changes in the proportion of infants who either died or survived handicapped ($P < .0005$). From 1961 through 1977, the proportion of healthy survivors approximately tripled, while the proportion of handicapped survivors remained low (6% to 8%) (Fig 9–1). When the proportions of infants who died and survived handicapped were compared with the proportions of infants who survived healthy in all 7 quinquennia, a highly significant increase in the proportion of healthy survivors over the 32 years of study was observed ($P < .0005$). The same trends seemed to be emerging for infants weighing 1,000 gm or less.

It is concluded that the improved chances of healthy survival for

Fig 9–1.—Data pooled by quinquennium to show percentage of VLBW infants (<1,500 gm) who died, survived handicapped, or survived healthy. (Courtesy of Stewart, A. L., et al.: Lancet 1:1038–1040, May 9, 1981.)

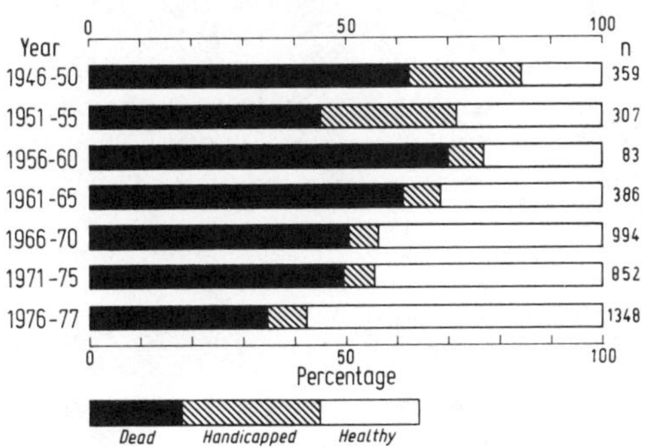

(9–1)   Lancet 1:1038–1040, May 9, 1981.

VLBW infants can be attributed primarily to improved medical interventions, rather than to social or demographic factors.

▶ [We do not usually include review articles in the YEAR BOOK but this one was selected because it represents an excellent summary of the changing prognosis during the past 35 years of the infant weighing less than 1.5 kg. Survival has essentially tripled over this period (actually during the past 20 years) and the proportion of handicapped infants has remained constant at 6%–8%. Infants of very low birth weight are the major users of neonatal intensive care units and this review documents that their utilization is effective.] ◀

9–2 **Changing Trends of Neonatal and Postneonatal Deaths in Very Low Birth Weight Infants.** Maureen Hack, Irwin R. Merkatz, Paul K. Jones, and Avroy A. Fanaroff (Case Western Reserve Univ.) documented all deaths among 427 very low birth weight (less than 1.5 kg) infants admitted during 1975–77. The study was done to determine the current relevance of neonatal mortality results as indicators of outcome for very low birth weight (VLBW) infants managed in a tertiary care center. Gestational age ranged from 24 to 36 weeks. Of the 427 infants, 145 (34%) died during the first year of life. Ninety deaths (62%) occurred during the early neonatal period (0–6 days), 35 (24%) in the late neonatal period (7–27 days), and 20 (14%) in the postneonatal period. Seventeen of the 20 infants in the postneonatal group died from conditions directly related to complications of prematurity, such as bronchopulmonary dysplasia, necrotizing enterocolitis, or infection. Sixteen of the 20 infants never left the hospital. Thus, only 83% (66/79) of the VLBW infants who survived the first week lived to age 1 year.

Until recently, all perinatal-related deaths could be anticipated to occur before age 28 days. Advances in perinatal care have yielded a decline in neonatal mortality rates, but also an extension of the period during which the VLBW infant remains at risk of death. This is particularly true for infants weighing 1,001–1,500 gm at birth. Thus, the early neonatal period can no longer be considered adequate for any evaluation of neonatal or perinatal mortality data in this high-risk group, because approximately 20% of infants who die of complications of premature birth are excluded. A corrected definition of the neonatal period should be used in the evaluation of regional or center results in VLBW infants. The period from birth until discharge from the hospital is the most appropriate parameter. This will allow for an improved assessment of newer methods of care and of the iatrogenic complications characteristic of VLBW infants.

▶ [The definition of neonatal death is death within the first 28 days of life, although some statistics are based on only the first week after birth. These may have been adequate formerly when premature infants who died almost always did so within a few days of birth, but modern neonatal intensive care sometimes prolongs the life of very small infants, and figures based on even 28 days may be misleading. In this survey of infants with birth weights less than 1,500 gm during 1975–1977, 38% of the deaths occurred on or after the seventh day; 14% took place after 27 days and thus were not, strictly speaking, neonatal deaths. These data point out that the interests of accurate vital statistics require some modification in the traditional definition. Because premature infants dying beyond the neonatal period usually (80% in this series) have not been discharged from the hospital, the authors propose that the interval from birth to

(9–2) Am. J. Obstet. Gynecol. 137:797–800, Aug. 1, 1980.

hospital discharge be used to tabulate mortality data for very low birth weight infants.] ◄

9–3 School Achievement and Behavior of Children Who Were Small for Dates at Birth. Infants small for dates (SFD) are more likely to have neurologic and behavioral abnormalities, poor developmental test scores, and learning difficulties at school, but it is not clear which infants will have later difficulties. Christine E. Parkinson, Sheila Wallis, and David Harvey (London) report a schoolteacher assessment of achievement and behavior at school by 45 SFD children, defined as having a birth weight below the tenth percentile for gestational age after correcting for sex, birth order, and the mother's height and midpregnancy weight. All were single births after gestations lasting 37 weeks or longer. Slow intrauterine head growth began at or before 26 weeks' gestation in 9 cases, at 27–34 weeks in 14, and after 35 weeks' gestation in 4; it was not evident in 18 cases. Nineteen control subjects also were evaluated. The mean age at the time of study was 7.2 years.

Study children whose head growth had slowed before 26 weeks' gestation showed less achievement at school than those with no evidence of slow intrauterine head growth. They appeared to be less able to concentrate. Boys but not girls whose head growth had slowed at 27–34 weeks' gestation also had problems at school. No significant differences in atypical behavior were found between the study and control children.

Children who at birth were small for dates may have difficulties at school, and the achievement and behavior of these children are related to the severity of slow prenatal growth as well as to sex and social class. It is not possible at present to identify at birth which SFD infants are most likely to have problems at school. Current efforts should be directed to helping these children during their developmental years.

► [These authors previously have reported that the effects of fetal growth retardation on subsequent stature of the child were more marked the earlier in intrauterine life that growth (of the head) was slowed. The present study notes a similar relationship with respect to assessment of school performance and behavior—the earlier the onset in utero, the more marked the later effect. A sex difference was also apparent, with boys being apparently more vulnerable than girls, in addition to the well-known relation of school performance to social class.] ◄

9–4 Intravenous Dexamethasone for Prevention of Neonatal Respiratory Distress: Prospective Controlled Study. Bruce K. Young, Steven A. Klein, Miriam Katz, Stephen J. Wilson, and Gordon W. Douglas (New York City) report results of a trial of intravenous dexamethasone PO_4 for prevention of neonatal respiratory distress syndrome (RDS). There were 112 treated and 188 control patients, matched for gestational age, birth weight, time of rupture of membranes, and antepartum diagnosis. All patients in early labor without premature rupture of the membranes (PROM) were given alcohol intravenously to arrest labor. In addition, 12 mg of dexameth-

(9–3)   Develop. Med. Child. Neurol. 23:41–50, February 1981.
(9–4)   Am. J. Obstet. Gynecol. 138:203–209, Sept. 15, 1980.

TABLE 1.—EFFECT OF LOW 5-MINUTE APGAR SCORE ON INCIDENCE AND SEVERITY OF RESPIRATORY DISTRESS SYNDROME AMONG STEROID AND CONTROL GROUPS

	Steroids			Control		
	5-min Apgar	*5-min Apgar*		*5-min Apgar*	*5-min Apgar*	
	6 or less (%)	*7 or more* (%)	*p*	*6 or less* (%)	*7 or more* (%)	*p*
RDS	11/15 (73)	25/84 (30)	<0.05	28/35 (80)	83/140 (59)	<0.05
Severe RDS	6/15 (40)	4/84 (4.7)	<0.001	21/35 (60)	38/140 (27)	<0.01

asone PO_4 was given by intravenous infusion for 15 minutes. The dosage was repeated in 24 hours. Additional courses of treatment were given if delivery had not occurred by 7 days and the pregnancy was of less than 34 weeks' duration. Patients with maternal or fetal indications for early delivery in the absence of labor were treated with the same infusions of dexamethasone and were delivered 1–7 days

TABLE 2.—INCIDENCE AND SEVERITY OF RESPIRATORY DISTRESS
SYNDROME IN STEROID-TREATED AND CONTROL GROUPS

	Steroid (%)	No steroid (%)	p
26-27 weeks			
RDS	5/8 (63)	7/12 (58)	N/S
Severe RDS	2/8 (25`	3/12 (25)	N/S
28-33 weeks			
RDS	29/71 (41)	80/108 (74)	<0.001
Severe RDS	8/71 (11)	50/108 (46)	<0.0001
34-36 weeks			
RDS	2/20 (10)	25/55 (45)	<0.02
Severe RDS	0/20 (0)	6/55 (11)	N/S
Total RDS	36/99 (36)	112/175 (64)	<0.001
Total severe RDS	10/99 (10)	59/175 (34)	<0.001

after the last dose unless membranes were ruptured. Patients with
PROM who were not in labor were given 12 mg of dexamethasone
intravenously on admission, which treatment was repeated in 12
hours. Delivery efforts began 12 hours after the second dose.

No short-term deleterious effects on mother or infant were demonstrable. Premature rupture of the membranes occurred in 51 (46%) of
the treated patients and in 62 (33%) of controls; the difference was
not significant. Of 312 infants delivered, 274 were appropriate for
gestational age and were without major malformations. Neonates in
treated and control populations were well matched: birth weight for
gestational age was closely matched from 26 to 36 weeks, and the
frequency of low Apgar scores was similar (15.2% in the steroid-
treated group, 16% in controls). The occurrence of neonatal depression (a 5-minute Apgar score below 7) significantly increased the risk
and severity of RDS in both groups, compared with neonates having
Apgar scores of 7 or more ($P < .01$) (Table 1). The uncorrected mortality rate was 127/1,000 in the treated group and 175/1,000 in controls. Between 28 and 33 weeks, steroid treatment reduced perinatal
mortality significantly. There was no statistically significant difference in mortality at 26–27 weeks or 34–36 weeks between the two
groups. Dexamethasone reduced the frequency and severity of RDS
among 71 treated fetuses compared with 108 control fetuses delivered
between 28 and 33 weeks. No reduction in RDS risk was noted prior
to 28 weeks, and only a limited reduction in RDS frequency (but not
severity) was observed after 33 weeks (Table 2). There was increased
infectious morbidity among treated patients (28% vs. 15%), but no
increase in severe infections, compared with controls. Cesarean section was performed more often in the treated group, especially in patients with PROM. Cesarean section (40%) and PROM beyond 24
hours (65%) were associated with the most significant incidences of
maternal infection regardless of steroid treatment. These factors are
more related to each other and to the high-risk patients studied than
to therapy. Intravenously administered dexamethasone appears to be
effective in reducing perinatal mortality from RDS in premature in-

fants delivered between 28 and 33 weeks of gestation. Long-term follow-up studies are needed to evaluate long-term risks.

▶ [Certain findings in this study are consistent with commonly held views. Low Apgar scores predisposed the neonate to RDS; prolonged ruptured membranes may have been protective in this regard; incidence and severity of RDS in the steroid-treated group were significantly less from 28 to 33 weeks' gestation than in controls. Although this is a "controlled" study, assignment to the drug or no-drug groups was apparently not random. From 28 to 33 weeks, the steroid was used in 52% of patients with ruptured membranes and 28% of patients with intact membranes. Cesarean section was significantly more common in the steroid group. Were the chances of receiving the drug equal in the two participating hospitals? While this and other studies have noted the apparent benefits of steroids in reducing the prevalence and severity of RDS in the neonate at 28 to 33 weeks' gestation, and the absence of short-term adverse effects, we believe that antenatal steroid therapy must still be regarded as under clinical investigation.] ◀

9–5 **Betamethasone and the Rhesus Fetus: Effect on Lung Morphometry and Connective Tissue.** Jeanne C. Beck, Wayne Mitzner, John W. C. Johnson, Grover M. Hutchins, Jean-Michel Foidart, William T. London, Amos E. Palmer, and Rachel Scott treated pregnant rhesus monkeys *(Macaca mulatta)* at 67%–85% of term pregnancy with 1 mg of betamethasone phosphate and 1 mg of betamethasone acetate intramuscularly daily for 3 days and then delivered them by cesarean section.

The treated fetuses had larger maximal lung volumes (V_{max}, 32.6 ± 1.8 ml/kg of body weight) than gestational age-matched control animals (22.9 ± 3.2 ml/kg of body weight, $P < .025$) but no alterations in surfactant properties as measured by amniotic fluid L/S ratios, alveolar deflation stability, or lung phosphatidylcholine. The findings suggest that betamethasone effects an increase in fetal lung volume by some method other than alteration in alveolar surfactant concentrations. An 11% increase in the collagen-to-elastin concentration in treated fetuses as compared with control animals ($P < .01$) was also demonstrated, suggesting alterations in lung connective tissue. Morphometric studies on the air-fixed inflated lung demonstrated a decreased number of alveoli per unit volume of lung among treated animals ($0.95 ± 0.07 \times 10^6$) compared with control animals ($1.19 ± 0.08 \times 10^6$, $P < .025$) and a reduction in the mean surface area of the lungs in the treated animals (506 ± 10 sq cm/cu cm) compared with control animals (561 ± 9 sq cm/cu cm; $P < .005$).

The findings suggest that at least part of the increased V_{max} is related to increased alveolar distensibility (but increased number of alveoli cannot be excluded) and that a major effect of betamethasone on the rhesus fetal lung is to alter connective tissue characteristics. The disparity between these findings and other animal studies might be due to differences in species, the preparation, or method of glucocorticoid administration. The increased lung weight-body weight ratio (13%) in treated animals versus control animals was not found in previous studies, and its significance is unclear. In this species, there is no statistically significant difference in V_{max}/kg of body weight or residual lung volume between male and female animals; both types

---

(9–5) Pediatr. Res. 15:235–240, March 1981.

of fetuses exhibit approximately the same percentage change after betamethasone. Further studies are in progress to determine whether the hyperinsulinemia observed in this model might account for the apparent minimal effect of glucocorticoids on pulmonary surfactant.

▶ [Dr. Johnson and his associates at Johns Hopkins University have reported several studies of glucocorticoid effects on the fetal macaque that seem to cast doubt on the commonly held belief of surfactant induction, indicating instead more of an action on lung volume and structure. This study confirms and extends these observations by documenting the increased collagen-to-elastin ratio of lung connective tissue and increased alveolar distensibility. If the glucocorticoid effects on fetal lung are more mechanical (as indicated by these observations) than functional (i.e., enzyme induction), then long-lasting or late effects on the lung become of even greater concern.

The possibility of a heretofore unrecognized adverse effect of glucocorticoids on the fetus is suggested by a study by Momma and associates (*Pediatr. Res.* 15:19, 1981). Fetuses of pregnant rats treated with hydrocortisone, prednisolone, or betamethasone demonstrated a dose-related constriction of the ductus arteriosus.] ◀

9–6 **Lung Volumes and Lung Mechanics in Babies Born Vaginally and by Elective and Emergency Lower Segmental Cesarean Section.** Compression of the thoracic cage during vaginal delivery results in elimination of fetal lung liquid. The crying vital capacity has been reported to be reduced in infants born by cesarean section. A. W. Boon, A. D. Milner, and I. E. Hopkins (Nottingham, England) made serial measurements of lung volume and lung mechanics in 25 vaginally delivered infants, 15 born by elective cesarean section, and 7 born by emergency section following established labor for 3 to 27 hours. Mean gestational ages were similar in all groups of infants.

Striking differences in thoracic gas volumes were found in the first 6 hours of life between the infants vaginally born and those born by elective cesarean section, with higher values in the former group. Infants born by emergency section had intermediate values. Midvolume total pulmonary resistance was significantly higher in the elective cesarean section group than in the vaginally born infants. Dynamic compliance was lower in the emergency section group than in the other groups. The differences gradually disappeared over the first 72 hours after birth. No significant difference in thoracic gas volumes was present at 48 hours.

The differences in thoracic gas volumes observed in this study probably are attributable to the presence of unresorbed lung fluid in infants born by cesarean section. The intermediate values found in infants born by emergency cesarean section in established labor suggests that the process of labor itself may aid the clearance of lung fluid. The 48 hours required for thoracic gas volumes in infants born by elective cesarean section to reach the values found in vaginally born infants presumably represents the time taken for excess lung liquid to be cleared by the pulmonary lymphatics. This closely parallels the time course for the resolution of transient tachypnea in the newborn infant.

▶ [Infants born by cesarean section have usually, though not always, been found to have a somewhat increased risk of respiratory distress. Earlier studies have indicated some effects of cesarean delivery on lung volumes and mechanics—less compliance,

(9–6) J. Pediatr. 98:812–815, May 1981.

greater pulmonary resistance, lower lung volume, and increased respiratory frequency. This report confirms these findings and indicates further that about 48 hours are required for the findings in the two groups to be equal. In general, the effects of emergency cesarean section were intermediate between those of vaginal birth and elective cesarean section, suggesting a combined influence by labor and cesarean section. It is tempting to conclude that these effects result from a "thoracic squeeze" with pelvic delivery that is lacking with cesarean section birth, leading to residual lung fluid. However, other factors (anesthesia, different management of cord clamping, etc.) also could be responsible.] ◄

9-7 **Technical Aspects in Management of Meconium Aspiration Syndrome With Extracorporeal Circulation.** J. C. German, C. Worcester, A. B. Gazzaniga, R. F. Huxtable, R. N. Amlie, N. Brahmbhatt, and R. H. Bartlett (Orange, Calif.) treated 18 patients who had severe respiratory failure from meconium aspiration syndrome by means of extracorporeal circulation with a membrane oxygenator (ECMO), a technique of venoarterial bypass with a membrane oxygenator that can support cardiopulmonary function during severe but reversible pulmonary failure. Other steps in the technique included parenteral hyperalimentation into the pump circuit, systemic antibiotics, preventive maintenance on the pump circuit, and coagulation control based on frequent measurements.

All 18 patients weighed more than 2 kg (average birth weight, 3.67 kg; average gestational age, 41.4 weeks). They had a mean PA_{O_2} of 25 mm Hg, pH of 7.08, and PA_{CO_2} of 70 mm Hg. None had improved with conventional support, and all had pulmonary insufficiency scores indicating 90%–100% mortality. None had contraindications such as birth weight under 1 kg, intracranial or pulmonary bleeding, chromosomal anomalies, ventilator dependency of more than 7 days, or evidence of bronchopulmonary dysplasia. The typical patient course of ECMO was stabilization for the first 12 hours followed by improvement on high bypass flow rates for 12–24 hours to maintain a PA_{O_2} of 50–60 mm Hg with minimal ventilator settings with an FI_{O_2} of 0.3–0.4. Bypass flow rates were reduced to maintain adequate PA_{O_2} with similar ventilator settings for another 24 hours. Survivors were taken off bypass and decannulated while on similar ventilator settings.

Of the 18 patients, 11 survived (61%) and 7 died (39%). Mean age at onset of ECMO was 20 hours for nonsurvivors and 33 hours for survivors. Mean total perfusion time was 69 hours. Only one technical malfunction occurred. Of the most recent 9 patients, 8 survived. All survivors were extubated 24–48 hours after ECMO decannulation. Of the 11 survivors, 1 has brain damage and 10 are normal. Nonsurvivors stabilized or improved but usually exhibited signs of intracranial hemorrhage by 48 hours. Intracranial hemorrhage appeared to be related to the degree of prebypass acidosis.

Successful ECMO support reduces the mortality from severe meconium aspiration syndrome by 50%. Its early institution, before acidosis worsens, should reduce the morbidity of conventional ventilator management and prevent intracranial hemorrhage from severe prebypass acidosis.

(9–7) J. Pediatr. Surg. 15:378–383, August 1980.

▶ [Extracorporeal circulation was moderately successful in improving the survival rate of neonates with severe pulmonary failure due to meconium aspiration. Mean perfusion time was about 3 days. With appropriate obstetric care (clearing of the hypopharynx prior to delivery of the shoulders and laryngoscopy prior to assisted ventilation), severe meconium aspiration syndrome should be rare.] ◀

9–8 **Growth and Development in Children Recovering From Bronchopulmonary Dysplasia.** Bronchopulmonary dysplasia (BPD) is a serious complication of ventilation in newborn infants, with reported mortality as high as 39%. Little is known of the prognosis for surviving patients. T. Markestad and P. M. Fitzhardinge examined growth patterns, cardiopulmonary status, and neurodevelopment in 20 survivors of BPD, who were followed prospectively from birth for at least 2 years. All had required positive-pressure ventilation for primary lung disease in the first 3 days of life and oxygen supplementation to maintain PA_{O_2} of more than 50 mm Hg beyond age 30 days. All had alternating areas of focal emphysema and atelectasis lasting at least 30 days. The 20 patients were among 26 who developed BPD at the Hospital for Sick Children, Toronto, in 1974–1977.

Pulmonary symptoms and lower respiratory tract infections declined markedly in the first 2 years of life. Chest films showed that all patients were improving at last follow-up, although most still had residual changes in the second year of life. Three of 10 patients had ECG evidence of right ventricular hypertrophy, but only 1 had signs of heart failure. Linear growth usually did not accelerate until there was marked improvement in the resting respiratory rate and clearing of the chest on auscultation. Four patients were growth retarded at age 2 years. Growth delay was associated with more severe lung disease. One patient had hydrocephalus, but there were no other major neurologic defects. Five patients had mean Bayley scores less than 85, and 2 were severely retarded. Low scores were associated with a prolonged need for oxygen supplementation and with recurrent apnea in the neonatal period. One patient had severe myopia following retrolental fibroplasia in the neonatal period. None had sensorineural hearing loss.

Infants who survive the acute stage of BPD have a prognosis comparing favorably with that of ventilated infants without this complication. Aggressive support of affected infants is indicated unless there is evidence of massive intraventricular hemorrhage. Neurodevelopmental status should be assessed only after respiratory function has improved markedly.

▶ [Longer-term studies are necessary for us to achieve a good understanding of the ultimate prognosis of bronchopulmonary dysplasia. Children with this disease, a complication of ventilator therapy, would have died as neonates in the pre-intensive care era. It is encouraging that pulmonary function generally improves during the first 2 years of life and that some catch-up in growth occurs coincident with this improvement; however, the fact that most of these children still have abnormal chest films at age 2 years is worrisome.] ◀

9–9 **Intracranial Hemorrhage in the Premature: Its Predictive Features and Outcome.** Intracranial hemorrhage is an increasingly

(9–8) J. Pediatr. 98:597–602, April 1981.
(9–9) Am. J. Dis. Child. 134:855–859, September 1980.

recognized cause of death with improvement in respiratory support of the preterm infant. Niki Kosmetatos, Colleen Dinter, Margaret L. Williams, Herbert Lourie, and Alfred S. Berne (Syracuse, N. Y.) examined the occurrence of intracranial hemorrhage in a series of 64 infants with birth weights of 500–1,500 gm. Those clinically suspected of having had intracranial bleeding had computed tomography (CT) scanning as soon as possible, and the other infants underwent scanning at age 7–10 days. Surviving infants with hemorrhage were followed up by weekly CT study for 4 weeks.

Thirty-seven infants (58%) were found to have intracranial hemorrhage. The diagnosis was made at autopsy in 7 cases, by postmortem ventricular tap in 3, and by CT scanning in the rest. Infants with hemorrhage had lower gestational ages and birth weights than the others. Twenty-two infants with hemorrhage and 2 other infants died. Ventricular and parenchymal involvement carried a worse prognosis than subarachnoid or subependymal hemorrhage only. Only 2 infants had progressive hydrocephalus that required shunt placement. Hemorrhage could not be related to maternal or pregnancy factors, but was associated with a low Apgar score, the need for ventilation after birth, hypoxia, metabolic acidosis, apnea, hypotension, and seizures. The most significant factors were low gestational age and respiratory distress syndrome. Twelve infants with hemorrhage had seizures. These infants had the most extensive hemorrhages, often with parenchymal involvement, and the highest mortality. Only 1 infant with seizures survived, compared with 14 of 25 without seizures.

Very low birth weight infants should be considered at risk for intracranial bleeding, which can be diagnosed by CT scanning. However, only infants at high risk should be examined because of questions of safety in terms of radiation exposure of the retina. Infants with intracranial bleeding are at maximum risk for later neurologic, developmental, and behavioral problems.

▶ [This systematic search, by means of CT scanning, for intracranial hemorrhage in small premature infants (500–1500 mg) revealed that 58% had hemorrhages and 60% of these died. Shorter gestations, the presence of respiratory distress syndrome, and lower Apgar scores were the strongest predicting factors. The importance of managing premature labor and delivery in order to prevent or minimize asphyxia is again apparent. The authors suggest that cesarean section may be protective, but they admit that more data are needed to answer this question.] ◀

9–10 **Subgaleal Hematoma: Complication of Instrument Delivery.** Subgaleal hematoma (SGH) is a rare but potentially fatal condition in the newborn that develops when blood accumulates in the loose areolar tissue between the pericranium and the galea aponeurotica of the scalp. Warren C. Plauché (Louisiana State Univ.) reviewed 123 cases of SGH reported in the literature.

Sixty cases of SGH were associated with vacuum extraction delivery, 35 with spontaneous vaginal delivery, 17 with midforceps delivery, and 11 with cesarean section delivery. The principal factors associated with an increased risk of SGH were difficult instrument delivery (intrapartal hypoxia) and neonatal coagulopathies. Other

(9–10) JAMA 244:1597–1598, Oct. 3, 1980.

predisposing factors included prematurity, fetal macrosomia, extensive molding of the skull, positional dystocia, and prolonged labor. The mortality rate in this review series was 22.8%.

Close observation of infants at risk, early recognition, differentiation from benign cephalohematoma, and prompt transfusion and correction of coagulopathies are essential for successful management of SGH.

▶ [This article nicely emphasizes the serious nature of a rare problem in the neonate. Subgaleal hematoma must be distinguished from the much more common (and relatively benign) cephalohematoma.] ◀

9–11 **Birth Injuries of the Brachial Plexus: Incidence and Prognosis.** A. E. Hardy (Auckland, New Zealand) reviewed data on 36 infants who sustained birth injuries to the brachial plexus at one hospital in 1969–1978, an incidence of 0.87 per 1,000 live births. Three infants had bilateral palsies. Fourteen had other associated birth injuries. Seventeen children were born to primiparous mothers. Four infants were delivered by breech and 2, by cesarean section. Eighteen of 30 cephalic deliveries were assisted with Kielland's forceps and 6 were assisted with other types of forceps. Shoulder dystocia was noted in 10 instances. The mean birth weight was 4,071 gm, and the mean gestational age was 40 weeks.

Six of 21 infants observed by others were recovering at the time of discharge, 10 had recovered by age 4 months and 4 recovered at ages 4–13 months. One child was not seen since age 6 weeks, when a residual deficit was present. Eight of the 15 infants followed up by the author were essentially normal, while 7 had residual signs at follow-up. Five of these infants had extensive lesions involving the C5–8 roots. Two infants had obvious gross weakness of the serratus anterior or other parascapular muscles. Shoulder abduction splintage with cloth splints was used for up to 3 months in 11 cases, but only once among the infants with residual deficit. The latter infant was the only one to have a medial rotational contracture of the shoulder.

Nearly 80% of infants in this series with birth injury to the brachial plexus recovered completely by age 13 months. None of those with significant residual deficits had severe sensory or motor deficit of the hand at follow-up. The author does not believe in using abduction splintage. The parents should place all the upper limb joints through a full range of motion when the child is fed after the first week of life. The prognosis of birth-induced palsy of the brachial plexus is less severe than previously thought.

▶ [This article written by an orthopedic surgeon offers useful information. Eighty percent of newborns with brachial plexus injury recovered over time. No child with signs at age 13 months recovered completely and no improvement was seen after age 2 years. Of the 6 children with residual damage who were delivered vaginally from cephalic presentation, 5 had been delivered with Kielland's forceps. The mean birth weight in these 6 cases was 4,576 gm! Careful management of labor and judicious use of cesarean section should minimize brachial plexus injury.] ◀

9–12 **Effectiveness and Safety of Prenatal Phenobarbital for Prevention of Neonatal Jaundice.** T. Valaes, K. Kipouros, S. Petme-

---

(9–11) J. Bone Joint Surg.[Br.] 63–B:98–101, April 1981.
(9–12) Pediatr. Res. 14:947–952, August 1980.

zaki, M. Solman, and S. A. Doxiadis (Inst. of Child Health, Athens) assessed the effect of 100 mg of phenobarbital at bedtime during the last few weeks of pregnancy (34–36 weeks of gestation) on the incidence and severity of neonatal hyperbilirubinemia. Newborns on the island of Lesbos and in Athens were enrolled in a controlled blind trial from 1968 to 1971. Phenobarbital was taken for a variable period (maximum 8 weeks) depending on the interval between the prenatal visit at 34–36 weeks of gestation and delivery. The control group received placebo tablets (phase I). After the efficacy of phenobarbital and the absence of immediate untoward side effects were demonstrated, all women in the last 4–6 weeks of pregnancy were given the drug in phase II of the study. Children of phase I patients were designated for follow-up.

No effect was observed in the newborns of mothers who took less than 10 tablets of phenobarbital. In the 1,310 newborns of adequately treated mothers (phenobarbital $\geq$ 1 gm), the incidence of marked jaundice (bilirubin >16 mg/dl) and the need to perform an exchange transfusion were reduced by a factor of 6 in relation to the incidence in 1,553 control infants. In infants with ABO fetomaternal incompatibility, the incidence of marked jaundice was reduced by a factor of 3, whereas exchange transfusion was reduced by a factor of 10. Of 3,075 newborns total, there were 2 with hemorrhagic manifestations, but both recovered after transfusion and administration of vitamin K. Both infants were in the phenobarbital group. These were the only instances in which phenobarbital administration in the mother could be considered responsible for complications in the newborn. No infant with symptoms suggestive of the withdrawal syndrome was observed.

A randomly selected group of 415 children (182 controls, 233 phenobarbital-treated) were reexamined at 61–82 months of age. There was no difference in overall morbidity and mortality between the control and the treatment groups. A detailed neurologic assessment failed to reveal any differences between the two groups. In the Visuo-Motor Integration test, the phenobarbital group scored significantly higher than the control group. In the Draw-A-Woman and the Verbal Intelligence tests, the difference was in the same direction but was not statistically significant. The degree of jaundice did not significantly influence performance in the neurologic examination and intelligence tests. In physical growth, the sex, social class, and place of residence were important variables, particularly for height; an advantage conferred by phenobarbital reached the level of statistical significance only for height. Sensorineural hearing deficit was significantly more common in children with moderate or marked neonatal jaundice (9.2%) than in those with slight or no jaundice (1.1%).

These findings suggest that prenatal phenobarbital administration is a practical, effective, and safe method for decreasing the incidence of neonatal hyperbilirubinemia. Clinical results should be ascribed to the action of the drug on the liver enzymatic mechanism of bilirubin elimination. The high incidence of marked jaundice and the need for infants from Lesbos to be transferred to Athens for its management make the financial benefits from prenatal phenobarbital administration considerable. Many substances (e.g., alcohol and pesticides) share phenobarbital's ability to induce liver enzymes. It is possible that part of the variability in newborn elimination of bilirubin is due to the differences in exposure during fetal life to environmental inducing agents.

▶ [Previous studies have demonstrated that maternal phenobarbital administration in late pregnancy diminishes neonatal jaundice by inducing the hepatic enzymatic mechanism, specifically glucuronyl transferase, involved in bilirubin metabolism. While this type of pharmacologic therapy has certain obvious benefits, the inevitable question of long-term safety must be raised. This study addresses that issue, and the results are reassuring. Children were examined by a battery of physical and neuropsychologic tests at ages 5 to 7 years, and those exposed prenatally to phenobarbital exhibited no adverse effects, compared with control children. In fact, according to one of the indexes, the Visuo-Motor Integration test, the phenobarbital-treated group scored significantly better than the control group. The authors conclude that routine prenatal phenobarbital treatment is a simple and safe method of decreasing the incidence of neonatal hyperbilirubinemia. It should be noted, however, that jaundice is a common problem in the Greek population studied. Whether this approach is advisable as a routine in lower-risk populations is uncertain at present. Finally, without belaboring the obvious, it should be pointed out that studies 5 to 7 years after birth, though reassuring, do not rule out long-term risks absolutely.] ◀

9–13 **Enhanced Activity of Pituitary-Gonadal Axis in Premature Human Infants.** J. Tapanainen, M. Koivisto, R. Vihko, and I. Huhtaniemi (Univ. of Oulu, Finland) studied postnatal pituitary-gonadal function in full-term and premature infants (mean gestational age, 40 and 32 weeks, respectively) between birth and 25 weeks of age.

Serum follicle-stimulating hormone (FSH) and luteinizing hormone (LH) values were significantly higher in premature than in full-term girls between birth and 10 weeks of age; mean FSH and LH levels in full-term girls varied between 0.6–6.2 and 3.8–4.7 mIU/ml, respectively. In premature girls, the peak FSH level was 63.1 and that of LH was 16.9 mIU/ml. In contrast, no difference in serum gonadotropin levels was observed between premature and full-term boys. No significant differences were seen in prolactin levels between the sexes or between premature and full-term infants. Postnatal testosterone levels between birth and age 5 weeks were similar in premature and full-term boys. From 6 to 15 weeks of age, serum testosterone values in premature boys (mean, 2.95 ng/ml) increased to a significantly higher level than in full-term boys (1.45 ng/ml). By 21–25 weeks of age, the serum testosterone level decreased to similar low levels in both groups. Mean serum testosterone levels in premature and full-term girls approximated 0.5 ng/ml immediately after birth, but decreased rapidly to very low levels. Serum FSH and LH values (girls) and testosterone levels (boys) were not significantly different between control premature infants and those given phototherapy for neonatal hyperbilirubinemia.

Elimination of placental steroids at birth is largely responsible for postnatal activation of the hypothalamic-pituitary-gonadal unit, as the gonadotropin levels of premature children reach their maximum after the first week of life following elimination of placental steroids (and possible other inhibitors) from the circulation. The magnitude of

(9–13) J. Clin. Endocrinol. Metab. 52:235–238, February 1981.

changes is evidently dependent on the extent of hypothalamic maturation in utero and, therefore, on length of gestation at birth. The dramatic postnatal elevation of serum gonadotropins in premature girls indicates that progressive sensitization of the hypothalamic gonadostat to sex steroid negative feedback occurs during the last few weeks of gestation. This sensitization continues after birth in premature girls, reaching the same set point as in full-term girls by about 6–10 weeks of age. Since full-term infants exhibit a transient, though much smaller, increase in gonadotropin levels, it is likely that progressive gonadostat sensitization extends into the immediate postnatal period. The nadir of postnatal gonadotropin levels reportedly is not reached until the second year of life. The fact that mean gonadotropin levels in premature and full-term boys were not significantly different could be due to testosterone levels in premature boys high enough to suppress pituitary gonadotropin secretion. The reason for the increased testosterone levels in premature boys aged 11–15 weeks is not clear.

▶ [Although the clinical significance, if any, of these findings is unknown, the observed differences between pituitary-gonadal axis function in full-term and premature infants are interesting. Apparently, in late fetal life the hypothalamus becomes more sensitive to the negative feedback of low levels of circulating sex steroids. It's no surprise, but again, we are reminded that there is more to fetal maturity than lungs that are resistant to the development of respiratory distress syndrome. Does prenatal corticosteroid administration to the mother affect neonatal sex steroid or gonadotropin levels?] ◀

9–14　**Cord Blood Tyrosine Levels in Full-Term Phenylketonuric Fetus and "Justification Hypothesis."** The justification hypothesis of Bessman (1972, 1979) attributes the mental retardation in phenylketonuria (PKU) to an inability of the heterozygous mother to deliver an appropriate amount of tyrosine to the fetus with PKU who, in turn, is unable to correct for this deficiency because of its genetic constitution. This hypothesis indicts tyrosine deprivation rather than excessive accumulation of phenylalanine as the important event in the pathogenesis of mental retardation in PKU.

Charles R. Scriver, David E. C. Cole, Sally A. Houghton, Harvey L. Levy, André Grenier, and Claude Laberge tested this hypothesis by measuring concentrations of tyrosine and phenylalanine in cord blood obtained at delivery from 14 infants with persistent postnatal hyperphenylalaninemia and from 56 control infants shown to be euphenylalaninemic. Of the 14 infants with hyperphenylalaninemia, 9 had PKU with blood phenylalanine levels above 1 mM while they consumed a normal diet and 5 had persistent (non-PKU) hyperphenylalaninemia (PHP) with blood phenylalanine levels below 1 mM while they consumed a normal diet.

The PKU and PHP groups were similar with respect to cord blood tyrosine and phenylalanine values. There was no deficiency of tyrosine in cord blood of the pooled PKU and PHP groups, compared with controls (54 vs. 61 µM, respectively). Phenylalanine levels in cord blood of the pooled PKU and PHP groups were somewhat greater

---

(9–14)　Proc. Natl. Acad. Sci. U.S.A. 77:6175–6178, October 1980.

than controls (144 vs. 128 μM, respectively). The magnitude of the differences in cord blood tyrosine and phenylalanine levels between control and PKU subjects was so small, however, that they probably did not have any consequence for physical and mental development. The justification hypothesis, as it pertains to blood tyrosine levels at term, was not upheld. Cord blood phenylalanine levels were higher than normal in infants with postnatal hyperphenylalaninemia. The phenotype was an excess of phenylalanine rather than a deficiency of tyrosine.

Maternal rather than fetal genotype appears to influence blood phenylalanine levels in the term fetus, and this influence is seen more in phenylalanine excess than in tyrosine deficiency. The fact that maternal serum tyrosine levels are normally depressed in pregnancy suggests that it may be further depressed in the obligate heterozygote during pregnancy. The fetus at term apparently reflects the maternal tyrosine enviroment. Normal infants and those with PKU do not differ in this respect.

▶ [An article abstracted in the 1979 YEAR BOOK (p. 182) suggested that mental retardation associated with phenylketonuria might be related to prenatal tyrosine deficiency rather than to phenylalanine excess. Not likely, according to this study. Although cord blood phenylalanine levels were higher in affected neonates than in control infants, there were no statistically significant differences in tyrosine concentrations.] ◀

9–15 **Hemodynamic Significance of Vasopressin in the Newborn Infant.** Maija Pohjavuori and Frej Fyhrquist (Univ. of Helsinki) measured plasma arginine vasopressin (AVP) levels in the newborn infant and investigated its relation to the course of delivery and hemodynamic status in 38 deliveries. Three groups were delineated: normal vaginal delivery (21); cesarean section after onset of labor (8); and elective cesarean section (9). Apgar scores, gestational age, and mean birth weight did not differ significantly among subgroups. Vaginal deliveries were induced with oxytocin, 0.5–1.0 IU/hour in 5% glucose intravenously. The plasma AVP concentration was measured by radioimmunoassay. Samples were obtained from the cord artery and vein immediately after birth and from a maternal vein at delivery. At delivery, early clamping of the umbilical cord was performed. Blood pressure (BP) of the infant was measured by the Doppler technique in the left arm of the infant 10 minutes after delivery. Rectal and heel temperatures and heart rate were measured at the same time.

Blood pressures of the infants were highest in the vaginal delivery group and lower in both cesarean section groups. There was a positive correlation of systolic BP with the difference between rectal and heel temperature ($r = 0.79$, $P < .01$). Figure 9–2 depicts this difference and systolic BP in infants delivered normally or by cesarean section. There was a negative correlation of systolic BP with heel temperature ($r = -0.87$, $P < .001$) in vaginal delivery. In normal deliveries, umbilical artery AVP concentrations were increased up to several hundred-fold above those in peripheral maternal blood or in infants 3

(9–15) J. Pediatr. 97:462–465, September 1980.

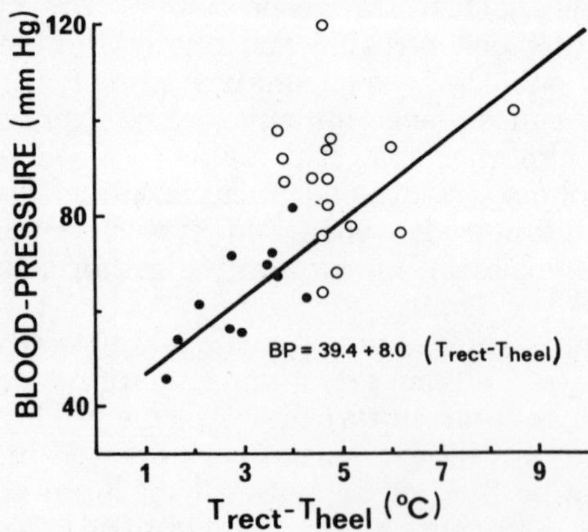

Fig 9–2.—Difference in rectal (T_{rect}) and heel temperature (T_{heel}) and systolic BP in infants delivered normally *(open circles)* and by cesarean section *(closed circles)*. (Courtesy of Pohjavuori, M., and Fyhrquist, F.: J. Pediatr. 97:462–465, September 1980.)

days later, and the mean umbilical arterial AVP level was sixfold higher than mean AVP concentration of the umbilical venous blood. In cesarean section after onset of labor, much lower cord blood AVP values were found, albeit clearly higher than in infants delivered by elective cesarean section. The mean umbilical artery AVP level was higher than that in the umbilical vein also in cesarean section after onset of labor, but not in elective cesarean section. Plasma AVP blood concentrations of mothers were not different from those of infants 3 days after delivery. There was a weak, but significant, correlation between umbilical artery AVP concentration and systolic BP when all deliveries were considered.

It is concluded that the massive release of vasopressin is associated with normal delivery and with peripheral vasoconstriction. Findings reflect favorable hemodynamic adaptation to the hypoxia and stress of delivery, intended to redistribute cardiac output to vital organs. The severalfold higher AVP values in cord arterial than in venous blood indicate the fetal origin of AVP. Reduction of placental blood flow during uterine contractions, causing fetal hypoxia, appears to be the main reason for fetal AVP release. Other nonosmotic factors associated with stress of delivery also may be involved.

▶ [The authors of this report make the interesting suggestion that the fetus responds to stress (hypoxia?) by secreting vasopressin. This increases peripheral resistance and blood pressure and perhaps redistributes the cardiac output to vital organs (heart, brain, adrenal glands). The association noted between the systolic blood pressure in the neonate and the rectal-heel temperature difference (see Fig 9–2) is consistent with this hypothesis.] ◀

9–16 **Single-Dose Penicillin Prophylaxis Against Neonatal Group B Streptococcal Infections: A Controlled Trial in 18,738 Newborn Infants.** Neonatal group B streptococcal infections do not always respond to antimicrobial therapy, and mortalities of 50% or

(9–16) N. Engl. J. Med. 303:769–775, Oct. 2, 1980.

INCIDENCE OF SEPSIS AND MENINGITIS DURING STUDY PERIOD*

	Penicillin Group (9439) †		Tetracycline (Control) Group (9299) †		P Value	
	Early-onset	Total	Early-onset	Total	Early-onset	Total
Pathogen						
Penicillin-susceptible organisms	1 (0.11)	6 (0.64)	15 (1.61)	21 (2.26) ‡	0.003	0.005
Penicillin-resistant organisms	8 (0.85)	23 (2.33) §	2 (0.22)	13 (1.40) ‡	0.11	0.19
Total	9 (0.95)	29 (3.07)	17 (1.83)	34 (3.66)	0.16	0.57
Group B streptococci	1 (0.11)	6 (0.64)	12 (1.29)	16 (1.72)	0.003	0.05
Deaths	2 (0.21)	12 (1.27) §	0	5 (0.54) ‡	0.5	0.15

*Values denote number of cases, with rate per 1,000 live births in parentheses.
†Number of live births in group.
‡One infant with late-onset, dual infection (isolation of *Streptococcus viridans* from lumbar cerebrospinal fluid and ventricular fluid and *Escherichia coli* from blood at the time of meningitis).
§One infant with early-onset, dual infection (isolation of *E. coli* and *Staphylococcus epidermidis* from blood, peritoneal fluid, and scrotal abscess).

greater have been reported. Jane D. Siegel, George H. McCracken, Jr., Norma Threlkeld, Bonnie Milvenan, and Charles R. Rosenfeld (Univ. of Texas Health Science Center, Dallas) evaluated the effect of a single intramuscular dose of aqueous penicillin G on the incidence of group B streptococcal colonization and disease rates in a prospective study of 18,738 newborn infants over a 25-month period. During the study period, 9,439 neonates were treated with penicillin and a control group of 9,299 infants was treated with tetracycline ointment.

A mean colonization rate of 26.6% was ascertained for the mothers. The concordance rate for neonates treated with penicillin was significantly ($P < .001$) lower than that for tetracycline-treated infants (12.2% vs. 50%). The incidence of early-onset and total disease caused by penicillin-susceptible organisms was significantly greater in tetracycline-treated infants than in penicillin-treated infants (table). However, the incidence of disease and the associated mortality caused by penicillin-resistant organisms was increased in the penicillin-treated group, but the difference between the tetracycline-treated infants and this group was not statistically significant (table).

It is concluded that routine intramuscular administration of penicillin at birth cannot be recommended until it is demonstrated that such treatment does not predispose to invasive disease caused by penicillin-resistant organisms. However, pencillin prophylaxis may be used temporarily to limit an outbreak of group B streptococcal disease within a nursery.

▶ [As faithful YEAR BOOK readers will recall, despite intense interest and several different approaches to the problem in recent years, just what to do about group B streptococci is not at all clear. The present report describes a "no free lunch" situation. Penicillin prophylaxis was effective in decreasing, but not eliminating, infections caused by group B streptococci and other penicillin-susceptible organisms; however, those infections caused by penicillin-resistant organisms were more frequent in the infants who received penicillin. Alas, still no answer!] ◀

9–17 **Iron Absorption From Human Milk and Formula With and Without Iron Supplementation.** It has been suggested that introduction of solid foods to breast-fed infants at about age $3^{1/2}$ months reduces the high bioavailability of iron from human milk. Philip J. Garry, George M. Owen, Elizabeth M. Hooper, and Barbara A. Gilbert studied iron absorption during the first 6 months of life on the basis of changes in total body iron determined from body weights, hemoglobin concentrations, and plasma ferritin values. Of 232 healthy infants enrolled in the study, 90 received human milk and 142 received proprietary formula containing only trace iron. Of the 90 breast-fed infants, 42 received another 10 mg of iron daily in a vitamin supplement containing ferrous sulfate beginning at age 4 weeks. Of the 142 formula-fed infants, 73 were given an iron-fortified formula containing 12 mg of ferrous sulfate per L beginning at age 4 weeks, and 69 remained on the nonfortified formula.

Total body iron was calculated from the sum of hemoglobin iron and body storage iron as described by Saarinen and Siimes. Iron absorption was then determined from the increments of total body iron; estimated daily iron loss from desquamated cells of skin, urinary tract, and intestinal mucosa; and estimated iron intake from human milk, supplemental iron, and iron-fortified and nonfortified infant formula.

From birth to age 3 months the increments of total body iron were

(9–17) Pediatr. Res. 15:822–828, May 1981.

49 mg for breast-fed infants who received no iron supplement (B), 59 mg for breast-fed infants receiving supplemental iron (B$^+$), 24 mg for infants receiving nonfortified formula (F), amd 28 mg for infants receiving iron-fortified formula (F$^+$). Between ages 3 and 6 months increments of total body iron were: B, -3 mg; B$^+$, 26 mg; F, 7 mg; and F$^+$, 23 mg. The percentage of iron intake that was absorbed during the first 3 months was calculated for each feeding group: B, 81%; B$^+$, 10%; F, 97%; and F$^+$, 6%. Between ages 3 and 6 months percentages of iron intake that were absorbed were: B, 10%; B$^+$, 4%; F, 22%; and F$^+$, 3%.

Although these data suggest, as do those of Saarinen and Siimes, that the bioavailability of iron in human milk is high, a different interpretation is offered as to why breast-fed infants do not appear to gain total body iron between ages 3 and 6 months. The present findings show that exclusive breast-feeding without iron supplementation is no certain means of preventing iron deficiency in midinfancy.

It has been reported that introduction of solid foods to breast-fed infants during the first 3 to 6 months inhibits iron absorption from human milk, resulting in a negative iron balance during this period. The infants in this study did not receive appreciable amounts of solid food until after age 5 months and then only in limited quantities. The negative iron balance observed in these breast-fed infants from age 3 to age 6 months can be explained by lack of sufficient iron in human milk to meet demands, even though nearly all iron in human milk may be absorbed. This finding suggests that even without the introduction of solid foods before age 6 months, some exclusively breast-fed infants might deplete their iron reserves rather rapidly after that age unless supplemental iron is provided.

▶ [The question of whether the breast-fed infant should receive supplemental iron is controversial among pediatricians. In this study, calculated total body iron increased to similar degrees (49 mg and 59 mg in infants not given and those given iron supplements, respectively) over the first 3 months of life. Over the succeeding 3 months, however, infants not given iron supplements lost an average of 3 mg, whereas those given iron supplements gained 26 mg. The iron concentration in human milk is low and, although the levels present are well absorbed, exclusive breast-feeding may lead to iron deficiency in the latter part of the first year of life.] ◀

9–18 **Comparative Newborn Anthropometric Data in Symmetric Versus Asymmetric Intrauterine Growth Retardation.** There are two basic patterns of intrauterine growth retardation (IUGR). In symmetric IUGR, all body organs are proportionately reduced in size; etiologic factors include maternal smoking, drug exposure, congenital anomalies, and intrauterine infection. In asymmetric IUGR, some body organs (e.g., liver) are affected more than others (e.g., brain); the cause is uteroplacental insufficiency. The "brain-sparing" concept of asymmetric IUGR has led to the suggestion that ultrasonic measurement of biparietal diameter is of limited value in detecting IUGR because biparietal diameter is an indirect reflection of head and brain size.

James P. Crane and Mazie M. Kopta (Washington Univ., St. Louis)

(9–18)   Am. J. Obstet. Gynecol. 138:518–522, Nov. 1, 1980.

studied the effects of asymmetric and symmetric IUGR on head circumference, birth weight, length, and ponderal index in 33 consecutive growth-retarded infants, of whom 20 had asymmetric IUGR and 13 had symmetric IUGR. The measurements were compared with those of normal infants of the same gestational ages.

No parameter studied was useful in distinguishing between symmetric and asymmetric IUGR. Approximately equal percentages of infants in each group had ponderal indexes below the tenth percentile for gestational age. Mean reductions in birth weight, body length, and head circumference were also similar. The percentage decrease in head circumference was about 8.5% in infants with asymmetric IUGR and 6.3% in those with symmetric IUGR ($P = .1$).

The concept of absolute "brain-sparing" in asymmetric IUGR is erroneous. Ultrasonic measurement of biparietal diameter can be of value in detecting this form of IUGR.

▶ [In this comparison, anthropometric data were similar in infants with symmetric and asymmetric IUGR. The latter, reflecting uteroplacental insufficiency, generally has been credited with a "brain-sparing" effect. A problem exists in the selection of the symmetric IUGR cases. Six of the 13 were related to maternal smoking and 1 to anemia. Smoking and anemia can result in uteroplacental insufficiency and, therefore, are probably not ideal choices for the symmetric group. It is curious that abdominal circumferences were not recorded in these neonates, given the current ultrasonographic interest in this dimension. The authors emphasize an important point: the "brain-sparing" effect in asymmetric IUGR is, at best, relative!] ◀

9–19 **Noise Pollution in Neonatal Units: A Potential Health Hazard.** The damaging effect of high-intensity noise on the human cochlea is well known. There is evidence that high noise levels stimulate the hypophyseal-adrenocortical axis and cause peripheral vasoconstriction. D. Anagnostakis, J. Petmezakis, J. Messaritakis, and N. Matsaniotis (Athens Univ.) measured hospital noise levels for 4 consecutive days every 2 hours throughout the day in a neonatal intensive care unit (NICU), a normal nursery room, and inside infant incubators associated with different types of life-support equipment.

There was a difference in noise level between the normal nursery and the NICU, and a considerable noise increase occurred when the infant received oxygen, was under a ventilator, or when an air compressor was in operation (table). High noise levels were similar in A.M. and P.M. hours in the NICU; highest noise levels corresponded to admission of a high-risk baby.

Noise levels in incubators were above a level that has a 25% probability of seriously affecting sleep in adults. Although noise levels were below the hearing damage risk criteria for adults, the safe sound level for babies is unknown. There is evidence based on animal studies that infants may be more susceptible to noise-induced hearing loss than adults. Damage risk criteria for adults are based on intermittent noise exposure, whereas newborns in incubators are exposed to continuous noise for days to months, with no recovery time. Another concern is the increased susceptibility to noise damage induced by ototoxic drugs. It is recommended that a special attempt be made

(9–19) Acta Paediatr. Scand. 69:771–773, November 1980.

Mean (±1 SD) Noise Levels in the Normal Nursery, the NICU Room, and Inside Incubators

Source	Noise level (dBA)	No. of measure- ments
Normal nursery	44±1.6	48
NICU room	51±2.0	48
Inside the incubator		
At the middle of the mattress	53±0.9	20
At the sides of the mattress	55±1.0	20
Opening the sleeves of the incubator	63±0.8	20
Under the hood (with O_2 5 l/min)	70±1.8	15
Under the hood (with O_2 through humidifier)	75±1.5	15
Respirator in operation	65±1.7	10
Air compressor in operation	67±1.8	10
During baby's cry	75±85	10

to limit unnecessary noise in the NICU; that if an infant receives ototoxic drugs, noise levels of the incubator and other devices should be regularly measured; and that noise-producing devices should be positioned as far from the newborn's head as possible. Since many high-risk infants spend a long time in a NICU, there is need for further evaluation of noise levels and their effect on outcome of infants.

▶ [This study demonstrates that noise levels in a neonatal intensive care unit exceed those in a normal nursery by approximately 25%. Whether this level of "excessive" noise is harmful to the newborn is unknown, but one could speculate that the sick premature infant might be especially sensitive to adverse influences on hearing or other physiologic systems.] ◀

PART TWO

GYNECOLOGY

10. Operative Gynecology

^{10–1} **Incidence, Trends, and Risks of Ectopic Pregnancy in a Population of Women** were analyzed by L. Weström, L. Ph. Bengtsson, and P.-A. Mårdh (Univ. of Lund). In women in Lund, Sweden, aged 15–39 years, the rate of tubal ectopic pregnancy per 1,000 diagnosed conceptions increased from 5.8 during 1960–1964 to 11.1 during 1975–1979. The mean annual incidence of ectopic pregnancy per 1,000 women increased from 0.6 to 1.2 during the same period. The increase was most pronounced in women aged 20–29. The numbers of ectopic pregnancies per 1,000 diagnosed conceptions increased with increasing age of the women (4.1 in teenagers, 6.9 in those aged 20–29, 12.9 in those aged 30–39). From 1970 on, the mean annual incidence of ectopic pregnancy per 1,000 women in those aged 20–29 became higher than in those aged 30–39.

Intrauterine contraceptive devices (IUCDs) were not used in Sweden before 1965. Among 20- to 29-year-old sexually active women at risk of pregnancy who had never had acute salpingitis, the rates of ectopic pregnancy per 100 woman-years were the same (0.3) in those who did not use contraceptives as in those using nonmedicated or copper-medicated IUCDs. The risk of an ectopic pregnancy increased sixfold to sevenfold after acute salpingitis. It was calculated that if the 20- to 29-year-olds who used IUCDs had used oral contraceptives instead, the increase from 4.6 to 9.7 in ectopic pregnancy rate per 1,000 conceptions from 1960 to 1979 would have stopped at 5.0.

The findings confirm the increased risk of ectopic pregnancy after salpingitis. The use of IUCDs—at least among women aged 20–29 years—seems to account for a substantial proportion of the increased rate of ectopic pregnancy in Lund during the past 2 decades.

▶ [A number of reports have called attention to an apparent increase in the frequency of tubal pregnancy during the past 20 or 25 years. This one from Sweden is particularly important because of the well-defined nature of the population. Except for patients with early spontaneous abortions who do not seek medical attention, all pregnancies in the city of Lund are under the care of the authors' clinics. Thus, the virtual doubling of the total ectopic pregnancy rate (5.8 to 11.1 per 1,000 conceptions) from 1960–1964 to 1975–1979 is undoubtedly real. The data show a close correlation with both salpingitis and the use of intrauterine contraceptive devices, leading the authors to conclude that the intrauterine contraceptive device is at least partially responsible for the increase in tubal gestations.] ◀

^{10–2} **β-Human Chorionic Gonadotropin as a Diagnostic Aid for Suspected Ectopic Pregnancy.** Early diagnosis of ectopic pregnancy is complicated by the fact that no single laboratory test is sufficient for differential diagnosis. Radioimmunoassay (RIA) of the serum β-subunit of human chorionic gonadotropin (β-hCG) is recog-

---

(10–1) Br. Med. J. 282:15–18, Jan. 3, 1981.
(10–2) Obstet. Gynecol. 56:197–203, August 1980.

SERUM β-hCG AND URINE PREGNANCY TESTS FOR PATIENTS WITH
SUSPECTED ECTOPIC PREGNANCY

No. of patients ($N = 86$)	Urine pregnancy test*	Serum β-hCG (positive > 1 ng/ml)	Urine test false positive or negative (%)
39	Negative	Negative	
14	Positive	Positive	
14	Negative	Positive	15
19	Positive	Negative	22

*Tests were performed in the hospital clinical laboratories (2-hour tube tests) or in the emergency room (2-minute slide tests).

nized as a rapid and unequivocal test for assessing trophoblastic viability. Ronald O. Schwartz and David L. Di Pietro (Vanderbilt Univ. Med. Center, Nashville, Tenn.) evaluated the results of RIA determination of β-hCG in a retrospective study of the hospital records of 234 patients who were tested because of signs and symptoms suggestive of ectopic pregnancy.

One hundred eighty-eight patients (80%) had negative serum β-hCG tests (less than 1 ng/ml); no patient was subsequently found to have an intrauterine or ectopic pregnancy. The most common symptoms were abdominal pain (91%), amenorrhea (76%), irregular bleeding (68%), and adnexal mass (55%). A final diagnosis of ectopic pregnancy was made in 22 patients. All had positive serum β-hCG assays, although 10 did not show the classic triad of symptoms (pain, uterine bleeding, and adnexal mass). There were no false negative β-hCG RIA results, whereas there were 15 false negative and 22 false positive urine pregnancy test results (table). A protocol for diagnosis of ectopic pregnancy is outlined.

The use of β-hCG RIA is recommended in cases of suspected ectopic pregnancy.

▶ [This report concerns the role of a sensitive pregnancy test (radioimmunoassay of β-hCG) in the diagnosis of ectopic pregnancy. Although standard urine pregnancy tests are not helpful in this situation, the serum β-hCG test can be. No patients with ectopic pregnancies had "negative" tests, and all patients with "positive" tests had pregnancies somewhere. Only half of the patients with ectopic pregnancies during the study period had the test performed. Presumably, the others were sick enough or symptoms were clear-cut enough that surgical intervention was indicated immediately and the several hours delay in waiting for the test result was inappropriate. We wonder how many of the positive test results in this series actually were reported "after the fact" to the clinicians involved. A sensitive serum pregnancy test can be helpful in diagnosing ectopic pregnancies, especially in those patients who one is "quite sure" are not pregnant. A positive test result, of course, does not discriminate between an intrauterine and extrauterine location of the pregnancy.] ◀

10–3 **Rh Immunoglobulin Utilization After Ectopic Pregnancy.** The fetomaternal hemorrhage associated with ectopic pregnancy can sensitize Rh-negative women at risk, and it has been suggested that unsensitized women with ectopic pregnancy should be protected with

(10–3) Am. J. Obstet. Gynecol. 140:246–249, June 1, 1981.

immune globulin. David A. Grimes, Franklyn H. Geary, Jr., and Robert A. Hatcher assessed the use of Rh immunoglobulin (RhIG) after ectopic pregnancy in a series of 305 patients treated in 1975–1978 who had a histologically confirmed ectopic pregnancy. They were compared with 389 patients having spontaneous abortion and treated at the same hospital in 1975.

The rate of ascertainment of Rh type was significantly higher for patients with ectopic pregnancy than for the comparison group. Only 1.6% of the former patients with ectopic pregnancy had no record of Rh type, compared with 4.9% of the group having spontaneous abortion. Candidates for receiving RhIG after ectopic pregnancy received it significantly less often than patients having spontaneous abortion. The difference persisted and was greater than threefold when women who were sterilized at the time of surgery for ectopic pregnancy were excluded. Rates of use of RhIG in presumably fertile candidates were not significantly influenced by race or age.

If ectopic pregnancy sensitizes 3%–4% of women at risk, an estimated 150–200 women may be sensitized each year as a result of ectopic pregnancy, although a lower fertility rate for these patients may reduce the impact of Rh sensitization. The advisability of administering RhIG to candidates who are sterilized at the time of laparotomy for ectopic pregnancy is unclear. If the present data are representative of national practices, patients with ectopic pregnancy are an important part of the "Rh immune globulin gap." Creative use of Rh prophylaxis is necessary if patients with ectopic pregnancy are to be protected from Rh sensitization.

▶ [We are not surprised that failures to utilize Rh immune globulin are more frequent after ectopic pregnancy than after other pregnancy episodes, but we are surprised by the high failure rate (64%) reported here. As we have commented previously (1979 YEAR BOOK, p. 435), protocols for Rh immune globulin utilization are generally in effect in the postpartum nursing unit and in the abortion clinic. In other pregnancy events, e.g., spontaneous abortion and ectopic pregnancy, the "system" is less likely to identify the patient who requires Rh immune globulin. *Individuals* must remember to pay attention to the Rh status of the patient. Therein lies the rub. Solutions? A more conscientious effort by all of us as individuals and the development of policies in our emergency rooms and on our gynecology wards are required to insure that Rh-negative patients with spontaneous abortions or ectopic pregnancies receive appropriate prophylaxis.] ◀

10–4 **Natural History of Diethylstilbestrol-Associated Genital Tract Lesions: Cervical Ectopy and Cervicovaginal Hood.** To describe the natural history of cervical ectopy and cervicovaginal hood (CVH), Donald A. Antonioli, Louis Burke, and Emanuel A. Friedman (Harvard Med. School) reviewed 2,563 colpophotographs taken at initial and follow-up examinations of 173 women who had been exposed to diethylstilbestrol in utero. The subjects were observed for as long as 5 years, and 23.1% had three or more follow-up examinations.

At initial examination, cervical ectopy was found in 121 patients and CVH in 123; both were present in 104. A dramatic devolution in cervical ectopy was observed over time; 91 women (75.2%) showed a decrease in extent and 38 (31.4%) showed complete eradication (Figs 10–1 to 10–3). Cervicovaginal hood diminished in 65 patients

(10–4) Am. J. Obstet. Gynecol. 137:847–853, Aug. 1, 1980.

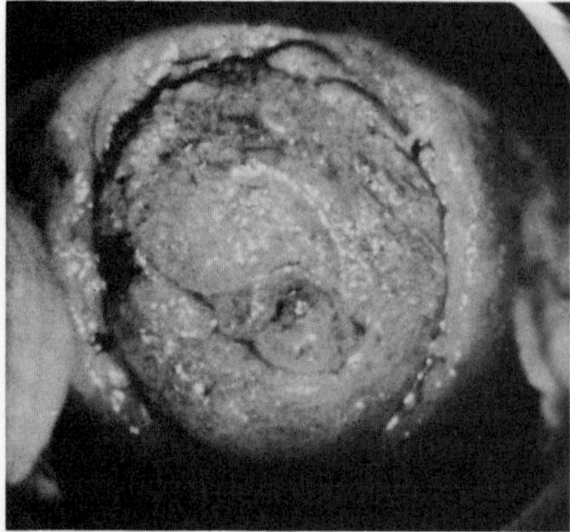

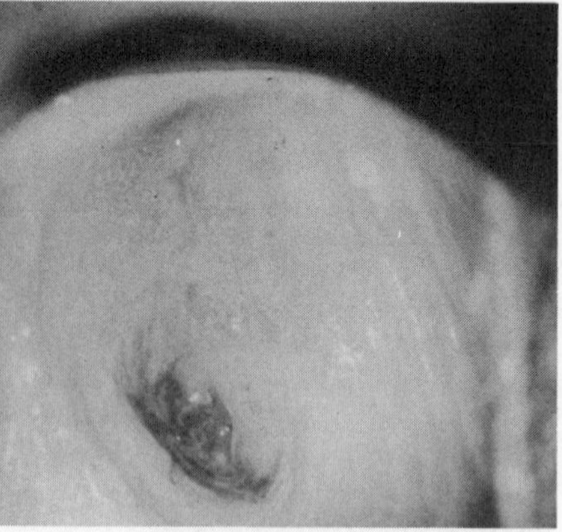

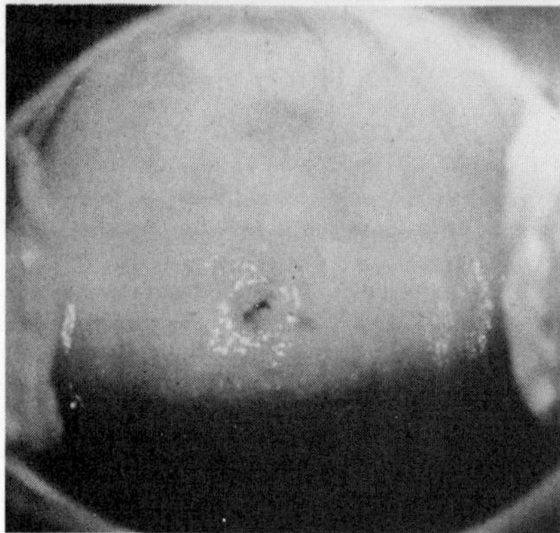

Fig 10–1 (above left).—Colpophotograph of cervix and CVH. Portio of cervix has complete ectopy. The CVH is circumferential and coverd with columnar epithelium. Groove demarcating CVH from portio is prominent; original magnification ×8.

Fig 10–2 (above).—Colpophotograph 24 months after first examination. All CVH mucosa and 70% of ectopy have been replaced by metaplastic tissue. Groove of CVH is obliterated between 9 and 4 o'clock; original magnification ×8.

Fig 10–3 (left).—Forty-two months after first observation. Entire portio is covered by metaplastic tissue and groove of CVH is completely obliterated.

(Courtesy of Antonioli, D. A., et al.: Am. J. Obstet. Gynecol. 137:847–853, Aug. 1, 1980.)

(52.8%) and completely disappeared in 35 (28.4%). The likelihood of devolution of these lesions increased with the duration of follow-up. Only 3.4% of those with cervical ectopy failed to show any change from the initial observation after 3 years. Women with both cervical ectopy and CVH showed parallel decreases in the extent of the lesions.

Diethylstilbestrol-related cervical ectopy and CVH are labile lesions that tend to diminish with time and may disappear altogether.

▶ [This report demonstrates for the first time a distinct tendency for diethylstilbestrol-associated cervicovaginal lesions to regress spontaneously. Both of the two major lesions, cervical ectopy and cervicovaginal hood, tended to decrease with time and actually to disappear in a substantial proportion, as illustrated in Figures 10–1 to 10–3. Ectopy seems to disappear somewhat more rapidly than a hood. Perhaps because of this tendency toward resolution of these changes, particularly ectopy, the incidence of cervical epithelial neoplasia has not been increased any more than it has in diethylstilbestrol-exposed women.] ◀

10–5 **Relation Between Measured Menstrual Blood Loss and Patient's Subjective Assessment of Loss, Duration of Bleeding, Number of Sanitary Towels Used, Uterine Weight, and Endometrial Surface Area.** T. H. Chimbira, Anne B. M. Anderson, and

(10–5) Br. J. Obstet. Gynaecol. 87:603–609, July 1980.

A. C. Turnbull (John Radcliffe Hosp., Headington, Oxford) investigated the relation between measured menstrual blood loss during two consecutive periods and the patient's subjective assessment of blood loss, the number of days of bleeding, and the number of sanitary pads and tampons used. The subjects were 92 women with the complaint of heavy but regular periods for which no cause was found. In 40 patients who had a hysterectomy 2 to 9 months after menstrual blood loss assessment, the uterus was weighed and the endometrial surface area measured by planimetry. All 92 women had been examined at least 2 months before the study; uterine curettage and general examination had excluded an organic cause of the menorrhagia.

There was no correlation between menstrual blood loss and the parameters investigated. The patient's judgment of blood loss showed no correlation with measured loss; there was a wide scatter of menstrual blood volumes in the three categories (light, medium, heavy). Thus, the parameters used in gynecology clinics to assess the amount of menstrual blood loss are not very precise in many women. An individual woman can only assess the amount of blood loss in relation to her previous pattern. In the women with hysterectomy, all uteri appeared normal with no evidence of fibroids, adenomyoma, or malignancy. In these women, no correlation was found between uterine weight and blood loss.

It seems possible that many women could be persuaded against therapy for menorrhagia if they knew that their menstrual blood loss was within normal limits. The mechanism of heavy regular menstruation remains unsolved, but the evidence presented in this study does not rule out the possibility that the problem lies within the uterus. In the absence of any obvious abnormality of pituitary-ovarian function, the cause of heavy menstruation could be an abnormality in function of the endometrium or myometrium or in their blood supply, a defect in prostaglandin synthesis or metabolism or both, or a defect in fibrinolytic activity.

▶ [The amount of menstrual blood loss on these patients without anatomical uterine abnormalities was unrelated to endometrial surface area, the patient's subjective assessment, or the number of pads or tampons used. Hemoglobin concentrations were not helpful either, although, in fairness, 12 patients were taking iron orally and others showed morphological evidence of iron deficiency. Our impression is that the hematocrit is of help in evaluating these patients. Perhaps, as the authors suggest, an objective measurement of menstrual blood loss such as that utilized in this study will find its way into clinical practice in order to permit better quantification of this common complaint.] ◀

10–6   **Cul-de-Sac Insufflation to Induce Pneumoperitoneum: Analysis of Rare Problems.** Various approaches to induce pneumoperitoneum for laparoscopy have been described. Kees J. van Schie, Dirk A. F. van Lith, Willem Beekhuizen, and Marijke du Plessis-Alblas (Center for Human Reproduction, Leiden, The Netherlands) believe that the vaginal route via puncture of the posterior fornix has the following advantages, which can reduce the potential for certain complications inherent to the abdominal route: it enables laparoscopic ex-

(10–6)   Int. J. Gynaecol. Obstet. 18:245–247, 1980.

amination to be offered to the severely obese patient; it is easy to use; it eliminates the possibility of vessel or organ perforation with the Veress needle since, in the midline, the cul-de-sac is virtually empty; and it reduces operating time because it can take place while a peri-umbilical block is given. Since 1977, cul-de-sac insufflation routinely has been performed to create pneumoperitoneum in patients under-going elective female sterilization with local anesthesia, and techni-cal failure rates of 3.6% in an initial series of 195 patients and 1.9% in a series of 155 patients have been reported; the failure rate in the last additional 220 patients was 1.4%, giving an overall rate of 2.1% (12 failures) for the total 570 patients.

It is believed the decline in technical failures is reflected by better recognition of contraindications, increased surgical experience, intro-duction of the modified Hulka intrauterine manipulator in combina-tion with a Trelat self-retaining speculum and a double-channeled insufflation needle, and limiting the depth of insertion of the pneu-moperitoneum needle to about 1 cm; this depth establishes the correct position of the needle tip in the cul-de-sac and prevents problems re-lated to obstruction of gas flow because of direct contact with the co-lonic wall or surrounding organs. Four reasons for failure of the tech-nique (Fig 10–4) are incorrect site of entry of the pneumoperitoneum needle directly into the lower posterior part of the uterine cervix, in-correct entry of the pneumoperitoneum needle too far below the true cul-de-sac so that the tip impinges on the rectum or coccyx, improper direction or depth of needle insertion after correct entry into the cul-de-sac, and malfunctioning or blocked insufflation needle. A double-barreled insufflation needle facilitates easy flow of gas while permit-ting use of a manometer to monitor continuously intra-abdominal pressure, which is particularly important in obese patients or pa-tients given general anesthesia. The procedure described may be of

Fig 10–4.—Recurrent reasons for failure in establishing pneumoperitoneum via the posterior vaginal fault: *(1)* site of entry of Veress needle too ventral, *(2)* site of entry of Veress needle too dorsal, *(3)* improper direction or depth of insertion of Veress needle once entry has been made at the proper site. (Courtesy of van Schie, K. J., et al.: Int. J. Gynaecol. Obstet. 18:245–247, 1980.)

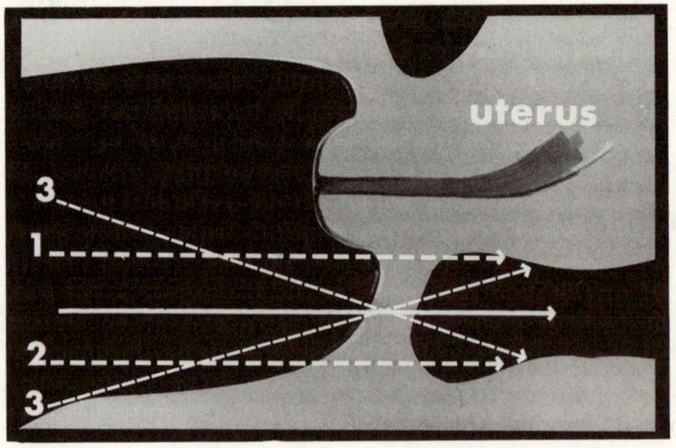

assistance in patients with multiple abdominal scars from prior surgeries.

▶ [The authors advocate the cul-de-sac route routinely for inducing pneumoperitoneum. While we have not used it on a routine basis, we have found it advantageous in patients with extensive previous abdominal surgery (such as a colostomy) or massive obesity.] ◀

10–7 **Combined Laparoscopic Surgery and Danazol Therapy for Pelvic Endometriosis.** James F. Daniell and Cathy Christianson (Vanderbilt Univ.) reviewed the treatment of pelvic endometriosis in 66 patients diagnosed by laparoscopy at evaluation for infertility. All implants that could be fulgurated without risking injury to vital structures were treated at laparoscopy. Peritubal and periovarian adhesions were lysed where possible. Endometriomas smaller than 3 cm were aspirated, fulgurated, and irrigated with saline for aspiration. Patients with mild or moderate residual disease and no residual adhesions received danazol in a dose of 800 mg daily for 25 days, followed by 600 mg daily. Treatment lasted 4 months in mild cases and 6 months in moderate cases. Six patients with severe endometriosis received 800 mg of danazol daily for 4 months before conservative surgery was performed.

Mild endometriosis was present in 35 patients and moderate disease was present in 25. The duration of infertility ranged from 1 to 14 years. Of the patients having laparoscopy and danazol therapy, 54% conceived, and 92% of them were delivered of a live infant. The corrected fertility rate of patients with mild and moderate disease was 68%. One of 5 patients who had conservative surgery after danazol therapy for severe endometriosis was delivered of a normal child. There was 1 ectopic pregnancy. Most pregnancies occurred within 6 months after danazol therapy was stopped. No complications resulted from laparoscopy. Two patients stopped taking danazol because of muscle cramps. Three of 19 patients with mild or moderate disease who had a second-look laparoscopy required further conservative surgery. No adhesions attributable to initial laparoscopy were observed.

A combination of laparoscopic surgery and danazol therapy can be effective in infertile patients with endometriosis. Second-look laparoscopy permits an accurate reappraisal of the pelvis and an opportunity for repeated conservative surgery if indicated.

▶ [This paper reports the use of laparoscopic surgery (cautery of endometriotic implants and lysis of adhesions) followed by danazol in 66 patients with endometriosis. The results (conception rates of 54% overall and 68% when corrected for other causes of infertility) seem comparable to those obtained with conventional (i.e., open) surgery and hormonal therapy. However, it is not possible to be certain of this point in the absence of a randomized trial.] ◀

10–8 **Preparation of Vagina for Surgery: Comparison of Povidone-Iodine and Saline Solution.** Marvin S. Amstey and Albert P. Jones (Univ. of Rochester) assigned patients undergoing major vaginal surgery to treatment with prophylactic antibiotics (ampicillin sodium, 1 gm, or cefazolin sodium, 500 mg, beginning at midnight before surgery and every 6 hours until 24 hours after surgery). Then, the effec-

(10–7) Fertil. Steril. 35:521–525, May 1981.
(10–8) JAMA 245:839–841, Feb. 27, 1981.

tiveness of preoperative vaginal preparation with 10% povidone-iodine solution as a douche the night before and on the morning of surgery in 17 patients was compared with that of saline douches in 16 patients. In the operating room, vaginas and perineums were scrubbed with the same solution as in the douche.

Preoperative cervicovaginal cultures after vaginal preparation showed more organisms per patient in the saline group. Postoperative cultures showed no qualitative difference in the type of organisms in each patient. Six patients treated with povidone-iodine and 3 treated with saline had febrile morbidity due to cuff cellulitis; all 9 patients were treated satisfactorily with penicillin G sodium (or ampicillin sodium) and kanamycin sulfate. Offending organisms in saline-treated patients were *Escherichia coli* (1 patient) and *Enterococcus* (2 patients). Offending organisms in the povidone-iodine-treated patients included *Proteus mirabilis, E. coli,* β-*Streptococcus* group B, and *Pseudomonas* (1 patient each); cultures revealed no growth in 2 patients. There was no statistical difference between the two groups.

Prophylactic antibiotics probably were of real benefit in reducing infection in both groups. Perhaps a more important factor in reducing infection, particularly in the saline-treated group, was the dilution effect of the solution. It was concluded that minimal infection occurs after using prophylactic antibiotics and only saline solution for vaginal preparation. No additional benefit could be demonstrated by using povidone-iodine instead of normal saline solution.

▶ [The results of this study seem to indicate that the ritual of preoperative vaginal preparation makes little difference with respect to the agent used, at least in patients treated with systemic antibiotic prophylaxis.] ◀

10–9 **Cefoxitin Sodium: Double-Blind Vaginal Hysterectomy Prophylaxis in Premenopausal Patients.** Cefoxitin sodium is a new semisynthetic cephamycin antibiotic derivative of cephamycin C. It has a broad antibacterial spectrum in vivo and in vitro that includes all strains of cephalosporin-sensitive bacteria and the majority of cephalosporin-resistant bacteria. Abe Mickal, David Curole, and Carter Lewis (Louisiana State Univ., New Orleans) undertook a double-blind (cefoxitin and placebo) study in premenopausal women undergoing vaginal hysterectomy. Of 152 patients, 125 completed the study, the objective of which was to determine the clinical effectiveness of cefoxitin as a safe prophylactic antibiotic. There were no major clinical differences among patients, since both placebo and cefoxitin groups were from the authors' clinic. Preoperatively, each patient received two injections, one deep in each buttock or lateral thigh muscle. Each syringe contained 1 gm of cefoxitin sodium or a similar-appearing placebo. No adverse reactions were noted in either group.

Anaerobic organisms and aerobic organisms showed no significant difference between placebo and treated groups preoperatively. There was no significant variation in the number of organisms per culture in the preoperative and postoperative cefoxitin group. However, there was a 37% increase in the number of organisms per culture in the

(10–9) Obstet. Gynecol. 56:222–225, August 1980.

postoperative placebo group, a possible reason for the higher postoperative morbidity in the placebo group. Complications related to postoperative respiratory tract infections, fever of undetermined origin, breakdown of the vaginal incision, and infection of the lower urinary tract were classified as minor morbidity; these did not differ between groups (53% in placebo and 47% in the cefoxitin group). Hospital stays and recovery were not altered by minor morbidity. Major morbidity was defined as general sepsis with a high index of suspicion for bacteremia. These complications included moderate to severe pelvic cellulitis or abscess formation, pelvic thrombophlebitis, and temperature of 39.4 C or above. There were 17 patients (29.8%) with early major morbidity in the placebo group and 7 (10.3%) in the cefoxitin group. One patient in the placebo group had late major morbidity (pelvic abscess).

The vagina, cervix, endocervix, and postoperative vaginal cuff harbor many aerobic and anaerobic organisms. It is difficult to isolate specifically the organisms causing the morbidity from cultures taken from these sites. The present study and a review of the literature lead to the conclusion that prophylactic antibiotic therapy is beneficial in premenopausal women undergoing vaginal hysterectomy.

▶ [Several previous studies have demonstrated the efficacy of short-term antibiotic prophylaxis in premenopausal women undergoing vaginal hysterectomy. Cefoxitin, a broad-spectrum cephamycin with activity against a wide range of organisms, including *Bacteroides* species, was associated with significantly less major morbidity than was placebo in this study. Whether this drug does a better job than others more frequently used in these patients (e.g., ampicillin or other cephalosporins) remains to be determined.] ◀

10–10 **Experience in Series of Fimbriectomies.** Selwyn Oskowitz, Albert D. Haverkamp, and Walter L. Freedman (Univ. of Colorado) reviewed 247 consecutive sterilizations by fimbriectomy performed by residents in obstetrics and gynecology during 1969 to 1971, of which 220 were bilateral and 27 were unilateral with a different type of tubal ligation performed on the other side. The surgical techniques included 4-to 6-cm suprapubic transverse incisions, 4-cm subumbilical vertical incisions, semilunar periumbilical incisions in postpartum patients, or 4-cm incisions in the typical culdotomy vaginal approach. Two 0 silk sutures were used on the tube. A first-stick suture was placed in the mesosalpinx and tied around the tube. The second suture was similarly placed, just distal to the first, and tied on both sides. The fimbriae were then resected. Microscopic examination confirmed fallopian tube tissue in all cases.

There were 6 failures (2.4%), all of which occurred in operations with limited exposure (table). Excluding the unilateral fimbriectomies, the failure rate was 2.7%. Of the 6 failures, 3 had fimbrial tags and 1 had an accessory ostium. Four of the failures occurred within 12 months of surgery, but 1 occurred as late as 59 months. Patient age was not related to fimbriectomy failure. Morbidity rates were higher for postpartum patients (14.5%) than for interval patients (3.4%), but this difference may not be related to surgery.

(10–10) Fertil. Steril. 34:320, October 1980.

FAILURE RATES BY SURGICAL APPROACH

Surgical approach	No. of cases	No. of failures	Failure rate
Postpartum periumbilical	121	5	4.1%
Interval vaginal	56	1	1.8%
Interval abdominal	18	0	0
Cesarean section	29	0	0
Hysterotomy (therapeutic abortion)	21	0	0
With ectopic pregnancy	2	0	0
Total	247	6	2.4%

Fimbriectomy has a high failure rate, which makes it unacceptable as an operative form of sterilization. Modifying the technique to include removal of most of the tube reportedly yields better results, but this detracts from the original purpose of fimbriectomy, i.e., minimal interference in the tubo-ovarian vasculature. Acquired tuboperitoneal fistulas, not seen in this series, have been described in other fimbriectomy failures, and it is not clear how these may be avoided. Fimbriectomy should not be regarded as the method of choice unless wide surgical exposure and complete removal of fimbriae, including the fimbria ovarica, can be insured.

▶ [The failure rate for sterilization by fimbriectomy noted here, 2.4%, is quite similar to the figure of 1.8% found by Metz in an article abstracted in the 1978 YEAR BOOK (p. 269). Clearly, it is time to lay to rest this operation as a means of female sterilization.] ◀

10–11 **Endometriosis and Development of Tuboperitoneal Fistulas After Tubal Ligation.** John A. Rock, Tim H. Parmley, Theodore M. King, Leonard E. Laufe, and Brian C. Su (Johns Hopkins Hosp.) detail gross and histologic findings of 79 previously ligated fallopian tubes from three groups of patients.

Of 20 oviducts removed after documented sterilization failure (group I), 6 revealed a process compatible with endometriosis. India ink was successfully injected in 4 of 9 previously ligated fallopian tubes removed at the authors' institution from patients having pelvic surgery (group II). In 2 patients, histologic examination demonstrated the India ink in epithelium-lined spaces that lay in and beyond the muscle of the tubal wall, extending from the tubal lumen to the serosal surface; many of these spaces were apparently foci of endometriosis, in which gland lumina provided the fistulous tract.

Fifty oviducts were studied in 25 patients requesting reversal of sterilizations (group III). By preoperative histerosalpingography, 8 patients and 11 tubes showed evidence of a fistula at the tip of the proximal segment of the tube. At operative injection of indigo carmine dye, all radiographically demonstrated fistulas were confirmed, and three unsuspected fistulas in 3 additional patients were documented. Five of the fistulas extended into the broad ligament but did not reach the peritoneal surface. At operation there was no evidence

(10–11) Fertil. Steril. 35:16–20, January 1981.

STERILIZATION REVERSAL (GROUP III): PERCENTAGE OF FISTULA
FORMATION AND ENDOMETRIOSIS VS. LENGTH OF REMAINING
PROXIMAL TUBAL SEGMENT

Length of remaining proximal tubal segment	No. of fistulas/ no. of tubes studied		No. of tubes with endometriosis/ no. of tubes studied	
cm				
<4	13/29	(45%)	20/27[a]	(74%)
≥4	1/21	(5%)	4/21	(20%)

*One tube was not subjected to pathologic examination.

of ovarian or peritoneal endometriosis, but in 15 patients, apparent endometriosis was observed at the tip of the proximal segment of the ligated fallopian tube; in 1, neither a fistula nor endometriosis was identifiable microscopically. Similar foci were not seen on the distal segment of the fallopian tube. Microscopically, all but 1 of 14 tubes with a fistula appeared to have endometriosis at its tip extending through the tube wall; 1 of these tubes was not studied microscopically. In 10 patients, endometriosis without fistula was seen microscopically, but it was not extensive and was not seen to extend through the tube wall. A higher percentage of fistulas and endometriosis was demonstrated in patients with less than 4 cm of remaining proximal tube segment (table). Most fistulas were demonstrated in patients for whom 3 years had elapsed since the sterilization procedure. Patients sterilized by laparoscopic cautery methods had a higher percentage of fistula formation and histologic demonstration of endometriosis at the sterilization site, as compared with patients sterilized by other methods. Although no fistulas were demonstrated in tubes ligated with a Silastic ring, 4 revealed endometriosis.

These findings suggest that oviduct ligation within 4 cm of the uterine cornu may predispose to development of endometriosis and subsequent fistula formation in the tip of the ligated oviduct. Prior to fistula development, the tube appeared to have been dilated. It is speculated that regurgitated menstrual fluid may be responsible for the development of endometriosis and tube dilatation. Observations suggest that the Pomeroy procedure, performed more than 4 cm from the cornu, results in fewer fistulas. As the process appears to develop within 1–4 years of tubal ligation, it is of interest to consider what role it may play in the so-called posttubal ligation syndrome. It is conceivable that pain and irregular bleeding might be concomitant symptoms.

▶ [Although we have used the term "recanalization" to explain tubal sterilzation failures, we may have misspoken. The authors of this article point out that they have not seen reestablishment of the tubal lumen as such. Rather, tuboperitoneal fistulas explain the rare failures. These fistulas apparently result from endometriosis and occur more commonly if the remaining proximal tubal segment is short.] ◀

10–12 **Luteal Function After Tubal Sterilization.** Jacques Donnez, Michel Wauters, and Karl Thomas (Univ. of Louvain, Brussels) eval-

(10–12) Obstet. Gynecol. 57:65–68, January 1981.

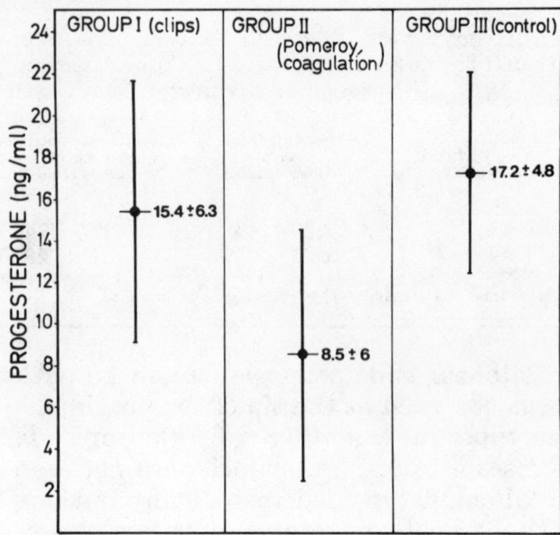

Fig 10–5.—Mean ± SD midluteal serum progesterone levels in groups 1, 2, and 3. (Courtesy of Donnez, J., et al.: Obstet. Gynecol. 57:65–68, January 1981.)

uated luteal function in 35 women sterilized by Hulka-Clemens clips (group 1). Evaluation was done by measurement of serum progesterone levels and endometrial dating. Blood samples and endometrial biopsy specimens were obtained 5 to 10 days before the next menstrual period, in the midluteal phase. The findings were compared with those for 23 women who had been sterilized by tubal ligation or electrocoagulation (group 2) and those for 65 fertile women who served as controls (group 3).

Women in group 2 had a significantly ($P < .001$) lower mean midluteal serum progesterone level (8.5 ± 6.0 ng/ml) than those in group 1 (15.4 ± 6.3 ng/ml) and group 3 (17.2 ± 4.8 ng/ml) (Fig 10–5). Comparisons among the three groups on days 19 and 20 of the menstrual cycle and also on days 21 and 22 yielded the same statistical data as the comparison of mean progesterone levels. Serum progesterone levels less than 10 ng/ml were found in 54% of group 2 women, but in only 20% of group 1 and 12% of group 3. Nine of the 35 women in group 1 and 11 of 20 in group 2 showed an endometrial development that was retarded by 2 days or more. In group 2, 6 endometrial specimens were in the proliferative phase, with progesterone levels less than 3 ng/ml, and 3 specimens showed a tendency to glandular cystic hyperplasia, with progesterone levels less than 3 ng/ml.

The results suggest that the application of Hulka-Clemens clips does not alter luteal function. The observed differences between the two sterilized groups (1 and 2) may be explained by the fact that the Hulka-Clemens technique preserves the continuity of the uteroovarian artery.

▶ [We expressed surprise at an earlier report that suggested that luteal insufficiency not uncommonly followed tubal sterilization by electrocautery or the Pomeroy technique (Radwanska et al.: *Obstet. Gynecol.* 54:189, 1979; and 1980 YEAR BOOK, pp. 415–416). Our surprise notwithstanding, the current study is confirmatory and suggests that use of the Hulka clip obviates this problem. Most internal sterilizations on our service are done with cautery. Clips are chosen in certain young patients if we have concerns about the permanence of the patient's decision. Our aim is to make reanastomosis easier, should it later be required. This report suggests an added advantage of the clip in this situation. We use the Pomeroy technique for puerperal sterilizations. Should we be clipping rather than "tying" the tubes in young women who request sterilization post partum?] ◄

10–13 **Microsurgical Tubal Reanastomosis: Role of Splints.** David R. Meldrum (Univ. of California, Los Angeles) describes a microsurgical technique of tubal reanastomosis in which splints are not used during or after the repair. Thirty-two patients were operated on between 1976 and 1979 and subsequently attempted conception for at least 1 year. In 25 cases tubal occlusion was due to previous sterilization. Tubal ligation and resection had been done at laparotomy in 21 of these. Repair was done after menstruation had ceased but before the expected time of ovulation under coverage with cefazolin. Iris scissors were used to make a small opening in the center of the point of occlusion as the lumen was distended with indigo carmine. The opening was matched to the proximal segment as far as was possible. The submucosa and inner muscularis were approximated with 8–0 nylon sutures under 10 to 15 powers of magnification. Patency was verified by transfundal dye irrigation before closure of the serosa and outer muscularis and the mesosalpinx.

All but 4 of the 25 patients undergoing repair for reversal of sterilization achieved an intrauterine pregnancy, and no ectopic pregnancies occurred. Mean time from operation to estimated date of conception was about 26 weeks. Threatened abortion was seen in 1 case that was not followed further. Four of the 7 patients treated for occlusion due to disease achieved an intrauterine pregnancy. One had an early spontaneous abortion. Patency has been confirmed in all 7 patients. One patient had an ectopic pregnancy that was not due to the reanastomosis.

Use of a splint is unnecessary to assure accurate suture placement or to aid in assuring postoperative tubal patency in patients undergoing reanastomosis. The approach described avoids most intraluminal manipulation. No evidence of luteal insufficiency has been obtained in previously sterilized women who have had this procedure. Newer methods of sterilization involving less tubal destruction and further experience with microsurgical methods may make female tubal sterilization essentially reversible.

► [Two points: (1) This series indicates a high success rate for microsurgical reanastomosis in the absence of splints, and (2) in contrast to reports both above and in the 1980 YEAR BOOK (pp. 415–416), luteal insufficiency as indicated by low progesterone levels was not a consequence of tubal sterilization. This latter issue is an important one and apparently is not yet resolved.] ◄

10–14 **A Comparison of Treatment for Bilateral Fimbrial Occlusion.** Alan H. DeCherney and Nathan Kase (Yale Univ.) divided 18 patients with bilateral tubal occlusion, without other causes of infertility demonstrated, alternately into two groups. Nine women under-

---

(10–13) Obstet. Gynecol. 57:613–619, May 1981.
(10–14) Fertil. Steril. 35:162–166, February 1981.

COMPARISON OF STUDIES UTILIZING VARIOUS SURGICAL TREATMENTS TO CORRECT FIMBRIAL OCCLUSION

Study	No. of patients	Patency rate	No. of patients conceiving	Term pregnancy rate	Ectopic pregnancy rate
Prosthetic device					
Young et al.[6] (1970)	24		37.5%	25%	4%
Sovak technique					
Garcia and Aller[7] (1974), hood	36	90%	26%	18.2%	0%
Roland and Leisten[11] (1972), stent	130	95%	25%	23%	0%
Terminal salpingostomy (microsurgical technique)					
Swolin[1] (1975)	33			24%	18%
Gomel[2] (1978)	41		44%	27%	12%
DeCherney[a] (1981)	54	90%	44%	26%	17%

[a]Present study. Other superscript numbers refer to references in original paper.

went a two-stage surgical procedure utilizing a Rock-Mulligan Silastic hood prosthesis; the other 9 underwent terminal neosalpingostomy with microsurgical technique, defined as use of microcautery, vigorous normal saline lavage, and careful handling of tissues with the operating microscope employed. Both groups received preoperative, intraoperative, and postoperative antibiotics, Decadron, and Phenergan.

Hysterosalpingography 4 months postoperatively revealed 89% of both groups had one or two patent tubes. Term intrauterine pregnancy rates were 22.2% (2 patients) in the hood group and 44.4% (4 patients) in the microsurgical group. There were no complications, ectopic pregnancies, or early pregnancy wastage. Of the 12 patients who did not conceive, 1 in each group showed bilateral hydrosalpinges on postoperative hysterosalpingograms. Four of the other patients had recurrent hydrosalpinx and peritubal adhesions documented on laparoscopy 1 year after surgery. No factor was found to account for the recurrence. No patient conceived after laparoscopic terminal salpingostomy (as reported by Gomel, 1977). In 54 patients subsequently treated by terminal salpingostomy, hysterograms showed a 90% patency rate 4 months later. There were no complications. Of 24 patients (44.4%) who conceived, 4 (7.4%) had tubal ectopic pregnancies and 6 (11.1%) had early abortions; 14 patients (25.9%) carried to term. No statistical difference was found in comparing the hood group with the two microsurgical groups.

It was concluded that Rock-Mulligan hoods offer no advantage over microsurgical salpingostomy, but have the disadvantage of requiring two surgical procedures. Various surgical methods of correction of hydrosalpinges are reviewed (table). The high failure rate in salpingostomy stems from previous intrinsic damage to tubal epithelium; failure to identify the end of the tube when neosalpingostomy is performed; the questionable essential role of the fimbria ovarica; damage to the fimbriae and blood supply by any technique; and postoperative scarring.

▶ [The use of Rock-Mulligan hoods and their required second laparotomy did not offer any advantages over microsurgical terminal salpingostomy in this study. All patients had hydrosalpinges and none required only fimbriolysis. Note the disparity between the patency and term pregnancy rates given in the table. This undoubtedly reflects intrinsic tubal damage. If this is so, does the microscope really make a difference?] ◀

10–15 **Prevention of Abdominal Wound Disruption Utilizing the Smead-Jones Closure Technique.** Darryl Wallace, Wilfredo Hernandez, J. B. Schlaerth, R. N. Nalick, and C. Paul Morrow (Los Angeles) evaluated the Smead-Jones technique for abdominal wound clo-

Fig 10–6.—Smead-Jones closure technique. (Courtesy of Wallace, D., et al.: Obstet. Gynecol. 56:226–230, August 1980.)

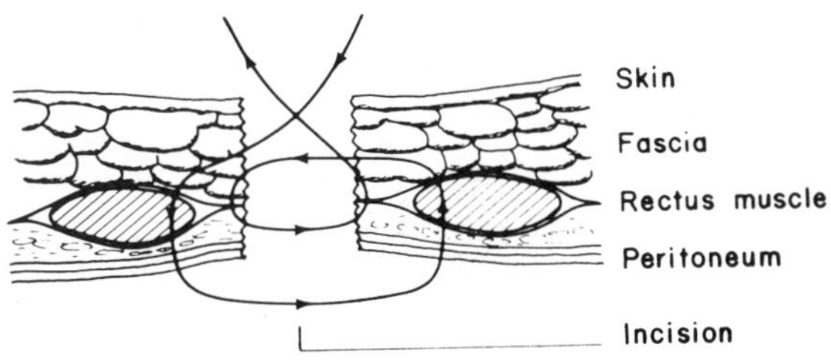

FACTORS IN WOUND DISRUPTION

Preoperative patient predisposition
    Nutritional—hypoproteinemia, anemia, advanced age
    Metabolic—diabetes, uremia, steroid therapy
    Prior irradiation
    Malignancy
    Obesity
    Pulmonary disease
    Chemotherapy
Intraoperative technique
    Incision choice
    Suture—tensile strength, knot strength
    Closure technique—suture cutting through fascia
    Pressure necrosis
Postoperative increased tension on suture line
    Increased intraabdominal pressure: ascites,
       ileus, bowel obstruction, vomiting
    Pulmonary disease—coughing
    Mesomorph—nulliparous
Wound infection

---

sure (Fig 10–6) in a retrospective study of 747 patients undergoing surgery in a gynecologic oncology service. The findings were compared with those for 545 lower-risk procedures using layered wound closure.

No dehiscences occurred with the Smead-Jones technique, while 5 occurrences of wound disruption were recorded for surgical wounds closed in layers. The overall infection rate for the Smead-Jones technique was 14%. Preoperative, operative, and postoperative high-risk factors for wound dehiscence are listed in the table.

The results indicate that the Smead-Jones technique was superior in the prevention of wound disruption.

▶ [The efficacy of the Smead-Jones closure in preventing wound disruption is clearly demonstrated in this series of high-risk patients. The authors used prolene or nylon sutures. Although we don't think this closure is necessary in every gynecologic laparotomy through a vertical incision, it should be considered in patients who are predisposed to wound dehiscence. If a layered closure is selected in other patients, the fascia should be closed with interrupted sutures of a material other than catgut.] ◀

11. Gynecologic Urology

11–1 **Urine Culture After Treatment of Uncomplicated Cystitis in Women.** Follow-up urine culture for urinary tract infection (UTI) is recommended widely, but is done relatively infrequently. Richard N. Winickoff, Susan I. Wilner, Gail Gall, Thomas Laage, and G. Octo Barnett (Boston) made a retrospective study of 141 women with culture-proven ($\geq 10^5$ organisms per ml urine) symptomatic lower UTI treated with an antimicrobial agent. Excluded were patients judged to be at high risk for renal complications of UTI and those with symptoms at first follow-up culture (after completion of antimicrobial drug treatment, within 3 months of the initial positive culture).

There were 80 patients (56.7%) who had a follow-up culture and 61 (43.3%) who did not. The two groups were comparable in important risk parameters for UTI and its complications. Mean ages were 28.7 years in the "no follow-up" (NFU) group and 29 years in the "follow-up" (FU) group. *Escherichia coli* accounted for 80.8% of infections. Sulfisoxazole was prescribed for 83.7% of initial UTIs. Morbidity in the FU group in the first 3 months after infection was excluded from analysis. In the FU group, 12 (15%) of the 80 women had a subsequent UTI; 5 (8.2%) of 61 had a subsequent UTI in the NFU group. The relative risk of a subsequent symptomatic UTI was 0.5 for women who did not obtain a follow-up urine culture (95% confidence interval = 0.2–1.5, not significant); thus, such women were not at greater risk for the development of a subsequent UTI. Excluding cultures obtained in the first 3 months after initial infection, 13.1% of women in the NFU group and 16.2% in the FU group had asymptomatic bacteriuria over the year. Only 3 (3.8%) asymptomatic patients of the FU group had positive initial follow-up cultures ($\geq 10^5$ organisms/ml of any type, or $\geq 10^4$ organisms/ml if they were of the same species and sensitivities as initially). This is the group that would have been expected to benefit from follow-up cultures. One patient had a subsequent symptomatic cystitis with the same organism 5 months after initial infection and 4 months after the positive culture, which had not been treated. The positive follow-up culture in 1 patient was negative 9 days later when repeated, and no subsequent infection occurred. A third patient was treated and never had symptoms. Most recurrences (11 of 12) could not have been prevented by follow-up cultures, because these were negative.

Several studies have shown that, in nonpregnant women with unobstructed urinary tracts, asymptomatic bacteriuria does not lead to chronic renal failure or to an increased incidence of pyelonephritis. Studies have concluded that antimicrobial therapy does not prevent

(11–1) South. Med. J. 74:165–169, February 1981.

further symptomatic episodes and may lead to more subsequent symptomatic UTIs, often with different organisms; the inconvenience and risk of drug reactions also must be considered. With routine follow-up cultures eliminated, patients with untreated asymptomatic bacteriuria would be allowed to reappear with recurrent UTIs. Patients with several symptomatic infections in a year would undergo further diagnostic evaluation. The findings support the ineffectiveness of follow-up urine culture in asymptomatic, healthy women in reducing subsequent urinary tract infections.

11–2 **Excretory Urography, Cystography, and Cystoscopy in Evaluation of Women With Urinary Tract Infection: A Prospective Study.** Jackson E. Fowler, Jr., and E. Thomas Pulaski studied 104 women with symptomatic urinary tract infection without historical or clinical evidence of other urologic disorders or bacteriologic evidence of persistent urinary tract infection. Fifteen (14%) had 1 infection, 61 (59%) had 2 or 3 infections, and 28 (27%) had more than 3 infections. Gross hematuria associated with symptoms of bacteriuria or with culture-proved bacteriuria occurred in 30 (29%) women.

No patient had more than 1 abnormal finding in a single diagnostic study, or more than 1 abnormal finding among 3 studies (excretory urography, cystography, cystoscopy). No abnormalities influencing treatment of the infections were found among 104 excretory urograms, which uncovered 12 abnormal findings apparently unrelated to urinary tract infection. Only 1 of these abnormalities, renal cell carcinoma, required therapeutic intervention. Five other abnormalities, apparent sequelae of renal or upper urinary tract infection, did not alter treatment decisions; the latter were based on the frequency of bacteriuria and clinical extent of recent infections (none of these patients had had clinically suspected renal infection within 6 months). Among 75 cystograms and 74 cystoscopies the only abnormalities that altered treatment of infections were 3 instances of urethral diverticula. Of 2 patients who underwent surgical repair of the diverticula, 1 was asymptomatic during 18 months of postoperative observation and the other was lost to follow-up. Cystography revealed vesicoureteral reflux in 1 patient; however, normal ureteral orifices at cystoscopy and an unremarkable excretory urogram suggested that the reflux might have resulted from recent bacteriuria, and the finding did not influence therapy. Among 3 incidental findings on cystoscopy, only a transitional cell carcinoma required treatment.

Approximately 99% of women with "recurrent" urinary tract infection are thought to have reinfections, as opposed to persistent infections. It is concluded that radiographic and endoscopic investigations of the urinary tract rarely provide information important in the management of single urinary tract infections, or urinary tract reinfections, in women.

▶ [This article and the preceding one suggest that certain interventions commonly performed in women with urinary tract infections may not be worthwhile. The preceding report concerns the posttreatment follow-up culture. After the elimination of cer-

(11–2) N. Engl. J. Med. 304:462–465, Feb. 19, 1981.

tain patients at high risk for renal complications, the routine posttreatment culture in asymptomatic women wasn't very helpful. Only 4% of tested patients had positive cultures, and a negative culture didn't reduce the chance for the recurrence of symptomatic infection within the 1-year observation period, compared with those patients who did not have posttreatment cultures.

The second report suggests that cystoscopy and an intravenous pyelogram will only rarely influence the treatment of patients with recurrent rather than persistent infection. We think the authors are too pessimistic. Urethral diverticula were diagnosed in 3 patients, urinary tract cancers in 2 others, and renal calculus in yet another 2. Urinary tract infections are common in women and recurrent infections are certainly not unusual. All patients with recurrent infections don't require urologic evaluation. If the recurrences are frequent, severe, or associated with signs or symptoms that suggest underlying urologic abnormality, however, we think radiologic and cystoscopic examinations are indicated.] ◄

11–3 **Meatal Colonization and Catheter-Associated Bacteriuria.** Richard A. Garibaldi, John P. Burke, Michael R. Britt, William A. Miller, and Charles B. Smith (Univ. of Utah) examined meatal colonization and catheter-associated bacteriuria in patients who required an indwelling catheter for the urinary bladder. A urine specimen was collected at the time of catheter placement or during the first 24 hours thereafter. A swab sample from the urethral meatus was obtained from most patients within the first 24 hours of catheterization. Specimens of urine from the catheter were cultured each day thereafter throughout catheterization. The 1,213 patients who comprised the final study population did not have bacteriuria at catheterization, did not acquire bacteriuria on the first day of catheterization, and remained catheterized for at least 24 hours after meatal culture.

Patients with positive meatal cultures acquired bacteriuria significantly more frequently than did patients with negative ones (table). A study of population subgroups showed that 72% of female patients had positive meatal cultures as compared with 30% of male patients; 59% of patients who did not receive systemic antibiotics had positive cultures as compared with 45% of those who did receive them; and 61% of patients whose underlying disease was treated medically had positive cultures as compared with 45% of those whose disease was treated surgically. The rates of positive meatal cultures were the

INCIDENCE OF BACTERIURIA IN 1,213 CATHETERIZED PATIENTS, ACCORDING TO MEATAL CULTURE

	MEATAL CULTURE	
	POSITIVE	NEGATIVE
Number of patients with cultures	612	601
Number of patients with bacteriuria (incidence)	110 (18%)	28 (5%)
	$P<0.0001$ *	
Number of days at risk	1470	1390
Incidence per day	7.5%	2.0%
	$P<0.0001$ *	

*By chi-square test.

(11–3) N. Engl. J. Med. 303:316–318, Aug. 7, 1980.

same in the subgroup of patients aged 50 years or older as in the younger subgroup. No difference in the mean duration of catheterization was noted between patients with positive meatal cultures and those with negative ones. An association between positive meatal cultures and subsequent acquisition of bacteriuria was observed in all subgroups. Of 110 patients, 94 (85%) with positive meatal cultures who acquired bacteriuria were infected by the same species of bacteria previously recovered from the urethral meatus.

The findings confirm previous observations that female patients aged 50 or older who are not receiving antibiotics or who have conditions not treated by surgery have an increased risk for the development of catheter-associated bacteriuria. The findings suggest that the use of methods to block urethral colonization might prevent infection. These techniques should be identified and evaluated.

▶ [With the use of closed urinary drainage systems, the acquisition of catheter-associated bacteriuria relates in part to meatal colonization by pathogenic bacteria, according to this report. While this is helpful in improving our understanding of the pathogenesis of catheter-associated bacteriuria, what to do in order to prevent the problem is not clear. The authors cite examples from the literature where attempts at decreasing the rate of catheter-associated infections by means of cleaning the meatal area with antiseptic solutions have not been successful.] ◀

11–4 **Urethral Diverticulum in Females.** C. R. J. Woodhouse, J. T. Flynn, E. A. Molland, and J. P. Blandy (London Hosp.) report the features of 13 cases of urethral diverticulum in women and describe a new operative approach for the excision of these diverticula.

Of the 13 patients, 9 presented with urinary abnormalities, 6 of which were detected on vaginal examination; 2 presented with infection in previously undiagnosed diverticula, and 2 presented with vaginal swelling. In all 7 cases in which micturating cystourethrography was performed, the diverticulum clearly was demonstrated; in no case was intravenous urography of diagnostic value. Palpation of the sac on vaginal examination was the most important physical sign. In 9 cases, the opening of the diverticulum was seen in the midline posteriorly on urethroscopy.

Two women with suppuration underwent incision and drainage into the vagina, and 10 women, including 2 with recurrences, were treated by excision of the sac and primary closure of the urethral defect. In 1 patient in whom stones were detected in the diverticulum, an operative technique involving a laterally based vaginal flap incision was used with a successful outcome (Fig 11–1). The outcome was also successful in 8 of 10 patients who underwent simple diverticulectomy. Pathologic material from 11 patients showed smooth muscle in addition to fibrous tissue, which suggests a congenital rather than an acquired origin. In 1 patient the mucosa was part squamous and part transitional, and an adenocarcinoma, deeply invasive of the diverticular wall, with a well-differentiated papillary component, was found.

The laterally based vaginal flap incision technique was used successfully in a total of 7 patients. The technique makes full exposure of the diverticulum easy and covers the urethral defect with intact

---

(11–4) Br. J. Urol. 52:305–310, August 1980.

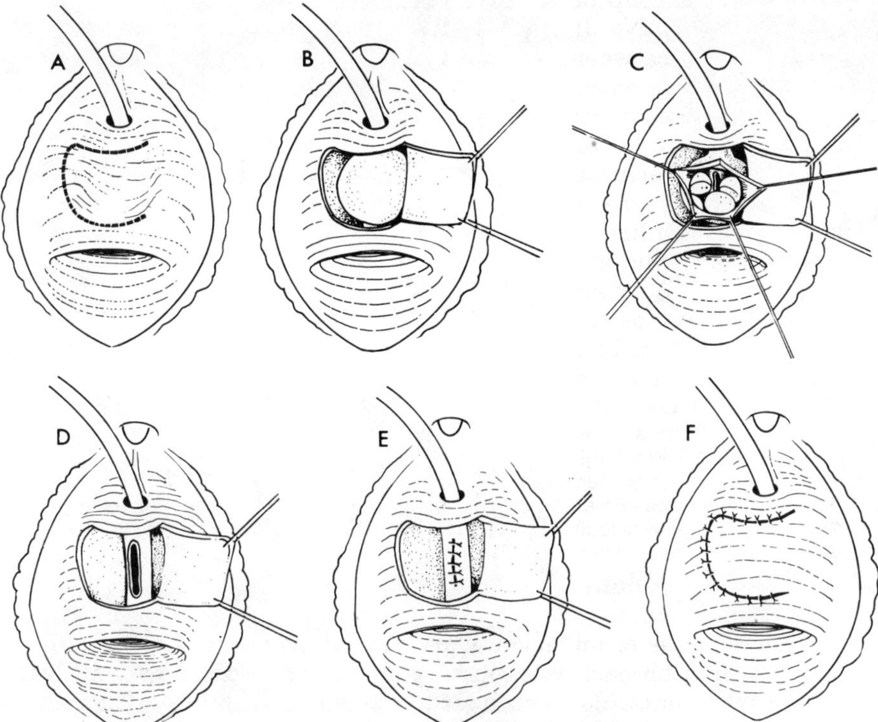

Fig 11–1.—**A,** incision in the anterior wall of the vagina (a catheter has been passed into the urethra). **B,** the vaginal flap has been raised to reveal the diverticulum. **C,** the diverticulum has been opened and four stones are seen inside. **D,** the sac has been removed and the small opening into the urethra is left. **E,** closure of the urethra. **F,** closure of the vaginal flap. (Courtesy of Woodhouse, C. R. J., et al.: Br. J. Urol. 52:305–310, August 1980.)

vaginal wall. It is not difficult to perform, even in recurrent cases, and was without complications in this series.

▶ [This article serves as a nice review of an uncommon, but not rare, problem. Although "stress incontinence" is often listed as a symptom, in our experience the urine loss is more apt to be postvoiding dribbling or to occur when the patient gets up from sitting rather than after a cough or sneeze. The diverticulum may fill with voiding or at rest and then be emptied with changes in position unrelated to increases in intra-abdominal pressure as such. We, too, have seen pregnant patients with diverticula present with acute infection and suburethral abscess formation. If a patient has recurrent "urinary tract infections," it is important for the gynecologist to examine the urethra carefully in an attempt to identify a diverticulum. In a recent case on our service, although the diverticulum could not be identified as such on physical examination (or its orifice seen on urethroscopy), it was suspected because of what seemed like a very long urethra on vaginal examination. At operation, it was apparent that the finger-like diverticulum had distorted the surface anatomy of the anterior vaginal wall.] ◀

11–5   **Causes of the Acute Urethral Syndrome in Women.** Walter E. Stamm, Kenneth F. Wagner, Richard Amsel, E. Russell Alexander, Marvin Turck, George W. Counts, and King K. Holmes (Seattle) investigated the cause of acute urethral syndrome in 59 women with

(11–5) N. Engl. J. Med. 303:409–415, Aug. 21, 1980.

AGENTS ASSOCIATED WITH ACUTE URETHRAL SYNDROME

FEATURE	CYSTITIS	ACUTE URETHRAL SYNDROME			ASYMPTO-MATIC WOMEN
		BLADDER BACTERIURIA	STERILE PYURIA	NO PYURIA	
	(N = 35)	(N = 27)	(N = 16)	(N = 16)	(N = 66)
		number of subjects			
Bladder bacteriuria					
Coliforms	31	24	0	0	NA *
S. saprophyticus	2	3	0	0	NA *
C. trachomatis infection	1	1	10	1	3
Isolates from first-void urine					
U. urealyticum	20	12	10	11	39
M. hominis	10	4	5	2	10
Cytomegalovirus	1	0	0	1	0
Isolates from urethra					
Herpes simplex virus	1	1	0	2	0
N. gonorrhoeae	0	0	0	0	0

*NA denotes not available.

dysuria and frequent urination whose voided urine was sterile or contained less than 10^5 microorganisms per ml, in 35 women with typical cystitis, and in 66 women without symptoms of urinary tract infection.

None of the women with urethral syndrome had more than 3.4×10^4 bacteria per ml in either of two successive midstream urine specimens. However, samples of bladder urine obtained by suprapubic aspiration or catheterization from 24 of these 59 women contained coliforms, and samples from another 3 contained *Staphylococcus saprophyticus* (table). A sample from 1 woman contained *Klebsiella*. Of these 27 women, 26 also had pyuria. Of 32 women with sterile bladder urine, *Chlamydia trachomatis* was present in 10 of 16 with pyuria and 1 of 16 without pyuria. The incidence of chlamydial infection was significantly ($P < .01$) higher in women with urethral syndrome and pyuria (11 of 42) than in those without symptoms (3 of 66) and those with cystitis (1 of 35). On the whole, 42 of 59 patients with urethral syndrome also had abnormal pyuria and 37 of these were infected with coliforms, *S. saprophyticus,* or *C. trachomatis;* few women without pyuria had demonstrable infections.

Bacteriuria greater than 10^5/ml may be an insensitive diagnostic criterion for symptomatic infection of the lower urinary tract and patients who have urethral syndrome with either bladder bacteriuria or *C. trachomatis* infection will most likely respond to antimicrobial therapy.

11–6 **Treatment of Acute Urethral Syndrome.** Walter E. Stamm, Kate Running, Mary McKevitt, George W. Counts, Marvin Turck,

(11–6) N. Engl. J. Med. 304:956–958, Apr. 16, 1981.

CLINICAL AND MICROBIOLOGIC RESPONSE TO THERAPY

RESPONSE	DOXYCYCLINE GROUP (N = 32)	PLACEBO GROUP (N = 30)	P VALUE *
	no. cured/no. treated		
Clinical cure			
Bladder bacteriuria †	11/12	4/10	0.016
Sterile pyuria ‡	10/10	3/9	0.003
No pyuria	7/10	8/11	0.63
All cases	28/32	15/30	0.002
Microbiologic cure			
Esch. coli/Staph. saprophyticus	11/12	3/10	0.005
C. trachomatis	4/4	0/3	0.03
Resolution of pyuria			
Bladder bacteriuria	8/12	3/10	0.09
Sterile pyuria	9/10	2/9	0.005

*Fisher's exact test, one tailed.

†Urine obtained by suprapubic aspiration or catheterization contained *Escherichia coli* or *Staphylococcus saprophyticus,* although two consecutive clean-catch, midstream urine specimens contained less than 10^5 uropathogens per ml.

‡Urine obtained by suprapubic aspiration or catheterization was sterile but contained at least 8 WBCs per cu mm; 11 of the 19 women were infected with *C. trachomatis,* as measured by microimmunofluorescence assay.

and King K. Holmes (Seattle) conducted a randomized, double-blind comparison of the effectiveness of doxycycline and placebo in the treatment of 62 women, aged 19 to 73 years, who had acute urethral syndrome without bacterial cystitis or vaginitis.

Patients received treatment for 10 days with either doxycycline (100 mg twice daily by mouth) or placebo (1 tablet twice daily). They were examined periodically for 3 months after completion of treatment.

Clinical cure occurred in 28 of 32 women given doxycycline but in only 15 of 30 given placebo (table). Doxycycline was significantly more effective than placebo in eradicating urinary tract symptoms, pyuria, and the infecting microorganism among women with the urethral syndrome due to coliforms, staphylococci, or *Chlamydia trachomatis.* In women with acute urethral syndrome and no pyuria, however, no benefit could be ascribed to antibiotic therapy. Side effects were infrequent and mild in both treatment groups.

► [Women with dysuria and increased urinary frequency who do not have vaginitis may have "infected" urine in the absence of the traditional 10^5 organisms per ml. Those patients with pyuria (defined as 8 or more white blood cells per cu mm of unspun urine) and colony counts $<10^5$ tended to have either lower numbers of bladder bacteria or evidence of chlamydial infection. Our standard criteria for evaluating patients with these symptoms may well require revision.

If the symptoms are due to infection, antimicrobial therapy should help. Doxycycline was more effective than a placebo, according to this article by Stamm et al., except in patients who did not have pyuria. Another view emphasizing psychodynamic rather than microbiologic factors follows.] ◄

11–7 Evaluation and Treatment of Female Urethral Syndrome.
Women with irritative bladder symptoms (frequency, urgency, and

(11–7) J. Urol. 124:609–610, November 1980.

dysuria) but no evidence of organic disease or urinary infection are said to have urethral syndrome. C. C. Carson, J. W. Segura, and D. M. Osborne (Mayo Clinic) reviewed findings in the 160 women seen since 1974 with this syndrome. They were aged 20 to 45 years (mean, $34^1/_2$ years), only 6 were unmarried, and most had been pregnant. Symptoms included dysuria in 139 patients, frequency in 159, urgency in 144, and all 3 symptoms in 118. Only 18 patients had nocturia. Other common complaints included fatigue, malaise, back pain, and abdominal discomfort.

Routine urinalysis was negative in 103 of the 160 women but showed white blood cells in 42 and red blood cells in 18. Urine culture was positive in only 5 of the 160 patients. Urine cytology was negative in all 160 women. Excretory urography was normal in 134 of 145 patients, but none of the findings required medical or surgical treatment. Cystoscopy was normal in 89 of 160 women but showed urethrotrigonitis in 49, pseudomembranous trigonitis in 16, urethral diverticula in 3, acute cystitis in 2, and vesical neck hypertrophy in 1.

The Minnesota Multiphasic Personality Inventory was completed by 56 patients. Compared with normal women, those with urethral syndrome scored higher on the hypochondriasis, hysteria, and schizophrenia scales. High scores on the hypochondriasis and hysteria scales combined with normal depression scores is known as the conversion-V, a configuration found in patients who manifest psychophysiologic reactions and who gain from these symptoms by escaping stressful or anxiety-producing situations.

Slightly fewer than half the patients received no treatment, and slightly fewer than half received local instillations of silver nitrate and urethral suppositories. The success rate was about 85% in each group (follow-up, 4–38 months; mean, 22 months). Four women were treated surgically, with good results in all. Two patients required intermittent self-catheterization. Psychiatric treatment was successful in 13 of 15 patients.

Because lower tract infections and urinary tract anatomical anomalies are rare causes of urethral syndrome, the extent of investigation of a woman with this syndrome may be safely limited to a general physical examination, urinalysis, and urine culture. If no abnormalities are found and the history suggests no additional symptoms, no further diagnostic procedures are necessary. Some women may require further investigation for reassurance. Treatment should consist of patient reassurance, with psychiatric consultation when necessary.

▶ [In this large series of patients with the urethral syndrome (frequency, urgency, and dysuria in the absence of urinary "infection"), psychometric testing revealed high hysteria and hypochondriasis scores. This Mayo Clinic population is undoubtedly largely referred and may not be typical. We remain confused as to the "cause" of the urethral syndrome; we are encouraged that expectant therapy was usually effective.] ◀

11–8 **Controlled Trial of Bladder Drill for Detrusor Instability.** The treatment of detrusor instability with drugs is often unsatisfactory, with an incidence of side effects as high as 43% and cure rates generally less than 60% having been reported. In a controlled trial, G. J.

(11–8) Br. Med. J. 281:1322–1323, Nov. 15, 1980.

SYMPTOMS OF PATIENTS BEFORE AND SIX MONTHS AFTER TREATMENT

SYMPTOMS	BLADDER DRILL GROUP (n = 30)		CONTROL GROUP (n = 30)	
	Before	After	Before	After
Diurnal frequency	30	5	30	23
Nocturnal frequency	27	3	25	20
Urgency	30	4	30	23
Urge incontinence	30	3	30	23
Stress incontinence	21	3	20	16

Jarvis and D. R. Millar (Jessop Hosp. for Women, Sheffield, England) investigated the effectiveness of an inpatient bladder drill in the treatment of detrusor instability. Sixty women, aged 27 to 79 years, with urinary incontinence due to idiopathic detrusor instability participated in the study; 30 served as controls. The drill requires the patient to pass urine at a specific interval, usually every $1\frac{1}{2}$ hours initially, until the target is met. The interval is then increased by 30 minutes daily until the patient can remain continent for 4 hours. The frequency of micturation at night is not taken into account. The patient is encouraged to maintain her normal fluid intake and to keep a fluid balance chart. Patients are introduced to someone who has been treated successfully by the method.

After treatment, 27 of the 30 patients in the bladder drill group were continent and 25 were symptom free, whereas only 7 of the 30 control patients were continent and symptom free (table). The results were significant for all symptoms. In all cases, the subsidence of symptoms was confirmed by a normal cystogram. In patients who remained incontinent, cystometrograms obtained after treatment were closely similar to those obtained prior to treatment.

The mode of action of bladder drill is, presumably, psychological. Because of the safety and efficacy of bladder drill, it is concluded that it is the method of choice in the treatment of detrusor instability in women.

▶ [The assignment of patients to treatment or control groups in this study is stated to have been random. The reported results are striking! We hope others systematically evaluate bladder training in patients with urgency incontinence. It is interesting that coincident with symptomatic improvement was a normalization of bladder pressure-flow studies.] ◀

11–9 **Sexual Dysfunction Associated With Urinary Incontinence.** Symptoms related to sexual intercourse are particularly important to young women with incontinence. John Sutherst and Malcolm Brown (Univ. of Liverpool) obtained information on marital life and sexual habits from 208 women attending an incontinence clinic. Mean age was 46.1 years. In 40 cases sexual activity had been disturbed by other illnesses. Ninety women reported that their urinary symptoms had affected their sexual lives adversely. In 73 instances intercourse was less frequent than before, and in 17 it had ceased. Dyspareunia was the most common cause. Wetness at night, embarrassment, leak-

(11–9) Urol. Int. 35:414–416, 1980.

age during coitus, and marital discord also were mentioned. Women with detrusor instability appeared to be affected more than the others, particularly by dyspareunia and bed-wetting before and during coitus. The dyspareunia was related to constant wetness and soreness. Unsatisfactory sexual relations due to incontinence were more common in patients with unstable bladder than in those with simple sphincter weakness.

Women with urinary incontinence commonly have associated sexual dysfunction. This is especially likely if incontinence is due to detrusor instability. In this study, patients whose sexual lives had been affected by other illnesses more often had genuine stress incontinence than bladder instability, suggesting that lack of sexual fulfillment is not a major cause of bladder instability.

▶ [More than 40% of women attending a urinary incontinence clinic answered affirmatively when asked whether their condition had affected sexual activity adversely (i.e., coital frequency had diminished). A number of possible reasons come to mind, some physical, some psychological, and some esthetic. The most common reason stated was dyspareunia; unfortunately, this article gives no data about previous surgery that might be related. It is interesting that the frequency of sexual problems correlated significantly with the type of incontinence (as determined by urodynamic studies)—29% with "genuine stress incontinence," 60% with detrusor instability, and 26% with mixed type. Effects of treatment of the incontinence on sexual function would be of interest.] ◀

11–10 **Comparative Study of Symptoms and Objective Urodynamic Findings in 214 Incontinent Women.** T. J. Cantor and C. P. Bates (City Hosp., Nottingham) used videocystourethrography to investigate urinary incontinence in 214 women who were suspected of suffering from detrusor instability or were having this possibility excluded before surgery. Intravesical and rectal pressures were measured. The detrusor pressure was obtained by electronically subtracting the latter from the former. Of 96 patients with stable bladder, 69% had frequency of micturition, 34% had nocturia, 13% had enuresis, 75% had urgency (motor and/or sensory), and 55% had urge incontinence. Of 118 unstable patients, 86% had frequency, 67% had nocturia, 30% had enuresis, 96% had urgency, and 91% had urge incontinence. The small differences in incidence between stable and unstable bladder groups makes frequency and urgency poor symptoms for distinguishing between the two groups.

Three key symptoms of detrusor instability were therefore identified, namely nocturia, nocturnal enuresis, and urge incontinence. The presence of one of these symptoms was associated with a 64% incidence of detrusor instability. When two or three of these symptoms were present, the incidence of detrusor instability rose to 76% and 81%, respectively. Thus, if a woman has any of these key symptoms, she should be assumed to have an unstable bladder until cystometry shows otherwise. Two patients in the unstable bladder group who had none of the three key symptoms had atypical incontinence. One had incontinence without prior warning while she was standing. She was a 22-year-old nullipara. The other, a 36-year-old multipara, complained of dribbling incontinence after voiding. Urodynamic investi-

---

(11–10) Br. J. Obstet. Gynaecol. 87:889–892, October 1980.

gation as well as neurologic assessment is recommended in all women with atypical incontinence.

Patients participating in this study were selected for referral because they had ambiguous symptomatology. This bias would tend to reduce rather than exaggerate the differences in symptoms between stable and unstable bladder groups.

It is recommended that all women with nocturia, nocturnal enuresis, urge incontinence, or atypical incontinence should be offered urodynamic assessment before surgery for incontinence. Such assessment is not required for incontinent women whose only other symptoms are daytime frequency of voiding or urgency.

11–11 **Assessment of Urodynamic Examination in Incontinent Women.** G. J. Jarvis, S. Hall, S. Stamp, D. R. Millar, and A. Johnson (Jessop Hosp. for Women, Sheffield, England) performed urodynamic investigation in 100 consecutive incontinent women. Each woman was asked to void in private immediately before the examination. A 12 F filling catheter was inserted per urethram alongside a 2-mm fluid-filled catheter attached to a transducer that measured intravesical pressure. Rectal pressure was measured by catheter as well. The bladder was filled with saline at a rate of 100 ml/minute, the filling volume being measured continuously. Bladder and rectal pressures were measured throughout; detrusor pressure was estimated by electronic subtraction of the rectal from the intravesical pressure. The provocation cystometry technique was used. The woman was asked to retain bladder contents; the volume at which she felt the desire to micturate was noted. The patient, who was supine, was asked to cough, strain, stand, and cough and strain again. The catheter was removed, and the patient then coughed, strained, and voided into a flowmeter. Flow rate, detrusor pressure, and volume passed were recorded.

Detrusor muscle instability was indicated by detrusor contraction exceeding 15 cm H_2O during filling or standing erect or on coughing. Genuine stress incontinence was indicated by involuntary leakage in the absence of a detrusor contraction. Sensory urgency was diagnosed if the women felt the desire to void before 50 ml of fluid had entered the bladder and the detrusor muscle was stable. The initial clinical diagnosis, made before urodynamic examination, agreed, at least partly, with final diagnosis in only 65 of 100 women, detrusor instability being overdiagnosed at the expense of genuine stress incontinence and sensory urgency. Twenty-two women complained of stress incontinence without urgency or urge incontinence; 20 of these had genuine stress incontinence. Fifty-one women complained of stress incontinence and either urgency or urge incontinence; 19 of these had genuine stress incontinence alone, and only 8 were diagnosed correctly. Five patients with undiagnosed detrusor muscle instability had cough-induced detrusor contractions.

Treatment based on careful history and clinical examination alone would have been inadequate in 31 women. Sphincter weakness was

(11–11) Br. J. Obstet. Gynaecol. 87:893–896, October 1980.

suspected in 30 of 48 patients who had genuine stress incontinence, while 11 women without genuine stress incontinence were suspected of having this condition. Without routine urodynamic examination, 18 women whose condition warranted surgical treatment might have been treated for urge incontinence. Eleven women might have undergone unnecessary surgery of the bladder neck. Urodynamic examination offered the clinician the option to treat at one hospital admission 7 women who had both genuine stress incontinence and detrusor muscle instability. Routine pressure flow studies are therefore recommended in all cases.

▶ [This article and the preceding one address the question of whether sophisticated urodynamic studies are necessary for correct diagnosis in patients presenting with urinary incontinence. In other words, can stress incontinence be differentiated from detrusor instability on the basis of clinical findings? This is a question of great importance, for the proper treatment of the two conditions is so different. The two studies seem to come down on opposite sides. Cantor and Bates found that certain key symptoms—nocturia, enuresis, and urge incontinence—were much more likely to be associated with detrusor instability. If any of the three were present, urodynamic studies were indicated; in their absence, one could forego these studies. Jarvis and associates, on the other hand, found that the clinical diagnosis coincided with the urodynamic diagnosis in 65%, and urodynamic studies significantly altered management in 31%.] ◀

11–12 **The Standing Cystometrogram.** Preoperative recognition of uninhibited bladder contractions may permit a medical cure and obviate unnecessary surgery. Stuart A. Weprin and Frederick P. Zuspan (Ohio State Univ.) report their experience with a simple office test for the diagnosis of uninhibited bladder contractions in 91 female patients with symptomatic urinary incontinence and 11 continent female patients without urologic symptoms who served as controls. Both standing and supine filling cystometrograms were used to evaluate all patients. Uninhibited bladder contractions of 30 mm Hg or greater were considered clinically significant. The tests were considered to be complete when the third segment of the cystometrogram was reached or the patient became too uncomfortable.

Of the 91 patients studied, 15 were found to have uninhibited bladder contractions. Ten of these cases were diagnosed in the standing position only. There were no false negative findings with the standing test. There was no significant association between uninhibited bladder contractions and previous surgical repair. Histories of patients with uninhibited bladder contractions and those with stress incontinence showed significant differences for symptoms of urgency, enuresis, and incontinence (table). However, because most patients with stress incontinence had at least two or more abnormalities frequently associated with uninhibited bladder contractions, these differences had little diagnostic value. Cystometrography of several patients treated nonsurgically tended to correlate with the posttreatment clinical response.

Because standing filling cystometrography eliminates the need for provocative maneuvers, simplifies the study of bladder dynamics, and

(11–12) Am. J. Obstet. Gynecol. 138:369–373, Oct. 15, 1980.

COMPARISON OF HISTOLOGIC FINDINGS IN PATIENTS WITH UNINHIBITED BLADDER CONTRACTIONS AND IN PATIENTS WITH STRESS INCONTINENCE

Patient category	Frequency (%)	Urgency (%)	Nocturia (%)	Enuresis (%)	Two or more infections of Urinary tract (%)	Incontinence characterized by a continuous stream of H_2O (%)
Uninhibited bladder contractions (N = 15)	80	100	80	47	47	27
Stress incontinence (N = 76)	69	72	80	16	22	1
	$P > 0.05$	$P \leq 0.05$	$P > 0.05$	$P \leq 0.05$	$P \geq 0.05$	$P \leq 0.05$

produces findings significantly different from those seen on supine cystometrography, it is the procedure of choice.

► [By the simple approach of performing cystometrograms with the subject standing, these authors feel they are able to identify uninhibited bladder contractions, characteristic of the condition known variously as detrusor dyssynergia and unstable bladder, which otherwise require sophisticated urodynamic studies for diagnosis. As is well known, it is extremely important to recognize this condition because it usually should be treated medically rather than surgically. Also of interest in this report is the distribution of symptoms in patients with uninhibited contractions and those with stress incontinence (table).] ◄

11-13 **Effects of Estrogens and Gestagens on the Urethral Pressure Profile in Urinary Continent and Stress Incontinent Women.** T. Rud (Norwegian Radium Hosp., Oslo) investigated the urodynamic effects of hormones on the lower urinary tract in women. Twenty-four stress incontinent and 6 continent women were randomly given estrogen (estriol and estradiol) orally in doses of 4–8 mg/day for 3 weeks (group I); another group of 8 women was given a single intramuscular injection of 1,000 mg gestagen (17-hydroxyprogesterone caproate). All members of group II suffered from cystic glandular hyperplasia; 5 were continent and 3 were stress incontinent. All the women were examined with simultaneous urethrocystometry, including urethral pressure profile (UPP) measurement before and after treatment. Patients were requested to cough after every 100 ml of saline had been infused, to simulate a stress situation. Calculations of resting pressures were done at a bladder volume of 200 ml.

The maximum urethral pressure (MUP) at rest increased in group I after estrogen therapy from a mean of 59 cm H_2O to a mean of 63 cm H_2O. There was no difference between continent and stress-incontinent patients. There was a nonsignificant increase in bladder pressure (BP), or maximum intravesical pressure, after estrogen treatment. Urethral closure pressure also did not change significantly after estrogen therapy. The functional urethral length (FUL), the part of the urethra where the intraurethral pressure exceeds the BP, increased significantly in patients in group I after estrogen, from a mean of 25 mm to a mean of 28 mm. There was no difference between estriol- and estradiol-treated patients or between continent and incontinent patients. The absolute urethral length (AUL), the part of the urethra where the intraurethral pressure exceeds the atmospheric pressure, increased significantly, from a mean of 33 mm to a mean of 37 mm, after estrogen.

Seventeen of 24 patients suffering from stress incontinence reported subjective improvement of symptoms. There was no correlation between subjective improvement and improvement of MUP, AUL, FUL, or closure pressure. The pressure transmission ratio, the percentage of intra-abdominal pressure transmitted to the urethra in relation to the bladder pressure on coughing, was measured in 18 group I patients. It was considerably improved in 6 after therapy; this correlated with subjective improvement. No recorded parameters changed significantly at rest after progesterone treatment in group II patients. Subjective improvement in group I may be related to the fact that estrogen treatment causes a trophic mucosa; therefore, urinary leakage may be less painful or even disregarded.

It may be concluded that estrogens in high doses over a long period improve female stress incontinence, mainly by an improved pressure

(11–13) Acta Obstet. Gynecol. Scand. 59:265–270, 1980.

transmission of intra-abdominal pressure to the urethra. Considering possible adverse effects, however, it is debatable whether such therapy is justified.

▶ [Postmenopausal women with urinary incontinence sometimes note improvement with estrogen treatment either topically or systematically, and this study was designed to see if urodynamic effects could be responsible. Whereas there were some estrogen-induced changes of the type that should promote continence (increased absolute and functional urethral length, increased maximum urethral pressure), the magnitudes were so small as to make it dubious that they could be responsible for symptomatic improvement. Perhaps it is primarily a placebo effect.] ◀

11-14 **Retropubic Urethrocystopexy: Vaginal Approach.** L. C. Powell, Jr. (Univ. of Texas, Galveston) describes a modification of the classic Marshall-Marchetti-Krantz (MMK) operation for retropubic urethrocystopexy by the vaginal approach and evaluated the technique in 25 patients with symptomatic pelvic relaxation, usually accompanied by stress incontinence. The results were compared with those for a group of 25 selected, matched control subjects who underwent the classic abdominal MMK procedure.

TECHNIQUE.—The vaginal mucosa and pubovesical-cervical fascia are incised and dissected laterally so that the operator can palpate the underside of the pubic ramus (Figs 11–2, A and B). A nonabsorbable suture is then placed on a curved general closure needle and a stitch is placed through the periosteum, with the index and middle fingers of the left hand used to push the bladder up and the urethra laterally (Fig 11–2, C and D). After penetration of the periosteum, the needle is redirected from a 90-degree to almost a 180-degree angle (Fig 11–2, E). The proximal needle tip is grasped while the distal end is released and the needle is carefully pulled through the periosteum following the curvature of the needle. The same procedure is performed on the other side of the urethra.

Traction on the Foley catheter is used to identify the urethrovesical angle, and a good bite of the periurethral tissues, including the pubourethral ligament, is taken on each side under direct vision (Fig 11–2, F). If a bladder puncture is identified, the suture must be removed and replaced. The sutures on both sides are tied and the urethrovesical angle is pulled up behind the symphysis (Fig 11–2, G). At this time, further reconstructive repair can be performed if necessary, and the urethra is then plicated with three sutures of the Kelly type.

At 6 weeks after operation, 96% of the study patients and 92% of the control group were cured or improved. At the end of 1 year, cure and improvement rates had dropped to 92% for the study group and 88% for the control group. Patients who underwent the modified MMK operation had less morbidity, a 1-day decrease in hospital stay, and 1½ fewer days of catheter drainage compared to control patients. There was 1 failure in the study group and 2 failures in the control group.

This modification of the classic MMK retropubic urethrovesical suspension offers the advantages of a shorter operating time, lack of an abdominal incision, and concomitant repair of other pelvic anatomic defects through the vagina. The initial results were at least equal to, or better than, those obtained with the conventional MMK technique.

(11–14) Am. J. Obstet. Gynecol. 140:91–98, May 1, 1981.

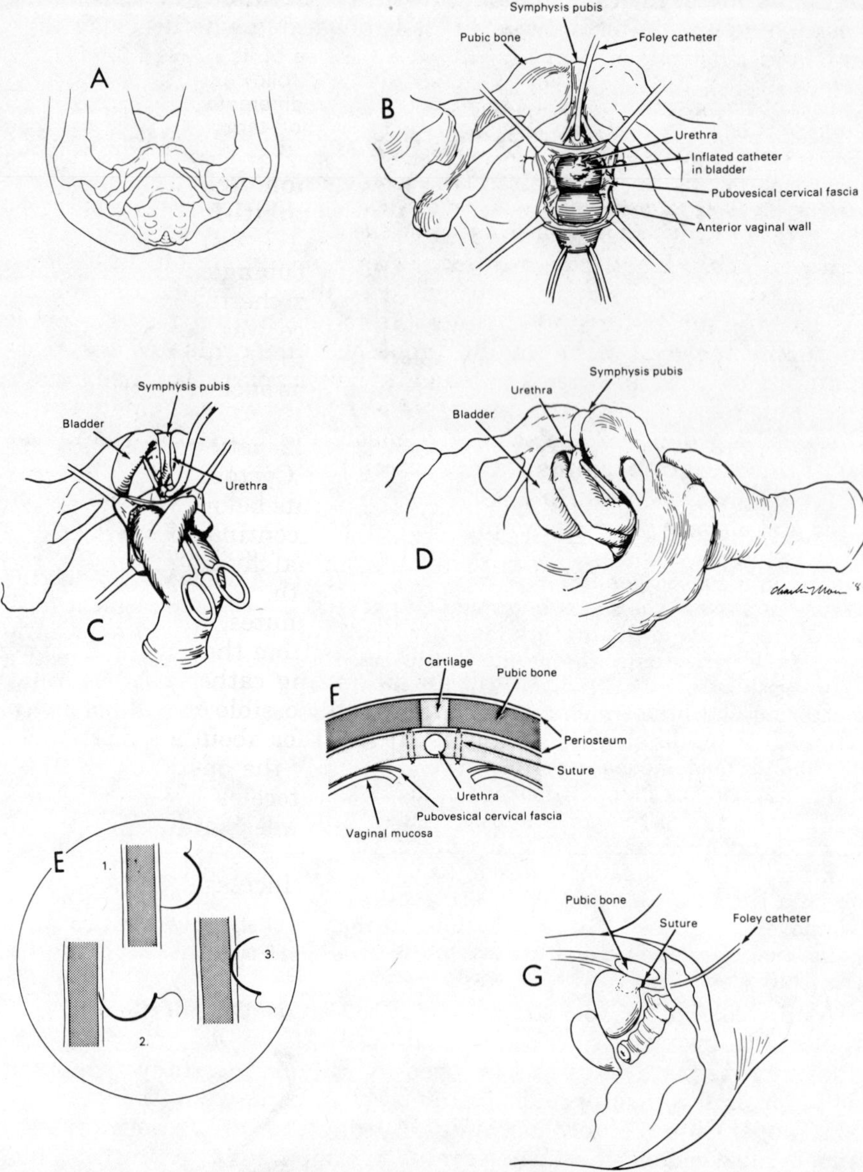

Fig 11–2.—Retropubic urethrocystopexy (MMK type) by the vaginal approach. **A,** orientation of bony pelvis at surgery. **B,** initial dissection to expose bladder neck. **C,** placement of pubic bone periosteal stitch (inferior view). **D,** placement of periosteal stitch (superior view). Note displacement of urethra and bladder by index and middle fingers. **E,** detail of periosteal stitch placement. Note change of angle necessary to lift periosteum from underlying bone. **F,** schematic drawing of cross-sectional anatomy at end of urethrocystopexy. **G,** sagittal view of pelvic support after completion of operation. (Courtesy of Powell, L. C., Jr.: Am. J. Obstet. Gynecol. 140:91–98, May 1, 1981.)

Further evaluation is necessary to determine whether these initially good results will hold up.

▶ [This is an interesting and appealing idea because of its simplicity. It should be noted, however, that the series is relatively small and follow-up assessment was at 6 weeks postoperatively. It seems that each of the many different kinds of operations for urinary stress incontinence give 95% cure rates on short-term follow-up. Later recurrences may vary considerably, however.] ◀

11–15 **Initial Clinical and Cystourethral Tonometric Results With a New Modification of the Marshall-Marchetti-Krantz Operation** was investigated by R. C. Briel, R. F. Frick, G. B. Frick, K. Gassner, F. D. Peters, and H. A. Hirsch (Univ. of Tübingen). From January 1976 to July 1978, a modified Marshall-Marchetti-Krantz procedure for correction of urinary stress incontinence was performed on 260 patients. With the new operation of fixing the neck of the bladder to the obturator fascia (Fig 11–3), complications such as cartilage necrosis, periostitis or osteomyelitis do not occur.

A follow-up examination was done in 132 patients 6 weeks after the operation and in 96 patients after 1 year. Cystourethral tonometric measurements were carried out in 66 patients before and 1 year after operation. In 247 of 260 cases (95%) the incontinence operation was performed in connection with an abdominal hysterectomy. All patients had incontinence or a cystocele, or both.

On the average, the operation took 9 minutes, the intraoperative blood loss was 10.5 ml, and the blood loss from the cavum retzii was 90 ± 63 ml. All patients had an indwelling catheter for 3–4 days, after which spontaneous micturition was possible in 92% of the patients; 15% had a residual urine of 100 ml for about $2^{1}/_{2}$ days.

There was no incontinence 6 weeks after the operation in 97% of the patients and after 1 year in 80%. Cystoceles were corrected by the procedure and remained so in 91% at 6 weeks after operation and in 87% at 1 year after.

The urodynamic evaluations showed an increase of the maximal

Fig 11–3.—Fixation of the neck of the bladder to the obturator fascia. (Courtesy of Briel, R. C., et al.: Geburtshilfe Frauenheilkd. 40:784–790, September, 1980.)

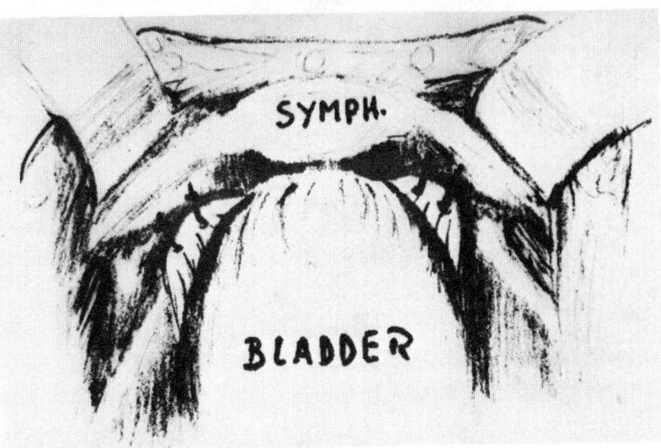

(11–15) Geburtshilfe Frauenheilkd. 40:784–790, September 1980.

urethral closure pressure and above all, a marked and significant improvement of the urethral stress profile.

Apart from elevated temperatures for $2^{1}/_{2}$ days in 18% and infections in 60% of the patients, the intraoperative blood loss (2.3%) was the most frequent complication. All other complications were less than 2%, including severe complications of less than 0.5%.

According to the unanimous opinion in the literature, motor and sensory urge-incontinence and hypertonic bladders are no indication for incontinence surgery. Improvement cannot be expected, and in some cases the condition may deteriorate. The surgery itself caused iatrogenic urge-incontinence in 10%–20% of the patients. In 6 patients a motor urge incontinence was found for the first time at the follow-up examination 1 year after operation.

The results of the new modification of the Marshall-Marchetti-Krantz procedure are similar to those described in the literature after other operations for urinary stress incontinence. At later studies, tonometric examinations with refined urologic measuring systems (e.g., microtransducers) as well as radiologic examinations should be used in addition to the clinical findings and subjective records.

▶ [The classic Marshall-Marchetti-Krantz operation utilizes the periosteum of the symphysis pubis for suspension of the urethrovesical angle. In order to avoid the occasional complication of osteitis pubis, Burch proposed Cooper's ligament as the "anchor." Cooper's ligament can sometimes be a long reach, so the technique described here in which the periurethral sutures are anchored to the obturator internal muscle and fascia was developed. The results seem quite good. We recently had occasion to see this procedure first hand. Hirsch of the University of Tübingen visited us and demonstrated it on a patient with two previous failed vaginal repairs.] ◀

12. Tumors

12-1 **Surgical Approach to Multifocal Carcinoma In Situ of the Vulva.** Vulvar intraepithelial neoplasia may occur in younger women as well as in postmenopausal subjects. Local excision, unlike topical chemotherapy, will reveal lesions with microinvasive foci, but may be impractical for patients with multiple, confluent vulvar lesions. Rutledge and Sinclair described a "skinning" vulvectomy with skin grafting for use in these cases. Philip J. Di Saia and William M. Rich (Univ. of California, Irvine) used a modification of the Rutledge procedure in 39 patients with multifocal disease in at least three quadrants of the vulva. Most patients had 20 or more lesions or large confluent areas of disease on the vulvar skin. Nineteen patients were aged 35 years or younger. Fewer than half of the patients had pruritus. More than one third of the patients had a history of cervical or vaginal intraepithelial neoplasia. En bloc removal of involved skin was followed by application of a split-thickness skin graft to the surgical defect. The clitoris was preserved even with disease present on the glans.

Patient acceptance of the procedure was good. Most patients were able to resume coitus in 8 weeks, and complete sensation in the graft was present by 6 months. In general, sexual response was reported to be comparable with that in the predisease period. One third of the patients had recurrences on follow-up for 12–90 months. All recurrent lesions were on preserved skin. All recurrences were excised locally. One patient had a keloid in part of the donor site. In no case was invasive disease found in the operative specimen.

Recurrences of intraepithelial vulvar carcinoma are frequent after en bloc removal of involved skin and split-thickness skin-grafting, but recurrences are not within the grafted area. Dyspareunia and seriously altered sexual function are not reported after this procedure. Patients have been pleased with knowing that the very troublesome area of skin at greatest risk has been removed and replaced in an esthetic manner.

▶ [Carcinoma in situ of the vulva seems to be increasing in frequency, particularly among young women. It is typically of multifocal origin, and for this reason some have advocated topical 5-fluorouracil as therapy. Unfortunately, its efficacy is questionable and side effects are a problem, so there seems to be a distinct place for surgery. The approach described here is the "skinning vulvectomy and skin graft" originally suggested by Rutledge. The results in cosmetic and functional terms were quite satisfactory. Of some concern is the fact that more than one third of patients developed recurrences, all on skin areas not operated on (i.e., none on grafted skin). This underscores the need for long and careful follow-up. As pointed out by the discussants of this article, all that is needed is careful inspection with a good light after application of 3% acetic acid.] ◀

(12–1)   Am. J. Obstet. Gynecol. 140:136–145, May 15, 1981.

12–2 Progressive Histobiologic Alterations in the Development of Vulvar Cancer: Report of Five Cases. Identification of patients at risk for the development of cancer and the precursory histopathologic changes has led to improvement in the 5-year survival rate among patients with cancer of the cervix and endometrium. In contrast, there has been controversy as to the precursory factors in vulvar neoplasia. Joseph Buscema and J. Donald Woodruff (Johns Hopkins Hosp.) report data on 5 patients in whom invasive cancer developed after treatment for in situ disease and attempt to define risk factors, including the specific area at which 3 of the 5 malignancies subsequently developed. Three of the 5 patients in whom in situ disease progressed to invasive disease were in the late third or early fourth decade of life when the initial lesion was discovered. The initial treatment in 2 of the 3 was vulvectomy; only wide local excision was performed in the final case. Two patients had received local 5-fluorouracil cream therapy. The third patient had immunosuppressive therapy; recurrent disease at the anal orifice was treated with radiation. Consequently, the local vulvar disease was controlled by surgical therapy or chemotherapy, or both. In all 3 patients, invasive cancer subsequently developed in the *perianal area,* suggesting that this skin is the tissue at risk.

Two patients in the eighth and ninth decades of life with vulvar in situ disease were initially treated, 1 each, by vulvectomy and wide local excision. Invasive cancer developed in both at the excisional area within a period of 5 years postoperatively. The unique histologic pattern was characterized by abnormal maturation of the tissues with the formation of intraepithelial pearls at the rete tips. Individual cell anaplasia was not a feature in these cases, as it was in the younger patient.

In the young patient treated for in situ neoplasia of the anogenital canal, invasive disease rarely develops. If malignancy does occur, it appears at the anal orifice, probably because of many irritants and traumas to which that area is subjected. This critical transformation zone at the anal orifice may respond to viral agents with atypical proliferations similar to those seen at the cervical os. The common finding of condylomata acuminata in association with neoplasia of the anogenital canal supports this thesis. In 1 patient in the present series, the area was also subjected to radiation, a known skin carcinogen, and the patient received long-term steroid immunosuppressive therapy. Most importantly, the physician must maintain a high degree of suspicion in follow-up of these patients, local irritants must be removed, and biopsy examination must be used freely.

▶ [The lesson here is that although recurrence of carcinoma in situ of the vulva is common, progression to invasive disease is not. If the latter should occur, the perianal area often is involved.] ◀

12–3 Microinvasive Carcinoma of the Vulva: A Clinicopathologic Evaluation. Alfonso E. Barnes, John D. Crissman, Helmut F. Schell-

(12–2) Am. J. Obstet. Gynecol. 138:146–150, Sept. 15, 1980.
(12–3) Obstet. Gynecol. 56:234–238, August 1980.

has, and Ramez S. Azoury (Univ. of Cincinnati) describe two types of neoplasms as superficially invasive or microinvasive carcinoma of the vulva. One type, which can be treated by conservative surgery, is commonly associated with extensive overlying intraepithelial neoplasia. Usually, one focus of microinvasion, but occasionally more, invades less than 2 mm into the underlying stroma. The infiltrating cells comprise one or more isolated cords, and confluency is never present. The second and less common form tends to metastasize early to lymph nodes and should be treated by a radical approach. This type seldom is associated with overlying intraepithelial neoplasia. It tends to be poorly differentiated and is confluent.

Records were reviewed of patients treated for vulvar cancer during the past 7 years. Eighteen cases had been diagnosed as superficial or early invasive carcinoma of the vulva. Microscopic slides and tissue sections were reviewed. Only patients with identifiable squamous cell carcinoma invasive to a depth of less than 5 mm were included in the study. Two patients underwent wide local excision of the cancer and had not experienced recurrence after 30 months of follow-up. Seven patients underwent vulvectomy; 1 of these had metastasis to an ipsilateral inguinal lymph node 13 months after surgery. She was treated with radiation therapy and remains free of disease after 2 years. Six patients underwent radical vulvectomy and bilateral inguinal-femoral lymphadenectomy. Three patients underwent vulvectomy followed by radiation therapy to the groin area; all 3 remain free of disease after more than 3 years of follow-up. The 2 patients in whom inguinal metastases developed had confluent invasion. Neither patient had identifiable vascular invasion; in both, the inguinal node metastasis was in the ipsilateral groin.

Two distinct histologic patterns of invasion emerged in the series. The first group of 15 patients had associated overlying intraepithelial neoplasia. The invasive component in 7 of these patients consisted of one or more isolated foci of single cords of groups of cells infiltrating the adjacent stroma. Extent of invasion was usually less than 2 mm from the limiting basement membrane of the epithelial site of origin. Epithelial changes varied from the classic bowenoid type to the intermediary form of undifferentiated cell proliferation. In the remaining 8 patients with associated epithelial neoplasia, a prominent epithelial maturation was observed. The pattern consisted of diffuse epithelial atypia with prominent keratinization and focal areas of well-differentiated microinvasive squamous cell carcinoma. The microinvasive component pattern was the verrucoid form of squamous cell carcinoma. The second recognized pattern of invasion consisted of 3 invasive carcinomas of the confluent or "spray" type, consisting of a single focus of invasive neoplasm infiltrating into the stroma in a symmetrically expanding pattern.

In the authors' opinion, depth of invasion is inadequate as the single parameter for selection of the therapeutic approach to patients with early invasive carcinoma of the vulva. Confluent carcinomas are capable of regional lymph node metastasis regardless of the level of infiltration, and therefore, a more radical approach is required. However, the vast majority of cases of microinvasive squamous cell carcinoma of the vulva can be treated by conservative surgery.

▶ [This is an attempt to clarify the confusion concerning microinvasive carcinoma of the vulva (1979 YEAR BOOK, pp. 267–268; and 1981 YEAR BOOK, pp. 275–276). The suggestion is that groin node metastases are associated with a lack of extensive intraepithelial carcinoma and with the presence of a confluent or "spray" pattern, rather than an isolated pattern, of invasion. The number of cases is too small to make definite statements, but we applaud this attempt to further characterize microinvasive carcinoma of the vulva.] ◀

12–4 **Individualized Treatment of Stage I Carcinoma of the Vulva.** Radical vulvectomy and bilateral lymphadenectomy has been the standard treatment for squamous cell carcinoma for some time. To determine whether it is safe to treat patients with small vulvar carcinomas on an individualized basis, T. Iversen, V. Abeler, and J. Aalders (Norwegian Radium Hosp., Oslo) collected a series of 117 patients with stage I squamous cell carcinoma of the vulva. The patients had follow-up for 3 to 21 years.

The carcinomas were classified as large cell keratinizing (73.5%), large cell nonkeratinizing (19.7%), and small cell nonkeratinizing (6.8%). Four patients were treated by local excision, 2 by hemivulvectomy, 35 by vulvectomy, 54 by radical vulvectomy with inguinal lymphadenectomy, and 22 by radical vulvectomy with inguinal and pelvic lymphadenectomy. There was no clear relationship between the depth of infiltration and vessel invasion, recurrence, or death. Of 76 patients who underwent radical vulvectomy and lymphadenectomy, 6 of 15 with vessel invasion had lymph node metastases, whereas only 2 of 61 without vessel invasion had lymph node metastases (Table 1). Of 8 groin lymph node metastases, 7 were located on the same side as the primary tumor and 1 was bilateral. The frequency of inguinal recurrence and of death was significantly higher in those with vessel invasion than in those without (Table 2). There were no cases of multiple primary lesions. The overall 5-year crude survival rate was 79% for the whole series and 52% for those with vessel invasion.

Since the most important prognostic factor in this series was vessel invasion, examination of excision biopsy specimens for evidence of vessel invasion is recommended before deciding on final therapy.

TABLE 1.—CARCINOMA OF THE VULVA: CORRELATION OF
VESSEL INVASION WITH LYMPH NODE METASTASIS IN
WOMEN TREATED WITH LYMPHADENECTOMY

Status of vessels	Mean age (range) in years	Total	Lymph node metastases
Invasion	65.9(40–78)	15	6
No invasion	63.6(34–83)	61	2
Total	64.8(34–83)	76	8

(12–4) Obstet. Gynecol. 57:85–89, January 1981.

TABLE 2.—CARCINOMA OF THE VULVA: CORRELATION BETWEEN VESSEL INVASION AND CLINICAL OUTCOME

Status of vessels	Mean age (range) in years	Total	Recurrence Vulva/ vagina	Inguinal	Distant	Deaths of cancer
Invasion	63.7(33–78)	19	3	5		6
No invasion	62.8(18–83)	98	9	2	1	4
Total	63.3(18–83)	117	12	7	1	10

When the depth of tumor infiltration is less than 1 mm and there is no evidence of vessel invasion, hemivulvectomy is proposed as the primary treatment; if the infiltration is deeper than 1 mm, ipsilateral or, in some case, bilateral inguinal-femoral lymphadenectomy should also be performed. Radical vulvectomy with inguinal-femoral lymphadenectomy is indicated in patients with stage I lesions and vessel invasion.

▶ [Histologic type and depth of invasion were not important prognostically in this series of patients with stage I carcinoma of the vulva. The presence or absence of vessel invasion was very important, as indicated in Tables 1 and 2. We imagine that others would disagree with the authors' suggestion that with a unilateral vulvar lesion only ipsilateral groin lymphadenectomy is required if the nodes on that side are negative for metastases. The vulvar lymphatic drainage is bilateral (1979 YEAR BOOK, p. 267).] ◀

12–5 **Multiple Primary Neoplasms of the Anogenital Region.** The anogenital region, comprising the cervix, vagina, vulva, perineum, and anus, has the potential for the development of multicentric and multiple primary neoplasms. Yew-Cheong Choo and George W. Morley (Univ. of Michigan) reviewed data from the University of Michigan Tumor Registry on all patients with multiple primary neoplasms of the female genital tract during a 20-year period from 1957 to 1977. Fifteen cases with 3 or more primary neoplasms involving the anogenital region were identified. There were 8 patients with synchronous carcinomas. Of these, 4 patients had multiple primary tumors of in situ origin and the other 4 had both in situ and invasive lesions. Their mean age was 54.3 years. Six of the 8 patients had only vulvar symptoms, 1 had vaginal bleeding, and 1 was asymptomatic. The large vulvar lesion often led to an erroneous initial diagnosis of single primary tumor. Five patients had associated carcinoma in situ of the vagina. Two patients with carcinoma in situ of the anus had a lesion identical to, but noncontiguous with, the vulvar lesion. Among the 8 patients with multiple synchronous primary tumors, the initial diagnosis was correct in only 3. The treatment program varied, and some methods were seemingly too radical by current standards. Patients with cancer in situ were all successfully treated, but 2 patients required additional surgical excision for recurrent tumor in situ of the vagina. Two patients died of postoperative sepsis and 1 died of probable cerebral metastases from the invasive cervical cancer.

(12–5)   Obstet. Gynecol. 56:365–369, September 1980.

Seven patients had sequential multiple primary tumors. Intervals between diagnosis of neoplasms ranged from 3 to 17 years. Only 1 patient had all 3 primary malignancies of in situ origin; the other 6 had combined in situ and invasive lesions. In all instances, the initial primary tumor was cervical. It may be significant that 4 patients had undergone radiation therapy 3–15 years previously. In 1 patient, 2 other nongenital primary tumors developed, and the patient died of an invasive vulvar carcinoma. Two other patients died, 1 from an initial vaginal cancer and the other from the subsequent simultaneous tumors.

It has become increasingly apparent that multiple primary malignancies may develop in the female reproductive tract. The malignancy should be considered a regional disease. There appears to be an embryologic predisposition to multiple malignancies in this region. A viral agent may act on this common epithelium. Irradiation and chemotherapy as possible carcinogenic stimuli cannot be dismissed. In this series, multiple neoplasms occurred in patients beyond the fifth decade of life. In primary malignancies in this area, a thorough clinical examination coupled with liberal use of diagnostic aids is necessary to detect synchronous or subsequently occurring tumors. Use of cervical cytology, Schiller iodine staining of the cervix and vagina, toluidine blue staining of external genitalia, and colposcopy are advocated. In treatment of multiple primary tumors, questions arise as to whether a more radical approach is justified in view of the entire anogenital region's being at risk. A conservative approach is acceptable only if all lesions are eradicated or if the surgical margins are free of tumor. Furthermore, possible persistence of carcinogenic stimulus places these patients at greater risk for the development of subsequent malignancies; follow-up care should be outlined accordingly.

▶ [A number of reports have called attention to multiple primary neoplasms of the lower genital tract occurring in the same patient and presumably reflecting the multicentric origin of squamous tumors in this area. This article describes 15 patients seen during 20 years at the University of Michigan in whom squamous neoplasia, usually in situ but sometimes invasive, was present in at least 3 of 5 (cervix, vagina, vulva, perineum, and anus) sites. In 8 cases the carcinomas were synchronous (i.e., were all present when the patient was first seen) and in 7 the tumors developed sequentially. Two messages seem clear: (1) in any woman presenting with a tumor in one of these sites (especially the vulva), coexisting neoplasia in another site must be ruled out, and (2) follow-up of patients treated for carcinoma in one location (especially the cervix) should include screening for subsequent development of another neoplasm.] ◀

12–6 **Screening Strategies for Cervical Cancer and Cervical Intraepithelial Neoplasia.** Ralph M. Richart and Bruce A. Barron (Columbia Univ.) observe that squamous carcinoma of the cervix has certain features that make it ideally suited for screening programs designed to detect it in its earliest stages. There is overwhelming evidence that eradication of cervical intraepithelial neoplasia (CIN) prevents squamous carcinoma and reduces mortality from cervical cancer. Cervical cancer is a venereally transmitted disease, and women who have had several partners are at high risk. The transition time

---

(12–6) Cancer 47 [Suppl.]:1176–1181, Mar. 1, 1981.

from development of a precursor lesion to invasive cancer is an important variable in screening strategies. A combination of os aspiration or an applicator stick sample of the canal and a cervical scraping results in the optimal detection rate. In routine clinical practice the false negative rate is about 33%.

Once an abnormal Papanicolaou smear is obtained, histologic verification of neoplasia is necessary before treatment is given. Colposcopy and cervical biopsy, with endocervical curettage, are indicated where available. The risk of invasion in patients with undetected CIN 3 increases exponentially as the interval between cytologic examinations increases. It is possible that if screening intervals are increased substantially, mortality will also increase, and the regular Papanicolaou smear again will be highly cost-effective. It will take 15 years to determine whether changing the screening interval from 1 year to 3 years, as recommended by the American Cancer Society, is the correct decision, and that also is a risk. The American College of Obstetricians and Gynecologists recommends annual smears for all sexually active women, but this is appreciated less widely than the recommendations of the American Cancer Society.

▶ [It is apparent that the authors of this article are not enthusiastic about the proposed 3-year interval between Papanicolaou smears. They point out both the "false negative" problem and the variable time involved in the progression from carcinoma in situ to invasive disease. Although the authors estimate a mean duration of carcinoma in situ of 10 years, they suggest that in 5% of patients this interval is less than 3 years. Finally, they emphasize that what is assumed to be the least costly for society in dollar terms may not best serve the individual patient. In our institution, annual cytologic screening of the cervix continues to be recommended.] ◀

12–7 **Cryosurgery of Cervical Intraepithelial Neoplasia.** Kenneth D. Hatch, Hugh M. Shingleton, J. Max Austin, Jr., Seng-Jaw Soong, and Dorothy H. Bradley (Univ. of Alabama, Birmingham) used cryosurgery to treat 968 patients with cervical intraepithelial neoplasia (CIN), including 722 with a colposcopic diagnosis of CIN I or CIN II and 246 with a diagnosis of CIN III (severe dysplasia to carcinoma in situ). Cryotherapy was offered to patients interested in further childbearing who had ectocervical lesions and in whom the entire transformation zone was visualized and there was no colposcopic indication of invasion. The cytologic and directed biopsy findings agreed. Presently, a freeze-thaw-refreeze technique with temperatures of −40 to −60 C is used. Median follow-up was 1 year.

Tissue confirmation of CIN was obtained in 6% of patients with CIN I and CIN II initially. After a negative first smear, 2% of patients had histologic confirmation of CIN, and subsequent follow-up showed confirmed CIN in 1.6% to 2% of cases. A total of 44 patients have had CIN confirmed to date. No patient had abnormal cytologic findings after five negative smears. Not all patients required conization for evaluation of recurrent abnormal cytology.

Cervical intraepithelial neoplasia was confirmed in 12.3% of patients with CIN III at initial follow-up. Thirty-three patients have had CIN confirmed to date. Seventeen of these patients required conization for evaluation. One patient had invasive cancer.

(12–7) Obstet. Gynecol. 57:692–698, June 1981.

Only 2 of 66 patients with endocervical curettage indicative of CIN I or CIN II had histologic confirmation of failure. Failure after cryosurgery was confirmed in 5 of 8 patients whose endocervical evaluations showed CIN III.

Cryosurgery is an acceptable treatment for CIN I and CIN II, but better results can be obtained by conization in patients with CIN III. Cryosurgery is acceptable treatment for CIN III if good follow-up can be assured, but conization or hysterectomy is preferable if follow-up is unlikely.

12–8 Cryosurgical Treatment of Cervical Intraepithelial Neoplasia. Cryosurgery commonly is used in the treatment of all grades of cervical intraepithelial neoplasia (CIN). Donald R. Ostergard reports his experience with cryosurgery in the treatment of 354 patients with CIN during an 8-year period. Treatable patients were selected on the basis of colposcopic impression, colposcopically directed biopsy, and endocervical curettage.

The therapy failure rates were 6.3% for cases prediagnosed as CIN I, 7.5% for CIN II, and 19.6% for CIN III (table). The failure rates for severe dysplasia and carcinoma in situ were 7.1% and 38.8%, respectively. Posttreatment diagnosis of therapy failures revealed a more advanced stage of disease in 4 of 13 CIN I treatment failures (31%), 2 of 7 CIN II failures (29%), and 1 of 9 CIN III failures (11%) (table).

It is concluded that cryosurgery is no longer appropriate or effective for the treatment of CIN III.

▶ [The success of cryosurgery in the treatment of cervical intraepithelial neoplasia has led some to choose this modality in patients with CIN III (severe dysplasia and carcinoma in situ) over the more traditional cone or hysterectomy. This article and the preceding one suggest that cryosurgery is not adequate therapy for advanced CIN. A freeze-thaw-freeze (3, 5, and 3 minutes technique, respectively) was used. Perhaps the length of freezing or some other factor explains the failure rates in patients with CIN III described here. Until or unless other studies clearly demonstrate the efficacy of cryosurgery in CIN III, however, we will continue the more traditional approach of treating these lesions in the operating room.] ◀

12–9 Significance of Atypical Vessels and Neovascularization in Cervical Neoplasia. Frederick Sillman, John Boyce, and Rachel Fruchter (SUNY, Downstate Med. Center) quantitatively studied the

POSTTREATMENT DIAGNOSES OF THERAPY FAILURES

Pretreatment diagnosis	No. treated	I	II	III	Stage Ia	Total
CIN I	205	9	2	1	1	13(6.3%)
CIN II	93	2	3	2	0	7(7.5%)
CIN III	46	3	1	4	1	9(19.6%)
Severe dysplasia	28	1	0	1	0	2(7.1%)
Carcinoma in situ	18	2	1	3	1	7(38.8%)
						29(8.4%)

CIN diagnosis after therapy

(12–8) Obstet. Gynecol. 56:231–233, August 1980.
(12–9) Am. J. Obstet. Gynecol. 139:154–159, Jan. 15, 1981.

Histology	Patients examined	Atypical vessels		Frequency of atypical vessels (%)
		Absent	Present	
Moderate dysplasia or less	1,481	1,481	0	0
Severe dysplasia	487	487	0	0
Carcinoma in situ	390	379	11	2.8
Microinvasion	8	4	4	50
Frank invasion	49	4	45	92
Total	2,415	2,355	60	2.5

relationship between atypical vessels seen colposcopically and dysplasia, carcinoma in situ (CIS), microinvasion, and frank invasion in 2,415 patients (table) seen over 3 years. Atypical vessels are defined as being two to ten times wider than normal capillaries and irregular in width, shape, and course; they have a horizontal component, abruptly appear and disappear, and are separated from each other (often widely) without forming a regular pattern, although occasionally they may simulate a deranged network. They can be confused with "bizarre" vessels, which may be prominent and tortuous but have less abrupt irregularities and less intercapillary distance. Bizarre vessels are not accompanied by other colposcopic indications of cancer.

No atypical vessels were found in patients with dysplasia, but atypical vessels were found in 2.8% of patients with CIS, half of those with microinvasion, and all of those with frank invasion in whom the entire zone of transformation was viewed. Of the 60 patients who had atypical vessels, all had either CIS or invasive cancer; 82% had invasion. Data did not suggest a correlation between atypical vessels and depth of invasion when invasion was less than 3 mm.

Conclusions are: (1) Atypical vessels are not present with dysplasia and rarely present with CIS. (2) Atypical vessels may be associated with microinvasion but are required for frank invasion. (3) Because atypical vessels are usually associated with invasion, which can be in or near the field of atypical vessels, diagnostic cone biopsy should be performed if such vessels are seen and colposcopic biopsy specimens do not show frank invasion. (4) Microinvasion without atypical vessels may be a localized disease.

▶ [The authors of this report make a strong case for performing cone biopsies in patients with atypical vessels on colposcopic examination unless the initial punch biopsies reveal frank invasion.] ◀

12-10 **Histologic Grade and Prognosis of Carcinoma of the Cervix.** C. K. Chung, John A. Stryker, Samuel P. Ward, William A. Nahhas, and Rodrigue Mortel (Pennsylvania State Univ.) used a histologic grading system based on tumor differentiation to correlate grade with course of disease in 122 patients with stage IB and stage IIA squa-

(12–10) Obstet. Gynecol. 57:636–642, May 1981.

INCIDENCE OF RECURRENCE BY SIZE OF PRIMARY LESION AND TREATMENT*

Treatment	Large tumor[†]			Small tumor[‡]		
	Grade 1	Grade 2	Grade 3	Grade 1	Grade 2	Grade 3
Group A (RT)	0/1	1/5	2/3	0/6	2/18	0/2
Group B						
B1) RT	—	3/3	4/4	0/2	0/2	0/1
B2) Surgery and RT	—	1/1	—	—	2/9	1/2
B3) Surgery	—	0/1	0/1	0/11	3/43	2/7
Total	0/1(0%)	5/10(50%)	6/8(75%)	0/19(0%)	7/72(10%)	3/12(25%)

*Both local recurrence and distant metastasis.
†Primary lesion at least 4 cm.
‡Primary lesion less than 4 cm.

mous carcinoma of the cervix. Tumors were graded on the basis of epithelial pearls, mitotic activity, nuclear pleomorphism, and amount of tumor cell cytoplasm. Thirty-five patients received definitive radiotherapy (RT); the other 87 were operated on and their para-aortic nodes were sampled. Twelve patients had unresectable disease and received RT. If diseased nodes or resection margins were found, RT was given after radical hysterectomy.

The more dedifferentiated the primary tumor, the larger was the primary lesion. Pelvic node metastasis was found in over half the patients with grade 3 tumors and in 17% of those with grade 1 and grade 2 lesions. Eleven patients had pelvic recurrences and 10, distant metastases. Nearly 90% of recurrences were found within 2 years of treatment. Local recurrence and distant metastasis were more frequent in patients with grade 3 tumors. Recurrences are related to both treatment and size of the primary in the table. Each patient with a well-differentiated primary tumor lived to 2 years without disease, regardless of stage or type of treatment. Patients with grade 3 tumors had significantly poorer survival at 2 years than those with grade 1 or grade 2 lesions.

Histologic grade correlates well with both the size of the primary tumor and pelvic node metastasis in patients with invasive cervical carcinoma. Patients with poorly differentiated tumors have large primary lesions, an increased rate of tumor recurrence, and lower survival without disease 2 years after treatment, compared with those who have well- and moderately differentiated lesions. Histologic grading is an important adjunct to clinical evaluation and treatment planning in squamous carcinoma of the cervix.

▶ [Histologic grading in general correlates with prognosis for most malignancies, though the correlation is probably less with carcinoma of the cervix than with endometrial cancer. This review of stage IB and stage IIA cervical lesions indicates that well-differentiated tumors respond better to treatment than do more anaplastic ones. The data are confounded by the fact that the more poorly differentiated tumors tended to be larger in size (40% of grade 3 were $\geq$ 4 cm compared with only 11% of grades 1 and 2). However, as indicated in the table, histologic grade appears to be important when the data are broken down by large and small size, so that grading seems to be something to be taken into account in planning the treatment regimen.] ◀

12–11 **Combined Radiation and Surgical Treatment of Stages IB and IIA and B Carcinoma of the Cervix.** P. Marziale, G. Atlante, V. Le Pera, T. Marino, M. Pozzi, and A. Iacovelli (Rome) reviewed the results of combined surgical and radiation therapy of stages IB, IIA, and IIB cervical carcinoma in 757 patients treated between 1965 and 1979. Intracavitary radium therapy was used preoperatively to deliver a total dose of 6,000 mg/hour. Radical hysterectomy was performed 3 to 4 weeks after radiotherapy. If diseased nodes were found at adenectomy, telecobalt therapy was delivered.

Survival was analyzed in 526 patients treated through 1975. Operative mortality was 0.5%. Complications included 11 ureterovaginal fistulas, 3 vesicovaginal fistulas, 18 cases of prolonged bladder atony, and 7 cases of stress urinary incontinence. A total of 69 recurrences were observed. With ideal treatment, survivals at 5 to 14 years were 94.8% among stage IB cases, 83.1% among stage IIA cases, and 58.8% among stage IIB cases. The primary lesion was sterilized in 63% of patients given preoperative radium therapy. Node status was an important determinant of survival. When the primary lesion was sterilized by radiotherapy, survival improved from 54.2% to 86.8%.

Combined radiotherapy and surgery appears to be the most effective treatment for cervical cancer. Preoperative radiotherapy sterilized the primary lesion histologically in nearly two thirds of cases in this series. Surgical failures from spread of tumor cells at operation are thus reduced. Radiotherapy alone sometimes fails. Excessive radicality in either surgery or radiotherapy has few advantages and may produce serious complications. The most suitable management for each patient can be achieved by collaboration between radiotherapists and oncologic gynecologists at a well-organized center.

▶ [The trend in recent years has been away from radiation therapy prior to radical hysterectomy because it seems to be associated with an increased complication rate, particularly urinary fistulas, and no clear-cut improvement in survival. In this large series from Rome treated by intracavitary radium, radical hysterectomy 3–4 weeks later, and teletherapy if positive nodes were found, the survival rates are excellent—95% for stage IB, 83% for stage IIA, and 59% for stage IIB. Moreover, there were only 11 ureterovaginal and 3 vesicovaginal fistulas, an incidence of about 2%. The authors state that they take great care with the ureter and "prepare the mesoureter according to Palmrich." Something must work!] ◀

12–12 **Adenocarcinoma of the Cervix: I. Clinical Evaluation and Pathologic Features.** Hugh M. Shingleton, Hazel Gore, Dorothy H. Bradley, and Seng-Jaw Soong (Univ. of Alabama, Birmingham) reviewed the findings in 137 patients with invasive cervical adenocarcinoma, 17 of whom had recurrent disease. The overall incidence of adenocarcinoma was 9.3%. The patients were slightly younger than those with squamous cell carcinoma and were more often nulliparous. A marked increase in adenocarcinoma occurred in 1979–1980. Stage I disease was present in 77% of primary cases. The median age was 47 years, but patients with stage II–IV disease were significantly older.

Nearly two thirds of stage I patients and 54% of all patients under-

(12–11) Gynecol. Oncol. 11:175–183, April 1981.
(12–12) Am. J. Obstet. Gynecol. 139:799–814, Apr. 1, 1981.

went total or radical hysterectomy, with or without adjunctive irradiation. Radiotherapy usually consisted of combined external beam therapy and intracavitary cesium therapy. Two thirds of patients had other than endophytic lesions. No positive nodes were found in stage I patients with lesions of 1 cm or less, whereas 10.7% of subjects with squamous cell carcinomas of this size had positive nodes. In all, 20.4% of stage I adenocarcinoma patients had positive nodes, compared with 13.5% of patients with stage I squamous cell carcinoma. The most common subpatterns of disease were the endocervical and papillary types. Survival at 3 years is comparable in adenocarcinoma patients and control subjects. Stage I lesions of 3 cm or larger appeared to have a prognosis similar to that of stage II lesions.

Surgery and radiotherapy both appear to be effective forms of treatment for adenocarcinoma of the cervix. Radiotherapy appears to be preferable to radical surgery for bulky stage IB lesions. Patients with adenosquamous lesions seem to have as good a prognosis as those with adenocarcinoma. Further follow-up of patients may give more insight into the efficacy of various forms of treatment as related to stage, size, grade, and histologic type of disease.

▶ [This is a large and well-analyzed series of adenocarinoma of the cervix. The results emphasize the importance of stage, histologic grade, and tumor size in prognosis. In patients with bulky central lesions (i.e., the "barrel-shaped" cervix), radical surgery did not seem very effective; radiation, perhaps with the addition of a simple hysterectomy, may be a better alternative. There was no evidence of difference in biologic behavior between squamous and adenomatous lesions of the cervix and, in contrast to the situation with endometrial tumors, patients with adenosquamous tumors and those with pure adenocarcinomas had similar outcomes.] ◀

12–13 **Carcinoma of the Cervix: Effect of Age on Survival.** C. Robert Stanhope, Julian P. Smith, J. Taylor Wharton, Felix N. Rutledge, Gilbert H. Fletcher, and H. Stephen Gallager (Wayne State Univ.) compared survival in 265 patients younger than age 35 who had invasive cervical carcinoma with that of similar patients older than age 35. Irradiation was used most frequently as the primary treatment. Of those patients younger than age 35, 216 received irradiation, 42 had surgery alone, and 7 had chemotherapy alone or with irradiation. In patients older than age 35, 806 received irradiation, 14 had surgery alone, and none had chemotherapy.

The 5-year survival for both groups is shown in the table. A significant decrease in 5-year survival was found in the younger patients compared to that in patients older than age 35 in all cancer stages except for stages IA and IV. Only 6 of the older patients had stage IA disease, and all with stage IV disease died. The greatest number of failures occurred in stage IIB patients in whom, despite central control of disease, distant metastases developed. In the younger group of patients, 42 had small volume cancer with early invasion of the cervical stroma; they were treated with surgery alone. There was only 1 treatment failure in this group. In 6 younger patients, adjunctive conservative extrafascial hysterectomy was performed after a less radical dose of irradiation. In 3 of these patients distant metastases devel-

---

(12–13) Gynecol. Oncol. 10:188–193, October 1980.

Squamous Carcinoma of the Cervix in Intact Uterus: Five-Year Survival (FIGO Staging)

	35 Years and less		Over 35 years		
	(Surv. %)	(No.)	(Surv. %)	(No.)	*P*
Stage I-A	98.0	(42)	100.0	(6)	—
Stage I-B (low volume)	85.7	(49)	96.3	(62)	0.05
Stage I-B (high volume)	76.4	(52)	91.3	(208)	0.005
Stage II-A	51.4	(37)	83.6	(160)	0.005
Stage II-B	40.0	(42)	65.6	(176)	0.005
Stage III	25.5	(35)	47.1	(207)	0.05
Stage IV	—	(8)	—	(1)	—
Total		265		820	

oped, leading to death; the other 3 survived. Sixteen (11.4%) patients with stage I cancer had recurrence. Regional failures occurred with greater frequency in patients younger than age 35 with stage IIA lesions than in those with stage IIB lesions. Distant metastases occurred in nearly 80% (19 patients) of stage IIB lesions in which treatment failed. Of these 19 patients, 12 had infiltrating exocervical lesions and 7 had endocervical barrel-shaped lesions. In patients with stage III involvement, central disease was controlled in all but 1. Forty-four (17%) of 265 patients younger than age 35 were pregnant or within 3 months post partum when treatment was begun. The number of pregnant patients was too small for accurate comparison of survival with nonpregnant patients stage by stage.

In an attempt to explain the decreased survival of patients younger than age 35, the original pathology of 194 of these patients was reviewed and grouped according to cell types. Of 194 patients, 65 (31.9%) had large cell keratinizing cancer, 110 (53.9%) had large cell nonkeratinizing cancer, and 19 (9.3%) had small cell cancer. The 5-year survival of these three groups was 70.8%, 49.0%, and 52.4%, respectively. The presence of keratin resulted in improved survival in patients younger than age 35.

Results suggest that pretreatment evaluation of younger patients, especially those with stage IIB cancer, should be more aggressive in attempts to detect cancer beyond the usual treatment fields. The poorer prognosis for patients younger than age 35 cannot be explained on the basis of cell type.

▶ [Age ≤ 35 years adversely affected the prognosis of patients with cervical cancer in this large, stage-adjusted series. Mann et al. (*South. Med. J.* 73:1186, 1980), in contrast, did not find age to be of prognostic significance in a smaller series of patients with stage I disease.] ◀

12-14 **Scalene Node Biopsy in Advanced Carcinoma of the Cervix Uteri.** Berkeley Brandt, III, and Samuel Lifshitz (Univ. of Iowa) reviewed data on 40 patients with advanced cervical cancer who underwent left scalene node biopsy as part of a pretreatment evaluation

(12–14) Cancer 47:1920–1921, April 1981.

because of para-aortic node metastasis identified at celiotomy (25), palpable scalene nodes (2), or other evidence of metastasis or unresectability.

Scalene node metastases were documented in 11 patients (27.7%); only 2 had palpable scalene nodes. Of those with para-aortic node metastasis, 7 (28%) had scalene node metastasis; none was palpable preoperatively.

Because scalene node involvement indicates that the disease is beyond the scope of both surgical and radiation treatment, routine left scalene node biopsy is recommended in patients with para-aortic node metastasis. Patients with positive para-aortic nodes but negative scalene nodes are treated with extended-field radiation. Those with positive scalene nodes are considered candidates for chemotherapy. Prognosis for patients with scalene node metastases is extremely poor. Review of the literature showed that overall incidence of scalene node metastasis in most series is low.

► [Preradiotherapy operative evaluation of patients with advanced carcinoma of the cervix was considered in two articles in the 1979 YEAR BOOK (pp. 278–281). The present report makes a good point. Scalene lymph nodes are sometimes positive for tumor in patients with positive para-aortic nodes. Scalene node biopsy is a simple surgical procedure that can identify patients whose disease is beyond the confines of even extended-field irradiation.] ◄

12–15 **Ovarian Endocrine Function in Young Women Undergoing Radiotherapy for Carcinoma of the Cervix.** The main treatment of early cervical cancer in Sweden is a full course of intracavitary and external radiotherapy or intracavitary radiotherapy combined with radical surgery. Both approaches involve castration and premature menopause in young women. Per Olof Janson, Inge Jansson, Asbjörn Skryten, Jan-Erik Damber, and Göran Lindstedt examined endocrine function in 14 women, aged 24 to 38 years, who underwent standard radiotherapy for cervical carcinoma stages IB and IIA. Radical hysterectomy and lymphadenectomy were carried out 3 to 4 weeks after radiotherapy. Four women had three combined intrauterine and vaginal applications of radium, and the other 10 had afterloading therapy with radiocobalt. The ovaries removed at operation were perfused, one of each pair with chorionic gonadotropin.

No significant changes in serum testosterone concentrations were found. Progesterone concentrations were low and variable in all cases, but values during radiotherapy were higher than those found the day before operation. Estradiol concentrations were continuously reduced during treatment, particularly at operation. Gonadotropin concentrations were inversely proportional to those of estradiol, reaching postmenopausal values at the time of operation. Addition of chorionic gonadotropin to the ovarian perfusion medium had no effect on estradiol release, but testosterone release was significantly increased. No release of progesterone was detected in the perfusion studies.

Ovarian follicular function deteriorated at an early stage of treatment in this study. Luteal function appeared to be less vulnerable to

(12–15) Gynecol. Oncol. 11:218–223, April 1981.

radiotherapy. Androgen production by the ovarian stroma was observed. There is no reason to preserve the ovaries if radical hysterectomy follows radiotherapy, since estrogen replacement will be necessary and because a remaining ovary may elicit virilizing symptoms. In early stage IB cases the cure rate is as good with operation alone as with radiotherapy, and by this approach ovarian function may be preserved and estrogen replacement avoided for a long period.

▶ [These results are interpreted as indicating that pelvic radiation essentially ablates ovarian follicular function (i.e., estrogen production), while not affecting ovarian stromal function (i.e., testosterone production). If this is true, the radiated ovary doesn't produce the good stuff and should therefore be removed at the time of subsequent surgery. To a considerable extent, these conclusions are based on the perfusion studies and, in the absence of any parallel studies on normal (i.e., unradiated) ovaries, we find these data not entirely convincing. Nevertheless, most gynecologic oncologists probably include oophorectomy with radical hysterectomy in a previously irradiated patient.] ◀

12–16 **Postradiation Ureteral Obstruction: A Reappraisal.** David Muram, Harry Oxorn, R. H. Curry, P. Drouin, and Jack H. Walters (Univ. of Ottawa) reviewed data on 34 patients who received radiation therapy for carcinoma of the cervix and in whom hydronephrosis later developed. Most patients were treated by intracavitary radiation (Manchester technique), supplemented by external radiation, cobalt-60 beam, aimed to deliver 7,500–8,000 R at point A and 5,000–5,500 at point B.

Twelve (35%) patients had no evidence of pelvic malignancy histologically; obstruction in these patients was caused by periureteral fibrosis. The incidence of obstructive uropathy due to periureteral fibrosis not associated with recurrent tumor increased when the obstructing lesion was unilateral, the clinical staging of carcinoma prior to therapy was stage IB (associated with the highest incidence of postradiation fibrosis) or stage II rather than stage III or IV, and the obstructing lesion developed 2 or more years after completion of radiation therapy. In 96% of patients with recurrent disease, the malignancy was diagnosed within 5 years after therapy. After 5 years, periureteral fibrosis was almost always the cause of ureteral obstruction. In 7 patients, ureteral obstruction was diagnosed 5 or more years after completion of therapy; 6 had periureteral fibrosis. In patients with periureteral fibrosis, the location of ureteral obstruction was within 5 cm from the ureteral orifice to the bladder in all but 1. Hydronephrosis associated with ipsilateral leg edema and sciatic pain strongly suggests recurrent tumor with poor prognosis.

The low incidence of postradiation fibrosis leading to ureteral obstruction reported in the literature derives from the fact that most series express the incidence as a fraction of the total number of patients treated. Because all but 1 of the patients studied received similar amounts of radiation within the acceptable therapeutic range, local factors were probably responsible for the different responses to therapy. Two local factors, pelvic inflammatory disease, and tumor infiltration, are well documented as increasing ureteral susceptibility

---

(12–16) Am. J. Obstet. Gynecol. 139:289–293, Feb. 1, 1981.

to radiation damage. Newer techniques using high-energy radiation increase the cure rate, but they also increase the complication rate, including ureteral obstruction due to postradiation fibrosis. The diagnosis of periureteral fibrosis should be considered in all patients in whom urinary tract obstruction develops after radiation for carcinoma of the cervix. If all other methods of investigation fail to confirm the presence of a malignant lesion, laparotomy and direct biopsy of the obstructing lesion is indicated; such investigations should be performed in an environment in which ureteral obstruction by a benign process can be managed surgically.

▶ [In a report abstracted in the 1979 YEAR BOOK (p. 310), ureteral obstruction after radiation therapy nearly always meant recurrent tumor. Not so, according to this study. Posttherapy hydronephrosis was often due to radiation fibrosis if the initial cervical cancer was stage I or stage II, the involvement was unilateral, or the interval between treatment and ureteral obstruction was more than 2 years. The message is that recurrent disease should be proved by biopsy and not merely suspected on the basis of findings on the intravenous pyelogram.] ◀

12-17 **Recent and Past Use of Conjugated Estrogens in Relation to Adenocarcinoma of the Endometrium.** It has been suggested that conventional studies associating estrogen use and endometrial cancer may have had a built-in selection bias because estrogens provoke uterine bleeding in women with otherwise asymptomatic disease. Samuel Shapiro, David W. Kaufman, Dennis Slone, Lynn Rosenberg, Olli S. Miettinen, Paul D. Stolley, Neil B. Rosenshein, Watson G. Watring, Thomas Leavitt, Jr., and Robert C. Knapp (Boston Univ.

RELATION OF TIME OF LATEST USE OF CONJUGATED ESTROGENS AND
DURATION OF USE TO RISK OF ENDOMETRIAL CANCER

TIME ELAPSED SINCE LATEST USE *	DURATION OF USE			χ_1^2 TEST FOR TREND †
	<1 yr	*1–4 yr*	*≥5 yr*	
<1 YEAR				
Cases	—	6	27	44.1
Controls	—	4	15	(P<0.01)
Rate ratio ‡	—	7.9	8.8	
≥1 YEAR				
Cases	2	6	14	8.5
Controls	14	16	13	(P<0.01)
Rate ratio ‡	0.9	1.6	3.6	
TOTALS				
Cases	2	12	41	41.9
Controls	14	20	28	(P<0.01)
Rate ratio ‡	0.9	2.6	6.0	

*For 5 patients and 5 control subjects, exact time of latest use was unknown.
†Computed with age and geography taken into account by an extension of Mantel-Haenszel procedure.
‡Adjusted for decade of age and geographic area by Mantel-Haenszel procedure and computed with 81 cases and 305 control subjects who never used conjugated estrogens as the reference category (rate ratio = 1.0).

(12–17) N. Engl. J. Med. 303:485–489, Aug. 28, 1980.

Med. Center) evaluated this hypothesis by comparing 149 patients with endometrial cancer and 402 control subjects with various conditions, but not uterine bleeding, with regard to the last time they used noncontraceptive conjugated estrogens and the duration of use. Rate-ratio estimates were computed for various categories of estrogen use, with 1.0 as the rate ratio for control subjects who had never used estrogens.

When estrogens were used for less than 1 year, there was no evidence of an association between endometrial cancer and estrogen use. However, when the duration of estrogen use exceeded 5 years, the rate-ratio estimates were 8.8 (95% confidence interval, 4.4–17) for recent use (less than 1 year since discontinuation) and 3.6 (1.6–8.4) for past use (table). When long-term use had been discontinued 2 or more years previously, the rate-ratio estimate was 3.3 (1.4–8.0).

The results suggest that the rate of endometrial cancer is increased in women who use conjugated estrogens and the risk increases with duration of use. It is concluded that this association cannot be accounted for by biased selection of cases according to estrogen use.

▶ [A few years ago, the suggestion was made that the apparent association between exogenous estrogens and endometrial cancer might be spurious, i.e., that estrogens, by causing symptoms (bleeding), might lead to the diagnosis of uterine cancer that otherwise would not have been recognized. This study suggests otherwise. The "rate ratio" was elevated in patients who had stopped estrogen use at least 1 year prior to diagnosis. Estrogen-induced uterine bleeding leading to diagnosis could not be implicated in these patients. Therefore, the association between exogenous estrogen and endometrial cancer remains.] ◀

12–18 **Predominance of Early Endometrial Cancers After Long-Term Estrogen Use.** The risk of endometrial cancer among women who use exogenous estrogens appears to be greatest for the noninvasive type of lesion. Barbara S. Hulka, David G. Kaufman, Wesley C. Fowler Jr., Roger C. Grimson, and Bernard G. Greenberg (Univ. of North Carolina) evaluated the risk of endometrial cancer associated with estrogen use for each histologic grade, cell type, clinical stage, and extent of invasion in 256 women with histologically confirmed endometrial cancer and 321 community control subjects matched for age and race.

The use of estrogens for less than $3^{1}/_{2}$ years did not markedly increase the risk of endometrial cancer for any stage, grade, histologic type, or extent of invasion. The use of estrogens for $3^{1}/_{2}$ years and longer, however, significantly increased the relative risk of stage IA (7.6), histologic grade I (5.5), and endometrial invasive (5.2) endometrial cancers. The increased relative risks were seen with both high-dose (greater than 0.625 mg) and low-dose (0.625 mg and less) estrogen preparations. The relative risk of stage IA endometrial cancer was 8.5 for the high-dose preparation. For the most part, the risks for the more advanced cancers were only slightly increased, although the long-term use of estrogens did increase the risk of advanced cancer when the preparation was taken continuously rather than cyclically. The long-term use of estrogens was not preferentially associated with the increased risk of adenocarcinomas and adenoacanthomas.

(12–18) JAMA 244:2419–2422, Nov. 28, 1980.

The results confirm the absence of endometrial cancer risk with short-term estrogen use.

▶ [While it is virtually certain that exogenous estrogen therapy increases the risk of endometrial cancer, the risk largely is limited to that of early (i.e., stage IA) disease. This is important to keep in mind, because 5-year survival rates with appropriate treatment of stage I well-differentiated endometrial cancers typically run to 80% or 90%. Such considerations should not allay concerns about estrogens and uterine cancer, but they are important in placing the risk in perspective. Other findings of interest in this report are the relationship with time (≥3.5 years) and with continuous versus cyclic therapy, but not with dose. The prognosis of estrogen-induced endometrial cancer is considered in further detail in the following article.] ◀

12–19 **Estrogen Use and Survival in Endometrial Cancer.** In studies that relate estrogen use to endometrial cancer, estrogen use is associated with favorable tumor characteristics. Although the superior survival rate of women with endometrial cancer who have been exposed to estrogen may be explained by this association, no study has controlled for the effect of the favorable factors to determine whether there remains a primary association between prior estrogen use and survival. J. Collins, L. H. Allen, A. Donner, and O. Adams (London, Ont.) conducted such a study in the 860 new patients with endometrial cancer referred to a regional cancer treatment center during 1967 to 1976. Of the 860 women, 259 (30%) who gave a history of noncontraceptive estrogen use for 6 months or more at some time before diagnosis were classified as users, and 568 (66%) who denied estrogen use, used it for less than 6 months, or used it only in oral contraceptives were considered nonusers.

Estrogen use was associated with younger age, earlier stage, lower grade of tumor, less common myometrial invasion, and preferred treatment including radiation and hysterectomy. Five-year survival was 92% for estrogen users and 68% for nonusers. Further analysis controlling for differences in distribution of variables associated with survival showed that for women with endometrial cancer, the risk of any death for nonusers was some 2.7 times greater than for estrogen users and the risk of death from endometrial cancer was 5.4 times greater for nonusers. Thus, the strong association between estrogen use and superior survival remained when the influence of other factors was held constant. A history of estrogen use was not associated with superior survival of women with poorly differentiated tumors or myometrial invasion.

Earlier diagnosis is not a sufficient explanation for the superior survival shown in this study because estrogen use also conferred superior survival on women with advanced disease. Tumors that appeared after estrogen use may have the pathologic appearance but not the biologic aggressiveness of malignant tumors. This does not imply that estrogen use is safe because of superior survival. Case-control studies have shown a three- to eightfold higher risk of endometrial cancer developing in the average estrogen user. Although the risk of death from other causes and from cancer is apparently less for

(12–19) Lancet 2:961–964, Nov. 1, 1980.

estrogen users than for nonusers, there remains for estrogen users a risk of development of endometrial cancer, a tumor that requires major surgery with or without radiotherapy.

▶ [The all-but-completely accepted relationship between exogenous estrogen and endometrial cancer is recognized generally as involving tumors with favorable prognostic signs—earlier stage, lower histologic grade, and less frequency of myometrial invasion. This study was designed to control for such features in order to permit a determination of whether estrogen use per se influences prognosis. The results indicate that it does; in other words, estrogen-associated endometrial cancers seem to be of lesser biologic aggressiveness than those unassociated with previous estrogen usage.] ◀

12-20 **Serum Sex Hormone–Binding Globulin Capacity and Percentage of Free Estradiol in Postmenopausal Women With and Without Endometrial Carcinoma: New Biochemical Basis for Association Between Obesity and Endometrial Carcinoma.** J. A. Nisker, G. L. Hammond, B. J. Davidson, A. M. Frumar, N. K. Takaki, H. L. Judd, and P. K. Siiteri studied the sex hormone-binding globulin (SHBG) capacity and percentage of free estradiol in the serum of 20 postmenopausal women with endometrial carcinoma and in 58 normal postmenopausal women. Special attention was paid to the relationship of serum SHBG capacity to patient weight.

Mean percentage of free estradiol in serum was 1.92% in women with cancer and only 1.65% in controls. This significant difference was probably due to a lower SHBG capacity in women with cancer (26 pmol/ml) than in controls (35 pmol/ml), because highly significant inverse correlations between serum SHBG capacity and percentage of free estradiol were found in both groups. Mean excess body weight was 69 lb in cancer patients and 25 lb in controls. Serum SHBG capacity was inversely related to excess body weight. When 11 cancer patients were individually matched with controls for deviation from ideal body weight, no differences in SHBG capacity and percentage of free estradiol were found.

In addition to the well-known above-normal peripheral production of estrogen associated with obesity, it also appears that higher concentrations of free estradiol are available to target cells because of a depression in serum SHBG capacity in obese postmenopausal women. These findings provide further evidence that endogenous estrogens may account for the epidemiologic link between obesity and the increased incidence of postmenopausal endometrial cancer. Because a reduction in weight in postmenopausal women reportedly normalizes serum levels of estradiol and SHBG capacity, obese postmenopausal women should be advised to lose weight.

▶ [The conventional explanation for the well-known association between obesity and endometrial cancer involves chronically high estrone levels as a result of aromatization of adrenal androgens in fat tissue. These observations suggest an additional endocrinologic mechanism. Endometrial cancer patients had lower sex hormone-binding globulin levels than controls, with amounts inversely related to excess body fat. Lower sex hormone-binding globulin leads to higher free estradiol levels available to stimulate the endometrium.] ◀

(12–20) Am. J. Obstet. Gynecol. 138:637–642, Nov. 15, 1980.

12–21 **Postoperative External Irradiation and Prognostic Parameters in Stage I Endometrial Carcinoma: Clinical and Histopathologic Study of 540 Patients.** Jan Aalders, Vera Abeler, Per Kolstad, and Mathias Onsrud (Norwegian Radium Hosp., Oslo) present the results of a 3- to 10-year follow-up of 540 patients with stage I adenocarcinoma of the corpus uteri. All of the patients entered a prospective clinical trial from 1968 to 1974 to evaluate the effect of postoperative external pelvic irradiation. Treatment protocol is shown in Figure 12–1. Primary treatment consisted of abdominal hysterectomy and bilateral salpingo-oophorectomy. Postoperatively, all patients received intravaginal radium irradiation; 6,000 rad was delivered to the surface of the vaginal wall. Of 540 patients, 277 were allocated to group A (control group) and 263 to group B in a randomized fashion. Group B received 4,000 rad to the pelvic lymph nodes with central shielding at 2,000 rad. Irradiation was given over a course of 4 weeks, 5 fractions per week.

No significant difference in survival was found between treatment group A (91%) and group B (89%) after 5 years; after 9 years, survival was 90% and 87%, respectively. In 3–10 years of follow-up, a significant reduction in vaginal and pelvic recurrences was found in group B as compared with group A (1.9% versus 6.9%, $P < .01$). However, more patients in group B had distant metastases than those in group A (9.9% versus 5.4%). The death and recurrence rate was increased in patients over 60 years of age; a higher percentage of these women had tumors infiltrating more than half the depth of the myometrial wall. Under weight and morbidly overweight patients had a poorer prognosis than normal or moderately overweight patients. A slightly higher death and recurrence rate was noted in groups A and B when the length of the uterine cavity exceeded 8 cm. Table 1 shows that a significantly higher death and recurrence rate was found in groups A and B for patients with tumor infiltration of more than half the myometrium. There was a higher frequency of death from cancer, vaginal and pelvic recurrence, distant metastasis, and poorly differentiated carcinomas in these patients. No positive effect was produced by pelvic irradiation in grade 3 (i.e., poorly differentiated) tumors in-

Fig 12–1.—Treatment protocol in patients with stage I carcinoma of the corpus uteri. (Courtesy of Aalders, J., et al.: Obstet. Gynecol. 56:419–427, October 1980.)

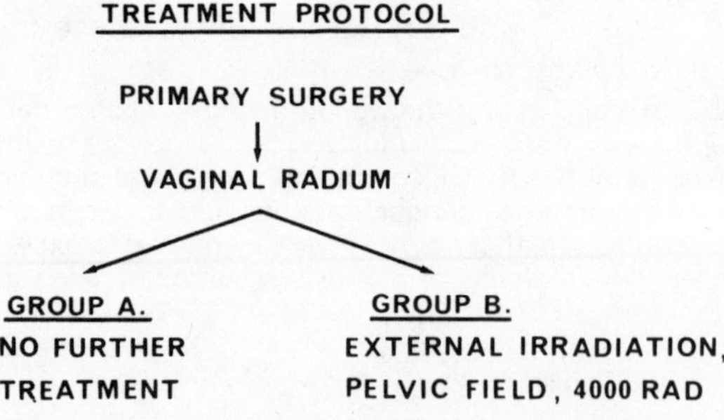

(12–21) Obstet. Gynecol. 56:419–427, October 1980.

TABLE 1.—RELATIONSHIP AMONG MYOMETRIAL INFILTRATION, RECURRENCE AND DEATH,* HISTOLOGIC GRADE, PELVIC RECURRENCE, AND DISTANT METASTASIS

Treatment group	Myometrial infiltration	No. of patients	DRR (%)	Deaths of cancer (%)	Histologic grade (%)			Vaginal and pelvic recurrence (%)	Distant metastasis (%)
					1	2	3		
A	≤ 0.5	162	6.8	3.7	15.4	62.3	22.2	4.3	2.5
	> 0.5	102	22.5	17.6	2.9	47.1	50.0	14.7	9.8
B	≤ 0.5	178	11.2	9.6	15.2	58.4	26.4	2.2	9.6
	> 0.5	76	17.1	14.5	3.9	36.8	59.2	6.6	11.8
Total		518	12.9	10.0	11.2	54.2	34.6	6.0	7.7

*DRR = death and recurrence rate.

filtrating less than half the myometrial wall (Table 2). Only patients with grade 3 tumors more than half the myometrial thickness bene- fited from additional external radiotherapy. Of the last consecutive 151 patients, 30 (19.9%) had tumor cells in endothelial lined spaces; the death and recurrence rate for these patients was 26.7%, signifi- cantly higher than in patients without vessel invasion. Therefore, pelvic irradiation is recommended in this group and in patients with

TABLE 2.—DEATH AND RECURRENCE RATE,* DEATH RATE, VAGINAL AND PELVIC RECURRENCE, AND DISTANT METASTASIS IN PATIENTS WITH HISTOLOGIC GRADE 3 TUMORS INFILTRATING LESS OR MORE THAN HALF THE MYOMETRIUM

| | Myometrial infiltration ≤ 0.5 | | | | | Myometrial infiltration > 0.5 | | | | |
Treatment group	No. of patients	DRR (%)	Deaths of cancer (%)	Vaginal and pelvic recurrence (%)	Distant metastasis (%)	No. of patients	DRR (%)	Deaths of cancer (%)	Vaginal and pelvic recurrence (%)	Distant metastasis (%)
A	36	11.1	8.3	5.6	5.6	51	31.4	27.5	19.6	15.7
B	47	21.3	17.0	2.1	17.0	44	18.2	18.2	4.5	13.6

*DRR = death and recurrence rate.

grade 3 lesions infiltrating more than half of the myometrial thickness. In a modified protocol, all other patients, irrespective of degree of differentiation or myometrial infiltration, should receive only postoperative intracavitary vaginal irradiation.

▶ [This randomized study involving a large number of patients treated at a single institution over a relatively short time span provides much useful information. Advanced age, undifferentiated tumor, vascular space involvement, and deep myometrial invasion adversely affected prognosis. Although external pelvic irradiation was associated with fewer pelvic recurrences, distant metastases were more common and survival rates were not improved. The 18% of patients with grade 3 tumors *and* deep myometrial invasion may have benefited from the external pelvic irradiation, although the relatively small number of patients in this category doesn't permit a definite statement.

12–22 **Endometrial Carcinoma in Women 40 Years of Age or Younger.** Endometrial carcinoma is uncommon in young women and is often associated with hormonal abnormalities, use of sequential oral contraceptives, and the clinical profiles of obesity, hypertension, infertility, and diabetes. John D. Crissman, Ramez S. Azoury, Alfonso E. Barnes, and Helmut F. Schellhas (Univ. of Cincinnati) reviewed 87 cases of endometrial cancer in patients aged 40 years and younger registered between 1960 and 1978 and representing 2.9% of all cases. The diagnosis was confirmed on pathologic review in 32 of 54 cases (table).

Mean age was 35.7 years. Twelve of the 32 patients had never conceived. Twelve patients were obese, 8 had documented hypertension, and 1 was diabetic. A large majority of patients had irregular vaginal bleeding. Two patients were infertile. Four patients had used oral contraceptives of unknown types for more than 3 years. Seven had received oral contraceptives or intramuscular estrogen injections sporadically for vaginal bleeding. One patient had a prolactin-secreting pituitary adenoma. All patients had well-differentiated adenocarcinomas. Twelve had adenoacanthomas. Six patients also had ovarian neoplasms, and 2 died of widespread ovarian carcinoma. Four of these tumors were endometrioid-type adenoacanthomas.

Most of these well-differentiated adenocarcinomas were associated with normal and hyperplastic endometrial changes. None of the patients in this series died of endometrial carcinoma. Currently patients with atypical endometrial hyperplasia and well-differentiated adenocarcinoma (clinical stage I) are managed by hysterectomy without radiotherapy.

▶ [This study confirms the generally good prognosis associated with endometrial carcinoma in the young patient. The tumors were well-differentiated and did not invade the myometrium. The patients, except for those with coexisting ovarian cancers, did well. The "bad news" here is that, on review, 22 of 54 (41%) cases originally diagnosed as endometrial cancer were given lesser diagnoses. Most disturbing is that the revised diagnosis was totally benign in 7 cases.] ◀

REVISED DIAGNOSIS

Endometrial diagnosis	No. of patients
Marked atypical hyperplasia	11
Adenomatous hyperplasia	4
Proliferative	4
Secretory	1
Menstruating	2
Total	22

(12–22) Obstet. Gynecol. 57:699–704, June 1981.

12-23 **Do Estrogen and Progesterone Receptors (E₂R and PR) in Metastasizing Endometrial Cancers Predict the Response to Gestagen Therapy?** The presence of specific cytoplasmic progesterone receptor protein is necessary for progesterone to exert its cellular effect in the treatment of advanced or recurrent endometrial carcinoma. In cases where the tumor is poorly differentiated or advanced age is involved, progesterone receptor content is reduced. Th. J. Benraad, L. G. Friberg, A. J. M. Koenders, and S. Kullander (Univ. Hosp., Lund, Sweden) prospectively studied biopsy specimens obtained from 150 women with primary, untreated endometrial cancer to determine the content of estrogen and progesterone receptors (E₂R and PR). Thirteen of these patients had metastases despite surgical and radiation treatment, and gestagen therapy was begun. The clinical effect of this treatment was studied to determine any correlation between the response to treatment and initial E₂R and PR contents.

Of the 13 patients, 8 (aged 61 to 71 years) were positive for E₂R (greater than 10 fmoles/mg of cytosolprotein), 2 did not show any PR, and 6 had PR in concentrations ranging from 7 to 892 fmoles/mg of cytosolprotein. Of 7 patients who showed a clinical response to gestagen therapy, the tumors were poorly differentiated in 3 and moderately differentiated in 4. Five of the women, 50 to 84 years of age, were negative for E₂R, did not show any PR, failed to respond to therapy, and died within 2 to 8 months after gestagen therapy was started. In these patients, the tumors were poorly differentiated in 2 and moderately differentiated in 3.

It appears that the determination of E₂R and PR is a clinically useful test for predicting the response of endometrial carcinoma to gestagen therapy.

▶ [Estrogen receptor analysis seems to be finding a clear place in management in breast cancer, and these results suggest that a similar situation may apply with endometrial cancer, at least with respect to the response to palliative progestational therapy. Of 5 patients whose primary tumor lacked estrogen receptors and who developed metastases, none responded to progestagens. However, among 8 patients with metastatic disease whose primary tumors contained estrogen receptors (and progesterone receptors in 6), all but 1 responded to progestational therapy.] ◀

12-24 **Significance of Positive Tubal Cytology in Patients With Endometrial Adenocarcinoma.** J. Menczer, M. Modan, and E. Goor (Tel Aviv Univ.) studied tubal cytologic features for 9 years in 47 patients with endometrial adenocarcinoma; malignant cells were demonstrated in the fallopian tubes in 10 (21.3%) of these patients.

Positive tubal cytologic features did not correlate statistically with age of the patients, grade and stage of tumor at diagnosis, preoperative radiotherapy, presence of residual tumor, or myometrial invasion. The 5-year survival in patients with positive tubal cytologic features (82%) did not differ significantly from that in patients with negative tubal cytologic features (74%). However, correlation of 5-year survival with stage at diagnosis was significant, being best in patients in stage I. There was also a trend, not significant, for im-

(12–23) Acta Obstet. Gynecol. Scand. 59:155–159, 1980.
(12–24) Gynecol. Oncol. 10:249–251, December 1980.

proved 5-year survival in patients with no residual tumor or myometrial invasion. Only 1 of 4 patients with malignant cells in the peritoneal fluid had positive tubal cytologic features.

The lack of correlation of positive tubal cytologic findings with factors considered to be of prognostic significance and with 5-year survival seems to indicate that the fallopian tube is not a major mode of endometrial cancer spread.

▶ [In this study, the presence of malignant endometrial cells in the fallopian tubes was associated with neither a lower survival rate nor any of the adverse prognostic factors studied. This is not to say that endometrial cancer cannot metastasize via this route, nor that occluding the tubes at the start of a hysterectomy done for endometrial cancer is the wrong thing to do, but rather, that the incidental finding of malignant cells in the tubal lumen by the pathologist is probably not very important.] ◀

12–25 **Endometrial Adenocarcinoma Arising in Adenomyosis.** Endometrial adenocarcinoma and adenomyosis are both fairly common abnormalities of the uterus in candidates for hysterectomy, though there are few reports of these two pathologic entities occurring in combination. Penetration of more than 50% of the myometrium by endometrial adenocarcinoma has been associated with an increased incidence of lymph node metastases and correspondingly reduced survival rates, regardless of the histopathology or size of the uterus. Since the differential survival between patients with myometrial invasion and those with malignancy arising in adenomyosis may have prognostic significance, Enrique Hernandez and J. Donald Woodruff (Johns Hopkins Hosp.) reviewed sections of uteri from the files of the Gynecologic Pathology Laboratory of The Johns Hopkins Hospital from 21 patients who underwent hysterectomy for endometrial adenocarcinoma with associated adenomyosis. The histopathologic features and outcome of treatment are reported.

Within the foci of adenomyosis, atypical endometrial hyperplasia was observed in 2 cases and adenocarcinoma in 6 cases. The atypical hyperplasia was characterized by the absence of intervening stroma as a result of aggressive epithelial proliferation, while individual cell atypia was not significant. In the 6 cases of adenocarcinoma in adenomyosis, the adenocarcinoma was well differentiated. Myometrial invasion was present to a depth of more than 50% in 2 cases and to a depth of less than 50% in the other 4. Individual cell anaplasia was not a significant feature. The prominent findings were pseudostratification of the epithelium, mitotic activity, and marked adenomatous crowding of the glands with papillary infolding into the lumina. The differential between direct myometrial invasion and adenocarcinoma arising from adenomyosis was based primarily on the presence of a direct transition from benign adenomyosis to malignancy and the presence of stroma with the epithelial elements (Fig 12–2). By contrast, the stromal element was classically lacking in metastatic or invasive foci. All of the patients were treated with abdominal hysterectomy and bilateral salpingo-oophorectomy; 3 cases were also treated with postoperative pelvic radiation. All of them are living and without evidence of disease 5 years or more after treatment.

(12–25) Am. J. Obstet. Gynecol. 138:827–832, Dec. 1, 1980.

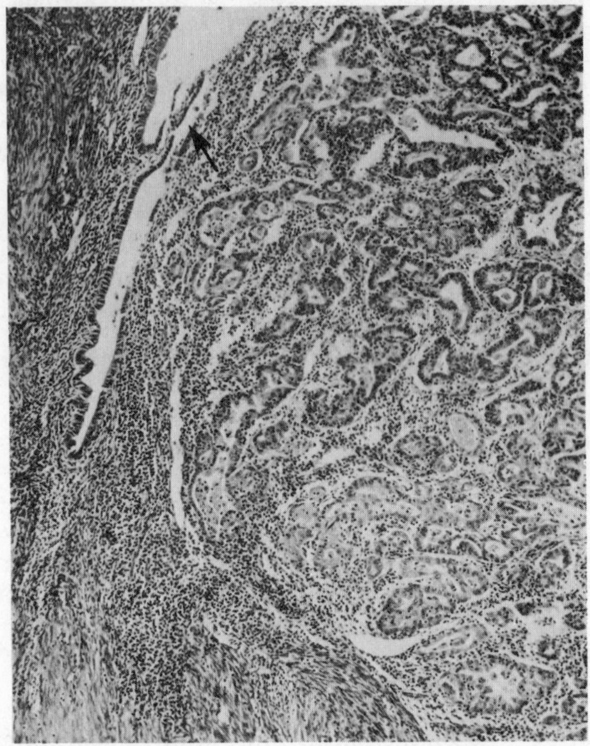

Fig 12–2.—Adenocarcinoma beginning in adenomyosis. *Arrow,* transition from benign adenomyosis to cancer. (Courtesy of Hernandez, E., and Woodruff, J. D.: Am. J. Obstet. Gynecol. 138:827–832, Dec. 1, 1980.)

The relatively high association of malignancy at separate sites in this series, compared with the few cases reported in the literature, is most likely attributable to differences in the interpretation of the myometrial disease. Although the number of cases in this series is small, it represents an approach to the differential diagnosis of metastatic and multifocal disease.

▶ [The point made here is that it is important to distinguish multifocal endometrial carcinoma involving both surface endometrium and adenomyosis from endometrial cancer with deep myometrial invasion, because the prognosis varies so greatly between the two conditions.] ◀

12–26 **Adenocarcinoma of the Uterine Corpus Following Irradiation for Cervical Cancer.** Tae H. Kwon, Thongbliew Prempree, Chik-Kwun Tang, Umberto VillaSanta, and Ralph M. Scott (Univ. of Maryland) review the literature and describe 8 patients with adenocarcinoma of the uterine corpus occurring 5 to 23 years after radiotherapy for cervical cancer (adenocarcinoma incidence in 830 patients so treated between 1941 and 1965, 0.96%). Patients with in situ adenocarcinoma and adenocarcinoma after radiotherapy for benign condi-

(12–26) Gynecol. Oncol. 11:102–113, February 1981.

tions were excluded, as were 2 patients who had mixed mesodermal uterine tumors.

Seven patients presented received external pelvic radiation in addition to radium application—5 by cobalt 60 and 2 by orthovoltage x-rays. Doses were not inconsistent with contemporary radiation treatment for cervical cancer. One patient received radium treatment alone. Four patients took 0.1 mg of Stilbestrol daily for 5 to 10 years; the other 4 received no hormones.

Abnormal vaginal bleeding was the presenting symptom in only 2 of 8 patients and in 30.7% of 27 collected cases. Abdominal pain or distention, back pain, pelvic mass, lethargy, and vaginal discharge were other presenting symptoms or signs; 3 patients were asymptomatic. Papanicolaou smears, performed in 7 patients, were abnormal in 4 and negative in 3. Dilatation and curettage established the diagnosis in 2 patients, but failed in 3 because of dense fibrotic obliteration of the upper part of the vagina. In none of the 8 patients was the cancer confined to the uterine corpus. Intra-abdominal spread or distant metastasis was documented in 5 of the 8 and in 12 of 26 collected cases (46%). The tumor showed moderate to poor differentiation in 7 of the 8 cases and focal malignant squamous components in 3. All 8 patients died of cancer. The longest survival was 5 years 1 month. Among 29 cases from the literature, only 3 patients survived 5 years or longer.

These unusual clinical features and the grave outcome are believed to be due to delay in diagnosis resulting from infrequent vaginal bleeding; postradiation cervical canal stenosis or obliteration of the upper part of the vagina appears to be the main obstacle.

▶ [This paper calls attention to an infrequent but significant problem—development of endometrial cancer many years after radiotherapy for cervical cancer. Eight such cases occurred among 830 patients treated with radiation over 25 years, an incidence of 1%. Four of the patients had received estrogen, which complicates any conclusions about etiology. Diagnosis seems to have been compromised by the previous radiotherapy—only 2 of the 8 presented with bleeding, and dilatation and curettage was possible in only 2 cases. All patients had advanced disease, which may reflect unusually aggressive behavior and/or early intra-abdominal spread due to a blocked cervical canal.] ◀

12-27 **Leiomyosarcoma of the Uterus: Clinicopathologic Study.** Joseph R. Vardi and Harold M. M. Tovell (Columbia Univ.) retrospectively reviewed the clinical behavior of uterine leiomyosarcomas in relation to their pathologic features in 32 consecutive patients seen during a 12-year period. Mean age was 55.5 years (range, 38–86 years). The mean interval from menopause to diagnosis was 6.7 years. Predominant symptoms were abnormal vaginal bleeding, pain or abdominal discomfort, or enlarged pelvic mass. Preoperative dilatation and curettage established the correct diagnosis in 5 (20.8%) of 24 patients. Uterine enlargement was common to all patients. There were 19 patients with stage I lesions (involving the uterine corpus), 2 patients with stage II lesions (involving the uterine cervix), 4 patients with stage III lesions (involving pelvic structures outside the

(12–27) Obstet. Gynecol. 56:428–434, October, 1980.

uterus), and 7 patients with stage IV lesions (involvement of upper abdomen or distant metastases). Ten of the 32 patients were obese, 7 had hypertension, and 4 had diabetes. Eight of 31 patients with recorded parity were nulliparous; 4 of the 8 had had 1 or more spontaneous abortions. Twenty-five patients had total abdominal hysterectomy (TAH) with bilateral salpingo-oophorectomy (BSO). Of these, 3 had external radiation therapy and intracavitary radium application; 2 patients were given adjuvant adriamycin. Four patients had external radiation therapy alone.

The single most important factor in treatment was the use of TAH and BSO. Of the total group, 25% survived for 5 or more years and 43.8% died within the first 3 years following diagnosis. The 5-year survival rates for patients with disease stages I, II, III, and IV were 36.8% (7 patients), 0%, 25% (1 patient), and 0%, respectively. Survival data according to mitotic count and histologic grade of tumor are shown in Tables 1 and 2, respectively. Grade I tumors maintained the general architecture of leiomyoma; grade II tumors had the most atypical cellular elements, pronounced necrosis, and hemorrhage; grade III tumors were the most anaplastic. Age at the time of diagnosis was an important prognostic indicator. Fourteen (43.7%) patients were premenopausal; the others were postmenopausal. Four of 11 patients younger than age 50 (premenopausal) died of the disease, whereas only 1 of 18 patients older than age 50 (postmenopausal) lived.

The most suggestive clinical feature of a uterine leiomyosarcoma is enlargement of a fibroid with or without vaginal bleeding in a postmenopausal patient. The clinical extent of disease at the time of initial surgery is thought to be the most important prognostic sign. A recurrence was clinically observed usually within 18 months after initial diagnosis and 31.3 months after onset of symptoms. The number of mitoses per 10 high-power field (HPF) is also a useful prognos-

TABLE 1.—RELATION OF 5-YEAR SURVIVAL TO MITOTIC ACTIVITY

No. of mitoses per 10 HPF	No. of patients	Alive at 5 years	Dead at 5 years
0–4	6	5	1
5–9	11	2	9
10 or more	15	1	14

HPF = high-power field.

TABLE 2.—RELATION OF TUMOR GRADE TO 5-YEAR SURVIVAL

Tumor grade	No. of patients	Alive at 5 years	Dead at 5 years
I	11	5	6
II	6	2	4
III	15	1	14

tic index. Survival rates are better at 2–5 mitoses/10 HPF than at 5–10 mitoses/HPF. The size of the uterus is of no prognostic value when the uterus bears a well-encapsulated tumor within large fibroids. The treatment of choice seems to be TAH and BSO alone. The best hope for cure is early removal of the leiomyosarcoma when it is still confined to a leiomyoma.

▶ [This study suggests that both mitotic activity and tumor grade are of prognostic importance in patients with leiomyosarcoma of the uterus. The authors state that it was frequently impossible to distinguish between leiomyosarcoma arising from myometrium and that arising within a preexisting myoma. It is not surprising that neither Papanicolaou smears nor dilatation and curettage were generally helpful in making the diagnosis prior to laparatomy.] ◀

12–28 **Benign Cystic Teratomas in Postmenopausal Women.** Benign cystic teratomas (dermoid cysts) are ovarian neoplasms derived from germ cells and composed of mature tissues representing two or more embryonic germ cell layers and usually containing hair, desquamated stratum corneum, and sebaceous material. Representing 15% to 20% of all benign ovarian tumors and 10% of all ovarian tumors, their peak incidence is in the third and fourth decades of life. Classically, then, they are tumors of young women. Alan Gordon, Neil Rosenshein, Tim Parmley, and Belur Bhagavan (Baltimore) studied the incidence of benign cystic teratomas in postmenopausal women.

Review of the files of two hospitals for the 6-year period of 1973 to 1978 showed 309 cases of benign cystic teratoma in patients aged 2 to 80 years. The largest group of cases (42%) occurred in women aged 20 to 29 years, but 16 (5%) occurred in postmenopausal women aged 49 to 80 years.

Of the 16 patients, 13 had an asymptomatic pelvic mass. In 3, the teratoma was discovered incidentally during operation for other gynecologic conditions. No patient had a preoperative clinical diagnosis of benign cystic teratoma, although calcifications within a pelvic mass were seen in 4 patients. The largest cyst measured $18 \times 15 \times 9$ cm. Of the 15 women who had not previously undergone an oophorectomy, 3 (20%) had bilateral dermoid cysts.

Histopathologic findings included "skin" consisting of stratified squamous epithelium with epidermal appendages (12 cases). In all cases the dermis was markedly scarred, having been replaced almost totally by dense collagen with obliteration of the loose reticular tissue of normal dermis. This indicates the prolonged presence of these tumors within the ovary, suggesting that they reposed within the young woman and were not detected until she reached menopause. The high rate of bilaterality also suggests that this is an end-stage disease when found in postmenopausal women.

Secondary neoplasms occurred in 3 (1%) of the 309 cases reviewed, all in postmenopausal women (19% of this group). One woman with mucinous cystadenocarcinoma is well 36 months after diagnosis, 1 with stromal carcinoid is well at 24 months, and 1 with squamous cell carcinoma died of primary adenocarcinoma of the colon.

All benign cystic teratomas in postmenopausal women should be

---

(12–28) Am. J. Obstet. Gynecol. 138:1120–1123, Dec. 15, 1980.

managed as if they were potentially malignant, with thorough staging procedures to evaluate the extent of disease and extensive sampling of the dermoid cyst.

▶ [The benign cystic teratoma is the most common tumor of women in the age range 20 to 40 years and is almost always benign. This collection of cases encountered in postmenopausal women indicates that in this age group the incidence of malignancy is appreciable (3 of 16).] ◀

12–29 **Functioning Ovarian Tumors in Postmenopausal Women.** Estrogenic symptoms have been observed in postmenopausal women with so-called nonendocrine tumors of the ovary. Robert M. Rome, Denys W. Fortune, Michael A. Quinn, and James B. Brown (Univ. of Melbourne) studied 80 postmenopausal patients with epithelial ovarian tumors seen from 1963 to 1979. All had been amenorrheic for over 6 months. No patient was receiving estrogen or progesterone.

Estrogen excretion was elevated in 55.2% of patients with benign tumors or proliferating tumors of low malignant potential and in 37.2% of those with primary malignant tumors (table). Significantly more patients with mucinous than with serous tumors had elevated estrogen excretion. Seventy-three percent of tumors associated with high estrogen excretion exhibited stromal luteinization, condensation, or both, compared with 15.8% of tumors associated with normal estrogen excretion. Postmenopausal bleeding was insignificantly

TUMOR EPITHELIUM AND ESTROGEN EXCRETION

Tumor type	Estrogen excretion (> 9 μg/ 24 hr)	$\bar{X}$	Range
Cystadenoma			
Mucinous	10/16	16.2	3.9–39.1
Simple serous cyst	0/1	4.1	4.1
Serous	0/3	3.5	2.2–6.0
Proliferating serous	0/1	4.8	4.8
Proliferating mucinous	2/2	22.3	11.2–33.4
Cystadenofibroma			
Serous	3/4	18.2	1.7–27.7
Mucinous	1/1	27.0	27.0
Mixed	0/1	5.6	5.6
Carcinoma			
Mucinous	7/9	28.7	1.5–61.0
Serous	1/20	3.0	0–9.8
Endometrioid	5/6	20.8	8.4–50.7
Clear cell	0/4	4.7	0.3–8.6
Mixed*	1/1	12.6	12.6
Undifferentiated	2/3	27.5	2.2–69.0
Metastatic†	8/8	69.8	20.0–138

*Serous, clear cell, and endometrioid elements.
†Primary neoplasms: stomach (2), colon (3), appendix (1), tube (1), and unknown (1).

(12–29) Obstet. Gynecol. 57:705–710, June 1981.

more frequent in patients with high estrogen excretion. Endometrial evidence of estrogen activity was obtained in 62.9% of patients with high and 16% of those with normal estrogen excretion. All but 3 of 16 patients with high estrogen excretion showed a fall to normal values after bilateral oophorectomy. One of the exceptions was obese, and the other 2 had incomplete removal of ovarian tumors. One patient with initially normal estrogen excretion had an elevation 2 years later when ovarian metastases from colon carcinoma were present.

The exact mechanism of increased steroid production by the stromal cells of ovarian tumors is unknown. Stromal changes in both the tumor and the other ovary correlated with high estrogen excretion in this series, suggesting a humoral basis for the phenomenon. There is growing evidence that endogenous chorionic gonadotropin is involved in the stimulation of tumor stroma to synthesize steroids. Residual primary tumor may be the source of persistently elevated estrogen excretion, but it has not been shown that metastases from primary ovarian malignancies can synthesize estrogen. Endocrine epithelial tumors of the ovary far outnumber the generally recognized functioning tumors of gonadal stromal origin.

▶ [As medical students, we learned about so-called functioning ovarian tumors. Although estrogen production by the stroma adjacent to "nonfunctioning" ovarian tumors has been recognized for several years, we had considered it to be an infrequent occurrence. This report suggests otherwise. Indeed, certain tumors (e.g., endometroid, mucinous) usually were associated with elevated urinary estrogen excretion. This may explain the fairly frequent presentation of postmenopausal bleeding with ovarian cancer.] ◀

12–30 **Cellular Fibromas and Fibrosarcomas of the Ovary: A Comparative Clinicopathologic Analysis of 17 Cases.** Most fibromatous tumors of the ovary are definitely benign, but fibrosarcomatous lesions may be seen. Jaime Prat and Robert E. Scully (Boston) reviewed the findings in 17 cases of atypical fibromatous tumor of the ovary. Follow-up ranged from 2 months to 13 years (average, 4 years).

Eleven patients (average age 49 years) had cellular fibromas, with 1–3 mitoses per 10 high-power fields. Seven patients were postmenopausal. Six had pelvic pain. Three tumors ruptured. Four patients had total abdominal hysterectomy and bilateral salpingo-oophorectomy. Four tumors had cystic elements which consisted chiefly of densely cellular tissue with few hypocellular fibrous areas. Two patients died with tumor present, 1 after incomplete resection. Six patients (average age, 58 years) had fibrosarcoma. One had radiation therapy and 2 received chemotherapy treatment. Four of these tumors were solid and 2 were cystic. Mitotic figures ranged from 4 to 25 per 10 high-power fields. Two tumors contained several abnormal forms. Four patients had pelvic recurrences, and 1 had evidence of hepatic metastases. Four patients died of tumor an average of 18 months postoperatively. Another patient died with tumor present; 1 was alive with metastatic disease at follow-up. The microscopic feature correlating best with the prognosis was the degree of mitotic activity.

(12–30) Cancer 47:2663–2670, June 1, 1981.

Cellular fibromas of the ovary can be managed by unilateral salpingo-oophorectomy in young women in whom the other ovary appears uninvolved. Adjuvant radiation therapy should be considered if tumor tissue persists postoperatively. Adjuvant chemotherapy appears to be indicated in cases of ovarian fibrosarcoma even when the tumor appears to be confined to the ovary. Radiation therapy may be useful if local disease persists postoperatively.

▶ [The situation here is apparently analogous to that of cellular myoma versus leiomyosarcoma in the uterus. In both situations, the mitotic count is an important predictor of subsequent behavior.] ◀

12–31   **Treatment of Epithelial Ovarian Carcinoma by Surgical Debulking Followed by Single Alkylating Agent Chemotherapy.** M. B. Hanson, D. E. Powell, E. S. Donaldson, and J. R. van Nagell, Jr. (Univ. of Kentucky, Lexington) retrospectively studied 52 patients with primary invasive epithelial ovarian carcinomas treated from 1966 to 1977 by exploratory laparotomy with debulking of tumor, followed by chemotherapy with a single alkylating agent. Alkylating agents used were L-phenylalanine mustard (Alkeran), 0.2 mg/kg orally on 5 consecutive days every 4 weeks; cyclophosphamide (Cytoxan), 6–8 mg/kg intravenously on 5 consecutive days every 4 weeks; or chlorambucil (Leukeran), 0.1–0.2 mg/kg orally every day as a maintenance dose. All surviving patients received 12 months of chemotherapy followed by second-look laparotomy. Patients with persistent tumor continued on an alkylating agent after a second surgical debulking. Patients were followed 2–12 years after initial therapy (mean 55.8 months) or until death.

Age of the patients was 40–70 years in 84%, under age 40 in 10%, and over age 70 in 6%. Patients under age 40 years had lower-grade tumors, lower-stage tumors, and better survival than other age groups. Patients over age 70 typically had poorly differentiated, advanced-stage disease and decreased survival. Sixty-five percent of the patients studied presented with stage III or IV disease (International Federation of Gynecologists and Obstetricians Staging System).

Prognosis was directly related to stage of disease at initial surgery. The 2-year survival was 92% in patients with stage I disease compared with 55% in patients with stage III disease. Degree of differentiation (grade) of the tumor was directly related to patient age; 93% of the patients with well-differentiated tumors, regardless of other prognostic factors, survived at least 2 years. Two-year survival was 59% in patients with serous tumors and 90% in patients with mucinous tumors, who often presented with earlier stage, well-differentiated lesions. Only 1 of 8 patients with anaplastic tumors of undeterminable cell type survived 2 years. Size of the largest residual tumor masses after initial surgery was most significant in patient survival. The 2-year survival was 95% in patients with tumor nodules less than 2 cm in diameter after initial surgery and 39% in patients with tumor greater than 2 cm in diameter after surgical debulking.

(12–31)   Gynecol. Oncol. 10:337–342, December 1980.

Average time required to complete 12 courses of chemotherapy was 14.6 months (average delay 2.6 months due to bone marrow depression). No hospitalizations required for toxicity due to chemotherapy, and no drug-related death occurred.

The findings suggest that excellent survival can be expected when single alkylating agent chemotherapy is used in patients with well-differentiated, early stage ovarian tumors completely excised at primary surgery. High-risk patients in whom primary combination chemotherapy is indicated include those with poorly differentiated tumors, residual tumor greater than 2 cm in diameter after surgical debulking, or stage III or IV disease.

▶ [This relatively small series of patients with ovarian cancer confirms the prognostic importance of stage and grade and indicates that good survival rates are attainable with single akylating agent chemotherapy in patients with well-differentiated stage I and stage II tumors, provided either no gross tumor or tumor masses < 2 cm in diameter remain after surgical treatment.] ◀

12–32 **In Vitro Clonogenic Assay for Predicting Response of Ovarian Cancer to Chemotherapy.** An in vitro soft agar human tumor stem cell assay for drug sensitivity that supports the growth of clonogenic ovarian tumor cells has been developed recently. David S. Alberts, H. S. George Chen, Barbara Soehnlen, Sydney E. Salmon, Earl A. Surwit, Laurie Young, and Thomas E. Moon (Univ. of Arizona) evaluated this drug sensitivity assay in 95 clinical trials with anticancer drugs in 40 patients with advanced ovarian cancer.

In vitro testing utilizing tumor biopsy specimens predicted sensitivity in 21 of the 40 patients. Of these 21, 15 showed a clinical response to drugs predicted to be effective in vitro; 2 had complete remissions of 1 and 12^+ months, 11 had partial remissions, and 2 showed a 25% to 49% reduction in tumor masses. In 73 of 74 trials in which drug resistance was predicted in vitro, there was no clinical response to treatment. The predictive accuracy of the assay for complete and partial remissions was 62%; this increased to 71% when those patients who showed objective improvement were included. The accuracy of the assay in predicting a lack of clinical response was 99%.

The human tumor stem cell assay can be an effective tool in planning a chemotherapy regimen for patients with ovarian cancer.

▶ [This is an interesting approach to the selection of particular chemotherapeutic agents for specific patients with ovarian cancer. In vitro drug resistance was highly predictive of a lack of patient response. More study is needed, but this technique looks promising.] ◀

12–33 **Role of Adjuvant Therapy in Stage I Ovarian Cancer.** Myroslaw M. Hreshchyshyn, Robert C. Park, John A. Blessing, Henry J. Norris, David Levy, Leo D. Lagasse, and William T. Creasman evaluated the role of adjuvant pelvic radiation and chemotherapy in 86 patients with stage I epithelial ovarian carcinoma; the disease was determined by exploratory laparotomy. Within 8 weeks after total abdominal hysterectomy and bilateral salpingo-oophorectomy, eligible patients were randomly assigned to one of three treatment regimens:

(12–32) Lancet 2:340–342, Aug. 16, 1980.
(12–33) Am. J. Obstet. Gynecol. 138:139–145, Sept. 15, 1980.

no further treatment (29 patients), pelvic radiation (23), or chemotherapy (34), without regard to substage of cancer, type of tumor, or degree of histologic differentiation. Radiation therapy consisted of 5,000 rad to the pelvis in 5–6 weeks, with a daily dose of 160–200 rad 5 times per week. The margins of radiation portals were the upper margin of the sacroiliac joint (superior), the upper third of the obturator foramen (inferior), and 1 cm beyond the lateral margins of the bony pelvis at the widest plane of the pelvis (lateral). The chemotherapy regimen consisted of melphalan (0.2 mg/kg) daily orally for 5 days every 4 weeks for 18 months if the leukocyte count was at least 3,000/cu mm and platelet count was at least 150,000/cu mm. The tumor grade was similar in all three postoperative treatment programs.

Among 86 patients, recurrence developed in 14 (Table 1): 6% of patients in the chemotherapy group, 17% of those receiving no treatment, and 30% of the radiation treatment group had recurrence. Radiation did not prevent pelvic recurrence (Table 2), because the incidence of pelvic recurrence was equal among all treatment modalities. Considering only recurrences outside the pelvis, lesions recurred in 3% of the chemotherapy group, 14% of those receiving no treatment, and 26% of those given radiation treatment. When recurrence was compared by substage, a definite trend became apparent: only 10% of patients with stage IA(1) lesions experienced recurrence, compared to 50% of those with stage IB(2) lesions. When substages were evaluated with regard to treatment categories, melphalan therapy was in each substage equal or superior to no treatment or radiation.

The difference in the rate of recurrence among the three treatment modalities ($P = .047$) is more meaningful when known prognostic factors are considered: 62% of the no-treatment group had stage IA(1) lesions, whereas 56% of the chemotherapy group and 48% of the radiation group had these lesions. Yet, within this category of lesions, patients with chemotherapy had the fewest recurrences. Analysis of

TABLE 1.—COMPARISON OF THERAPY AND RECURRENCE

Therapy	No. of patients	Recurrence No.	Recurrence %
No therapy	29	5	17
Radiation therapy	23	7	30
Chemotherapy	34	2	6

TABLE 2.—SITE OF RECURRENCE BY THERAPY

Site	No therapy	Radiation therapy	Chemotherapy
Pelvis	1 (3%)	1 (4%)	1 (3%)
Abdomen	0	2	0
Pelvis and abdomen	3 } (14%)	2 } (26%)	0 } (3%)
Distant	1	2	1

data on the 10% of patients with favorable cell types who experienced recurrence shows that melphalan produced the best results. Of 10 patients with stage IB lesions, all 4 treated with radiation had recurrence, whereas all 6 treated with chemotherapy remain free of disease. These results suggest that, with the exception of stage IA(1)g1 lesions, adjunctive therapy (melphalan) is beneficial in stage I carcinoma of the ovary. To date, leukemia has not developed in any patient treated with melphalan.

▶ [Single-agent chemotherapy was more effective than pelvic irradiation or no treatment in preventing recurrence after the initial surgical therapy for stage I ovarian cancer. Substage or grade considerations did not favor the chemotherapy group. Presumably, the pelvic irradiation was not successful in treating occult extrapelvic disease. Whether intraperitoneal radioactive phosphorus would yield results comparable to chemotherapy remains to be determined. Except *perhaps* for a stage IA(1)g1 lesion (a well-differentiated tumor confined to one ovary with an intact capsule without tumor on the external surface and negative peritoneal fluid cytology), the authors think that adjunctive therapy other than pelvic radiation is indicated in stage I ovarian cancer. We agree.] ◀

12–34   **Second-Look Operations in Ovarian Cancer.** Exploratory laparotomy after a planned course of chemotherapy, the "second-look" operation, is performed to assess the status of epithelial tumors of the ovary so that future management can be planned and any residual tumor removed. Peter E. Schwartz and Julian P. Smith evaluated second-look operations following chemotherapy in 186 patients with epithelial tumors of the ovary who were managed at the M. D. Anderson Hospital and Tumor Institute, Houston, over a 14-year period. The surgical technique used changed significantly during the period of study. Currently, laparotomy is performed through a vertical midline incision from the symphysis to approximately 6 cm above the umbilicus. If no gross tumor is present, cytologic washings from the pelvis and each paracolic space and multiple biopsy specimens from the abdominal and pelvic peritoneum are obtained. If gross tumor is present, an attempt is made to remove it.

At initial therapy, 27 patients had stage I disease, 31 had stage II disease, 105 had stage III disease, and 23 had stage IV disease. Of these 186 patients, 58 were found to have no evidence of disease at second-look and chemotherapy was discontinued, while 128 were found to have persistent cancer (table). There was no evidence of disease in 8 patients with advanced ovarian cancer 5 or more years after negative second-look operations; these patients presumably were

STAGE VERSUS FINDINGS AT SECOND-LOOK OPERATION

Stage	Total No. of patients	No. of patients with NED	No. of patients with persistent cancer	% NED
I	27	18	9	66.7
II	31	14	17	45.2
III	105	17	88	16.2
IV	23	9	14	39.1
Total	186	58	128	

(12–34) Am. J. Obstet. Gynecol. 138:1124–1130, Dec. 15, 1980.

cured by chemotherapy. A change in the mode of management was made in 7 patients who were found to have cancer at second-look operation; these patients were without evidence of disease 5 or more years later. All of the patients with stage IV disease who had no evidence of disease at second-look operation had been treated with melphalan. The most significant factors associated with negative second-look operations were the stage of disease, the amount of residual tumor remaining from the initial operation, and the number of chemotherapy treatments prior to the second-look operation. Survival rates after a positive second-look operation were related directly to the size of the tumor mass present at the time of operation and the amount of tumor remaining at the second-look operation. Those patients with positive second-look operations had a poorer survival rate when treated with radiotherapy than those treated with chemotherapy. Patients who received 12 or more cycles of chemotherapy had the best prognosis for survival.

▶ [This report from the M. D. Anderson Hospital and Tumor Institute represents a very large series of second-look operations after chemotherapy of ovarian cancer. More than half of the patients had had stage III disease originally, and single-agent therapy with melphalan was used in 87% of cases. The findings at second-look operation correlated closely with prognosis—with 5-year survival rates of 72% in those without evidence of disease, 38% in those with microscopic tumor, and 15% in those with macroscopic tumor. The principal advantage of the second-look operation is that it permits chemotherapy to be discontinued in those without evidence of disease. Less clear is whether a change in therapy benefits those with remaining tumor. Until some sensitive and specific technique of assessing tumor activity is developed, there will be a distinct place for second-look operation. For a nonoperative approach to monitoring ovarian cancer, read on.] ◀

12–35 **Early Primary Diagnosis of Ovarian Cancer and Detection of Recurrence by Serum Cystine Aminopeptidase Assay.** The absence of a method for the early diagnosis of ovarian cancer had led to numerous attempts to identify and quantify tumor-specific substances in blood, urine, or homogenized specimens of tumor tissue. Dimitre Kalinkov and Rudolph Buchholz (Univ. of Marburg, West Germany) measured serum cystine aminopeptidase (CAP) activity in 20 normal, nonpregnant women and 14 patients with fibromas of the uterus, 2 patients with ovarian sarcomas, and 27 patients with primary epithelial ovarian cancer or a recurrence.

Mean CAP activity values were 25 in normal patients, 25.5 in those with ovarian sarcomas, and 38 in patients with fibromas of the uterus (table). In the 27 patients with ovarian adenoneoplasm or recurrence, CAP activity corresponded to the size of the tumor mass (table). The highest mean CAP activity was observed in patients with a primary, untreated epithelial cancer of the ovary with diffuse peritoneal carcinosis. The relationship between CAP activity and tumor mass can be expressed as the function: $y = 4.5x + 36$, where y is the mean CAP activity and x is the mean tumor diameter in centimeters. Total hysterectomy plus bilateral adnexectomy in 11 of 13 patients with primary tumors resulted in a decrease in mean CAP activity from a pre-

---

(12–35) Am. J. Obstet. Gynecol. 138:1148–1150, Dec. 15, 1980.

CYSTINE AMINOPEPTIDASE ACTIVITY IN HEALTHY, NONPREGNANT PATIENTS, PATIENTS WITH FIBROMA OF THE UTERUS, AND PATIENTS WITH OVARIAN ADENOPLASM OR RELAPSE

	N	Mean value	Range	Standard deviation
Normal nonpregnant patients	20	25	10-41	11
Patients with fibromas of uterus	14	38	21-54	12
Patients with ovarian adenoneoplasm or relapse:				
Tumor mass				
3 cm	1	49	—	—
6 cm	4	62	47-78	12
Diffuse relapses	5	92	69-123	20
Diffuse primary tumors	12	108	73-155	24

operative mean value of 102 to 58 at 5 days postoperatively, to 37 after 10 days, and to 31 after 3 months. The other 2 patients with primary tumors and 14 patients with recurrent tumors received cytostatic treatment, which resulted in a 20% to 30% decrease in CAP activity from initial values in 12 of the 16; the other 4 patients showed a further increase in mean CAP activity.

It is concluded that assay of serum CAP activity is a quick and easily performed procedure that allows for qualitative and, in some cases, quantitative assessment of ovarian adenocarcinoma in nonpregnant women and may prove to be valuable in the follow-up of patients with ovarian cancer.

▶ [These preliminary results of serum cystine aminopeptidase levels in ovarian cancer are exciting. The correlation between serum level and presence and amount of tumor seems quite close. There appears to be a "gray zone" around 40 that might limit the usefulness of the test in early detection, but the possibilities of using a method such as this in following patients are obvious.] ◀

12–36 **Residual Trophoblastic Disease in Association With Partial Hydatidiform Mole.** A. E. Szulman, Ho-Kei Ma, L. C. Wong, and C. Hsu (Univ. of Hong Kong) reviewed the 138 cases of hydatidiform mole seen between 1968 and 1977. Strict morphological criteria were used to study the association of the partial mole syndrome with residual trophoblastic disease.

Of the 138 patients, 125 had classic complete moles. Twenty-one of these had residual trophoblastic disease (9 with metastases). Thirteen patients had partial moles associated with recent or prolonged fetal death, of whom 1 had residual trophoblastic disease (without metastasis), which required chemotherapy. Her lesion subsequently proved to be an invasive (partial) mole, the first example of its kind to be verified pathologically.

Woman, 22, had vaginal bleeding at 25 weeks' gestation. The uterus was only 14 weeks' in size. Urinary human chorionic gonadotropin (hCG) excretions were 30,000 to 50,000 IU per day. Hydatidiform mole was diagnosed and the uterus evacuated by suction curettage. Histologic examination confirmed molar pregnancy, now reassessed as a partial mole with long-standing fetal death. Irregular vaginal bleeding necessitated another curettage 4 weeks later; this yielded decidua only. The 24-hour urinary hCG excretions remained at 200 to 300 IU over the next 8 weeks. Gestational trophoblastic disease was suspected. Pelvic arteriography showed an enlarged uterus consistent with that diagnosis. No metastasis in the lungs, liver, or brain could be shown. Treatment with 15 mg of bleomycin weekly caused the hCG excretion to return to normal after 12 weeks.

Six months after original diagnosis of hydatidiform mole, severe abdominal pain and vaginal bleeding developed. A necrotic mass protruded from the cervical os. Emergency hysterectomy was performed. The mass was found to arise from the body of the uterus and to be an invasive mole of the partial type. It included necrotic but recognizable hyalinized chorionic villi matted together by maternal blood and reaching well below the level of the endomyometrial junction. The trophoblast of the intramyometrial part was virtually all necrotic, most likely as a result of chemotherapy. The trophoblast of the mole projecting into the endometrial cavity, however, was still focally viable and recognizable as typical of the original mole. The endometrium was low and showed no activity except for small islands of residual decidua. The postoperative course was uneventful. Bleomycin was continued for about a month. The patient was well 2 years later.

Many partial moles are probably lost to diagnosis. Products of conception aborted spontaneously or electively should be examined macroscopically for inconspicuous hydatidiform change and microscopi-

(12–36) Obstet. Gynecol. 57:392–394, March 1981.

cally for the presence of a partial mole. If disease is diagnosed, the patient should be followed clinically, with hCG surveillance.

▶ [A report abstracted in the 1979 YEAR BOOK (p. 306) characterized moles as being complete (no traceable embryo-46 XX karyotype) or partial (embryo present-triploid karyotype). The question then was whether or not persistent or metastatic trophoblastic disease followed the evacuation of partial moles. The present article indicates that at least persistent trophoblastic disease can occur in this situation. Therefore, patients with partial moles should be intensively followed after evacuation just as are patients with complete moles.] ◀

12–37 **Pretreatment Curettage: A Predictor of Chemotherapy Response in Gestational Trophoblastic Neoplasia.** Previous study has indicated that favorable responses of gestational trophoblastic neoplasms to chemotherapy are associated with the degree of trophoblastic growth, a plexiform pattern of trophoblastic growth, and fibrinoid deposition at the trophoblast-host tissue interface. Ross S. Berkowitz, Usha Desai, Donald P. Goldstein, Shirley G. Driscoll, Ann R. Marean, and Marilyn R. Bernstein (Boston Hosp. for Women) assessed the pathology of pretreatment endometrial curettings as an indicator of the response to chemotherapy in 37 patients in whom trophoblastic proliferation developed after molar evacuation.

Pretreatment dilatation and curettage did not yield trophoblastic tissue in 20 patients; only 1 of these patients required more than one course of chemotherapy to achieve complete remission (table). Among the other 17 patients, the trophoblastic histologic features were unchanged in 10 and worsened in 7. Multiple courses of chemotherapy were required by 4 of the patients with unchanged histologic features and by 6 of those with worsened findings. Three of the women with worsened histologic features were the only patients with human chorionic gonadotropin titers exceeding 50,000 mIU/ml; the excessive titers may represent a greater tumor burden.

It is concluded that pathologic analysis of trophoblastic tissue provides prognostically important information on the response of trophoblast proliferation to chemotherapy.

▶ [The pathologic findings at pretreatment dilatation and curettage in patients with persistent trophoblastic disease after molar pregnancy are prognostically important, according to this report. With so much attention justifiably placed on human chorionic gonadotropin levels in these patients, the poor pathologist may feel that he or she has

---

PATHOLOGIC FINDINGS AT PRETREATMENT DILATATION AND CURETTAGE AND
ENSUING THERAPEUTIC OUTCOME

Pathologic findings	Total No. of patients	No. of patients requiring > one course of chemotherapy
No trophoblastic tissue	20	1 (5%)
Trophoblastic tissue with unchanged histology	10	4 (40%)
Trophoblastic tissue with worsened histology	7	6 (86%)

(12–37) Gynecol. Oncol. 10:39–43, August 1980.

little to offer. This study suggests that there is a role for both a pretreatment dilatation and curettage and careful pathologic evaluation of the tissue obtained.] ◄

12–38 Isoelectric Heterogeneity of Human Chorionic Gonadotropin: Presence of Choriocarcinoma-Specific Components. Katsumi Yazaki, Chiaki Yazaki, Katsumi Wakabayashi, and Masao Igarashi (Gunma Univ., Maebashi, Japan) carried out comparative clinical studies on the isoelectric heterogeneity of serum human chorionic gonadotropin (hCG) in normal pregnancy and in trophoblastic disease by means of isoelectric focusing (IEF) and radioimmunoassay (RIA). Samples of 1 ml of blood were obtained from 10 healthy women between the 6th and 38th weeks of pregnancy, from 7 patients with intact hydatidiform mole, from 4 patients with intact destructive mole, and from 4 patients with choriocarcinoma who had not yet had chemotherapy. The homologous hCG, hCG-α subunit, and hCG-β subunit RIAs were carried out by the double-antibody method.

The immunoreactive hCG components in the serums of women with normal pregnancy were composed of 7 peaks with isoelectric points of 3.9, 4.1, 4.4, 4.7, 5.0, 5.8, and around 6.7. These components also were observed in the serums of patients with hydatidiform mole and invasive mole. However, in the serums of patients with choriocarcinoma, three additional components with isoelectric points of 3.2, 3.5, and 3.7 were observed in considerable amounts. These three additional components were immunoreactive with anti-hCG and anti-hCG-β. They were all significantly elevated from baseline levels at comparative pHs of patterns of hCG from serums of patients with normal pregnancy and hydatidiform mole. Moreover, the component of pI 3.9 (component A), which was a minor component in normal pregnancy, became a major component in all cases of choriocarcinoma.

In the management of trophoblastic disease, the early detection of choriocarcinoma is important; the assay of the three unique components (T_1, T_2, and T_3) will be useful for this purpose. After administration of combination chemotherapy, T_1, T_2, and T_3 were found in greater amounts than other components in the serum of a patient who responded well to chemotherapy, but the IEF pattern of hCG did not change in the serum of a patient who did not respond to the same combination chemotherapy. Results suggest that detection and quantitation of these three specific components might possibly constitute a new diagnostic procedure for choriocarcinoma. Further research may be needed to confirm this. In the 4 patients studied, these components were distinguished in considerable amounts (T_1, 12%; T_2, 7%; and T_3, 2%). It is also possible that the IEF pattern of hCG in serum may be correlated to responsiveness to chemotherapy.

► [Human chorionic gonadotropin apparently can no longer be considered as a single molecular species. Using "isoelectric focusing," the authors of this article describe three components in blood from 2 patients with choriocarcinoma not seen in samples from normal pregnant patients nor in those from patients with hydatidiform mole or invasive mole. Two patients won't pay the rent, but, if this holds up, the implications concerning the diagnosis of choriocarcinoma are apparent.] ◄

(12–38) Am. J. Obstet. Gynecol. 138:189–194, Sept. 15, 1980.

12–39 **Trophoblastic Disease Monitoring: Evaluation of Pregnancy-Specific β_1-Glycoprotein.** Timothy J. O'Brien, Eva Engvall, J. B. Schlaerth, and C. Paul Morrow (Univ. of Southern California) evaluated pregnancy-specific β_1-glycoprotein (SP_1) as a potential marker protein for monitoring trophoblastic disease in 12 patients. The SP_1 levels were compared with those of human chorionic gonadotropin (hCG). Study patients were divided into four groups for purposes of analysis: (1) postmolar pregnancy with spontaneous titer remission (4 patients); (2) postmolar nonmetastatic trophoblastic disease (3 patients); (3) metastatic choriocarcinoma (3 patients); (4) unusual cases (2 patients). In group 1, 2 patients had relatively low initial levels of hCG and SP_1, with a prompt decrease in both markers after molar evacuation. Levels of hCG before evacuation were higher than those of SP_1 and remained higher during the precipitate drop in both markers within 6 weeks of evacuation. The other 2 patients in this group had higher levels of hCG and SP_1 before evacuation, but both levels decreased rapidly after evacuation. Both patients showed fluctuating low levels of hCG, mostly in the absence of SP_1. In group 2, a plateau and/or rise in levels of both SP_1 and hCG were observed; thus SP_1 correlated closely with hCG as a marker. In 2 of the 3 group 3 patients, a discordant hCG and SP_1 profile were noted; hCG levels dropped at a regular rate during chemotherapy, but a rise in SP_1 occurred during the early phases of therapy. In group 4, 1 patient had a spontaneous remission, and 1 who previously had had choriocarcinoma was found to have low levels of hCG with higher levels of SP_1.

Results point favorably to the usefulness of SP_1 as an additional marker of trophoblastic disease. Possible deficiencies in the use of SP_1 lie directly in the present sensitivity limit of SP_1 assays. In several cases it was observed that low levels of hCG (5–10 mIU/ml) were not accompanied by detectable SP_1. More pertinent to the final evaluation of both markers will be the establishment of accurate background circulating levels. Another aspect of the SP_1-hCG analysis profile can be evaluated by attempting to relate the quantity of glycoprotein secreted to the number or type of trophoblastic cells. If SP_1 is produced by the syncytial trophoblast or the cytotrophoblast, or both, or some invasive predifferentiated form of the syncytial trophoblast, it would have unique value as a monitor of metastatic status. Data in the metastatic choriocarcinoma group indicate that metastasis or invasion of new tissue sites may be accompanied by increased levels of SP_1. Finally, the lack of cross reaction with other proteins and discordant expression, compared to hCG, are unique aspects of SP_1 that make further study worthwhile.

▶ [Pregnancy-specific β_1-glycoprotein (SP_1) measurement may be a useful adjunct in monitoring trophoblastic disease because, as demonstrated by this study, levels generally parallel human chorionic gonadotropin (hCG). The sensitivity of SP_1 is less than that of hCG, so its use as a sole method is not appealing. However, as suggested by 2 cases in this series, SP_1 may in some instances be more reliable in indicating new

(12–39) Am. J. Obstet. Gynecol. 138:313–320, Oct. 1, 1980.

metastatic disease. For its possible use in distinguishing benign from malignant disease, read on.] ◄

12–40 **Circulating Concentrations of Specific Placental Proteins (Human Chorionic Gonadotropin, Pregnancy-Specific β_1-Glycoprotein, and Placental Protein 5) in Untreated Gestational Trophoblastic Tumors.** Human chorionic gonadotropin (hCG) has been used extensively in diagnosis and management of trophoblastic tumors. However, serum levels of hCG do not distinguish between benign and malignant tumors.

Jau N. Lee, Hossam T. Salem, Abdullah T. M. Al-Ani, Tim Chard (St. Bartholomew's Hosp. Med. College, London), Su Cheng Huang, Pei Chuan Ouyang, Pin Yen Wei (Univ. of Taiwan), and Markku Seppälä (Univ. of Helsinki) measured serum levels of hCG, pregnancy-specific β_1-glycoprotein (SP$_1$), and placental protein 5 (PP$_5$) in 14 patients with hydatidiform mole and 9 patients with choriocarcinoma. The final diagnosis in each case was based on the histopathologic findings.

There were no obvious differences in serum hCG levels between patients with hydatidiform mole and those with choriocarcinoma (Fig 12–3). In contrast, all patients with hydatidiform mole had serum SP$_1$ levels greater than 2 mg/L, while all those with choriocarcinoma

Fig 12–3.—Levels of hCG, SP$_1$, and PP$_5$ in untreated gestational trophoblastic tumors. *H,* hydatidiform mole *(open circles); C,* choriocarcinoma *(solid circles).* (Courtesy of Lee, J. N., et al.: Am. J. Obstet. Gynecol. 139:702–704, Mar. 15, 1981.)

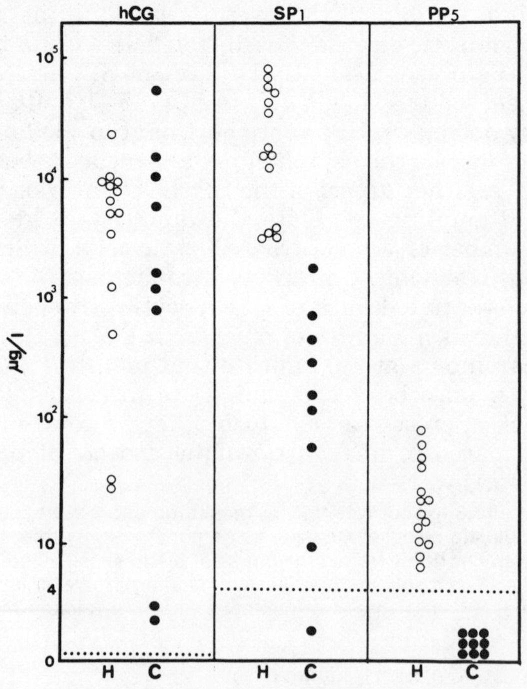

had levels below that value (Fig 12–3). Placental protein 5 was detectable in all patients with hydatidiform mole but not in any patient with choriocarcinoma (Fig 12–3).

The results demonstrate that the serum levels of SP_1 and PP_5, but not hCG, are quite distinct in patients with hydatidiform mole and choriocarcinoma. Measurement of serum SP_1 and PP_5 may provide an early approach to differentiation of benign and malignant trophoblastic disease.

▶ [These results seem to indicate that maternal levels of two of the recently discovered placental proteins (pregnancy-specific β_1-glycoprotein and placental protein 5) differ distinctly in hydatidiform mole and choriocarcinoma. The number of subjects is small (14 moles and 9 choriocarcinomas); if the findings are confirmed in a larger series, these blood tests might permit differentiation between benign and malignant trophoblastic disease.] ◀

12–41 **Pulmonary Resection in the Management of Metastases From Gestational Choriocarcinoma.** Pulmonary metastases occur in about two thirds of patients with choriocarcinoma. Cytotoxic chemotherapy remains the first-line treatment of pulmonary metastasis, but thoracotomy is indicated in certain situations. James D. Sink, Charles B. Hammond, and W. Glenn Young, Jr. (Duke Univ. Med. Center, Durham, N. C.) report data on 5 patients who had thoracotomy for pulmonary metastasis. They were among more than 350 patients treated for gestational choriocarcinoma since 1966. Most patients received additional cytotoxic chemotherapy after the first normal human chorionic gonadotropin (hCG) titer was obtained. All tumor was removed in 3 patients with no other site of active disease; these patients are alive with no evidence of recurrent disease. A patient from whom disease could not be completely excised because of involvement of contiguous structures died of progressive disease, as did a patient with liver metastases at the time of thoracotomy.

Pulmonary metastasis from choriocarcinoma in the form of a discrete nodule may be amenable to surgical removal. The present patients had metastatic lesions and elevated hCG titers resistant to multiple courses of combination chemotherapy. It is important to determine that no other areas of gross disease exist before thoracotomy. Excellent results can be expected from total excision of pulmonary metastases if no other areas of gross disease exist. Chorionic gonadotropin levels should return to normal within 10 days after operation. At least one course of chemotherapy should be given after excision of a metastatic pulmonary nodule, and patients should be followed up indefinitely by hCG assays.

▶ [Of these 5 patients with choriocarcinoma metastatic to the lung unresponsive to chemotherapy, pulmonary resection resulted in apparent cure in 3. Most patients with pulmonary metastases will respond to modern chemotherapy regimens, usually involving multiple agents, but in the occasional patient in whom pulmonary lesions persist and no other disease is apparent, thoracotomy seems to be indicated.] ◀

12–42 **Thyroid Function in Gestational Trophoblastic Neoplasia: Evidence That Thyrotropic Activity of Chorionic Gonadotropin Mediates Thyrotoxicosis of Choriocarcinoma.** Bruce C. Nisula

(12–41) J. Thorac. Cardiovasc. Surg. 81:830–834, June 1981.
(12–42) Am. J. Obstet. Gynecol. 138:77–85, Sept. 1, 1980.

and George S. Taliadouros (Natl. Inst. of Health) investigated thyroid function, human chorionic gonadotropin (hCG) levels, and thyroid-stimulating factors in 20 women referred for chemotherapy of gestational trophoblastic neoplasia. The study was undertaken specifically because of the controversy concerning whether hCG or some other factor accounts for acceleration of thyroid function in patients with metastatic choriocarcinoma. Many study patients had a history of molar pregnancy, but no patient undergoing initial treatment for hydatidiform mole was included.

Serum levels of thyroxine T_4, free T_4, and triiodothyronine (T_3) were normal in 15 patients whose serum hCG level was less than 100 international units (IU) per ml (range, 0.1–95 I/ml) prior to initiation of chemotherapy. The peak level of serum hCG rarely exceeds 100 IU/ml during normal gestation. Increased peripheral thyroid hormone levels were apparent only in those 5 patients whose serum hCG levels exceeded 100 IU/ml. In these 5, the degree of thyroid hyperfunction correlated closely with the serum hCG level; patients with higher levels of hCG had higher levels of serum T_3 and T_4. Signs and symptoms of thyrotoxicosis were apparent only in the 2 patients having the highest serum hCG levels. Both had widely metastatic choriocarcinoma and markedly increased levels of serum T_4 (21.4 and 27.7 µg/100 ml). In the other 3 of the 5 patients whose serum hCG levels exceeded 100 IU/ml, findings suggested euthyroidism. These patients had moderately increased levels of serum T_4 (13–17.1 µg/100 ml) and serum hCG (110–310 IU/ml).

Thyroid-stimulating activity in 27 urine kaolin-acetone concentrates and 18 unextracted serum samples obtained from 16 of the patients with trophoblastic neoplasia was examined using the mouse thyroid bioassay. There was detectable thyroid-stimulating activity in 9 of the urine concentrates and in 4 of the serum samples. The levels of hCG in these 13 specimens exceeded 2,000 IU/ml. No urine concentrate or serum sample which contained less hCG than 2,000 IU/ml had detectable thyroid-stimulating activity. Comparison of the qualitative nature of the thyroid-stimulating factor present in these 13 specimens with that of thyrotropin, long-acting thyroid stimulator, and purified hCG indicated that the biologic characteristics of the factor present in the 13 samples were identical with those of purified hCG. The level of hCG-like thyroid-stimulating activity in the patients' sera and urine correlated closely with the level of hCG in these specimens. No thyroid-stimulating factor other than hCG was apparent. Moreover, when tumors were responding to therapy in 3 patients and thyroid function was normal, no bioassayable thyroid-stimulating factor was detected in urine concentrates, and hCG levels were correspondingly reduced. These results provide evidence that the thyroid-stimulating activity intrinsic to the hCG molecule plays the central pathophysiologic role in choriocarcinoma-associated thyrotoxicosis.

▶ [Trophoblastic neoplasia is often accompanied by laboratory evidence of increased thyroid activity and, on occasion, by clinical hyperthyroidism. The explanation is controversial and depends on the question of whether the trophoblast produces a specific thyrotropic hormone (i.e., human calcitonin) or whether an inherent thyrotropic property of human chorionic gonadotropin (hCG) is involved. The findings of this study are consistent with the latter hypothesis, for there seemed to be quite good correlation between thyroxin and hCG levels, and bioassay studies found the characteristics of the thyroid-stimulating property to be those of purified hCG.] ◄

13. Infections

13–1 **The Course of Untreated Recurrent Genital Herpes Simplex Infection in 27 Women.** Genital herpes simplex infection affects an ever-increasing number of persons in the United States. Women, who are particularly burdened with this infection, may incur an increased risk of cervical cancer and may transmit herpes infection to their off-spring. Mary E. Guinan, Janet MacCalman, Earl R. Kern, James C. Overall, Jr., and Spotswood L. Spruance (Univ. of Utah) studied 27 women with a recurrence of genital herpes.

Seven women also had recurring oral herpes simplex, but none had concomitant oral and genital recurrences. Twenty-three patients usually had prodromal symptoms, which in 19 were itching, tingling, burning, or tenderness at the site of subsequent eruption; 5 described radiating pain consistent with neuralgia. Sixteen had recurrences every 2 months or more frequently, 7 had lesions every 3–6 months, and 3 had them once a year; 8 reported emotional stress, 5 reported menses, and 1 reported physical trauma as precipitating factors for recurrence. In 13 of 19 patients studied, the recurrence began 5–12 days before menses; assuming a random distribution of recurrences throughout 28 days, this was statistically significant. Seven women noted vaginal discharge coincident with the onset of herpes lesions. Twenty-one patients had only one lesion throughout the episode observed. Lesion location included the labia minora (9 patients), labia majora or perineum (5), mons pubis (4), perianal area (3), buttocks (1), and coccyx (1).

Maximum pain (usually mild), lesion size, and maximum viral titers in lesions (mean, $10^{3.2}$ plaque-forming units) occurred within 2 days of onset. Mean duration of virus shedding from lesions was 4.8 ± 2.7 SD days, and mean healing time was 8.0 ± 2.8 days (Fig 13–1); 16% of women shed virus from lesions after 6 days. A vesicle stage was not observed in 6 patients, and an ulcer stage was not seen in 12. Healing times were shorter in those with single lesions than in those with multiple lesions and shorter for lesions in moist skin areas, such as the labia minora, than for lesions on dry areas, such as the mons pubis. Persistence of virus was not associated with the number or size of lesions. Eighteen herpes simplex virus (HSV) isolates typed were all type 2. Cervical or vaginal lesions were not observed, but cervical shedding of HSV was noted in 33% of patients during recurrence. Between recurrences, only 1 of 64 cervical cultures was positive for HSV.

The rarity of internal lesions and the low viral titers in the absence of lesions suggest the risk of HSV transmission through sexual inter-

(13–1) N. Engl. J. Med. 304: 759–763, Mar. 26, 1981.

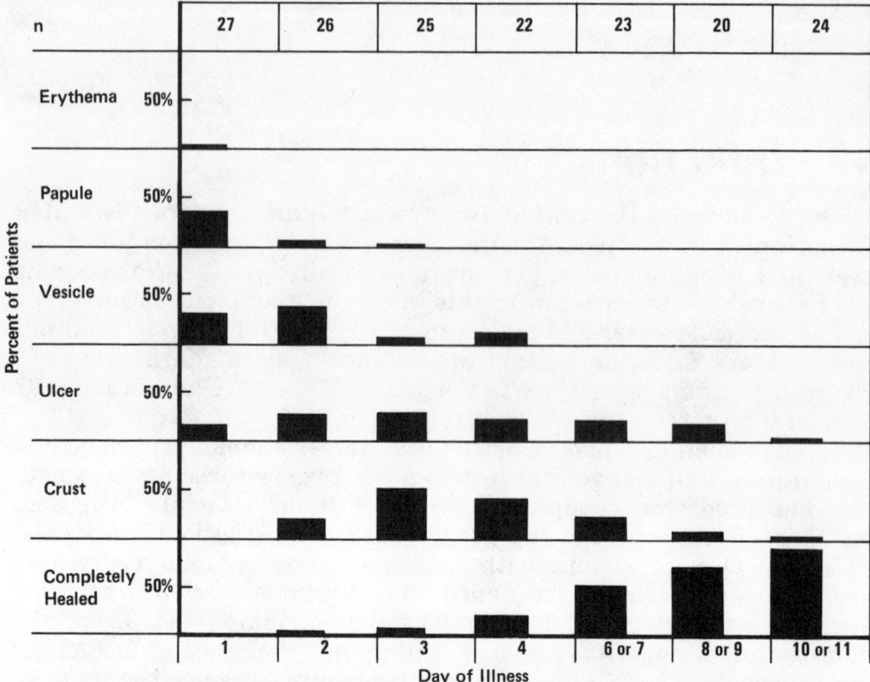

Fig 13–1.—Frequency of appearance of lesion stages during illness in women with recurring genital herpes simplex virus infection. Letter *n* denotes number of patients examined on day or days indicated. (Courtesy of Guinan, M. E., et al.: N. Engl. J. Med. 304:759–763, Mar. 26, 1981.)

course during asymptomatic periods is small. Recurrent genital herpes is sufficiently similar to recurrent oral herpes so that the guidelines developed for topical antiviral therapy of oral herpes may be applied to genital herpes.

▶ [This relatively small, but carefully done, study adds to our knowledge of the natural history of recurrent genital herpes infection. No vaginal or cervical lesions were noted during the acute episodes, but 30% of patients had positive viral cultures from the cervix on day 1. In contrast, only 1 of 64 cervical cultures was positive in the asymptomatic period between recurrences.] ◀

13–2 **Anaerobic Bacteria in Nonspecific Vaginitis.** Previous study has shown an increased prevalence of *Gardnerella (Hemophilus) vaginalis* and an increased concentration of anaerobic bacteria in the vaginal fluid of women with nonspecific vaginitis. To further assess the role of anaerobic bacteria in nonspecific vaginitis, Carol A. Spiegel, Richard Amsel, David Eschenbach, Fritz Schoenknecht, and King K. Holmes (Univ. of Washington, Seattle) quantitatively analyzed anaerobic cultures of vaginal fluid from normal women and women with nonspecific vaginitis before and after metronidazole therapy. Gas-liquid chromatography was used to analyze vaginal fluid for the nonvolatile and volatile organic acid metabolites of the microbial flora present before and after treatment (Fig 13–2).

(13–2) N. Engl. J. Med. 303:601–607, Sept. 11, 1980.

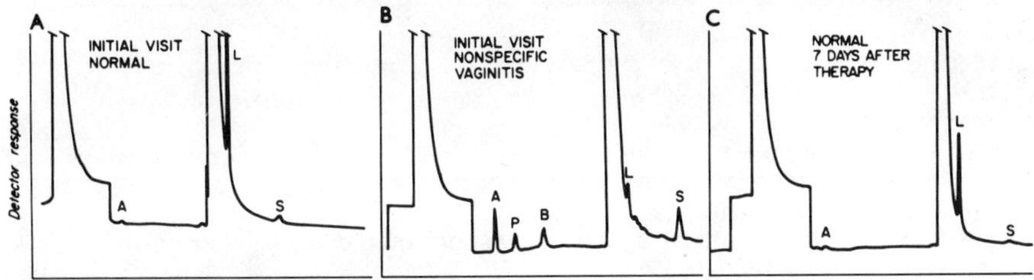

Fig 13–2.—Typical chromatographic pattern of vaginal fluid from a normal patient (**A**) and from a patient with nonspecific vaginitis before (**B**) and after (**C**) therapy with metronidazole. **A,** acetate is the only volatile acid present after the ether solvent peak, and lactate *(L)* and succinate *(S)* in a small amount are the only nonvolatile acids present after the chloroform solvent peak. The ratio of the peak height of succinate to that of lactate (S/L ratio) is 0.02. **B,** acetate peak is increased, proprionate *(P)* and butyrate *(B)* are present, and the lactate peak is decreased and the succinate peak increased, with an S/L ratio of 1.40. **C,** chromatographic pattern is normal after treatment with 500 mg of metronidazole twice a day for 7 days; the patient was clinically normal. (Courtesy of Spiegel, C. A., et al.: N. Engl. J. Med. 303:601–607, Sept. 11, 1980.)

Lactate was the predominant acid and lactobacilli and streptococci were the predominant organisms in normal vaginal fluid. Patients with nonspecific vaginitis showed a decrease in lactate levels and increases in levels of succinate, acetate, butyrate, and propionate. There was also a predominance of *G. vaginalis* and anaerobes, including *Bacteroides* species and *Peptococcus* species, in the vaginal fluid of patients with nonspecific vaginitis. The ratio of succinate to lactate was low in normal women and high in patients with nonspecific vaginitis (table). Treatment with metronidazole resulted in a clearing of the signs and symptoms of nonspecific vaginitis, the disappearance of butyrate and propionate, and the predominance of lactate and lactate-producing organisms.

GAS-LIQUID CHROMATOGRAPHIC ANALYSIS OF NONVOLATILE ORGANIC ACIDS IN VAGINAL FLUID

GROUP	NO. OF PATIENTS	LACTATE	SUCCINATE	PATIENTS WITH S/L ⩾0.4 †
		mean peak height (mm) *		*no. (%)*
College students				
Normal women	60	36 (5–115) *	4 (0–80)	1 (2)
Yeast vaginitis	15	59 (12–123)	9 (0–47)	2 (13)
Nonspecific vaginitis				
Asymptomatic	16	6 (0–29)	14 (0–49)	13 (81)
Symptomatic	6	5 (2–11)	27 (2–45)	6 (100)
Referred patients				
Nonspecific vaginitis, symptomatic	31	20 (1–180)	70 (8–240)	28 (90)
Normal clinical examination 7 days after drug	20	100 (10–224)	2 (0–7)	0

*Numbers in parentheses indicate range.
†S/L denotes ratio of succinate peak height to lactate peak height.

It is concluded that nonspecific vaginitis is caused by the interaction of certain anaerobes with *G. vaginalis* and that the succinate-lactate ratio is useful in the diagnosis of this condition.

▶ [The successful treatment of nonspecific vaginitis with metronidazole, discussed in the 1979 YEAR BOOK (pp. 258–259), makes more sense as a result of this study. It seems that anaerobes, in addition to *Gardnerella vaginalis* (formerly *Hemophilus vaginalis*), are involved. Polymicrobial infections are important in the vagina, just as they are in the upper genital tract. The gas-liquid chromatographic technique of identifying organic acid metabolites produced by the vaginal flora should be useful in studying other forms of vaginitis as well.] ◀

13–3 **A Double-Blind Study of the Value of Treatment With a Single-Dose Tinidazole of Partners to Females With Trichomoniasis.** It has been suggested that the chief reason for failure of tinidazole therapy for vaginal trichomoniasis is the untreated or inadequately treated partner. Jens Lyng and Jan Christensen (Copenhagen) carried out a double-blind study of single-dose tinidazole therapy of the partners of women with trichomoniasis. A total of 149 affected women, diagnosed by culture on Diamond's medium, received a single dose of 2 gm of tinidazole. Their partners received either four 500-mg tinidazole tablets or placebo tablets. The women had follow-up after 1–2 weeks and about 1 month after resuming sexual activity.

A total of 137 women with an average age of 34.9 years returned an average of 9.7 days after treatment. Five had positive cultures, for an overall primary cure rate of 96.4%. The failures received a repeated dose of tinidazole, and their partners were given the same dose; 3 had previously received placebo. Three of 4 patients were culture-negative at the second follow-up. The patient who remained culture-positive had had a conization shortly before initial treatment. A total of 118 women with initially negative cultures had follow-up an average of 60 days after treatment and 38 days after their first post-treatment coitus. The relapse rate was 14.4%. The relapse rate was 23.7% for women whose partners received placebo and 5.1% for those whose partners received tinidazole. Differences in sexual activity were not responsible. Nine of 12 women followed up after retreatment were culture negative. Side effects occurred in 3.7% of women, 7.4% of partners who received tinidazole, and 7.3% of partners who received placebo.

A single oral dose of 2 gm of tinidazole is an effective treatment for women with trichomoniasis. Treatment of their sexual partners is necessary to avoid relapse.

▶ [Most gynecologists probably prescribe simultaneous treatment of the sexual partner of patients with trichomonas vaginitis. This study makes a strong case for such an approach, for the relapse rate at 6 weeks was markedly lessened (23.7% to 5.1%) when the male partner was treated with active drug. The *Physicians' Desk Reference* is permissive, stating, "The decision to treat an asymptomatic male partner . . . for whom no culture has been attempted is an individual one."] ◀

13–4 **Metronidazole for Vaginal Trichomoniasis: Seven-Day Versus Single-Dose Regimens.** W. David Hager, Stuart T. Brown, Stephen

(13–3) Acta Obstet. Gynecol. Scand. 60:199–201, 1981.
(13–4) JAMA 244:1219–1220, Sept. 12, 1980.

J. Kraus, George S. Kleris, Goldie J. Perkins, and Musetta Henderson (Center for Disease Control, Atlanta) undertook a randomized double-blind evaluation of metronidazole therapy for trichomonal vaginitis to compare the efficacy and side effects of the single 2-gm dose and the standard 7-day (250 mg 3 times daily) regimens. The study group included women attending venereal disease clinics who had signs and symptoms of vaginitis and who had motile trichomonads in material obtained from the posterior vaginal fornix. Patients were requested to abstain from coitus and use of alcohol and to return 7–21 days after completing therapy. Patients with negative wet mounts and cultures were classified as cured.

Of 468 infected women who entered the study, 176 (37.6%) returned for reevaluation. Of these, 93 were assigned randomly to the 2-gm dose regimen and 83 to the standard 7-day regimen. There were 73 (79%) women in group A (single dose group) and 72 (87%) in group B (standard dose) who had symptoms of vaginal infection, e.g., discharge, pruritis, and dysuria. The remaining 31 women, examined because of histories of contact with men with gonorrhea or nonspecific urethritis, had abnormal vaginal discharges detected at that time. Eighty (86%) of the 93 women examined 7–21 days after therapy with the 2-gm regimen and 76 (91.6%) of 83 examined after the 7-day regimen were cured. These cure rates were not significantly different. In addition, symptom duration and the occurrence of side effects and yeast infection were not significantly different for the two groups. No significant difference was found in reports of sexual partner treatment with metronidazole between patients who failed treatment, compared with those who were cured. Nausea, vomiting, or both were reported by 22 patients (12%), but only 1 patient receiving the standard regimen had sufficiently severe problems to interrupt therapy. Whereas side effects between the treatment groups did not differ significantly, vertigo and headache were noted only in those taking the single 2-gm dose.

These findings support the single-dose regimen as a safe, effective treatment, but poor follow-up (38%) limits the confidence of this conclusion. More research on the safety and efficacy of this dose is required.

The vaginal pool wet mount is helpful in evaluating vaginitis; the test is rapid, simple, and highly specific, although its sensitivity is related to the number of organisms present. In the present study, the culture was positive in 466 (99.5%) of 468 women having a positive pretreatment wet mount; however, the wet mount was less useful as a test of cure, perhaps because of fewer organisms. Because patients will be more likely to comply with a single dose of medication than with 7 days of treatment, and because this regimen is less expensive, the 2-gm dose schedule is recommended.

▶ [Single-dose therapy was as effective as a standard 7-day metronidazole regimen in this placebo controlled, double-blind study of the treatment of vaginal trichomoniasis. Although there were no statistically significant differences in side effects, nausea and vomiting were more frequently reported by patients assigned to the single-dose regimen. The authors of this report acknowledge the high " lost to follow-up" rate (62%) in the study, which limits interpretation. Nonetheless, the results do suggest this matter should be looked at further; more convenient regimens using less total drug probably will replace the therapeutic plans most of us currently prescribe.

The efficacy of the single 2-gm dose was confirmed by Lossick (*Obstet. Gynecol.* 56:508, 1980). Side effects were reportedly not a problem.] ◄

13–5 **Prepubertal Gonorrhea: A Multidisciplinary Approach.** Over a 4½-year period, Michael K. Farrell, M. Elaine Billmire, Jerilyn A. Shamroy, and Jeanne G. Hammond (Univ. of Cincinnati) studied 43 girls and 3 boys aged 6 months to 11 years with gonorrhea by using a multidisciplinary team including physicians, social workers, and health department representatives.

Thirty-six patients presented because of vaginal or urethral discharge, 2 for alleged sexual assault, and 8 for "extragenital" complaints, including abdominal pain and gait disturbances. A history of exposure to gonorrhea was elicited during the initial emergency room interview in only 7 children. However, 25 of 34 children hospitalized eventually gave a history of exposure (P<.001). Criteria for hospitalization were a positive culture or positive Gram stain. Children often revealed incidents of sexual play or assault through drawings and doll play. Hospitalized children gave a history of exposure 5 times as often, identified twice as many contacts, and kept follow-up appointments 10 times as often as the 12 managed as outpatients. Extensive interviewing and routine culturing of contacts eventually identified the source of gonorrhea in 38 children (83%)—including 31 of those hospitalized. The primary contacts of 6 children were identified by routine culturing in the absence of a history. Gonorrhea was definitely acquired via some form of sexual contact by 63% of patients. Male contacts, both adult and preadolescent, were implicated as the source of gonorrhea almost twice as often as the child's mother. One half of all mothers and one third of all female siblings with gonorrhea had an infected male contact identified. Of 19 children who were sexual assault victims, only 4 had a hymenal orifice larger than 1 fingerbreadth. All alleged assailants were relatives or friends known to the child.

A Gram stain and culture for gonorrhea should be done in all children presenting with vaginal or urethral discharge, regardless of history. Hospitalization of children with suspected gonorrhea greatly facilitates contact identification. Prior to the discharge of a child from the hospital, the team must feel that he or she will be safe in returning home.

► [The authors make a good case for hospitalization of the prepubertal child with gonorrhea. In this protective environment, an accurate history of sexual contact is more likely to be elicited. It is sad that sexual assault by a male relative or acquaintance was implicated in more than 40% of the patients. Gonorrhea cultures should be done routinely on children presenting with vaginal discharge.] ◄

13–6 **Genital *Chlamydia trachomatis* Infection in Women.** Gunnar Johannisson, Gun-Britt Löwhagen, and Erik Lycke (Univ. of Göteborg, Sweden) examined 585 women who attended two venereal disease clinics for the first time between 1976 and 1978 and who had not received antibiotics during the previous 2 months. The isolation

---

(13–5) Pediatrics 67:151–153, January 1981.
(13–6) Obstet. Gynecol. 56:671–675, December 1980.

rates of *Neisseria gonorrhoeae, Chlamydia trachomatis, Candida albicans,* and *Trichomonas vaginalis* in women with and without genitourinary symptoms, the course of untreated chlamydial infection, the occurrence of chlamydial urethritis, and the response to antibiotic treatment were studied. Of the 585 women, 72% were younger than 25 years old.

Of 308 women with genitourinary symptoms, 11% showed *N. gonorrhoeae* only, 12% had *C. trachomatis* only, 15% had *C. albicans* only, 7% had *T. vaginalis* only, 19% had *C. trachomatis* combined with another organism, and 36% had none of the 4 organisms for which they were examined. Thus, *C. trachomatis,* observed in about a third of women with genitourinary symptoms, occurred as frequently as gonococcal infections.

Of 215 asymptomatic women examined because their partners had recently contracted a venereal infection, 27% had *N. gonorrhoeae* only, 13% had *C. trachomatis* only, 7% had *C. albicans* or *T. vaginalis* only, 12% had *C. trachomatis* and another organism, and 41% had no organisms.

Of 62 women with genital warts or recurrent herpes simplex virus infections, or who believed they had contracted a venereal disease, 8% had *N. gonorrhoeae* only, 8% had *C. trachomatis* only, 15% had *C. albicans* only, 2% had *T. vaginalis* only, 3% had *C. trachomatis* and another organism, and 65% had no organisms.

Examination of specimens from the cervix and urethra of 221 women with either gonococcal or chlamydial infection showed that whereas most gonococcal infections involved both the cervix and the urethra, chlamydial infections were restricted to one site or the other in 76% of patients.

Fifty-nine women with untreated chlamydial infections were observed a second time before antibiotics were administered. Of those observed after 2 to 4 weeks, about 50% had cultures still positive for *Chlamydia,* but of those observed after a 5 to 8-week interval, only 25% still had positive cultures.

Patients with *C. trachomatis* infection alone were treated with doxycycline (0.2 gm on day 1 and 0.1 gm/day on days 2–10), erythromycin (0.5 gm twice daily for 10 days), or a combination of trimethoprim (160 mg twice daily for 10 days) and sulfamethoxazole (800 mg twice daily for 10 days). After treatment with doxycycline, 43% still had symptoms but only 5% still demonstrated chlamydial infection. After treatment with erythromycin or trimethoprim-sulfamethoxazole, 27% had symptoms and 8% still had cultures positive for *Chlamydia.*

A third of women attending venereal disease clinics have chlamydial infection, an incidence about the same as that of gonorrhea. No support is found for the view that gonococcal infection facilitates colonization by chlamydia. If samples of urethral secretions are not obtained, 15% of chlamydial infections will be undetected. Chlamydiae may cause urinary infection. Untreated chlamydial infection may regress spontaneously. In view of reports of severe sequelae to chlamydial infection, active therapy with antibiotics is mandatory in women with such infections. Tetracyclines are considered the drugs of choice, but erythromycin or trimethoprim-sulfamethoxazole may also give satisfactory results.

▶ [This paper reports a large experience with chlamydial infections of the lower genital tract. Roughly one third of the patients attending a venereal disease clinic in Sweden had *C. trachomatis* isolated, an incidence similar to that for gonorrhea. The importance of urethral cultures in isolating chlamydial organisms is emphasized. Untreated chlamydial infections persist in about half of the cases and regress spontaneously in the other half. Treatment with doxycycline, erythromycin, or trimethoprim-sulfamethoxazole was effective.] ◀

13–7   **Toxic Shock Syndrome, A Newly Recognized Disease Entity: Report of 11 Cases.** Only recently has toxic shock syndrome been recognized as a disease entity. Ursula G. McKenna, J. Allen Meadows III, Nelson S. Brewer, Walter R. Wilson, and Jean Perrault (Mayo Clinic) report the clinical features and laboratory findings in 11 female patients with toxic shock syndrome seen at the Mayo Clinic since August 1975. The patients ranged in age from 13 to 43 years, with a median of 17 years; only 3 patients were 21 years of age or older. Four patients had 1 episode of toxic shock syndrome, 6 had 2 episodes, and 1 had 3 episodes. One patient died. All of the cases met the criteria for toxic shock syndrome (table.)

The syndrome was often life-threatening, developed shortly before or after the onset of menstruation, and was characterized by transient prodromal illness involving high fever, vomiting, diarrhea, conjunctivitis, headache, irritability, sore throat, myalgias, abdominal tenderness, and erythematous rash. The syndrome can progress to include hypotension or prolonged refractory shock, adult respiratory distress syndrome, diffuse intravascular coagulation with severe thrombocytopenia, and kidney failure. Pancreatitis developed in 2 patients, which may suggest an explanation for the persistent, generalized abdominal tenderness observed throughout the course of the illness and the intercurrent hypotension, hypocalcemia, and hyperglycemia. Pronounced desquamation and peeling of the skin occurred during convalescence. Numerous laboratory abnormalities were observed, including normocytic, normochromic anemia, hypokalemia, abnormal liver function tests, elevated creatine kinase levels, and metabolic acidoses. *Staphylococcus aureus* was isolated from the conjunctiva, throat, hard palate, nares, vagina, cervix, or stool in 5 of 11 patients. Vaginal or cervical cultures performed in 6 patients were

---

CRITERIA FOR TOXIC SHOCK SYNDROME*

All five of the following:
1. Hypotension (blood pressure <90 mm Hg)
2. Fever (≥38.9°C)
3. Erythematous rash followed by desquamation
4. Involvement of at least four organ systems
5. Reasonable evidence for absence of other well-known causes

*Note that these criteria have been modified slightly from those currently formulated by the Center for Disease Control.

(13–7) Mayo Clin. Proc. 55:663–672, November 1980.

positive for *S. aureus* in 4. A recently identified pyrogenic staphylococcal exotoxin was found in the isolates of 3 patients, though its etiologic significance remains unknown. Therapy consists mainly of supportive measures. Antistaphylococcal therapy did not appear to influence the course or outcome of the illness.

All of the patients in this series used tampons of various manufacture, although the role of vaginal tampons, if any, in the pathogenesis of toxic shock syndrome remains to be demonstrated.

▶ [No medical condition in recent times has received as much notoriety as has the toxic shock syndrome. This report of 11 cases from the Mayo Clinic is the largest series reported to date from a single institution, and it details the clinical and laboratory features.

These cases of toxic shock syndrome associated with tampon usage were reported by Watsky and Iannini (*Conn. Med.* 44:776, 1980). Vaginal cultures consistently grew *Staphylococcus aureus*. A similar association with *S. aureus* was made in a much larger series by Shareds and associates (*N. Engl. J. Med.* 303:1436–1442, 1980.)] ◀

13-8 **Pelvic Inflammatory Disease and the Intrauterine Device: Findings in a Large Cohort Study.** M. P. Vessey, D. Yeates, Rosemary Flavel, and Klim McPherson (Oxford) investigated the incidence of pelvic inflammatory disease among parous women in the Oxford-Family Planning Association contraceptive study.

Hospital admission rates for "acute definite" disease were 1.51/1,000 woman-years among those currently using an intrauterine device (IUD) and 0.14/1,000 woman-years among those using other birth control methods (age-standardized relative risk, 10.5 to 1 with 95% confidence limits of 5.4 to 1 and 32 to 1). There was also a suggestion that the risk might be slightly raised in ex-users. However, hospital admission for "chronic definite" disease was more common in ex-users of an IUD than in current users (table), women with "other" disease had no confirmatory evidence, and may have had noninflammatory pelvic or abdominal disorders. No disease category showed a strong relation to age, though rates declined in women older than age 40. Acute definite disease occurred somewhat more frequently in early months of IUD use than in later months, though a steady downward trend in incidence was interrupted by a high rate in those using an IUD for more than 6 years. While the rate of such disease was

INCIDENCE RATES PER 1,000 WOMAN-YEARS OF OBSERVATION FOR THE THREE CATEGORIES OF PELVIC INFLAMMATORY DISEASE (PID) IN RELATION TO IUD USE*

	Woman-years of observation	PID category		
		Acute definite	Chronic definite	Other
Current users of an IUD	20 482	1·51 (31)	0·54 (11)	0·54 (11)
Ex-users of an IUD	4 210	0·48 (2)	0·95 (4)	0·48 (2)
Non-users of an IUD	65 259	0·14 (9)	0·23 (15)	0·25 (16)

*Numbers in parentheses indicate number of patients with PID.
Note: current user vs. nonusers: acute definite $\chi^2_{(1)}$ = 60.27, $P < .001$; chronic definite $\chi^2_{(1)}$ = 3.89, $P = .05$; other, not significant. Ex-users vs. nonusers: acute definite, not significant; chronic definite $\chi^2_{(1)}$ = 5.11, $P < .05$; other, not significant.

(13–8) Br. Med. J. 282:855–857, Mar. 14, 1981.

increased in users of each type of device, the highest rate (8.1/1,000 woman-years) was observed in Dalkon shield users, but this rate was based on only 3 affected women. Chronic definite disease showed little relation to duration of use, but numbers were very small.

Since the "control" group consisted largely of women using the pill and diaphragm for contraception, and there is evidence that these methods may reduce the risk of pelvic inflammatory disease (compared with no method), this may in part explain the high relative risk of acute definite disease observed in current IUD users as compared with nonusers. Another possible reason for the high relative risk in this study were the stringent criteria applied in allocating cases to the acute definite disease category. Women in this study represented a selected group with a more positive attitude to health than average: at the time of the study, the participants were at least 25 years old, married, and had no known history of pelvic inflammatory disease; all these factors probably contributed to the generally low rate of disease and to the fact that little relation was observed between risk of disease and age or social class. The relative risk of acute pelvic inflammatory disease associated with IUD use has been found to be much higher in nulliparous than in parous women (Westrom et al. *Lancet*, 1976); the present study leaves little doubt of a substantially increased risk in parous women. The progressive decline in acute definite pelvic disease rates may reflect selective IUD discontinuation by women at risk. The possibility of an association between the apparent increase in acute definite disease risk in women using an IUD for more than 6 years and IUD replacement cannot be excluded.

▶ [This paper is representative of a number in the recent literature that strongly suggest a relationship between IUD usage and pelvic inflammatory disease. Acute infections were found significantly more frequently in users than in either ex-users or nonusers, whereas chronic disease occurred more often in ex-users than in the other two groups. The overall risk of acute pelvic inflammatory disease seemed to be increased about tenfold with the IUD, assuming that users and nonusers are otherwise similar.] ◀

13–9   ***Chlamydia Trachomatis* in Acute Salpingitis.** Classically, acute salpingitis has been divided into gonococcal and nongonococcal forms, based on recovery or nonrecovery of *Neisseria gonorrhoeae* from the lower genital tract. Recently, however, the most common cause of sexually transmitted diseases in many western societies has been *Chlamydia trachomatis*. Jorma Paavonen (Univ. Central Hosp., Helsinki) assessed the extent of chlamydial involvement in acute salpingitis in a prospective study of 228 women hospitalized with the disorder. Abscess formation was present in 86 cases.

Lower genital tract cultures for *C. trachomatis* and *N. gonorrhoeae* were positive in 69 and 60 patients, respectively (table). Seventeen patients had cultures positive for both microorganisms. Antichlamydial IgG antibody titers equal to or greater than 512 were found in 56 patients. The mean antibody titer was 264 in serums from patients with cultures positive for *C. trachomatis,* but only 49 in patients with negative cultures. In 167 patients with paired serums, marked

---

(13–9) Am. J. Obstet. Gynecol. 138:957–959, Dec. 1, 1980.

RESULTS OF CULTURES FOR *C. TRACHOMATIS* AND *N. GONORRHOEAE* FROM LOWER GENITAL TRACT OF 228 PATIENTS WITH ACUTE SALPINGITIS

	Culture for C. trachomatis		
Culture for N. gonorrhoeae	*Positive*	*Negative*	*Total*
Positive	17	43	60
Negative	52	116	168
Total	69	159	228

titer changes were observed in 17 of 54 (32%) with cultures positive for *C. trachomatis* and in 15 of 113 (13%) with negative cultures. Patients with abscess formation had a higher mean antichlamydial antibody titer (192) than those without pelvic mass (53), as well as a longer mean duration of symptoms. However, there was no correlation between a positive culture for *C. trachomatis* and abscess formation.

The results indicate that *C. trachomatis* is a common etiologic agent in acute salpingitis, which underscores the need to treat chlamydial cervicitis before it develops.

▶ [Cultures of the purulent peritoneal exudate in cases of acute salpingitis often indicate infection with several different species of aerobic and anaerobic organisms. *Neisseria gonorrhoeae* usually is recovered from only a minority of these patients. The polymicrobial nature of established pelvic inflammatory disease (PID) is generally accepted (1980 YEAR BOOK pp. 346–348). What remains somewhat controversial is the role of *N. gonorrhoeae* as the initiating agent. Some suggest that the gonococcus is nearly always the primary pathogen that paves the way for secondary infection by a variety of other organisms. Others think that nongonococcal salpingitis as a primary process is common. This latter view is prevalent in Scandinavia, where the number of cases of PID is increasing in the face of a decline in lower genital tract gonorrhea. *Chlamydia trachomatis* is considered by the author of this report to be a common etiologic agent in acute salpingitis. The significant titer changes in one third of tested patients with positive cervical cultures is suggestive. The relative importance of chlamydia versus gonococci in acute salpingitis may vary with the patient population being investigated.] ◀

13–10 ***Chlamydia trachomatis* Infection in Fitz-Hugh–Curtis Syndrome.** Perihepatitis, also known as Fitz-Hugh–Curtis syndrome (FHC), is usually thought to be a complication of gonococcal pelvic inflammatory disease (PID), although evidence of *C. trachomatis* infection in some cases of perihepatitis-peritonitis has been reported. San-Pin Wang, David A. Eschenbach, King K. Holmes, Gael Wager, and J. Thomas Grayston (Univ. of Washington, Seattle) examined 23 women with PID associated with symptoms of pleuritic upper abdominal pain characteristic of FHC, and two matched control groups, one with PID but no FHC, and one with no PID.

A fourfold or greater change in antibody titer to *C. trachomatis* was shown by microimmunofluorescence in 14 of the patients with FHC, and IgG antibody titer of at least 1:1,024 was seen in 13, and IgM antibody was demonstrated in 11. Of the 23 patients with FHC, 20

(13–10) Am. J. Obstet. Gynecol. 138:1034–1038, Dec. 1, 1980.

(87%), including all of the 12 with paired serums obtained at least 6 weeks apart, had serologic evidence of acute *C. trachomatis* infection. *Neisseria gonorrhoeae* was isolated from 7 (30%) of the 23 FHC cases and *C. trachomatis* from 3 of 10.

A larger proportion of patients with FHC had serologic evidence of acute *C. trachomatis* infection than either of the two control groups. Among those with antibody to *C. trachomatis,* the geometric mean antibody titer for the FHC group (1:724) was significantly higher than that for the PID group (1:138) or for the non-PID group (1:103). Therefore, FHC is not solely attributable to infection with *N. gonorrhoeae;* most cases are associated with acute *C. trachomatis* infection.

▶ [The results of this study confirm those in a report abstracted in the 1981 YEAR BOOK (pp. 326–327). No longer should we think of the Fitz-Hugh–Curtis syndrome as indicating *gonococcal* salpingitis exclusively. Indeed, in the present series, 87% of patients had serologic evidence of acute chlamydial infection.

That the Fitz-Hugh–Curtis can indicate gonoccal peritonitis was demonstrated by a case reported by Kornfleld and Worthington (*Am. J. Obstet. Gynecol.* 139:106, 1981).] ◀

13–11 Gonococcal Salpingitis is Less Likely to Recur with *Neisseria gonorrhoeae* of Same Principal Outer Membrane Protein Antigenic Type. T. M. Buchanan, D. A. Eschenbach, J. S. Knapp, and K. K. Holmes (Univ. of Washington, Seattle) hypothesized that if protective immunity were to develop after an episode of gonococcal pelvic inflammatory disease (or salpingitis), salpingitis should recur with organisms bearing antigens that do not react with these immune mechanisms. To test this hypothesis, gonococci from 15 women with gonococcal salpingitis, who experienced 19 subsequent episodes of gonococcal infection, were serotyped for their principal outer membrane protein (protein I) antigens.

Salpingitis recurred in none of 9 cases in which the initial and subsequent infections involved the same protein I serotype, but did recur in 5 of 10 cases in which the initial and subsequent infections involved different protein I types. Therefore, an episode of gonococcal salpingitis apparently produces some immunity to repeated episodes of salpingitis with the same protein I serotype while not necessarily preventing reinfection with the same protein I serotype. The immune response to protein I antigen may thus provide serotype-specific protection against gonococcal salpingitis.

▶ [This preliminary report suggests that a patient with gonococcal salpingitis may develop antibodies against specific gonococcal surface antigens. These antibodies may protect the patient from subsequent salpingitis caused by the same serotype, but not against mucosal colonization (i.e., lower tract gonorrhea). The implications here concerning a vaccine to protect against gonococcal pelvic inflammatory disease are apparent.] ◀

13–12 Microbiology and Pathogenesis of Acute Salpingitis as Determined by Laparoscopy: What is the Appropriate Site to Sample? *Neisseri gonorrhoeae* has been implicated as the cause of acute salpingitis in 33% to 80% of reported cases. However, a variable correlation between cervical and intra-abdominal cultures has been reported for specimens obtained from the peritoneal cavity and fallo-

---

(13–11) Am. J. Obstet. Gynecol. 138:978–980, Dec. 1, 1980.

(13–12) Ibid., pp. 985–989.

pian tube exudate by culdocentesis or laparotomy. Thus, the role of the gonococcus in the etiology and pathogenesis of acute salpingitis is controversial. R. L. Sweet, D. L. Draper, J. Schachter, J. James, W. K. Hadley, and G. F. Brooks (San Francisco) investigated the microbiologic etiology of salpingitis in 39 patients with laparoscopically confirmed acute salpingitis. Culture specimens were obtained from the endocervix, the cul-de-sac (by culdocentesis), and the fallopian tube exudate (by laparoscopy). In 10 patients, laparoscopy in addition to culdocentesis was used to obtain specimens from the cul-de-sac.

Although 49% of the patients had gonococci in the endocervix, the gonococcus could be recovered from the fallopian tube in only 8 (23%) of 35 patients and from the culdocentesis aspirate in 11 (30%). Anaerobic bacteria, of which *Peptostreptococcus* and *Peptococcus* species were the most prevalent, were the most frequently recovered organism from the fallopian tube exudate and were isolated in 10 cases (28.5%). With culdocentesis, anaerobic bacteria were recovered from the aspirate in 53% of the cases. In 10 patients in whom culture specimens were obtained from the cul-de-sac by both laparoscopy and culdocentesis, there was close agreement between fallopian tube exudate and cul-de-sac isolates obtained by laparoscopy (table). However, there was a poor correlation between these results and those for culdocentesis. Fifty percent more isolates were obtained from the culdocentesis aspirate; anaerobic bacteria, *Corynebacterium vaginale,* aerobic streptococci, and *Escherichia coli* were the major contributors. *Chlamydia trachomatis* was not isolated from the fallopian tube exudate or cul-de-sac in any patient, despite abundant serologic evidence of *C. trachomatis* infection. Five of 22 women with paired sera showed a fourfold increase in IgM and IgG titer, which is compatible with acute chlamydial infection.

The results confirm the polymicrobial etiology of acute salpingitis and suggest that gonococci do not necessarily initiate all primary episodes of salpingitis. Since the culdocentesis specimens yielded greater numbers of bacteria common to vaginal flora than did the fallopian tube isolates, vaginal contamination probably occurs with culdocentesis. To better understand the pathogenesis of acute salpin-

MICROBIAL ISOLATES FROM THE FALLOPIAN TUBES, CUL-DE-SAC, AND CULDOCENTESIS ASPIRATE OF ACUTE SALPINGITIS PATIENTS (N = 10)

Organism	Cul-de-sac by laparoscopy	Fallopian tube by laparoscopy	Culdocentesis
Aerobes	9	8	10
Anaerobes	4	6	12
Gonococcus	2	2	3
Ureaplasma urealyticum	2	1	2
Fungi	0	0	1
Chlamydia	0	0	0
Total	17	17	28

gitis, isolates must be obtained from the site of infection, that is, the fallopian tubes.

► [Since pelvic inflammatory disease is polymicrobial, some have advocated culturing the material obtained at culdocentesis in order to get information concerning the organisms involved in a particular patient. The data presented in the table indicate that vaginal contamination of the culdocentesis specimen must occur. While cultures obtained at laparoscopy might be helpful, those obtained at culdocentesis probably are not.] ◄

13–13 **Prospective, Randomized Comparative Study of Clindamycin, Chloramphenicol, and Ticarcillin, Each in Combination With Gentamicin, in Therapy for Intra-abdominal and Female Genital Tract Sepsis.** Mixed infections involving the *Bacteroides fragilis* group have been associated with high mortality rates. Clindamycin and chloramphenicol are, perhaps, the most effective antimicrobial agents known for the treatment of anaerobic infections involving *B. fragilis*, but they have been associated with significant and, on occasion, lethal toxicity. Recently, ticarcillin, a semisynthetic penicillin similar in structure to carbenicillin, has proved effective in the treatment of infections involving anaerobes.

G. K. M. Harding, F. J. Buckwold, A. R. Ronald, T. J. Marrie, S. Brunton, J. C. Koss, M. J. Gurwith, and W. L. Albritton (Winnipeg, Man.) conducted a prospective, randomized study to compare the efficacy and toxicity of clindamycin, chloramphenicol, and ticarcillin in the treatment of serious intra-abdominal and female genital tract infections with mixed aerobic-anaerobic bacteria. Each of the antimicrobial agents was administered in combination with gentamicin sulfate to provide more complete coverage against aerobic bacteria.

Of the 134 patients with intra-abdominal sepsis, 33 (79%) of 42 treated with clindamycin, 43 (81%) of 53 treated with chloramphenicol, and 35 (90%) of 39 treated with ticarcillin were cured. Of the 41 patients with genital tract sepsis, treatment was successful in 16 (94%) of 17 treated with clindamycin, 11 (100%) of 11 treated with chloramphenicol, and 12 (92%) of 13 treated with ticarcillin. The most common side effects were diarrhea in those treated with clindamycin, hematologic suppression in those treated with chloramphenicol, and hypokalemia in patients treated with ticarcillin.

The results indicate that the therapeutic regimens are equally effective in the treatment of intra-abdominal or female genital tract sepsis.

► [The infections included in this comparative study represent very much of a "mixed bag," but these problems should be minimized by the technique of random assignment. The three treatment regimens—ticarcillin (a new semisynthetic penicillin), chloramphenicol, and clindamycin—turn out to be essentially equivalent, as regards their efficacy. Toxicity is greater with chloramphenicol and clindamycin, so perhaps ticarcillin should be the first-time drug for intra-abdominal and genital anaerobic infections.] ◄

13–14 **C-Reactive Protein in Evaluation of Antibiotic Therapy for Pelvic Infection.** C-reactive protein (CRP), an acute-phase reactant not found in normal serum, has been shown previously, by qualitative

(13–13) J. Infect. Dis. 142:384–393, September 1980.
(13–14) J. Reprod. Med. 25:63–66, August 1980.

assay, to differentiate inflammatory from noninflammatory pelvic pathologic features. Neil S. Angerman, Mark I. Evans, William D. Moravec, Gebhard F. B. Schumacher, and Samir N. Hajj (Univ. of Chicago) obtained quantitative measures of serum CRP concomitantly with white blood cell (WBC) count and erythrocyte sedimentation rates (ESR) in patients admitted with the diagnosis of pelvic inflammatory disease (PID), by the standard criteria (increased temperature, WBC count, ESR, and pelvic tenderness with peritonitis). Antibiotic therapy was instituted according to the following criteria: for the first episode of infection, a single agent was used (penicillin); for an acute exacerbation of a chronic process, penicillin and an aminoglycoside were administered. Further antibiotics were added at 36-hour intervals if the temperature did not drop to a persistent value of < 37.5 C, or if the WBC count did not return to normal, or if pelvic tenderness and peritonitis did not improve. Clindamycin or chloramphenicol was the third antibiotic added to the regimen. Blood for quantitative CRP determinations was drawn at 12- to 24-hour intervals, and these results were not known to the treating physician.

Sixteen patients were treated successfully for PID with one antibiotic or with a combination. Half of the patients required 3 days or more of therapy to achieve remission. Five patients with acute PID required one drug only. One patient needed a second drug, and 10 who had a history of previous PID were initially given two-drug therapy. Three of these 10 patients required a third agent to achieve remission. Five of 16 patients had WBC values that decreased to within normal limits before remission was achieved. One of these patients and 3 others required the addition of another antibiotic after initial therapy to bring about clinical remission. In all 4 such patients the CRP values remained elevated, while in 3 of the 4 the WBC count was not helpful (falling more than 25% in 2, increasing 50% in the third, and remaining within normal values in the fourth). The ESR also did not proceed nor follow clinical changes reliably and therefore was of limited value in judging the course of therapy. Since CRP is not found normally in serum, there are no changes within normal limits that may confuse clinical interpretation of patients not showing rapid improvement. In all patients, the value at remission decreased to at least half that at admission. Following initiation of definitive therapy, CRP values fell at least 20% the first day and 40% the second day in 14 of 16 cases. Since percentage changes in CRP values were larger than those in WBC counts, they were therefore easier to interpret.

The successful use of single-agent therapy in most cases also suggests that the use of multiple antibiotics is unnecessary and that CRP levels can indicate when additional antibiotics are appropriate.

▶ [These results suggest that C-reactive protein levels may represent a good method of following the course of acute pelvic inflammatory disease and, in particular, of predicting the need to modify the antibiotic regimen.] ◀

13–15 **Surgical Treatment of Tuberculosis of the Female Genital Tract.** A. M. Sutherland (Glasgow) has made a study of 91 women

(13–15) Br. J. Obstet. Gynaecol. 87:610–612, July 1980.

with proved tuberculosis of the genital tract treated operatively between January 1951 and October 1979. In 77, the operation was performed during antituberculosis drug therapy, after the drug treatment was judged to have failed. The 14 patients diagnosed after the operation had had no drug treatments, but drug therapy was started as soon as possible after surgery. Indications for the operation were pain (40 patients), pelvic masses (36 patients), recurrence of endometrial tuberculosis (10 patients), uterine bleeding (3 patients), and suspicion of endometrial neoplasia (2 patients). Patients were admitted to hospital 1–2 weeks before the operation, which was timed for the middle of the menstrual cycle. Antituberculosis drugs were continued after the operation, usually for a total of 6 months, but for 1 year if activity was found in the tissues removed. Total hysterectomy with removal of both tubes and ovaries by the abdominal route was done in all but 2 patients, in whom pelvic clearance was not technically feasible. The ovaries were invariably unhealthy and adherent to surrounding structures.

The operations were less difficult to perform than had been anticipated, possibly due to the previous administration of antituberculosis drugs. Adhesions were invariably present and usually widespread, but they could be separated easily. Postoperative complications were relatively infrequent. There were 5 wound infections; 5 patients had deep venous thrombosis, and 3 patients required resuture of the vaginal vault because of bleeding. One patient had porphyria, and 1, a chest infection. There were no deaths and no fistula.

The average duration of follow-up was 6 years and 1 month. Late complications were infrequent. They included an upper abdominal adhesion in 1 patient, a pelvic cyst in 1 patient, and abdominal and pericardial tuberculosis 9 years after operation in 1 patient, who required a 2-year course of drug therapy. All 3 patients were well when last seen, as were the remaining 88. In all cases the vaginal vault was healthy.

▶ [Genital tuberculosis is rare in the United States. This large series is instructive concerning its surgical treatment.] ◀

14. Endocrinology

ESTROGEN THERAPY IN THE MENOPAUSE

Stanley J. Birnbaum, M.D.

Professor, Department of Obstetrics and Gynecology, Cornell University Medical College, New York

Introduction

"Never has so much conflicting information been disseminated by so few to confuse so many." This liberal paraphrase of Sir Winston Churchill's statement describes quite aptly the current status of reporting on estrogen replacement therapy for the postmenopausal woman. Each month, specialty journals expose gynecologists to various types of retrospective and prospective analyses of estrogen's benefits and risks, often reaching divergent conclusions.

Not only are the results of these studies in conflict, but iconoclastic statisticians have critically reanalyzed these data and further clouded the issue. Thus, the conscientious practitioner is unable to weigh properly the beneficial effects of estrogen in alleviating or preventing menopausal pathology against the risk of iatrogenic estrogen-related disease. The problem is further complicated by consumer pressure reacting to a lay press that by necessity reports incomplete and sensational data on estrogen therapy and has the public vacillating between the desire for perpetual youth and cancerophobia.

Any attempt to build a firm therapeutic edifice on this morass of conflicting data is doomed to failure. The goal of this article is to review the current information concerning the negative and positive aspects of estrogen therapy and to present a plan of therapy that in light of this information will tend to maximize benefits and minimize risks.

The use of any therapeutic modality should be evaluated as quantitatively as possible by considering its risk-benefit ratio. With some drugs, such as antibiotics, the risks are minimal with short-term therapy, whereas the benefits are considerable. With multiple-agent cancer chemotherapy the risks are great, but are still outweighed by the benefits of controlling a life-threatening disease. With estrogen therapy, quantitation of the ratio is not so easy. In the numerator (risks) appear major items such as genital cancer, breast cancer, gallbladder disease, and cardiovascular problems. In the denominator (benefits) appear the possible prevention or control of coronary artery disease, vasomotor symptoms, insomnia, genital atrophy, and osteoporosis.

Benefits, Risks and Uncertainties

BENEFITS

Vasomotor Symptoms

The only beneficial effects of estrogen replacement therapy agreed on by most investigators are those that relate to the early specific hormone deficiency symptoms of menopause. These include hot flashes, sleep disturbances, and vaginal atrophy. The effects of estrogen on the late, or nonspecific, manifestations of the menopause such as psychologic disorders and cardiovascular disease will be considered separately.

The hot flush as a manifestation of so-called vasomotor instability is the specific symptom "par excellence" of the menopause. Some concept of its incidence can be obtained from a Swedish study[1] that indicated that about two thirds of postmenopausal women suffered from this symptom through the sixth decade, after which the incidence fell to about 30%. The etiology of the vasomotor flush is still not clear, because not all women with low levels of estrogen develop this symptom and the administration of estrogen does not always ameliorate it. Recent studies suggest that a central mechanism resulting in the periodic disruption of temperature regulation is responsible for these sudden episodes of perspiration or flushing.[2] These studies point out certain objective findings that correlate beautifully with the subjective event of the "hot flush." There is an elevation of peripheral skin temperature with an increase of perspiration measured as a decrease of skin resistance. In addition, a pulsatile release of LH accompanies the flush and peaks about 13–14 minutes after the onset of skin temperature rise. Of interest is the fact that neither FSH nor estrogen levels correlate with the event.

Because hot flushes occur after hypophysectomy, it is clear that the flush is not due to LH release. The pulsatile release of gonadotropin-releasing hormone (GnRH) from GnRH neurons within the hypothalamus may be responsible. These GnRH neurons are in close proximity to the thermoregulating center in the preoptic anterior hypothalmus and may somehow manage to activate this center to initiate heat loss. Although hypoestrogenism does not appear to be a direct cause of vasomotor instability, a mechanism of increased hypothalmic activity resulting from a loss of steroid hormone feedback can be inferred on clinical grounds.[3]

With the objective criteria for the measurement of the vasomotor flush available, the value of estrogen in controlling this symptom can be verified readily when compared with a placebo. In general, estrogen replacement therapy almost always gives symptomatic relief to the patient with vasomotor flushes. The relief lasts as long as therapy is continued, but the vasomotor flushes reappear promptly in most cases when therapy is discontinued.

In addition to estrogen, other agents have been shown to be effective in treating the vasomotor flush. Thus, progestational agents like medroxyprogesterone acetate[4] and an α-adrenergic agonist-antagonist, clonidine,[5] have been found to be of significant value in the relief of this symptom.

Sleep Disturbance

The second problem clearly related to estrogen deprivation and relieved by estrogen replacement is sleep disturbance. Thompson and Oswald noted that estrogen therapy produced an objective decrease in sleep disturbances in menopausal women.[6] The beneficial effects of estrogen on sleep patterns include decreases of sleep latency, insomnia, and wakefulness episodes along with increases of sleep duration and rapid eye movement sleep.[7] More recently, a close temporal relationship was observed between the occurrence of menopausal hot flushes and waking episodes.[8] Skin temperature and resistance were used as objective markers of hot flushes. In this study, estrogen administration resulted in significant improvement of both the flushes and sleep disturbance, suggesting that at least part of the beneficial effect of estrogen on sleep disturbances in older women is the result of the diminution of hot flushes.

Genital Atrophy

The prevalent notion among women and some physicians that estrogen deficiency is synonymous with aging is difficult to quantitate at this time. The aging process is obviously multifactorial, and the role of estrogen in slowing or modifying this process is probably minimal and indirect.[9]

Because the genital tract is the primary target area for estrogen, it is here that estrogen deprivation should be related most directly to aging and here that estrogen replacement should have a maximal effect. There is no question that a significant minority of postmenopausal women develop symptomatic vulvar and vaginal atrophy that may be progressive. These patients may complain of vaginal dryness and itching. Occasionally, a foul discharge is present, particularly if there is secondary infection. If the patient is sexually active, dyspareunia is a prominent complaint. The administration of estrogen may dramatically reduce the symptoms associated with atrophic vaginitis in a short time.[10] It is important to remember in this context that vaginal administration of estrogen is probably effective in treating vaginal atrophy because of the rapid absorption of estrogen through the vaginal wall directly into the circulation.[11] Thus, the undesirable effects of estrogen are not avoided and the same contraindications to estrogen use should apply. In fact, vaginal administration of estriol results in less conjugation than the oral route and renders it even more active.[12] Vaginal administration of estradiol obviates its conversion to estrone and results in a higher estradiol to estrone ratio.[13]

Patients with genital atrophy may also complain of dysuria and the so-called urgency-frequency syndrome. Urologists have documented the fact that urethral mucosa is similar to vaginal mucosa in its response to estrogen deprivation,[14] and the administration of estrogen may correct the dysuria and frequency associated with urethral atrophy after secondary infection has been treated appropriately with antibiotics.

Another anatomical problem often attributed to atrophy of the pelvic supporting structures is uterine descensus and defects of vaginal wall support such as cystocele and rectocele. Unfortunately, there are no well-controlled studies relating estrogen use to the prevention of prolapse. There is evidence, however, that estrogen administration over several months will not alleviate the problem if increased vaginal tone, as measured by the perineometer, is used as the criterion for improvement.[15]

In summary, genital and urethral atrophy as manifested by atrophic vaginitis, dyspareunia, and dysuria does respond to estrogen administration, either parenterally or topically. Defects of vaginal wall support and prolapse do not seem to be altered by estrogen replacement once the anatomical defects are established.

Osteoporosis

Perhaps the greatest benefit of prolonged estrogen replacement therapy is the prevention or reversal of postmenopausal osteoporosis. That this problem is significant and overshadows all other aspects of estrogen replacement therapy is apparent from the shocking statistic that over 4,000,000 older Americans are affected by it. Furthermore, spinal compression fractures associated with osteoporosis afflict 25% of white women over age 60. In addition, 20% of white women will suffer a hip fracture by age 90 and 1 in 6 of these will die within 3 weeks of this injury.[16]

A woman reaching the menopausal age range has approximately 30 more years to live, during which there is a slow but steady loss of bone density of approximately 2.5%/year. This bone loss correlates strongly with the development of clinical fractures. Population surveys in the United States suggest that these fractures are more prevalent in small, fair-skinned women of northern European extraction.

There appears to be little doubt that estrogen deprivation plays a role in the development of osteoporosis in the postmenopausal woman. The biochemical rationale for this role has been studied extensively by Nordin and his associates at Leeds. They have shown a correlation between low androstenedione and estrone values and symptomatic osteoporosis.[17] This represents an expected finding because androstenedione is the substrate produced by the postmenopausal ovary and adrenal gland that is peripherally converted to estrone. In addition, long-term prospective studies of oophorectomized and postmenopausal women demonstrate that exogenous estrogen administration can protect to a great extent against both peripheral and central bone loss and reduce fractures.[18, 19] Furthermore, termination of estrogen therapy is followed by a rapid renewal of bone loss at the same rate as in the untreated patient.[20]

Estrogen is not the only factor necessary for the prevention or reversal of osteoporosis. There appears to be a small but significant resumption of mineral loss even after long-term estrogen therapy that probably reflects an estrogen-independent, age-dependent factor similar to that in aging men. There are also data that indicate that estrogen administration is relatively ineffective if started after bone loss is well established (3 to 5 years after menopause) or is used only a short period of time (less than 5 years).[16, 21]

A high calcium intake ($\pm$ 800 mg of Ca^+ daily) seems to retard postmenopausal bone loss even in the absence of estrogen, particularly if Vitamin D is given to enhance absorption.[22] It is of interest and therapeutic value to realize that smoking and its sequela of obstructive pulmonary disease interfere with this protective action of calcium, as does a high intake of caffeine.[23] A number of other non-hormonal substances have been found to affect bone metabolism and thus may be effective in the management of osteoporosis. Calcitonin prevents excessive or unwanted bone resorption[24] and its plasma level is increased by estrogen administration. This suggests that estrogen's effect on bone is at least partially mediated by calcitonin. Fluoride also has been studied widely in the management of osteoporosis, because it seems to stimulate osteoid formation and form a more stable, less soluble, mineral lattice.[25]

Another important aspect of osteoporosis prevention is exercise. There is invariably some component of disuse in osteoporotic patients. Women in societies where female labor is common or who partake of vigorous physical activity seem to avoid demineralization and fractures regardless of their endocrine status.

In summary, there is little question that estrogen administration can inhibit bone loss and osteoporosis in postmenopausal women if started before the disease is well established and if maintained long enough. Small doses of estrogen can protect young oophorectomized women against bone loss until well past the menopause. Once demineralization has been well established, even continuous estrogen therapy is only partially effective. Fortunately, nutritional factors such as high calcium and vitamin D intake, exercise and general "good health" habits (no smoking, avoidance of caffeine) can successfully minimize bone loss and fractures in the aging woman despite hypoestrogenism.

RISKS

Carcinoma of the Endometrium

The principal component of the numerator (risk) in the risk-benefit ratio for estrogen replacement therapy is the possibility of development of carcinoma of the endometrium. The role of estrogen has been suspected almost from the time of its isolation almost 69 years ago.[26] Clinicians have long been aware, for example, of the relationship between endometrial cancer and estrogen-secreting ovarian tumors and other "unopposed estrogen" disorders such as polycystic ovary syndrome. In the past few years, studies of endogenous estrogen and its role in the genesis of endometrial cancer have strengthened further the concept of a cancer-estrogen link. In postmenopausal women, the dominant plasma estrogen is estrone that is derived from androstenedione by peripheral conversion.[27] This conversion takes place in muscle and adipose tissue[28] and accounts for all of the estrone produced. This estrone is probably the major source of estradiol after the menopause, and both of these estrogens increase in parallel with percent of ideal weight.[29] The rate of peripheral conversion has been measured and is increased in postmenopausal women with adenomatous hyperplasia, a probable precursor of endometrial cancer.[30] This conversion rate also has been correlated with age and obesity, both important predisposing factors in endometrial cancer and, most convincingly, the conversion is elevated significantly in endometrial cancer patients. The chain of events has been summarized by Knab[31] as follows: Apparently, factors such as age and obesity increase the peripheral conversion of androgenic precursors to estrone (and ultimately to estradiol), creating a hormonal milieu that can lead to endometrial cancer over a long period of time in the patient made susceptible by genetic, immunologic, or other unknown factors.

The relationship between endometrial cancer and exogenous estrogen administration has been more difficult to evaluate. There have been numerous reports published since 1975,[32] often with conflicting results, probably due in part to differences in study design. The epidemiologic evidence has been summarized beautifully by Hulka,[33] who also added her own case-controlled study. In general, the accumulated evidence suggests an increased risk of endometrial cancer with exogenous estrogen therapy after the menopause that is proportional to duration of use and dosage. The factor of duration of estrogen use is the most consistent finding from all studies. Hulka's data indicated a significant increased risk after approximately 3½ years of estrogen intake. The "latency" period (the time interval from first use of estrogen to the diagnosis of cancer) varies from about 3 to 6 years, after which time the increasing risk becomes manifest. After about 10 years the risk remains elevated, but plateaus. An interesting finding is that studies of "recency" (the estrogen-free time between last estrogen use and cancer) demonstrate a drop in cancer risk to the level of nonusers after approximately 2 years. These extraordinarily short recency and latency intervals are suggestive of a promotional rather than a cancer-initiating role for exogenous estrogen.

Clinicians have long had the impression that carcinoma of the endometrium associated with postmenopausal estrogen administration was usually of low grade histologically and in an early clinical stage. This has been documented by Hulka et al.,[34] who found that long duration of estrogen use resulted in a striking increase in stage IAG1 disease without myometrial invasion. The lower or absent increase in risk for the more advanced and virulent tumors may be the result of earlier diagnosis or a biologically less aggressive cancer.

In addition to estrogen administration after the menopause, there are certain constitutional factors that appear to increase the risk of developing carcinoma of the endometrium. These recently have been reviewed singly and in various combinations by Davies and associates.[35] The characteristics usually associated with carcinoma of the endometrium include obesity and tallness, hypertension, diabetes, nulliparity, early menarche and late menopause, menstrual disorders, spontaneous abortion, gallbladder disease, polycystic ovaries, and other primary neoplasms. The evidence is not conclusive for most of these traits, but is most convincing for obesity and late menopause. The risk with polycystic ovary syndrome is also quite substantial, but most of the patients described are younger than age 40 and are not receiving estrogen replacement therapy. The administration of exogenous estrogen to a patient with one of these significant constitutional factors appears to increase the risk of endometrial neoplasm to a level appreciably higher than that due to estrogen alone.

In summary, there is an increasing body of evidence, both laboratory and clinical, linking postmenopausal estrogen use to neoplasia of the endometrium. The risk seems to be proportional to the duration of use and dosage and becomes manifest after a relatively short latent period of from 3 to 6 years. An estrogen-free interval of only 2 years returns the risk to the level of risk for nonusers. Fortunately, the estrogen-cancer link seems to hold only for well-differentiated, clinically early lesions. The prevalence of stage IAG1 lesions is either a tribute to good medical surveillance of these patients or a reflection of the fact that estrogen-promoted tumors are of inherently low virulence.

Gallbladder Disease

It is not possible to discuss a relationship between estrogen administration and gallbladder disease without considering other factors such as age, sex, obesity, and serum cholesterol levels. In general, cholesterol levels are higher in young men than in young women. Because the level in women tends to rise postmenopausally to a level even higher than that in men, it has been theorized that the lack of endogenous estrogen is responsible for this alteration. Unfortunately, results with estrogen replacement therapy are variable and do not consistently bring the cholesterol level down to premenopausal values.[10] Moreover, a recent retrospective study indicates a positive relationship between estrogen consumption and symptomatic cholesterol gallstones.[36] Over three times as many women receiving estrogen developed cholelithiasis as did control women. Although obesity was greater in the estrogen group, the increased incidence of stones was noted at all weight levels.

UNCERTAINTIES

Psychologic Effects

There are a group of symptoms often attributed to estrogen deprivation that relate to the psychologic status of the postmenopausal woman. These have been classified by Utian[9] as nonspecific or psychosociocultural symptoms and include such problems as depression, irritability, and frigidity. Numerous studies have been undertaken to distinguish the effects of estrogen deprivation from those of aging, preexisting psychologic, problems and environmental pressures, but these studies have been flawed by the lack of standardized testing methods and the unavailability of comparable control groups.

Two recent double-blind crossover studies, for example, reached opposite conclusions. One found no difference in psychologic problems in estrogen-treated or placebo-treated groups. The other study showed improvement in several parameters, such as memory, anxiety, and worry, when estrogen was administered.[37] Some of this improvement, however, might have resulted from the feeling of well-being associated with the elimination of vasomotor flushing.

Even studies of performance such as memory interpretation and reaction time give varying results depending on the type of test and the study population. It seems logical that hormone therapy would have little impact on cognitive findings because they are more dependent on learning and motivation.[10]

It is in the treatment of postmenopausal depression, or what was once called "involutional melancholia," that estrogen replacement has been advocated most frequently, yet the scientific evidence for this is not well established. Utian[9] described a highly stimulating "mental tonic" effect of estrogen significantly superior to a placebo in producing a feeling of well-being. Klaiber and his associates[38] also concluded that pharmacologic doses of estrogen seemed to ameliorate endogenous depression in both premenopausal and postmenopausal women. On the other hand, several studies have noted that estrogen therapy had no beneficial effect on depressed or neurotic subjects, but did improve the feelings of nondepressed and unneurotic women as measured by psychologic test scores.[39]

In summary, the beneficial effects of estrogen on the psychologic makeup of the postmenopausal woman are questionable, at best. Whatever improvement does occur may be due to the ability of estrogen to control vasomotor symptoms. There is a suggestion that estrogen may have an uplifting "mental tonic" effect on nondepressed patients, but this has defied verification and quantification because of a lack of proper study techniques.

Cardiovascular Disease

Demographic studies of the ratio of male to female deaths due to coronary artery disease (CAD) and the fact that the incidence of this problem increases in aging women seem to indicate that premenopausal endogenous estrogen exerts a protective influence on women. The ratio of male to female deaths from CAD in white patients at age 40 is 8 to 1. This ratio starts to diminish after age 55, ultimately to become unity after age 80.[40]

Several retrospective studies indicate this protective influence. Parrish and his associates[41] studied autopsy records of women who had been castrated premenopausally and compared them with a control group with intact ovaries. He found more evidence of arteriosclerotic heart disease in those women who had been castrated before age 40 than in controls. Another retrospective study by Johansson's group[42] reached a similar conclusion; in this series, women who were castrated before age 30 had an increased incidence of coronary artery disease through the eighth decade.

In attempts to find some biochemical rationale for the seemingly protective effect of estrogen, extensive studies of serum lipids have been made. Thus, it has been noted that cholesterol and low-density lipoprotein levels are higher in men than in premenopausal women and that these levels tend to increase in postmenopausal women. In addition, the administration of estrogen to postmenopausal women increases the level of high-density lipoprotein, which is associated with a decrease in myocardial infarction,[43] and diminishes the level of low-density lipoprotein.[44]

Unfortunately, there are some serious objections to the attractive theory that estrogen protects against CAD. The premenopausal high male-to-female ratio of CAD is not so striking in nonwhites and actually is close to 1 among the Japanese. The difference tends to disappear in white patients with hypertension or diabetes. Critical statistical analysis also indicates that it is the change in slope of the curve for men, rather than that of the curve for women, that accounts for the postmenopausal falloff of the sex-difference ratio.

Further disappointment results when studies of estrogen replacement therapy are reviewed. For example, the multicenter Coronary Drug Project in 1965 was a prospective, double-blind study of the effectiveness of estrogen in men with previous myocardial infarctions (MIs).[45] Not only was estrogen (in this case, Premarin) not protective, but high doses increased the number of nonfatal MIs, pulmonary emboli, and deaths! Other studies also have failed to demonstrate any association between estrogen therapy and myocardial infarcts in premenopausal and postmenopausal women.[46, 47]

The results of retrospective follow-up studies of estrogen use are even more confusing. Thus, Jick and associates[48] found that the relative risk for MIs was 7.5 when estrogen users aged 39 to 45 years were compared with nonusers. In agreement with this, the Framingham, Massachusetts, study found that estrogen use after the menopause increased the risk of CAD by a factor of 2.[49] On the other hand, Byrd[50] and Hammond[51] both reported a *lower* incidence of heart disease in estrogen users. Apparently, differences in the estrogen and control groups other than estrogen use, such as cigarette smoking, confound these studies and make their conclusions difficult to interpret. It has even been suggested that premenopausal hysterectomy, a common event in most studies of heart disease and estrogen use, predisposes to CAD regardless of ovarian status.[52]

It has been postulated that other cardiovascular diseases besides arteriosclerotic heart disease and MI may be associated with postmenopausal estrogen use. This has been suspected particularly since Vessey and Doll developed the convincing evidence linking oral contraceptives to thromboembolic disease.[53, 54] This relationship, fortunately, did not apply to postmenopausal estrogen use in a recent large collaborative study,[55] although one would have expected an even closer link because of the older age of the women studied.

The association of cerebrovascular accidents with estrogen use that appeared to be highly significant in several recent papers[56, 57] disappears when blood pressure is ruled out as a factor. Hypertension itself appears to be unrelated to estrogen use in this age group—at least at the usual clinical dosage range.[58]

In summary, there does not appear to be any conclusive evidence linking cardiovascular disease to estrogen use initiated in the perimenopause or postmenopause in either a negative or a positive way. There is some suggestion that estrogen replacement may protect against CAD in women surgically deprived of ovarian function years before their natural menopause.

Other Genital Malignancies

There does not appear to be any relationship between estrogen administration and any genital cancer other than carcinoma of the endometrium. The data are scarce for carcinoma of the cervix and vulva, although it is difficult to make even a theoretical case for either of these tumors. The incidence of cancer of the cervix and its precursors peaks before the menopause, whereas cancer of the vulva usually appears late in the menopause on a background of genital atrophy. There are some data, however, on carcinoma of the ovary, particularly the common epithelial tumors. The large Mayo Clinic case-controlled study of ovarian cancer was unable to find any relationship.[59] A similar, but less convincing, study from New York also failed to correlate estrogen use with ovarian cancer.[60] The Third National Cancer Survey also found the incidence of malignancy at all sites except endometrium to be within the expected range.[61]

Carcinoma of the Breast

The effect of exogenous estrogen administration on the breast deserves special consideration, because breast tissue resembles endometrium in that it, too, contains numerous estrogen and progesterone receptors and is thus hormonally dependent. There is also evidence that the absolute incidence of breast cancer in postmenopausal women slowly is increasing in developed countries, and this increase roughly parallels the sales figures for estrogen tablets.[62] Because of these disturbing suggestions, numerous case-controlled studies have been undertaken to clarify the possible association. These studies were summarized recently by Hulka,[33] and, in general, they do not support any increased risk of breast cancer associated with estrogen use. Further support for this conclusion can be drawn from a study by Bland and associates, who could find no shift toward malignant disease in mammographic parenchymal patterns after long-term estrogen therapy.[63]

Despite these reassuring studies, there is some cause for concern. Several retrospective studies have found an increased risk of breast cancer if estrogen therapy was prolonged at a high dosage. To cite two of these, Hoover et al.[64] reported that a dose of more than 0.625 mg of conjugated estrogens administered for over 10 years produced a risk of 2.7 compared with the expected risk projected by the National Cancer Survey. Ross and associates[65] also reported a risk of 1.8, compared with matched controls, if estrogen was used for over 7 years.

In conclusion, there appears to be no correlation between estrogen use and malignant disease of the genital tract other than carcinoma of the endometrium. The incidence of cancer of the breast—the other hormonally dependent tumor—apparently is not affected if the dose of estrogen is kept low and if therapy is not prolonged.

Therapeutic Considerations

When devising a therapeutic plan for estrogen replacement therapy, the physician must balance the assets and liabilities of the regimen. On the positive side of the ledger is strong objective evidence that estrogen can relieve the vasomotor symptoms and sleep disturbances of postmenopausal women. It also relieves the symptoms of genital and urethral atrophy, such as dyspareunia and dysuria. There may be some "mental tonic" effect on the personality of nondepressed patients over and above the relief of vasomotor flushes.

The belief that estrogen protects against coronary artery disease in postmenopausal women, based on theoretical and biochemical grounds, unfortunately is not supported by demographic studies. There is some evidence, however, that it may protect the younger woman prematurely deprived of ovarian function 10 to 20 years before her normal menopause.

The most important potential benefit of estrogen replacement is the prevention or reversal of osteoporosis—a major source of morbidity and mortality in aging women. There is little doubt that bone loss can be minimized if estrogen is started before osteoporosis is well established. Even small doses can protect young women until they are well past the normal menopause. Ultimately, bone loss resumes and normal bone density cannot be reestablished. Fortunately, other factors, such as exercise and high-calcium intake, can effectively inhibit this disease.

On the debit side of the ledger are several important negative features. Symptomatic gallbladder disease is significantly more common in women receiving estrogen replacement. A relationship between estrogen use and thromboembolic disease and cerebrovascular accidents also has been suggested by analogy to oral contraceptive use and on biochemical grounds. Again, this apparently does not apply to the postmenopausal patient when other factors such as hypertension are ruled out.

The most important reason for not initiating estrogen replacement therapy remains its link to carcinoma of the endometrium, particularly the well-differentiated, early lesions. The risk is proportional to duration of use and dosage with a latency of 3 to 6 years. The risk returns to unity after an approximately 2-year drug-free interval. There is a disproportionally large increase in risk when estrogen is administered to a patient with other constitutional predisposing factors, such as obesity and late menopause.

On balance, the risk of developing a potentially lethal disease such as endometrial cancer outweighs the symptomatic benefits of routine long-term estrogen replacement after the menopause. Remember that most of the alleged protective effects of estrogen against cardiovascular disease have not been proved by large clinical studies and the proven protection against bone loss can be at least partially substituted by activity and nutritional changes. Exceptions to this include the young woman deprived of estrogen 10 or more years before her natural menopause. She probably is protected against coronary artery disease and osteoporosis by small doses of estrogen and if this is discontinued at the usual perimenopausal period, there is little, if any, increased risk of uterine malignancy. In the patient who previously has had a hysterectomy, the risk-benefit ratio shifts and favors estrogen replacement after ovarian estrogen production ceases.

Which woman, then, with her uterus in situ in the postmenopausal period should be given estrogen replacement therapy? There are women whose tolerance to estrogen deprivation is exceedingly low. They are unable to pursue their usual life-styles because of debilitating vasomotor flushes, sleep disturbances, and dyspareunia. Other women, such as the small, fair, North European type, seem to be prone to rapidly progressive bone loss with its accompanying bone pain and fractures. These patients are candidates for estrogen replacement, particularly if they are free of other risk factors for endometrial cancer. Certainly, the presence of one or more of these constitutional predisposing factors is a relative contraindication to estrogen, and nonhormonal therapy should be used. Once the decision is made to initiate estrogen therapy, certain principles should be followed. The drug should be titrated down rapidly to the lowest dose that gives relief. The duration of treatment should not exceed $3^1/_2$ years, if possible, because there is a significant increase in risk after this period. If a drug-free interval of approximately 2 years is then achieved, the risk again approaches unity. Unfortunately, there are no data describing the risk of initiating a second course of treatment after this interval, but this type of interruption might be a consideration in long-term therapy. If a patient continues to receive therapy without interruption, it is necessary to sample the endometrium at yearly intervals for the duration of treatment and for at least 2 years after cessation, because the risk plateaus at an excess level after 10 years of latency and falls to normal only after 2 years of abstinence. If adenomatous hyperplasia is found at the time of endometrial biopsy, estrogen should be discontinued immediately and the patient should be given several courses of progestational therapy, such as medroxyprogesterone acetate (Provera), 10 mg daily for 7 days at monthly intervals for 2 or 3 months. The endometrium then should be rechecked; if the adenomatous hyperplasia still persists, hysterectomy is indicated.

Much has been written about the differences in safety of various estrogen preparations, particularly in light of the "estrone hypothesis" of endometrial cancer. Studies of intracellular activity of estrogen tend to dispute these differences.[66] All estrogens are bound to a cytoplasmic binding complex or receptor when they enter the target cell. These receptor complexes act on nuclear DNA and produce the characteristic estrogen effect on that cell. Because all estrogens act by first binding to this cytoplasmic receptor, there theoretically is no biologic difference other than binding ability, which is a function of dose and potency.

One way of comparing the relative potency of various estrogens is to measure the increase in sex hormone-binding globulin. With the use of this technique, 0.625 mg of conjugated estrogen (which is 51% sodium estrone sulfate) is equivalent to 0.01 mg of ethinyl estradiol. Both return sex hormone-binding globulin to premenopausal levels at this dosage. Estriol, which was once thought to be a safe form of estrogen, is now considered to have comparable risks if equivalent potency is used. It is not available in the United States.[10]

There may be some advantage to the vaginal or transdermal route of estrogen administration compared with its oral ingestion. These routes minimize estrogen's effect on the liver, and it is this effect that may initiate gallbladder disease, cardiovascular disease, and hepatic adenomas. They also may allow the use of lower doses to achieve correction of calcium metabolism and vasomotor instability. These routes are currently under evaluation.

In the past, estrogen replacement therapy was usually given continuously or in interrupted 3-week courses with a 1-week abstinence period. Recent studies indicate that the addition of a progestogen to these regimens for at least 10 days each month can reduce the risk of hyperplasia and perhaps carcinoma of the endometrium markedly, although the patient may notice withdrawal bleeding.[67] Progesterone apparently is able to diminish estrogen binding and is also capable of enzymatically decreasing the amount of intracellular estradiol.

Regardless of the therapeutic plan, patients receiving estrogen must have periodic smears and endometrial samplings. It is also important to measure blood pressure and occasionally triglyceride levels to screen out those patients at risk for cardiovascular complications.[29]

In summary, those patients who are candidates for estrogen replacement therapy can be treated with an oral estrogen (such as 0.625 mg of conjugated estrogens or 0.01 mg of ethinyl estradiol) for the first 21 days of each month. A progestational agent (such as 10 mg medroxyprogesterone acetate or 5 mg of norethindrone) is added to the estrogen for the last 7 to 10 days of treatment. If menopausal symptoms persist, the estrogen dose may be increased in small increments, with periodic attempts to return to the lowest dose possible. As long as any bleeding is confined to the withdrawal or abstinence period, routine sampling and follow-up are continued. If there is any departure from this pattern, endometrial sampling and immediate cessation of therapy are indicated.

With this type of therapeutic approach, no patient who is truly in need of estrogen replacement will be denied therapy. Close monitoring and use of a progestational agent will minimize risk. If any of the feared complications do threaten, they should be discovered during their precursor stages. There is then time to discontinue therapy with the hope of a reversion to normal.

REFERENCES

1. Rybo G., Westerberg H.: Symptoms in the postmenopause: A population study. *Acta Obstet. Gynecol. Scand.* (Suppl. 9) 50:25, 1971.
2. Tataryn I.V., Meldrum D.R., Lu K.H., et al.: LH, FSH, and skin temperature during the menopausal hot flush. *J. Clin. Endrocrinol. Metab.* 49:152, 1979.
3. Meldrum D.R., Tataryn I.V., Frumer A.M., et al.: Gonodotropins, estrogens, and adrenal steroids during the menopausal hot flush. *J. Clin. Endrocrinol. Metab.* 50:685, 1980.
4. Albrecht B.H., Schiff I., Tulchinsky D., et al.: Objective evidence that placebo and oral medroxyprogesterone acetate therapy diminish menopausal vasomotor flushes. *Am. J. Obstet. Gynecol.* 139:631–635, 1981.
5. Claydon J.R., Bell J.W., Pollard P.: Menopausal flushing: Double-blind trial of a nonhormonal medication. *Br. Med. J.* 1:409, 1974.
6. Thompson J., Oswald I.: Effect of estrogen on the sleep, mood, and anxiety of menopausal women. *Br. Med. J.* 2:1317, 1977.
7. Schiff I., Regestein O., Tulchinsky D., et al.: Effects of estrogens on sleep and psychologic state of hypogonadal women. *JAMA* 242:2405, 1979.
8. Erlik Y., Tataryn I.V., Meldrum D.R., et al.: Association of waking episodes with menopausal hot flushes. *JAMA* 245:1741, 1981.
9. Utian W.H.: Current status of menopause and postmenopausal estrogen therapy. *Obstet. Gynecol. Surv.* 32:193, 1977.
10. Schiff I., Ryan K.J.: Benefits of estrogen replacement. *Obstet. Gynecol. Surv.* 35:400, 1980.
11. Englund D.E., Johannson E.D.B.: Plasma levels of estrone, estradiol and gonadotropins in postmenopausal women after oral and vaginal admin-

istration of conjugated equine estrogens. *Br. J. Obstet. Gynaecol.* 85:975, 1978.

12. Schiff I., Wentworth B., Koos B., et al.: Effect of estriol administration on hypogonadal women. *Fertil. Steril.* 30:278, 1978.
13. Rigg L.A., Hermann H. and Yen S.S.C.: Absorption of estrogen from vaginal creams, *N. Engl. J. Med.* 298:195, 1978.
14. Smith P.: Age changes in the female urethra. *Br. J. Urol.* 44:667, 1972.
15. Stark M., Adoni A., Milwidsky A., et al.: Can estrogens be useful in treatment of vaginal relaxation in elderly women? *Am. J. Obstet. Gynecol.* 131:585, 1978.
16. Nachtigall L.E., Noditigall R.H., Nachtigall R.D., et al.: Estrogen replacement therapy: I. A 10-year prospective study in the relationship to osteoporosis. *Obstet. Gynecol.* 53:277–281, 1979.
17. Marshall D.H., Crilly R.G. and Nordin B.E.C.: Plasma androstenedione and estrone levels in normal and osteoporotic postmenopausal women. *Br. Med. J.* 2:1177, 1977.
18. Lindsay R., Hart D.M., Aitken J.M., et al.: Long-term prevention of postmenopausal osteoporosis by estrogen. *Lancet* 1:1038–41, 1976.
19. Lindsay R., Hart D.M., Forrest C., Baird C.: Prevention of spinal osteoporosis in oophorectomized women, *Lancet* 2:1151–1154, 1980.
20. Lindsay R., Hart D.M., MacLean A., et al.: Bone response to termination of estrogen treatment. *Lancet* 1:1325–1327, 1978.
21. Hutchinson T.A., Polansky S.M., Feinstein A.P.: Postmenopausal estrogens protect against fractures of hip and distal radius. *Lancet* 2:706, 1979.
22. Horsman A., Gallagher J.C., Simpson M., et al.: Prospective trial of estrogen and calcium in postmenopausal women. *Br. Med. J.* 2:789–792, 1977.
23. Daniell H.W.: Osteoporosis of the slender smoker. *Obstet. Gynecol. Surv.* 31:808, 1976.
24. Stevenson J.C., Hillyard C.J., MacIntyre I., et al.: A physiologic role for calcitonin: Protection of the maternal skeleton. *Lancet* 2:769–70, 1979.
25. Heaney R.P.: Diseases of Bone—The osteoporoses, in Beeson B.P., McDermott W. (eds.): *Cecil Textbook of Medicine.* Philadelphia, W.B. Saunders Co., 1971, vol. II, pp. 1860–1865.
26. Doisy E., Allen E.: An ovarian hormone. *JAMA* 81:819, 1923.
27. Grodin J.M., Siiteri P.K., MacDonald P.C.: Source of estrogen production in postmenopausal women. *J. Clin. Endocrinol. Metab.* 36:207, 1973.
28. Longcope C., Pratt H.J., Schneider S.H., et al.: Aromatization of androgens by muscle and adipose tissue in vivo. *J. Clin. Endocrinol. Metab.* 46:146, 1978.
29. Meldrum D.R.: Weighing benefits and risks of hormone therapy in the menopause. *Contemp. Obstet. Gynecol.* 17:157, 1981.
30. MacDonald P.C., Siiteri P.K.: The relationship between the extraglandular production of estrone and the occurrence of endometrial hyperplasia. *Gynecol. Oncol.* 2:259, 1974.
31. Knab D.R.: Estrogen and endometrial carcinoma. *Obstet. Gynecol. Surv.* 32:267, 1977.
32. Ziel H.K., Finkle W.O.: Increased risk of endometrial carcinoma among users of conjugated estrogens. *N. Engl. J. Med.* 293:1167, 1975.
33. Hulka B.S.: Effect of exogenous estrogen on postmenopausal women: The epidemiologic evidence. *Obstet. Gynecol Surv.* 35:389, 1980.
34. Hulka B.S., Fowler W.C., Kaufman D.G., et al.: Estrogen and endometrial cancer: Cases and two control groups from North Carolina. *Am. J. Obstet. Gynecol.* 137:92, 1980.

35. Davies J.L., Rosenstein N.B., Aretunes C.M.F., et al.: A review of the risk factors for endometrial carcinoma. *Obstet. Gynecol. Surv.* 36:107, 1981.

36. Honore L.H.: Increased incidence of symptomatic cholesterol cholelithiasis in perimenopausal women receiving estrogen replacement therapy. *J. Reprod. Med.* 25:187, 1980.

37. Coope J.: The Management of the Menopause and Postmenopausal Years: Double-Blind Crossover Study of Estrogen Replacement Therapy, in Campbell S. (ed.): *The Management of Menopause and Postmenopausal Years.* Baltimore, Univ. Park Press, 1976, pp. 159–168.

38. Klaiber E.L., Braverman D.M., Vogel W., et al.: Effects of estrogen therapy on plasma MAO activity and EEG driving responses of depressed women. *Am. J. Psychiatry* 128:1492, 1972.

39. Schneider M.A., Brotherton P.L., Hailes J.: The effect of exogenous estrogens on depression in menopausal women. *Med. J. Aust.* 2:162, 1977.

40. Ryan K.J.: Estrogens and atherosclerosis. *Clin. Obstet. Gynecol.* 19:805, 1976.

41. Parrish H.M., Carr C.A., Hall D.G., et al.: Time interval from castration in premenopausal women to development of excessive coronary atherosclerosis. *Am. J. Obstet. Gynecol.* 99:155, 1967.

42. Johansson B.W., Kaij L., Kullander S., et al.: On some late effects of bilateral oophorectomy in the age range 15–30 years. *Acta Obstet. Gynecol. Scand.* 54:449, 1975.

43. Bradley D.D., Wingerd T., Petitti D.B., et al.: Serum high-density-lipoprotein cholesterol in women using oral contraceptives: Estrogens and progesterins. *N. Engl. J. Med.* 299:17, 1978.

44. Tikkanen J.J., Nikkila E.A., Vartiainen E.: National estrogen as an effective treatment for type II hyperlipoproteinemia in postmenopausal women. *Lancet* 2:490, 1978.

45. The coronary drug project research group: The coronary drug project, initial findings leading to modification of its research protocol. *JAMA* 214:1303, 1970.

46. Rosenberg L., Armstrong B., Jick H.: Myocardial infarction and estrogen therapy in postmenopausal women. *N. Engl. J. Med.* 294:1256, 1976.

47. Pfeffer R.I., Whipple G.H., Kurosaki T.T., et al.: Coronary risk and estrogen use in postmenopausal women. *Am. J. Epidemiol.* 107:479, 1978.

48. Jick H., Dinan B., Rothman K.J.: Noncontraceptive estrogens and nonfatal myocardial infarction. *JAMA* 239:1407, 1978.

49. Gordon T., Kannel W.B., Hjortland M.C., et al.: Menopause and coronary heart disease: The Framingham study. *Ann. Intern. Med.* 89:157, 1978.

50. Byrd B.F., Burck J.C., Vaughn W.R.: The impact of long-term estrogen support after hysterectomy: A report of 1,016 cases. *Ann. Surg.* 185:547, 1977.

51. Hammond C.B., Jelovsek F.R., Lee K.L., et al.: Effects of long-term estrogen replacement therapy. I. Metabolic effects. *Am. J. Obstet. Gynecol.* 133:525, 1979.

52. Centerwall B.S.: Premenopausal hysterectomy and cardiovascular disease. *Am. J. Obstet. Gynecol.* 139:58, 1981.

53. Vessey M.P., Doll R.: Investigation of relation between use of oral contraceptives and thromboembolic disease, *Br. Med. J.* 2:199, 1968.

54. Vessey M.P., Doll R.: Investigation of relation between use of oral contraceptives and thromboembolic disease: A further report. *Br. Med. J.* 2:651, 1968.

55. Boston collaborative drug surveillance programs. Boston Univ. Med. Center: Surgically confirmed gallbladder disease, venous thromboembol-

ism and breast tumors in relation to postmenopausal estrogen therapy. *N. Engl. J. Med.*

56. Pfeffer R.I., Van Den Noort S.: Estrogen use and stroke risk in postmenopausal women. *Am. J. Epidemiol.* 103:445, 76.
57. Pfeffer R.I.: Estrogen use, hypertension and stroke in postmenopausal women. *J. Chronic Dis.* 31:389, 1978.
58. Pfeffer R.I., Kurosaki T.T., Charlton S.K.: Estrogen use and blood pressure in later life. *Am. J. Epidemiol.* 110:469, 1979.
59. Annegers, J.F., Strom H., Decker O.G., et al.: Ovarian cancer: Incidence and care-control study. *Cancer* 43:723, 1979.
60. Wynder E.L., Dodo H., Barber H.R.K.: Epidemiology of cancer of the ovary. *Cancer* 23:352, 1969.
61. Hammond C.B., Jelovsek F.R., Lee K.L., et al.: Effects of long-term estrogen replacement therapy: II. Neoplasia. *Am. J. Obstet. Gynecol.* 133:537, 1979.
62. Armstrong B.: Recent trends in breast cancer incidence and mortality in relation to changes in possible risk factors. *Int. J. Cancer* 17:204, 1976.
63. Bland K.I., Buchanan J.B., Weisberg B.F., et al.: The effects of exogenous estrogen replacement therapy of the breast: Breast cancer risk and mammographic parenchymal patterns. *Cancer* 45:3027, 1980.
64. Hoover R., Gray L.A., Cole P., et al.: Menopausal estrogens and breast cancer. *N. Engl. J. Med.* 295:401, 1976.
65. Ross R.K., Paganini A., Gerkins V.R., et al.: A case control study of menopausal estrogen therapy and breast cancer. *JAMA* 243:1635, 1980.
66. Lipsett M.B.: Estrogen use and cancer risk. *JAMA* 237:1112, 1977.
67. Sturdee O.W., Wade-Evans T., Paterson M.E.L., et al.: Relations between bleeding pattern, endometrial histology, and estrogen treatment in menopausal women. *Br. Med. J.* 1:1575, 1978.

14–1 Endogenous Opiates Modulate Pulsatile Luteinizing Hormone Release in Humans. To test the postulate that endogenous opioid peptides may be involved in the neuroendocrine mechanisms controlling the amplitude and frequency of luteinizing hormone (LH) pulses, J. F. Ropert, M. E. Quigley, and S. S. C. Yen (Univ. of California, San Diego, La Jolla) sequentially infused saline and an opioid receptor antagonist, naloxone (1.6 mg/hour), each for 6 hours, in 6 normal cycling women during the luteal phase of the menstrual cycle.

Naloxone infusion induced a significant (P <.01) increase in the frequency of LH pulses and in the amplitude of the first pulse compared with saline controls. The mean percent increment of LH during naloxone infusion was significantly greater than in saline controls by 75 minutes, reached a maximum of 119.5% ± 33% at 105 minutes, and thereafter progressively declined. Although follicle-stimulating hormone (FSH) pulses were not discernible, mean percent FSH increased significantly by 105 minutes of naloxone administration and remained significantly higher for the duration of the study.

The data strongly suggest that endogenous opiates, through an inhibition of hypothalamic luteinizing releasing factor (LRF), participate in the endocrine events leading to the low frequency of episodic LH secretion characteristic of the luteal phase of the human menstrual cycle; the precise mechanism(s) by which endogenous opiates

(14–1) J. Clin. Endocrinol. Metab. 52:583–585, March 1981.

modulate the frequency of LRF-LH pulsatile release must yet be elucidated.

14–2 Endorphins and the Regulation of the Human Menstrual Cycle. The findings that morphine can block ovulation in rats and that female narcotic addicts often have menstrual abnormalities suggest that endorphins (endogenous opiate-like substances) may affect gonadotropin secretion in women. J. Blankstein, F. I. Reyes, J. S. D. Winter, and C. Faiman (Univ. of Manitoba) studied the effects of intravenous administration of 10 mg of naloxone, a specific opiate antagonist, in 10 normal women, 13 women with amenorrhea or hyperprolactinemia or both, and 2 women with putative deficiency of gonadotropin-releasing hormone. In 13 subjects a saline control study also was performed.

In the normal women, naloxone failed to elicit changes in serum gonadotropin concentrations when it was administered during the early follicular phase of the menstrual cycle. However, significant increments of luteinizing hormone (LH) were noted 30 to 165 minutes after naloxone injection during the late follicular phase. Similar LH responses occurred in the amenorrheic and hyperprolactinemic women. There was a tendency toward a concomitant increment in follicle-stimulating hormone concentrations, which reached significance variably 60 to 105 minutes after naloxone injection. The LH response to naloxone in individual subjects showed a significant quadratic (U-shaped) relation to the log basal estradiol concentration. No response to naloxone was found in the 2 women with deficiency of gonadotropin-releasing hormone, despite a brisk response to an exogenous bolus of that hormone.

Central nervous system inhibitory opioid pathways may be involved in the regulation of LH secretion in normal women, and excessive production of endogenous opioids may play a role in the pathophysiologic changes of some amenorrheic conditions.

▶ [That the endorphins (endogenous opioid polypeptides) may be involved in the regulation of the menstrual cycle and in the pathogenesis of amenorrhea in certain patients is suggested by these neat studies utilizing the opiate antagonist naloxone.

In a related study, Grossman and associates (*Clin. Endocrinol.* 14:41, 1981) found that naloxone caused higher levels of LH and an increase in pulsatile LH release in menopausal women and in young adults of both sexes.] ◀

14–3 Pituitary Response to LHRH in Hypothyroid Women. Terrance S. Drake, William F. O'Brien, and Donald R. Tredway (Naval Regional Med. Center, Oakland, Calif.) investigated pituitary function in hypothyroid and euthyroid periods in 6 premenopausal women who had been treated with radioactive iodine for Graves' disease 6–18 months before diagnosis of hypothyroidism and who had basal thyroid-stimulating hormone (TSH) levels greater than 10 μu/ml and a thyroxine level less than 4.5 μg/dl. Pituitary function was evaluated by rapid infusion of 10 μg of luteinizing hormone-releasing hormone (LHRH) every 2 hours for a total of 6 hours. The concentrations of estradiol (E_2), prolactin (PRL), follicle-stimulating hormone (FSH),

(14–2) Clin. Endocrinol. 14:287–294, March 1981.
(14–3) Obstet. Gynecol. 56:488–491, October 1980.

BASAL ENDOCRINE STUDIES FOR 6 PATIENTS DURING THE 2 STUDY PERIODS

Hormone	Hypothyroid	Euthyroid	Significance
Estradiol	183 ± 46 pg/ml	169 ± 44 pg/ml	NS*
Prolactin	14.3 ± 1 ng/ml	12.5 ± 0.5 ng/ml	NS*
FSH	29.4 ± 4 mIU/ml	12.6 ± 3.6 mIU/ml	$P < .01$*
LH	34.9 ± 7.3 mIU/ml	14.4 ± 2.4 mIU/ml	$P < .01$*
Thyroxine	3.5 ± 0.16 mg/dl	9.6 ± 0.24 mg/dl	$P < .01$*
TSH	55.8 ± 16 µU/ml	< 3 µU/ml	$P < .01$*

NS = not significant.
*Paired t test.

and luteinizing hormone (LH) were measured by radioimmunoassay at 30, 15, and 0 minutes before infusion. Samples were obtained for FSH and LH every 30 minutes for the duration of the 6-hour study. After the initial study, when patients were hypothyroid, thyroid replacement was begun. The LHRH test was repeated in 6–8 weeks when patients were euthyroid.

The table compares the basal endocrine studies for the 6 patients during hypothyroid and euthyroid periods. Although there was no significant difference in basal E_2 and PRL levels, basal gonadotropin levels were significantly elevated during the hypothyroid period (P<.01). Expected differences were noted in thyroxine and TSH levels, which confirmed the diagnosis of hypothyroidism.

Pituitary sensitivity was defined as the increase in LH concentration above the baseline 30 minutes after the first LHRH injection. Pituitary reserve was defined as the integrated area under the LH response curve above the baseline for the 6-hour study. In all 6 patients, pituitary sensitivity and reserve correlated significantly with basal E_2 levels (P<.05) but were not altered by hypothyroidism.

The mechanism by which primary hypothyroidism induces increased basal gonadotropin levels is not known. It may be altered estrogen metabolism and/or increased neurotransmitter activity. No major alterations in pituitary responsiveness to LHRH stimulation were apparent in this investigation. Chronic elevation of basal gonadotropin levels may in part explain the anovulation that is seen so frequently in primary hypothyroidism. Three of the 6 subjects reported a change in duration of their menstrual periods and in menstrual flow with hypothyroidism, but none was amenorrheic.

▶ [Although basal levels of gonadotropins were increased in the hypothyroid study subjects, there were no significant alterations in the response of the pituitary to LHRH. The mechanism of increased levels of gonadotropins in hypothyroidism is unclear.] ◀

14-4 **Suppression of Prolactin Secretion in Normal Young Women by 2-Hydroxyestrone.** 2-Hydroxyestrone is a catechol estrogen that is the principal metabolite of estradiol in human beings. It has no apparent uterotropic activity, but it does affect the hypothalamic-pi-

(14–4) Science 210:73–74, Oct. 3, 1980.

tuitary axis, which indicates a dissociation between central and peripheral activities. Prolonged infusion of 2-hydroxyestrone has been shown to suppress serum prolactin levels in estrogen-primed postmenopausal women. J. Fishman (Rockefeller Univ.) and D. Tulchinsky (Harvard Med. School) investigated the effect of intravenous infusion of 2-hydroxyestrone on prolactin secretion in 12 normal, premenopausal women for a total of 16 studies; 80 μg of rigidly purified 2-hydroxyestrone in propylene glycol and saline per hour was infused for 3 hours. Blood samples were obtained at 30, 60, 120, and 180 minutes after infusion was begun.

Infusion of 2-hydroxyestrone caused a rapid and profound suppression of serum prolactin in most subjects. In 8 of the studies, serum prolactin fell to 59%, 26%, and 22% of baseline values at 30, 60, and 120 minutes, respectively. In another 5 studies, serum prolactin also was decreased, but to a lesser extent (50% of maximum).

It is not known whether 2-hydroxyestrone inhibits prolactin secretion at the pituitary or hypothalamic level. It appears that the regulation of prolactin secretion by estrogens is of a dual nature, however, with estradiol acting in a positive feedback mode and 2-hydroxyestrone acting in an inhibitory mode. A better understanding of the mechanism of prolactin secretion inhibition may make it possible to use 2-hydroxyestrone to differentiate between functional hyperprolactinemia and the hyperprolactinemia that results from pituitary tumors.

▶ [Exogenous estrogens increase prolactin levels. This study suggests that the relationship between estrogen and prolactin is not simple. 2-Hydroxyestrone (a catechol estrogen metabolite of estradiol that has central effects, but no effect on the uterus) given to premenopausal women resulted in a decrease in serum prolactin levels. Therefore, agents that affect the activity of the enzyme that converts estradiol to 2-hydroxyestrone may affect prolactin secretion by altering the ratio of stimulator (estradiol) to inhibitor (2-hydroxyestrone). The authors suggest that there may be clinical implications here in the treatment of hyperprolactinemia.] ◀

14-5 **Decreased Bone Density in Hyperprolactinemic Women.** Anne Klibanski, Robert M. Neer, Inese Z. Beitins, E. Chester Ridgway, Nicholas T. Zervas, and Janet W. McArthur (Mass. Genl. Hosp.) studied 14 women aged 20–40 years, who had hyperprolactinemic amenorrhea. Patients with hypopituitarism were excluded. Serum prolactin values ranged from 22 to 99 ng/ml (normal, <15 ng/ml). In all patients, basal serum prolactin concentrations failed to increase by more than 25% after thyrotropin-releasing hormone stimulation. Five patients had surgically confirmed pituitary adenomas, and 1 had a partially empty sella.

All patients had normal levels of serum calcium, inorganic phosphorus, albumin, alkaline phosphatase, parathyroid hormone, and 25-hydroxyvitamin D (25-OHD). There was no correlation between serum 25-OHD concentration and serum prolactin or estradiol values. Estradiol concentrations ranged from undetectable (<20 pg/ml) to 90 pg/ml; 6 women had serum estradiol concentrations <20 pg/ml, and in 8 patients median estradiol values were 59 pg/ml, comparable to

(14–5) N. Engl. J. Med. 303:1511–1514, Dec. 25, 1980.

those occurring in normal women during the follicular phase of the menstrual cycle. Serum estradiol levels did not correlate with duration of amenorrhea or serum prolactin concentrations.

Fourteen hyperprolactinemic patients had a significant reduction in bone density ($P<.001$) when compared with age-matched normal controls. There was a positive correlation between bone density and serum estradiol concentrations. Patients with serum estradiol values above 20 pg/ml had bone densities significantly lower than those of age-matched controls ($P<.05$). Women with undetectable levels of serum estradiol had bone densities strikingly lower than those of age-matched controls ($P<.001$) or of patients with estradiol concentrations above 20 pg/ml ($P<.01$). Also, these women had bone densities lower than those of postmenopausal controls aged 48–69 years ($P<.05$). There was no significant correlation between serum prolactin level and bone density.

Reduced bone density is probably secondary to the estrogen-deficient state that may accompany hyperprolactinemia. It appears unlikely that hyperprolactinemia exerts a direct effect on calcium metabolism or on bone mineral content. Surgical or medical normalization of the serum prolactin value usually restores normal gonadal function in hyperprolactinemic women. Bromocriptine is effective in establishing normal estrogen levels and ovulatory menstrual cycles in most such women. Low bone density and estrogen deficiency in hyperprolactinemic patients may be an indication for medical treatment.

▶ [This study indicates that women with hyperprolactinemia have decreased bone density, compared with that of normoprolactinemic controls. The degree of bone loss correlated inversely with serum estradiol levels, implying that relative estrogen deficiency is the mechanism responsible. Thus, prevention of osteoporosis may be an additional reason for treating hyperprolactinemia.] ◀

14-6 **Partial or Complete Regression of Hyperprolactinemic Amenorrhea-Galactorrhea Syndrome After Bromocriptine-Induced Pregnancy.** G. M. Molinatti, C. Campagnoli, L. Belforte, F. Massara, C. Peris, and N. Pinna (Turin, Italy) used bromocriptine to induce pregnancy in 20 women with hyperprolactinemic amenorrhea and then followed them for 6 to 15 months after delivery. Clinical or biologic variables, or both, were improved in 9 women, unchanged in 7, and made worse in 4.

Of the 9 women whose conditions improved, 6 had minor sellar alterations suggesting the presence of a prolactin-secreting microadenoma, 1 had a normal sella, and 2 had greater sellar abnormalities but had previously undergone surgery and [198]Au intrasellar implantation, respectively, without remission of the syndrome. In these 9 women the mean plasma prolactin concentrations were 116.9 ng/ml before bromocriptine treatment and 51.8 ng/ml after delivery. Ovulatory cycles occurred after delivery in 3 women (2 with sellar findings suggestive of pituitary microadenoma and 1 who had previously undergone intrasellar radiotherapy), and 2 of these had a spontaneous conception 8 to 9 months after the first delivery. In 4 women a few sponta-

(14–6) Panminerva Med. 22:125–130, July-Sept. 1980.

COMPARISON BETWEEN MAIN CLINICAL AND HORMONAL FINDINGS IN PATIENTS WITH PREVIOUS HYPERPROLACTINEMIC AMENORRHEA IMPROVED AFTER BROMOCRIPTINE-INDUCED PREGNANCY AND THOSE OF PATIENTS UNCHANGED OR WORSENED

	Age (years) (Mean±SEM)	Sella turcica* (plain X-rays and tomography)	Previous surgical therapy	PRL (ng/ml) before bromo-criptine therapy (Mean±SEM)	Weeks of medical therapy before conception (Mean±SEM)	Dose of bromo-criptine (mg/day) (Mean±SEM)	PRL (ng/ml) after bromo-criptine-induced pregnancy (Mean±SEM)
Improved 9/20 (45%)	30.3±2.2	++ 2/9 (22.2%) + 6/9 (66.7%) — 1/9 (11.1%)	2/9 (22.2%)	116.9±20.3	31.3±8.0	5.0±0.6	51.8±11.7
Unchanged 7/20 (35%)	29.6±1.7	++ 1/7 (14.3%) + 4/7 (57.1%) — 2/7 (28.6%)	1/7 (14.3%)	161.1±44.1	18.0±5.9	5.5±0.8	146.3±37.3
Worsened 4/20 (20%)	28.7±2.1	+ 3/4 (75%) — 1/4 (25%)	0/4 (0%)	113.0±39.3	28.2±1.4	4.7±0.3	161.0±51.3

*++, Distinct sellar alterations; +, slight sellar alterations; —, normal sella.

neous cycles were followed by the return of amenorrhea; 3 of these cases responded to progestogen. In the other 2 women, amenorrhea persisted after delivery.

There were no substantial clinical or radiologic differences among women whose conditions were improved, unchanged, or worse after bromocriptine-induced pregnancy (table). There were no significant differences in plasma prolactin values before treatment, duration of therapy before conception, or dosage of bromocriptine between women who improved and those who did not. However, basal prolactin concentrations after delivery were significantly lower in women who improved than in those whose condition was unchanged or worsened.

The improvement in the hyperprolactinemic amenorrhea-galactorrhea syndrome that sometimes follows a bromocriptine-induced pregnancy is probably due to regressive events that occur during pregnancy in adenomatous or hyperplastic prolactin-secreting structures. These changes may be due to hemorrhage or blood supply defects, or both, which result from alterations induced by raised estrogen concentrations.

▶ [As experience with bromocriptine treatment rather than surgery grows in patients with prolactin-secreting microadenomas who desire pregnancy, the impression of most investigators is that medical treatment is generally safe (1981 YEAR BOOK, pp. 341–343). In the present series, nearly half of the patients were improved post partum compared with their status prior to pregnancy. The authors speculate that the stimulation of the prolactin-secreting tissue by the high estrogen levels during pregnancy may result in vascularization defects or hemorrhage, leading to regression of the lesion.] ◀

14-7 **Induction of Ovulation in Patients With Normoprolactinemic Amenorrhea by Combined Therapy With Bromocriptine and Clomiphene.** Bromocriptine is known to be effective in treatment of women with hyperprolactinemic anovulation or normoprolactinemic amenorrhea-galactorrhea. Koji Koike, Toshihiro Aono, Akira Miyake, Hirohisa Tsutsumi, Keishi Matsumoto, and Keiichi Kurachi (Osaka Univ.) used a new schedule of combined treatment with bromocriptine and clomiphene citrate in 23 women with normoprolactinemic secondary amenorrhea without galactorrhea who failed to respond to treatment with clomiphene alone (3 treatment courses, 150 mg/day for 5 days). All patients had withdrawal bleeding in response to a single intramuscular injection of 50 mg of progesterone. Patients were treated with bromocriptine, 2.5 mg orally once daily for 2 days, from the second day of menstruation or withdrawal bleeding; 2.5 mg twice daily was given for 12 days. Clomiphene, 50 mg 3 times daily, was administered from day 5 of menstruation or withdrawal bleeding.

Ovulation was restored by treatment in 14 patients (60.9%), resulting in pregnancy in 3. Ovulation usually occurred within 2 weeks, approximately 8 days after the end of clomiphene treatment. Statistical comparison of prolactin, luteinizing hormone (LH), and follicle-stimulating hormone values before treatment revealed no significant difference between responders and nonresponders. Profiles of hormonal change revealed an ovulatory response in 1 woman studied daily and an anovulatory bleeding response in another. Treatment

(14–7) Fertil. Steril. 35:138–141, February 1981.

resulted in immediate suppression of serum prolactin levels (but a transient increase occurred after cessation of treatment) and a gradual increase in serum LH and estradiol levels followed by an LH surge.

Results indicate that bromocriptine-clomiphene combination therapy is effective in treatment of amenorrheic patients with normoprolactinemia who do not respond to treatment with clomiphene alone, and suggest that bromocriptine restores responsiveness of the hypothalamic-pituitary-ovarian system to clomiphene. Pregnancy rate was rather low, due in part to other factors, such as oligospermia in 4 husbands.

▶ [Bromocriptine alone probably is not effective in patients with normoprolactinemic amenorrhea (1980 YEAR BOOK, p. 351). In this study, the combination of bromocriptine and clomiphene successfully induced ovulation in most patients who were refractory to clomiphene alone. The reason for this apparent success is unknown. It may be because "normoprolactinemic" patients may not always be so. Read on.] ◀

14–8 **Rationale for Use of Bromocriptine in Patients With Amenorrhea and Normoprolactinemia.** The return of menses in amenorrheic normoprolactinemic women after treatment with bromocriptine is well documented. Bernard Corenblum and Patrick J. Taylor (Univ. of Calgary) investigated whether an increased pituitary prolactin-secreting capacity may be the underlying mechanism. Fourteen women aged 20–29 years who complained of secondary amenorrhea of 6–22 months' duration were studied. None was taking any medication or had a recent history of pregnancy. There was no history of weight loss or gain greater than 10% of body weight. None complained of galactorrhea, but in all 14 it was possible to express a few drops of milk from the nipple. Basal serum follicle-stimulating hormone and prolactin levels were normal, as were sellar tomograms in all 14 women. Serum luteinizing hormone level was normal in 10 and elevated in 4. Withdrawal bleeding was achieved with medroxyprogesterone acetate, 5 mg twice daily for 5 days. Stimulation of prolactin secretion was produced in the 14 women by means of thyrotropin-releasing hormone (TRH), and 7 patients were stimulated with chlorpromazine (CPZ) as well. The range of normal response to TRH and CPZ was established in 20 normally cycling women studied during the early follicular phase. After testing, all 14 patients were treated for a minimum of 3 months with bromocriptine, 2.5 mg twice daily by mouth.

Nine of the 14 patients had return of ovulatory menses as suggested by biphasic basal body temperature shifts and cyclic withdrawal bleeding associated with characteristic molimina. Of these 9, 7 desired pregnancy; at the time of writing, 5 had conceived. Five women did not experience return of menses. Clinical characteristics of both groups were similar with regard to age, previous parity, and previous oral contraceptive ingestion. The mean prolactin response to TRH was significantly greater in the 9 women who experienced return of menses, although there was individual overlap between the groups. The mean peak prolactin response of the 5 nonresponders to

---

(14–8) Fertil. Steril. 34:239–241, September 1980.

bromocriptine did not differ from that of the normal group. Of the 7 patients who underwent a CPZ test, 6 responders to bromocriptine showed greater stimulation than normal women.

Findings suggest that some amenorrheic patients, although apparently normoprolactinemic, will have enhanced prolactin secretory capacity. The excessive responses to TRH and CPZ suggest that the site of the disorder in these patients may be at the level of the lactotroph or may involve increased hypothalamic serotonergic activity. Results support a rationale for a therapeutic trial of bromocriptine in selected normoprolactinemic patients with amenorrhea and demonstrable galactorrhea.

▶ [This study suggests a mechanism for the finding of some—but by no means all—reports that bromocriptine is successful in treatment of normoprolactinemic amenorrhea. Those women who responded to bromocriptine by return of menstrual function did not differ from nonresponders in basal prolactin levels, but the response to the provocative stimulus of thyrotropin-releasing hormone given intravenously was nearly 3 times as great in responders as in nonresponders. Thus, it appears that some patients are normoprolactinemic in the basal state, but are relatively hyperprolactinemic with provocation.] ◀

14–9 **Galactorrhea-Amenorrhea Syndrome: Follow-up of 45 Patients After Pituitary Tumor Removal.** A prolactin-secreting pituitary adenoma is likely to be present in women with the galactorrhea-amenorrhea syndrome, and tumor removal reduces the serum prolactin level to normal in a high proportion of patients. H. St. George Tucker, Stephen R. Grubb, James P. Wigand, Alain Taylor, Harvey V. Lankford, William G. Blackard, and Donald P. Becker (Med. College of Virginia, Richmond) have followed 45 women for 1–8 years after transsphenoidal surgery for galactorrhea-amenorrhea syndrome and presumed prolactinoma. The mean follow-up time was 3.1 years. Pituitary tumor was confirmed histologically in all but 2 cases. Forty-two tumors were shown to be chromophobe adenomas; 3 were eosinophilic adenomas.

Selective total tumor removal was attempted in all cases. Pituitary function was preserved at the preoperative level in all but 1 patient, a woman with suprasellar extension. One patient who had had prior tumor removal continued to have hypopituitarism. Fifteen patients had transient diabetes insipidus, and 2 had transient sixth nerve palsy. The serum prolactin level fell to normal in 20 of 27 patients with microadenomas and in 6 of 10 with enclosed macroadenomas. Two of 5 patients with locally invasive tumors, but none of 3 with generalized invasion beyond the sella, appeared to be cured. A normal prolactin level 1 week postoperatively was not an indication of cure. Only 6 months after surgery was there a clear separation between patients whose prolactin level would remain normal and those whose levels would remain high. Fifteen patients of 20 who wished to conceive had 19 pregnancies, and all but 2 pregnancies were uneventful.

Higher cure rates are obtained in patients with galactorrhea-amenorrhea syndrome who have lower preoperative serum prolactin levels. Oral contraceptive use was not unusual in the present patient popu-

---

(14–9)   Ann. Intern. Med. 94:302–307, March 1981.

lation. A small proportion of patients with apparent tumor may actually have diffuse lactotropic hyperplasia and hypersecretion. The serum prolactin level 6 months after surgery appears to be a reliable measure of cure. Bromocriptine has not yet been used to allow pregnancy, but its use is safe in postoperative patients from whom a large part of the tumor has been removed.

▶ [Anthony A. Luciano, of the University of Iowa, reviewed this paper at our request and commented as follows:

"The surgical management of patients with prolactin-secreting pituitary adenomas has yielded consistent results from several different institutions. Surgical success, determined by resumption of regular menses and normalization of serum prolactin levels, is achieved in about half of the patients and, as expected, is inversely related to the preoperative serum prolactin concentration, the size of the tumor, or both. This report, in agreement with previous studies, found preoperative pituitary perturbation studies (gonadotropin-releasing hormone, thyrotropin-releasing hormone, insulin tolerance test, etc.) not to be useful in either estimating the extent of these lesions or in predicting the outcome of the surgical therapy. Normalization of prolactin levels by the sixth month after surgery was found to be an accurate predictor of "ultimate cure"; unfortunately, however, this information is of little value to those patients who are not cured by surgery.

"A relationship between the clinical presentation of patients with prolactin-secreting pituitary adenomas and the surgical outcome, which may be useful in predicting patient response, has been suggested by Schlechte et al. (*J. Clin. Endocrinol. Metab.* 52:785, 1981), who found that patients with onset of symptoms post partum or shortly after discontinuation of birth control pills (i.e., estrogen related) had a higher post surgical cure rate than those patients whose onset of symptoms was spontaneous and unrelated to estrogen (72% vs. 33%). Unfortunately, the present study did not address this potentially important variable. If a means of predicting surgical curability could be identified, it might be reasonable to consider primary bromocriptine therapy, which has been shown to be useful in alleviating symptoms, reducing the size and occasionally effecting complete regression, for patients with a limited chance of cure by surgery."] ◀

14–10 **Longitudinal Evaluation of Patients With Untreated Prolactin-Secreting Pituitary Adenomas.** C. M. March, O. A. Kletzky, V. Davajan, J. Teal, M. Weiss, M. L. J. Apuzzo, R. P. Marrs, and D. R. Mishell, Jr. (Univ. of Southern California, Los Angeles) examined the natural course of pituitary microadenomas in a series of 43 conservatively managed patients with galactorrhea, hyperprolactinemia, and radiographic evidence of pituitary adenoma who had follow-up for 3–20 years. Galactorrhea had been present for a mean of 51 months before initial evaluation. Thirty-four patients had had secondary amenorrhea for a mean of 49 months. Ten patients wished to conceive; 1 did so spontaneously, while 9 received ovulation-inducing drugs. All patients had definite radiographic evidence of a pituitary adenoma. Thyroid function was normal in all cases. Three amenorrheic women had evidence of ovarian failure.

Mean prolactin levels ranged from 177 to 218 ng/ml in women followed up for 4 years or longer; the values were not significantly different from the initial serum levels. In 3 women, prolactin levels returned to the normal range and have remained normal. These women now have normal menses and no galactorrhea. Visual fields have remained normal in all patients. Follow-up computed tomography (CT)

(14–10) Am. J. Obstet. Gynecol. 139:835–844, April, 1981.

studies showed progression of tumor in 2 patients. All 9 patients who received ovulation-inducing drugs conceived. Menstrual patterns remained unchanged in 40 of the 43 patients during follow-up.

Most patients with small prolactin-secreting pituitary adenomas can be followed up with annual CT scans, with or without medical treatment. Surgery should be reserved for patients with large tumors, those with visual field loss, and those with signs of tumor enlargement. Medical treatment may be with clomiphene citrate or bromocriptine. Patients with withdrawal bleeding during progesterone administration usually respond to clomiphene. Estrogen-deficient women require therapy with bromocriptine or human menopausal gonadotropin.

▶ [This is an important study because it gives considerable information about the natural history of prolactinoma. Of 43 patients with prolactin-secreting adenomas who had follow-up without treatment for a median period of 5 years after radiographic diagnosis, 2 underwent surgical removal because of tumor enlargement, 3 had spontaneous remission of symptoms and signs, and the others had no change. These results suggest, among other things, that simple observation (i.e., annual prolactin measurement, CT scan, perhaps visual field determination) is a reasonable approach in some patients. As a generalization, the management of this condition has become progressively more conservative. Several years ago, immediate surgery usually was advised. Then as bromocriptine became available, medical therapy was recommended increasingly. Now it appears that no treatment at all is a viable option.] ◀

14–11   **Preovulatory Follicular Size: A Comparison of Ultrasound and Laparoscopic Measurements.** Colm O'Herlihy, Lachlan Ch. De Crespigny, Alexander Lopata, Ian Johnston, Ian Hoult, and Hugh Robinson (Univ. of Melbourne) compared real-time or static ultrasound measurements of ovarian follicles in the immediate preovulatory period with the volumes of aspirated intrafollicular fluid obtained at laparoscopy in 36 patients (39 follicles) who were awaiting laparoscopic ovum aspiration prior to attempted in vitro fertilization. Ultrasound examination of the pelvis was performed within 12 hours of laparoscopy. Because of restricted oral intake prior to laparoscopy, fluid was instilled through a Foley catheter in order to achieve a full bladder, required for ultrasound examination. Twenty-nine patients (30 follicles) were examined during spontaneous cycles. Laparoscopy was timed 26–28 hours after the initial midcycle luteinizing hormone (LH) surge. In 6 patients, follicular development was stimulated by clomiphene citrate; on days 12–14 of the cycle, 5,000 IU of human chorionic gonadotropin (hCG) was given empirically. In stimulated cycles, laparoscopy was performed 30–34 hours after hCG had been given.

In each patient, the mean diameter was calculated from ultrasonic measurements of the follicle in 3 planes; the volume was derived using the formula $4/3\pi r^3$. The volume of aspirated follicular contents was used to calculate a diameter for comparison with the mean diameter measured by ultrasound. Follicular dimensions based on the volume of aspirated fluid corresponded well with the ultrasound measurements ($r = 0.847$; $P < .001$). The preovulatory mean follicular diameter calculated by both methods in 29 patients with spontaneous

---

(14–11) Fertil. Steril. 34:24–26, July 1980.

cycles was 21.1 mm, with ranges of 17–25 mm and 16–24.5 mm for the ultrasound and aspiration estimates, respectively. Mean volume was 5.1 ml. In 7 stimulated cycles, the mean diameter was 18.4 mm and mean volume was 3.5 ml. This study shows that an ultrasound estimate of follicular size correlates well with the aspirated follicular volume in the immediate preovulatory period. In most patients, the ultrasound estimate exceeded the aspirated volume by a small margin, possibly because of incomplete collection of follicular fluid at laparoscopy. Poor delineation of follicular margins might have resulted in overestimates of follicular size in ultrasound measurements. Systematic errors and bladder distention might have contributed to inaccuracy.

In this study, no definitive ultrasonic marker suggesting impending ovulation was found. The demonstrated variation in size of the preovulatory follicle is too wide to permit an accurate prediction of the actual day of ovulation on the basis of a single ultrasound examination.

▶ [A number of centers recently have reported ultrasound visualization of the developing follicle (see 1981 YEAR BOOK, pp. 333–334). The reliability of this technique, which has a number of obvious clinical uses in infertility patients, is further confirmed by this study demonstrating a high degree of correlation between ultrasonic and direct measurement of follicular size.

In a related study, Queenan and associates (*Fertil. Steril.* 34:99, 1980) confirmed the usefulness of ultrasound in detecting ovulation. Considerable variability in size of the preovulatory follicle was noted.] ◀

14-12 **Significance of FSH Elevation in Young Women With Disorders of Ovulation.** Approximately 10% of all patients with secondary amenorrhea have high serum follicle-stimulating hormone (FSH) levels consistent with ovarian failure. Recently, there have been several isolated reports of pregnancies occurring following a diagnosis of premature ovarian failure. A gonadotropin resistance syndrome has been proposed to explain these cases. C. O'Herlihy, R. J. Pepperell, and J. H. Evans retrospectively studied the progress of 67 young women, all younger than age 35, with secondary amenorrhea or oligomenorrhea and serum FSH levels greater than 20 U/L. Serum prolactin concentrations were normal in all patients.

Fifty of the women presented with secondary amenorrhea and 17 with oligomenorrhea. During the 4-year study period, 24 of the women remained amenorrheic, but 26 had further menstrual bleeding, and endocrinologic evidence of ovarian follicular development was apparent in at least 4 patients. Subsequent ovulation occurred in 17 women and conception occurred in 6 (twice in 2 women). There were no significant differences between those whose amenorrhea persisted and those in whom ovarian function returned with respect to age at menarche, parity, age at diagnosis of elevated FSH levels, or incidence of symptoms of estrogen deprivation. Patients who remained amenorrheic, those who later menstruated, and patients who subsequently ovulated showed significant differences with respect to total urinary estrogens and serum luteinizing hormone (LH) levels.

(14–12) Br. Med. J. 281:1447–1450, Nov. 29, 1980.

Generally, absolute FSH concentrations had little prognostic value, although few women with FSH values greater than 40 U/L ovulated or conceived. Mean LH concentration was significantly lower in the 17 patients who ovulated or conceived than in those who did not. No patient responded to treatment with estrogens, clomiphene citrate, human pituitary gonadotropin, or bromocriptine while FSH levels remained elevated. However, when FSH levels fell spontaneously, ovulation could often be induced with clomiphene or human pituitary gonadotropin. Four of the 8 pregnancies occurred without treatment.

The results suggest that a fair proportion of women of childbearing age with ovulatory disorders associated with FSH values reflective of menopause will spontaneously regain ovarian function, and some will conceive.

▶ [Although one might assume that, in a young woman with amenorrhea, vasomotor symptoms and elevated FSH levels meant that it was "curtains" as far as the ovaries were concerned, this is not necessarily the case. This series highlights a phenomenon noted in several recent case reports. Certain patients with an apparent premature menopause will subsequently resume ovulation. The ovarian show reopens! According to this study, patients who resumed ovulation were more apt to have higher estrogen and lower LH levels at the time of presumed "menopause" than those who remained amenorrheic, but FSH levels were not discriminatory. Therapy was ineffective until or unless FSH levels declined. The next time we diagnose a patient as having premature menopause, we will be more careful in advising her as to what this means.] ◀

14–13 **Abnormal Follicle-Stimulating Hormone and Luteinizing Hormone Patterns Contrasting With Normal Estradiol and Progesterone Secretion in Women With Long-Standing Unexplained Infertility.** Abnormal FSH and LH secretion has been associated with an inadequate rise in plasma progesterone (P) concentrations, which may be a cause of deficient follicular development and deficient corpus luteum function. However, normal cyclic estradiol (E_2) and P levels during regular menstrual cycles in the absence of normal FSH and LH secretion patterns has not been described before. W. P. Dmowski, P. Rezai, F. J. Auletta, and A. Scommegna (Chicago) studied 6 women with long-standing unexplained infertility and regular menstrual cycles. Plasma levels of FSH, LH, E_2, and P were determined daily or every other day during one menstrual cycle, and the results were compared with those found in 5 apparently normal women. All of the infertile women had luteal structures identified on normal-appearing ovaries at laparoscopy and normal plasma androgen levels.

All of the control subjects showed normal patterns of plasma FSH, LH, E_2, and P concentrations (Fig 14–1). All of the infertile women had normal patterns of E_2 secretion, with a typical midcycle increase, followed by a normal sustained elevation of plasma P concentration. However, secretory patterns of FSH and LH were grossly abnormal in 5 of these patients. One patient, aged 35, had FSH and LH levels that fluctuated between high normal and menopausal values without appreciable regularity or synchrony (Fig 14–2). This patient showed a moderate, but synchronous, midcycle rise in FSH and LH that co-

(14–13) J. Clin. Endocrinol. Metab. 52:1218–1224, June 1981.

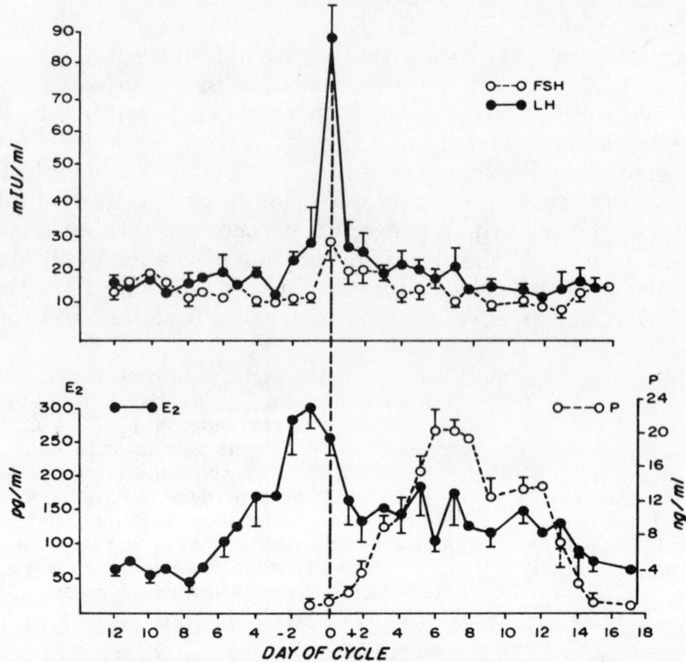

Fig 14–1.—Plasma FSH, LH, E$_2$, and P concentrations in 5 normal women during one menstrual cycle (mean ± SEM; all values were centered around the LH peak). (Courtesy of Dmowski, W. P., et al.: J. Clin. Endocrinol. Metab. 52:1218–1224, June 1981.)

incided with the rise in the E$_2$ concentration and which was followed by a sustained rise of the P concentration. These changes have been seen in women during the transition to menopause. In the other 4 infertile patients, plasma LH concentrations were consistently higher than FSH concentrations, and 3 patients had absolute LH concentrations greater than control levels. Midcycle LH surges could be identified in all 4 of these patients, but only 1 had an FSH surge. The ratio of LH to FSH was consistently greater than 2.

The results indicate that plasma E$_2$ and P secretory patterns characteristic of a normal ovulatory cycle may be associated with grossly abnormal FSH and LH secretion and suggest that these abnormal gonadotropin patterns may be causally related to the infertility in these patients.

▶ [This report nicely demonstrates that normal estradiol and progesterone levels do not indicate necessarily that the associated FSH and LH patterns also will be normal. As more is learned in this area, the hope is that specific therapies will evolve for certain "normal" infertile women. It is interesting that the patient with high, irregular gonadotropin levels (Fig 14–2) subsequently conceived after exogenous estrogen treatment during the follicular phase.] ◀

14–14 **Reproductive Endocrine System in Cystic Fibrosis: I. Basal Gonadotropin and Sex Steroid Levels.** The onset and progress of sexual maturation in children with cystic fibrosis can be delayed

(14–14) Am. J. Dis. Child. 135:422–426, May 1981.

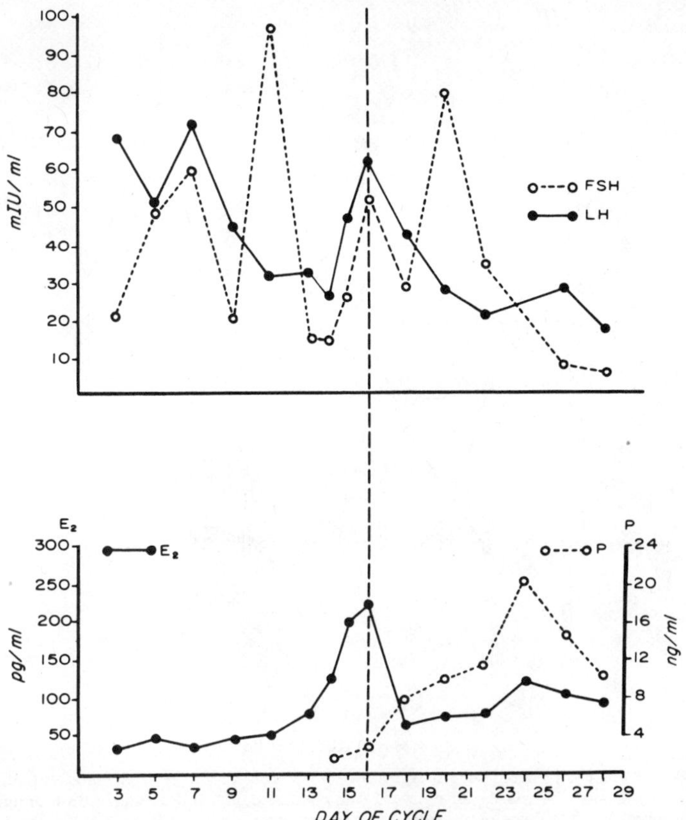

Fig 14–2.—Plasma FSH, LH, E₂, and P concentrations in patient A. M. during one menstrual cycle. (Courtesy of Dmowski, W. P., et al.: J. Clin. Endocrinol. Metab. 52:1218–1224, June 1981.)

markedly, but maturation of the reproductive endocrine system in such patients has not been studied. Edward O. Reiter, Robert C. Stern, and Allen W. Root measured gonadotropin and gonadal and adrenal sex steroid concentrations in 46 male and 60 female subjects, aged 8 to 24 years, who had cystic fibrosis.

The incremental pattern in serum LH and FSH concentrations was abnormal in male adolescents with cystic fibrosis, with a chronological delay of 2 to 4 years. In girls with cystic fibrosis, serum LH concentrations were similar to normal values at all ages and pubertal stages, but the pubertal rise in the FSH concentration was 2 to 4 years delayed. These data suggest that boys and, to a lesser extent, girls with cystic fibrosis have a chronological delay in usual age-related increments of serum gonadotropin concentration.

The pattern of the adolescent increase of serum testosterone concentrations in boys with cystic fibrosis mirrored, and was probably secondary to, the chronological delay seen in the rise of gonadotropin values. In late adolescence normal basal concentrations of serum testosterone were finally achieved. Concentrations of dihydrotestoster-

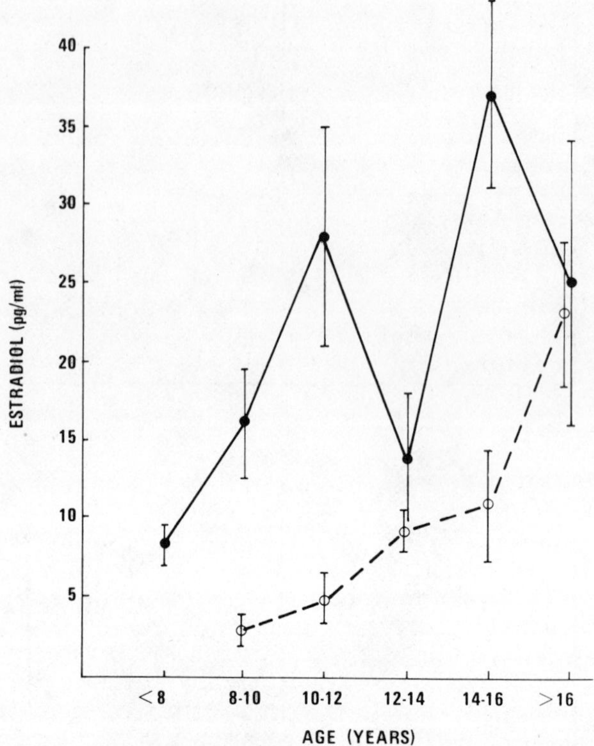

Fig 14–3.—Adolescent rise of serum estradiol concentrations for normal females *(solid circles)* and females with cystic fibrosis *(open circles)*. Age-related delay and normal late-teenage concentrations are apparent. Numbers of subjects in each age group ranged from 9 to 24 for normal females and 5 to 23 for females with cystic fibrosis. Means ± SEM are shown. (Courtesy of Reiter, E. O., et al.: Am. J. Dis. Child. 135:422–426, May 1981; copyright 1981, American Medical Association.)

one were lower than normal in both prepubertal and pubertal boys. Delayed initiation of pubertal hypothalamic-pituitary gonadotropic interactions may largely explain the slow sexual maturation of boys with cystic fibrosis.

In girls with cystic fibrosis the pattern of rise in serum estradiol concentration during adolescence differed from that of normal controls, especially in the early pubertal stages (Fig 14–3). Girls finally achieved normal estradiol values after age 16 years, but pubertal girls as a group had a mean estradiol concentration only 50% of the norm. In pubertal girls, concentrations of estrone, progesterone, and 17-hydroxyprogesterone were 40% to 60% of control values, consistent with impaired ovarian steroidogenesis. In girls with cystic fibrosis, as in boys, an abnormality may reside at the hypothalamic-pituitary level.

The finding of delayed maturation of both sex steroid hormone secretory systems in patients with cystic fibrosis is similar to that observed in normal patients with constitutional delay in growth and sexual maturation.

▶ [The survival with cystic fibrosis (CF) has improved dramatically in recent years, and many victims of this disease are presently living to adolescence and beyond. This cross-sectional study of gonadotropin and steroid hormone levels indicates that CF patients have some delay in maturation of their reproductive endocrine system. In girls with CF, FSH levels were lower than in control girls until about age 12 and estradiol levels were lower until age 16. By age 16, however, the two groups were indistinguishable. Thus, reproduction should be possible and, indeed, pregnancy complicated by CF is beginning to be seen. Last year we cared for such a patient; she had considerable difficulty during pregnancy and died of pulmonary complications within a few months post partum.] ◀

14–15 **Ovarian Failure in Long-Term Survivors of Childhood Malignancy.** Robert J. Stillman, Jay S. Schinfeld, Isaac Schiff, Richard D. Gelber, Joel Greenberger, Martin Larson, Norman Jaffe, and Frederick P. Li studied ovarian failure among 182 long-term survivors of childhood cancer. Mean age at diagnosis of cancer was 6.9 years and mean follow-up since diagnosis was 16.4 years. Ninety-four patients (52%) received fractionated external beam radiotherapy to the abdomen. Estimated mean ovarian tissue doses were approximately 3,200 rad (range 1,200–5,000 rad) for 25 patients with both ovaries inside the field, 290 rad (range 90–1,000 rad) for 35 patients with at least one ovary at the edge of the field, and 54 rad (5–150 rad) for 34 patients with at least one ovary outside the abdominal radiation field.

Twenty-two (12%) patients had ovarian failure, defined as amenorrhea accompanied by persistently elevated levels of both gonadotropins. Ovarian failure was found in 17 (68%) of 25 patients who had both ovaries within abdominal radiotherapy fields, in 5 (14%) of 35 patients whose ovaries were at the edge of the treatment field, and in none of 34 patients with at least one ovary outside the treatment field. The odds of ovarian failure developing in patients having both ovaries within the radiation field were 19.7 higher than those for other irradiated patients (95% confidence interval, 5.2–72.8). Covariate and multivariate analyses of tumor type, age at diagnosis, duration of follow-up, abdominal tumor surgery, abdominal radiotherapy, number of chemotherapeutic agents given, and cumulative doses of several drugs revealed that the location of ovaries relative to the radiation treatment field was the only risk factor for subsequent ovarian failure.

Less gonadal radiation exposure can often be accomplished by ovariopexy and lead shielding of the ovaries. Before puberty, the relative quiescence of ovarian stromal cells and oocytes may provide some protection against cytotoxic drugs with cell-cycle specific activity. Also, the larger number of oocytes in children may permit survival of sufficient oocytes to preserve adequate ovarian function during early adulthood. More intensive chemotherapy regimens in current use may have greater effects on fertility and ovarian function.

▶ [The results of this study indicate quite clearly that loss of ovarian function in survivors of childhood cancer relates entirely to radiation effects. When follow-up was done 14 years or longer after treatment, ovarian failure had occurred in 68% of those whose ovaries had been within the field of radiation, 14% of those with at least one ovary at the edge of the treatment field, and none with at least one ovary outside the

---

(14–15) Am. J. Obstet. Gynecol. 139:62–66, Jan. 1, 1981.

field. Efforts to minimize gonadal irradiation (shielding, field modification, ovariopexy, etc.) certainly merit consideration in treatment of children with radiation.] ◄

14–16 Pituitary-Adrenal Function in Women Treated With Low Doses of Prednisone. K. Fujieda, F. I. Reyes, J. Blankstein, and C. Faiman (Univ. of Manitoba) examined the response of plasma cortisol to insulin-induced hypoglycemia in 23 women treated with prednisone (5 mg /day) compared to that in 19 untreated women. Forty-two women with clinical (hirsutism or polycystic ovary syndrome) and biochemical (high serum testosterone levels) evidence of hyperandrogenism were studied. The average length of treatment in the treated group was 8.8 months (range 3–40 months). Insulin-induced hypoglycemia tests were performed by intravenous bolus injection of 0.1 U of regular insulin per kg body weight between 8 and 10 A.M. after an overnight fast.

Circulating testosterone concentrations declined during therapy from a mean of 79.9 to 34.6 ng/dl, but mean basal levels of plasma cortisol were similar (mean ± SE 11.2 ± 0.7 µg/dl in the nontreated group versus 11.6 ± 0.9 µg/dl in the treated group). Responses of the hypothalamic-pituitary-adrenal (H-P-A) axis after insulin-induced hypoglycemia in the two groups were comparable in the degree of hypoglycemia attained. Blood glucose level fell to less than 45 mg/dl in each subject, but the plasma cortisol increment after insulin stimulation was consistently lower in the treated group. This difference was significant only at 60 minutes (6.7 ± 1.0 versus 11.6 ± 1.2 µg/ dl). Comparable results were obtained in a subset of 10 women who were tested both before and during therapy. Seven of 10 patients showed a diminished cortisol response; 2 showed no change, and 1 had an enhanced response during treatment. Patients who received therapy for longer periods of time tended to have a greater diminution in the cortisol response. It is notable that 13 of the 23 women (56.5%) in the steroid-treated group, compared to 1 of 19 (5.3%) in the untreated group, showed a rise in plasma cortisol of less than 6 µg/dl at 60 minutes.

Results indicate that long-term administration of low-dose prednisone produces a small but significant suppressive effect on the H-P-A axis. Insulin hypoglycemia examines the integrity of the H-P-A axis and is recommended as the best clinical predictor of response to stress. The finding of a greater than 50% reduction in mean testosterone levels in the presence of unchanged basal cortisol levels during prednisone treatment strongly suggests that H-P-A axis suppression is not involved in the inhibitory effect of glucocorticoids on androgen production. The results suggest that although supplementary corticoid therapy during operation appears not to be required as a rule, it is recommended for anticipated or prolonged stress in patients who have received low doses of glucocorticoids.

► [Long-term administration of low-dose prednisone resulted in a slight but significant suppressive effect on the hypothalamic-pituitary-adrenal axis in this study. The marked drop in serum testosterone levels in the face of normal basal cortisol levels

(14–16) Am. J. Obstet. Gynecol. 137:962–965, Aug. 15, 1980.

suggests that the efficacy of prednisone in this situation is *not* based on the central suppression of ACTH, however.] ◄

14–17 Dehydroepiandrosterone Sulfate As an Indicator of Adrenal Androgen Function. There is some evidence that serum concentrations of dehydroepiandrosterone sulfate (DHEAS) reflect abnormal adrenal androgen secretion more accurately than do urinary 17-ketosteroid (17-KS) concentrations. To determine whether serum DHEAS assays could be used in place of urinary 17-KS measurements, Rogerio A. Lobo, Wellington L. Paul, and Uwe Goebelsmann (Univ. of Southern California) measured serum DHEAS and urinary 17-KS and creatinine levels in 71 women with and without signs of androgen excess who were attending the Reproductive Endocrinology/ Infertility Clinic. In another group of 26 women with possible androgen excess, serum DHEAS was measured and compared with fractionated urinary 17-KS (androsterone, etiocholanolone, and dehydroepiandrosterone [DHEA]) levels. Normal serum DHEAS values were established by measuring serum DHEAS in 41 nonhirsute, regularly menstruating women.

Serum DHEAS concentrations in normal women ranged from 0.3 to 2.8 µg/ml, with a mean of 1.78 ± 0.10 µg/ml. In the 71 women with and without signs of androgen excess, DHEAS levels did not correlate with body weight, body surface area, or ponderal indices. In these subjects, serum DHEAS concentrations were highly correlated ($P < .0005$) with total urinary 17-KS excretion adjusted for creati-

Fig 14–4.—Correlation between serum DHEA-S in µg/ml and total 17-KS in µg/24 hours, corrected for creatinine (assuming 20 mg creatinine per kg) in 71 women. (Courtesy of Lobo, R. A., et al.: Obstet. Gynecol. 57:69–73, January 1981.)

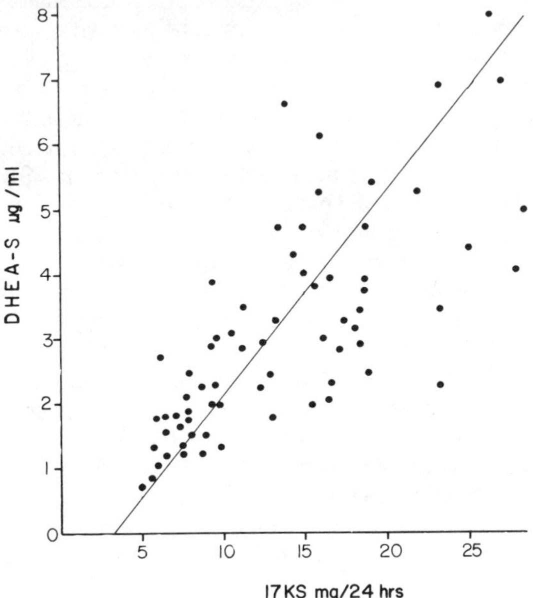

(14–17) Obstet. Gynecol. 57:69–73, January 1981.

nine excretion (Fig 14–4). However, the sum of the 17-KS fractions was less than that for total 17-KS. In 26 women with suspected androgen excess, urinary androsterone and DHEA, but not etiocholanolone, correlated well with serum DHEAS concentrations ($P < .001$). In 11 of these women, with elevated serum DHEAS concentrations and increased total 17-KS excretion, urinary levels of androsterone also were increased, but the etiocholanolone-androsterone ratio was less than 1; the inverse is normally the case.

It is concluded that measurement of serum DHEAS provides a more suitable estimate of adrenal androgen production than measurement of 17-KS excretion. However, additional serum androgens may have to be measured in the absence of 17-KS assays to obtain a more complete androgen profile.

▶ [Sensitive radioimmunoassay techniques have facilitated the measurement of hormones in blood rather than urine. Sample collection is certainly easier. Serum DHEAS and urinary 17-KS were highly correlated in this study. Therefore, the former can serve as an indicator of adrenal androgen production. A patient with apparent androgen excess should have blood testosterone and androstenedione levels determined (usually reflecting ovarian androgen production), as well as a test for the adrenal contribution.] ◀

14–18 Serum Levels of DHEAS in Gynecologic Endocrinopathy and Infertility. The serum concentration of dehydroepiandrosterone sulfate (DHEAS) has been a useful indicator of adrenal androgen secretion, and it is more convenient and reliable than urinary 17-ketosteroid (17-KS) determination. Rogerio A. Lobo, Wellington L. Paul, and Uwe Goebelsmann measured serum DHEAS concentrations in 32 infertile patients who were ovulatory, 37 oligomenorrheic women, and 52 hirsute women under basal conditions. Ten hirsute women also were studied in conjunction with ACTH stimulation and dexamethasone suppression. Forty-nine of the hirsute patients were oligomenorrheic, and 23 of them were considered to have polycystic ovary syndrome. In addition, 41 healthy, nonhirsute women with regular cycles were studied. Serum DHEAS was measured by radioimmunoassay.

All patient groups had significantly higher serum DHEAS concentrations than did controls. Values were elevated in 19% of the infertile patients and in 34% of the nonhirsute, oligomenorrheic women. The findings in hirsute patients are shown in the table. Serum DHEAS elevations were found in 59% of this group and unbound testosterone (T) elevations in 68%. Both concentrations were elevated in 45% of the patients. Only 11% of hirsute patients had no elevated hormone values. All the hirsute patients studied showed a fall in serum DHEAS concentration after dexamethasone and a rise after ACTH infusion. Ten patients given 0.5 mg of dexamethasone daily for 2 weeks showed a fall in mean serum DHEAS concentration from 4.6 to 0.6 µg/ml; all patients had a fall in DHEAS concentrations.

The serum DHEAS value is a clinically useful marker of adrenal C-19 steroid or androgen production. Elevations are found in a variety of states. Combined with clinical and other hormonal studies, the

---

(14–18) Obstet. Gynecol. 57:607–612, May 1981.

MEAN (± SE) DHEAS, T, UNBOUND T, ANDROSTENEDIONE (A),
AND 24-HOUR 17-KS VALUES IN 52 HIRSUTE WOMEN*

Hormones	Levels†	Percent elevated*
DHEAS	3.43 ± 0.23 µg/ml	59
T	0.55 ± 0.34 ng/ml	38
Unbound T	12.27 ± 1.41 ng/100 ml	68
A	3.11 ± 0.16 ng/ml	50
17-KS	15.1 ± 1.2 µg/24 hr	50

*Number of women in whom values exceeded 2 SD above normal mean is listed as percent of 52.

†All mean values were significantly greater than normal ($P < .01$).

serum DHEAS concentration is useful in gynecologic endocrinology and infertility investigations.

▶ [Reports in previous YEAR BOOKS have differed as to whether or not free testosterone is elevated uniformly in hirsute women. Sixty-eight percent of hirsute women had elevated free testosterone levels in the current study; an additional 14% had increased concentrations of DHEAS. A rational treatment for hirsute patients with elevated DHEAS levels in the presence of normal free testosterone and androstenedione levels would seem to be low-dose corticosteroids, because the adrenal gland is probably the culprit in this situation.] ◀

14–19 **Dexamethasone Suppression Test in Management of Hyperandrogenized Patients.** Guy E. Abraham, George B. Maroulis, Stephen P. Boyers, John E. Buster, David M. Magyar, and Carlene W. Elsner (Harbor-UCLA Med. Center, Torrance, Calif.) evaluated 86 hyperandrogenized women with measurements of serum cortisol, dehydroepiandrosterone sulfate (DHEAS), testosterone, and dihydrotestosterone levels in pooled sera before and after a dexamethasone suppression test. Androgen-producing ovarian and adrenal tumors were essentially ruled out by absence of virilization, absence of significant ovarian enlargement, a serum testosterone value below 2 ng/ml, and a serum DHEAS value below 7,000 ng/ml. The dexamethasone suppression test was considered inadequate when a postsuppression serum cortisol concentration greater than 40 ng/ml or DHEAS level greater than 400 ng/ml was found; the test was then repeated for a longer period. Patients having no significant suppression of serum cortisol values were evaluated for Cushing's syndrome. With adequate suppression of serum cortisol and DHEAS concentrations, the dexamethasone test was interpreted as follows: if the peripheral androgen concentration was elevated during the control period and suppressed to normal after dexamethasone treatment, its source was considered adrenal; if the androgen level was not suppressed to normal after dexamethasone treatment, and the difference between presuppression and postsuppression values equaled the normal adrenal contribution, its source was considered ovarian; if the androgen level

---

(14–19) Obstet. Gynecol. 57:158–165, February 1981.

was partially suppressed after dexamethasone treatment, and the difference between presuppression and postsuppression values was greater than the normal adrenal contribution, its source was considered mixed (adrenal and ovarian). If control androgen concentrations were normal, after dexamethasone suppression four categories were established: normal ovarian and adrenal contributions, and adrenal, ovarian, and mixed hyperandrogenism.

Of the 86 women, 70 (81%) had a major glucocorticoid suppressible component. The clinical responses were evaluated in 55 women who received endocrine therapy for 6–15 months as dictated by results of the dexamethasone test. In the 38 women with adrenal hyperandrogenism, dexamethasone was administered in a dose adjusted to maintain a serum cortisol concentration 20 ng/ml or more and a DHEAS value of 400 ng/ml or less. In the 3 with ovarian hyperandrogenism, an oral contraceptive containing 0.5 mg norgestrel and 0.05 mg ethinyl estradiol (Ovral) was given cyclically, or depomedroxyprogesterone acetate (Depo-Provera) was given intramuscularly, 150 mg every 3 months. In the 14 patients with mixed hyperandrogenism, dexamethasone was given initially; if response was poor, ovarian suppression therapy was added.

Of 29 patients with adrenal or mixed hyperandrogenism associated with abnormal menses, the menstrual status of 17 (59%) improved after dexamethasone therapy. Acne improved in all 39 women affected. Hirsutism improved to a moderate or marked degree in 40 (73%) of 55 women.

These findings indicate that endocrine suppression therapy, particularly with repeated low-dose dexamethasone prescribed on the basis of a dexamethasone suppression test, is effective in managing hyperandrogenism. When dexamethasone is discontinued after 1 year, the recurrence rate is 15%. In ovarian hyperandrogenism, however, the recurrence rate is 90%, thus most patients require longer treatment.

▶ [Doctor Abraham and his associates at Harbor Hospital, Torrance, California, have been the chief proponents of the view that adrenal hyperfunction is a common cause of androgenicity, whereas others have held that the ovary is nearly always the origin of excess androgen secretion. The issue hinges on the question of whether suppressibility by glucocorticoids means *ipso facto* that the adrenal is the source. In this study, long-term dexamethasone suppression yielded impressive clinical improvement in terms of restoration of menstrual function and lessening of acne and hirsutism.] ◀

14–20 **Obesity and Its Role in Polycystic Ovary Syndrome.** Recent findings have suggested that obesity may be a causative factor in polycystic ovary (PCO) syndrome. Stephen R. Plymate, Bruce L. Fariss, Martin L. Bassett, and Louis Matej (Madigan Army Med. Center, Tacoma, Wash.) examined the effect of obesity on ovulation in 55 patients with oligo-ovulation or anovulation and a 2-year history of infertility. They had normal husbands, no cervical or tubal problems, and normal serum prolactin levels. Sex steroid-binding globulin (SSBG) levels were measured by saturation analysis. Thirty patients weighing more than 145% of ideal body weight were considered obese, and 25 weighing less than 120% of ideal body weight were

(14–20) J. Clin. Endocrinol. Metab. 52:1246–1248, June 1981.

considered to be of normal weight. No patient weighed less than 90% of ideal body weight.

The obese and normal weight groups did not have significantly different testosterone or estradiol levels. Testosterone levels were elevated or at the upper limit of normal. The LH levels were higher and SSBG levels lower in obese patients than in those with normal weight. There were no group differences in FSH or prolactin levels. Correlation was noted between body weight and SSBG levels.

Obesity may be a factor regulating the SSBG level, independent of androgen or estrogen status. Whether the problem is a decreased response to estrogen or increased clearance is not known. In patients with PCO syndrome or an underlying tendency to develop the syndrome, a decrease in SSBG level or an increase in free testosterone level may permit the syndrome to become manifest. The change in SSBG level may not be the primary factor causing PCO syndrome, but it may be significant in those patients who have another defect that leads to PCO disease. A fall in SSBG level may be followed by an increase in testosterone level which, by inhibiting follicular maturation, may initiate the sequence of events seen in PCO syndrome.

▶ [Estrogens increase and testosterone decreases the level of sex steroid-binding globulin (SSBG). Although the significance of the reported inverse relationship between body weight and SSBG levels is unclear, it may well be important. Although testosterone and estradiol levels did not differ between the obese and normal weight patients studied here, the lower SSBG levels in the obese mean higher free or unbound hormone levels. Adipose tissue serves as a paraendocrine organ converting androstenedione to estrone and testosterone. This report suggests a separate role for, or at least association with, excess fat.] ◀

14–21 Novel Use of Spironolactone: Treatment of Hirsutism. Spironolactone has been used in the treatment of aldosteronism and low-renin hypertension or hypokalemia. German Shapiro and Shmuel Evron (Hadassah Univ. Hosp., Jerusalem) evaluated the antiandrogenic properties of spironolactone in 30 hirsute nonobese women. Most of the women received 100 mg of spironolactone twice daily from day 4 to day 22 of each menstrual cycle.

After 13 months of treatment, a clinically significant improvement in hirsutism was observed in 23 of the 30 women, with the first signs of improvement occurring 3 to 5 months after treatment was initiated (table). A therapeutic effect was seen in 8 of 11 women with normal pretreatment serum testosterone levels and in 14 of 19 with elevated testosterone concentrations. The effect of treatment varied with the site involved, with the lower abdomen and back being most resistant. Concomitant acne improved in 7 of 8 women. All patients showed a decrease in serum testosterone levels during treatment, with a mean decrease of approximately 80% being attained at 6 to 9 months after treatment was initiated. Though not as pronounced, women with normal pretreatment testosterone levels also showed a decrease. Serum estradiol concentrations increased in 25 women and decreased in 5; however, the mean overall level was significantly higher than before treatment. A significant decrease was observed in mean progesterone

(14–21)   J. Clin. Endocrinol. Metab. 51:429–431, September 1980.

GRADING OF HAIR DENSITY IN HIRSUTE PATIENTS BEFORE AND DURING SPIRONOLACTONE TREATMENT AND IN 24 NONHIRSUTE WOMEN

Patients	Before treatment	After 3 months of treatment	After 6 months of treatment	After 9 or more months of treatment
Hirsute	17.0 ± 4.6 (30)	16.4 ± 4.2 (30)[a]	11.8 ± 4.2 (30)[b]	10.8 ± 3.4 (26)[b]
Nonhirsute	2.5 ± 3.2 (24)[c]			

All values given as mean ± SD. Number of subjects given in parentheses.
[a]Not significant compared with pretreatment scoring.
[b]$P<.01$ compared with pretreatment scoring.
[c]$P<.01$ compared with hirsute group before treatment.

and follicle-stimulating hormone levels, although the decrease in serum luteinizing hormone was not significant. Although there were transient, mild side effects that disappeared without intervention, no patient had to discontinue treatment. Even when the treatment was considered a failure, there was a psychological benefit in that the hair became less coarse and did not grow as fast.

The results show that spironolactone is of value in the treatment of hirsutism. The absence of serious side effects with spironolactone and its effectiveness warrant its wider use in the treatment of hirsutism.

▶ [These results are consistent with those of a study abstracted in the 1981 YEAR BOOK (pp. 353–356). The mechanism for the fall in testosterone (T) concentration has not been established. The authors cite diminished activity of enzymes involved in T synthesis and displacement from binding proteins of T by spironolactone, leading to enhanced elimination of T, as possibilities. The intermittent treatment (day 4 to day 22 of each cycle) was not associated with severe side effects.] ◀

14–22 **Acute Adolescent Menorrhagia** is a much underestimated clinical problem, often requiring urgent medical intervention. In a 9-year case review by E. Anne Claessens and Carol A. Cowell (Univ. of Toronto) of 59 patients in whom genital tract pathology was excluded, 44 (74%) had dysfunctional uterine bleeding, 11 (19%) had a coagulation disorder, and 4 (7%) had other major contributing factors to menorrhagia, including endometrial stromal sarcoma in 1. About one third of those requiring transfusion, about 50% of those seen at menarche, and about 25% with severe menorrhagia had an underlying coagulation disorder.

Proper screening is essential in girls with menorrhagia. This includes medical and family history, physical examination, blood smear analysis, and coagulation screen; the latter should include, prior to transfusion or hormone therapy, determination of prothrombin time, partial thromboplastin time, platelet count, and bleeding time. On curettage, the yield of findings indicating significant abnormality was very low.

If bleeding is not heavy and the hemoglobin value is greater than 10 gm/100 ml, watchful expectancy is a reasonable approach. Oral iron replacement is required, and follow-up is undertaken. Patients with a known coagulation disorder were treated primarily with appropriate replacement therapy (blood, cryoprecipitate, platelet concentrates). Corticosteroids were given for idiopathic thrombocytopenic purpura when appropriate. To achieve initial hormonal hemostasis in acute menorrhagia, particularly with very heavy or prolonged bleeding, high-dose conjugated estrogens (Premarin), 40 mg intravenously every 4 hours for a maximum of 6 doses, were administered. Concurrently, a highly progestational combined estrogen-progestin oral preparation (containing 5 mg of progestin) was given. The initial loading dose was 2 tablets, followed by 1 tablet 4 times daily, the dose gradually tapered over the following month according to response. A patient requiring maximal doses of conjugated estrogens needs additional progestin to counteract estrogenic effects. It is unnecessary to continue parenteral estrogen therapy beyond 24 hours (or very occa-

(14–22) Am. J. Obstet. Gynecol. 139:227–280, Feb. 1, 1981.

sionally 48 hours); uncontrolled bleeding beyond this time indicates the need for examination with the use of anesthesia and diagnostic dilatation and curettage. Neither high-dose estrogen nor progestin works effectively alone. Following this intense therapy, 3 months of cyclic therapy with conventional combined oral contraceptive pills may be undertaken, and the patient then reassessed. If the anovulatory pattern recurs, a progestin (e.g., medroxyprogesterone acetate, 10 mg daily for 5 days every 40 days) can be given, as the drug is an excellent cycle regulator. Continued severe anovulatory dysfunctional bleeding merits endocrinologic evaluation.

In general, patients with acute adolescent menorrhagia have an increased incidence of anemia, transfusions, operations, subsequent infertility, spontaneous abortions, and risk of endometrial adenomatous hyperplasia and carcinoma. Ten years and more after the initial episode, bleeding problems continue in 30% to 40% of these patients. Those with menorrhagia developing at menarche have the worst prognosis. It has been necessary occasionally to induce prolonged suppression of menses in patients with "unstable" hematologic diseases.

▶ [Severe anemia, the need for transfusion, presentation at menarche, or some combination of these increases the possibility that acute adolescent menorrhagia is a manifestation of an underlying coagulation disorder. Although pregnancy and dysfunctional uterine bleeding are the first things that come to mind in this situation, the authors' point that coagulation disorders may first present in this fashion is a good one.] ◀

14–23 Menstrual Synchrony in Female Undergraduates Living on a Coeducational Campus. McClintock first observed an effect of social factors on the menstrual cycle in the form of menstrual synchrony dependent on social interaction. Other reports of synchrony have come from groups of women living in all-female communities. C. A. Graham and W. C. McGrew (Univ. of Stirling) sought to determine whether menstrual synchrony could develop in women living on a coeducational university campus. Seventy-nine women aged 17 to 21 years recorded their cycles for 4 months from the start of the autumn semester. The subjects lived in buildings with about 50% women, and there were no official restrictions on the access of either sex to the other.

A significant decrease in differences between pairs' onset dates, i.e., a trend toward synchrony, was observed for close friends (table), but there was no significant effect for neighbors or for random peers. There were no significant correlations between cycle length or duration of menstruation and the amount and nature of social interaction with men. Only 16% of subjects reported being aware of their close friends' cycles. The amount of time that subjects spent together, rather than similar living conditions, was the significant factor in synchrony.

Menstrual synchrony has been observed in women within 4 months of living in a mixed-sex community. The significant determinant appears to be the degree of association between women. The mechanism

(14–23) Psychoneuroendocrinology 5:245–252, September 1980.

MEAN DIFFERENCES BETWEEN MENSTRUAL ONSET DATES FOR
CLOSE FRIENDS, NEIGHBORS, AND RANDOM PAIRS FOR FOUR-
MONTH PERIOD, SEPTEMBER TO DECEMBER, ONE-WAY ANALYSIS OF VARIANCE

Source of variation	d.f.	S.S.	M.S.	F.	Prob.
Closest friends					
Subjects	17	1620.1			
Months	3	243.8	81.2	2.95	$\leqslant 0.040$
Months × subjects	51	1400.6	27.4		
Neighbours					
Subjects	17	1208.5			
Months	3	16.0	5.34	0.162	$\leqslant 0.920$
Months × subjects	51	1675.7	32.8		
Random pairs					
Subjects	17	2029.9			
Months	3	16.9	5.64	0.214	$\leqslant 0.886$
Months × subjects	51	1361.7	26.3		

and function of menstrual synchrony are unclear. A pheromone may be involved. Close friendship involves both physical proximity and emotional affiliation, and these variables should be examined individually in a larger sample. The finding in this study that neighbors exhibited no intermediate degree of synchrony between close friends and random peers suggests that affiliative attachment is more important than physical proximity.

▶ [Menstrual synchrony is a fascinating phenomenon. If we understood its mechanism, we would probably be able to solve many puzzles in neuroendocrinology.] ◀

14-24 **Gastrointestinal Transit: The Effect of the Menstrual Cycle.** Gastrointestinal disturbances such as heart burn, constipation, and abdominal distention are common in pregnant women. They have been attributed to compression by the enlarging uterus, the effects of sex steroids, and psychic factors, but the role of the menstrual cycle is unclear. Arnold Wald, David H. Van Thiel, Leah Hoechstetter, Judith S. Gavaler, Kimberly M. Egler, Raymond Verm, Larry Scott, and Roger Lester examined the effect of the menstrual cycle on gastrointestinal transit, using breath hydrogen analysis as a monitor of the delivery of lactulose, a nonabsorbable disaccharide, to the cecum. Studies were done in 15 women with a mean age of 29 years who had normal cycles and had not used oral contraception for at least 6 months. Studies were done in the follicular and luteal phases of the menstrual cycle. Four subjects were studied in three consecutive cycles.

Gastrointestinal transit times were 25% longer in the luteal phase than in the follicular phase of the cycle; the difference was highly significant. Eleven of the 15 subjects had longer transit times in the luteal phase. Changes in progesterone levels during the cycle were relatively small, but were significant. The findings were consistent in the subjects studied repeatedly when the timing of their cycles was taken into account.

The luteal phase of the menstrual cycle is associated with both in-

(14–24) Gastroenterology 80:1497–1500, June 1981.

creased progesterone levels and prolongation of the gastrointestinal transit time. It is not clear whether the effect of female sex steroids on gut motility is caused by an effect on gut membranes, antialdosterone activity, or a specific action mediated by classic progesterone receptors in the cytosol of progesterone-responsive tissues. Receptors for glucocorticoids and aldosterone are present in the gut, and estradiol receptors also have been identified in gastrointestinal tissues. The presence of progesterone receptors in these tissues would not be unexpected.

▶ [The standard teaching is that constipation, distention, and other common gastrointestinal complaints in pregnant women relate in part to a progesterone-mediated decrease in gut tone and motility. The prolonged transit time during the luteal phase of the cycle in these nonpregnant women is consistent with this teaching.] ◀

14–25 **Retrograde Menstruation in Women Undergoing Chronic Peritoneal Dialysis.** Michael J. Blumenkrantz, Nancy Gallagher, Richard A. Bashore, and Henry Tenckhoff reviewed the records of 11 female patients, aged 15 to 50 years (mean, 38.8), who had a history of menstrual bleeding after the start of maintenance peritoneal dialysis. In 8 patients menstruation had ceased before dialysis. One had primary amenorrhea. At the time of study, 5 women were no longer undergoing peritoneal dialysis; 3 had had successful renal transplantation and 2 were undergoing hemodialysis. Peritoneal fluid was collected from 3 women on several occasions.

Eight of the 11 women developed secondary amenorrhea when chronic renal failure developed, and all resumed menstruating after peritoneal dialysis was stated. The mean interval to resumption was 7.7 months. Five patients had regular menses after the start of dialysis. All patients but 2 had small amounts of blood in the peritoneal catheter, or in the effluent dialysate, or both, at the time of menstruation, a few days before onset of vaginal bleeding. The blood usually persisted during the first day of menstrual flow. None of the 6 patients operated on exhibited endometriosis. No patient required blood transfusions once stabilized on peritoneal dialysis. No definite evidence of endometrial or tubular epithelial cells in the peritoneal effluent or aspirate was obtained.

Retrograde menstrual bleeding into the peritoneal cavity appears to be the rule in women undergoing peritoneal dialysis and possibly occurs in all menstruating women. This tends to support Sampson's concept of retrograde menstrual bleeding as the likeliest and most frequent cause of pelvic endometriosis.

In an addendum, the authors report having treated more patients who menstruated while being maintained on peritoneal dialysis. All showed evidence of retrograde bleeding, except 1 patient who had undergone tubal ligation.

▶ [This article adds information in two areas, one clinical and one more basic. First, when one is asked about blood in the peritoneal dialysate in the premenstruum (as we recently were), reassuurance can be given that this is not only a common event, but apparently is usual. Second, retrograde menstruation is probably the rule, rather than the exception. It is interesting that the blood was noted *prior* to the appearance of vaginal bleeding and on the first day of menstruation.] ◀

(14–25)   Obstet. Gynecol. 57:667–670, May 1981.

14-26 **A Role for Prostacyclin (PGI$_2$) in Excessive Menstrual Bleeding.** S. K. Smith, R. W. Kelly, M. H. Abel, and David T. Baird (Univ. of Edinburgh) studied the synthesis of prostanoids from arachidonic acid incubated with endometrium (from the luteal phase of the menstrual cycle) alone or together with myometrium without obvious abnormality; endometrium was obtained from 6 women with excessive menstrual blood loss (range, 57–186 ml; median, 86 ml).

Production of prostaglandins (PGs) $F_{2\alpha}$, E_2, and D_2 was similar to that observed for the endometrium of 7 women with normal periods (range, 5–50 ml; median, 11 ml). However, production of 6-oxo-$PGF_{1\alpha}$, the stable metabolite of prostacyclin (PGI$_2$), by endometrium incubated with a control myometrium preparation (removed in the secretory phase of the menstrual cycle) was threefold greater in the group with excessive menstrual blood loss than in the control group. In both groups, the combined incubations synthesized more 6-oxo-$PGF_{1\alpha}$ than did endometrium incubated alone, but less $PGF_{2\alpha}$, PGE_2, or PGD_2.

That the synthesis of 6-oxo-$PGF_{1\alpha}$ is enhanced by combination of myometrium with endometrium suggests that endoperoxides synthesized from arachidonic acid by the endometrium are converted to 6-oxo-$PGF_{1\alpha}$ by myometrium that contains the enzymes necessary for the synthesis of PGI$_2$. The ability of the uterus to generate PGI$_2$, which is known to inhibit platelet aggregation and stimulate vasodilatation, may influence the degree and duration of menstrual bleeding.

▶ [Prostaglandin production differed if endometrium was incubated with normal myometrium rather than if it was incubated alone. In the presence of myometrium there were lower levels of $PGF_{2\alpha}$ and PGE_2, but higher levels of the metabolite of PGI$_2$ (prostacyclin). This last compound causes vasodilation and inhibits platelet aggregation. It is interesting that those patients with excessive menstrual bleeding had higher PGI$_2$ metabolite levels.] ◀

14-27 **Prostaglandins in Primary Dysmenorrhea: Comparison of Prophylactic and Nonprophylactic Treatment With Ibuprofen and Use of Oral Contraceptives.** W. Y. Chan, M. Yusoff Dawood, and Fritz Fuchs (Cornell Univ.) monitored menstrual prostaglandin release using tampon specimens in 14 dysmenorrheic subjects before and during treatment with a prostaglandin synthetase inhibitor, ibuprofen (Motrin), in a controlled double-blind, crossover trial, and in 2 dysmenorrheic subjects while they were taking combination-type oral contraceptives and while they were not (total of 89 ovulatory cycles studied). Prophylactic and therapeutic (nonprophylactic) regimens of ibuprofen were given. In the prophylactic regimen, 8 patients were instructed to take 1 tablet (400 mg) 4 times a day, beginning 3 days before expected onset of menses through 3 days after onset of menses, with therapy not to exceed 7 consecutive days in any cycle. In the therapeutic regimen, 6 patients were instructed to take 2 tablets at the first sign of menses, then 1 tablet 4 times a day for 3 days. Severity of dysmenorrhea was assessed by the patients and by a clinician

(14–26) Lancet 1:522–524, Mar. 7, 1981.
(14–27) Am. J. Med. 70:535–541, March 1981.

during an office visit between the second and third day of menstruation. Total prostaglandin bioactivity in menstrual fluid was monitored by bioassays.

Ibuprofen reduced menstrual prostaglandin release and significantly relieved dysmenorrhea, but placebo did not. The efficacy of the therapeutic regimen equalled that of the prophylactic regimen. Oral contraceptives decreased menstrual flow, reduced prostaglandin release, and alleviated dysmenorrhea. Radioimmunoassays showed that $PGF_{2\alpha}$ is the principal prostaglandin in menstrual fluid. In nearly all samples measured, prostaglandin activity determined by bioassays was 20%–40% greater than the sum total of $PGF_{2\alpha}$ and PGE_2 determined by radioimmunoassays. There was a positive correlation between the severity of dysmenorrhea and the level of menstrual prostaglandin released during the corresponding period. No side effects were noted in any patient receiving ibuprofen.

It is concluded that primary dysmenorrhea is related to a high level of menstrual prostaglandin release. Ibuprofen inhibits prostaglandin synthesis, whereas oral contraceptives inhibit ovulation and cyclic endometrial development. Ibuprofen is not known to suppress endometrial growth and does not reduce menstrual flow significantly. Thus, the two drugs suppress endometrial prostaglandin through different mechanisms. Reduction of menstrual prostaglandin release leads to alleviation of dysmenorrhea. The portion of bioassay activity that was in excess of radioimmunoassay activity could be active prostaglandin intermediates and metabolites or unknown prostaglandins. Problems with the prophylactic ibuprofen regimen include difficulty in accurately predicting date of onset of menses and potential danger of exposing an early embryo to prostaglandin synthetase inhibitors, should the patient become pregnant in that cycle. The therapeutic regimen should be preferred as it reduces treatment to 2 or 3 days per menstrual cycle. The long-term effect of ibuprofen in a young population is unknown. For patients with severe dysmenorrhea, or when adequate relief is not obtained by the therapeutic regimen, prophylactic therapy may make the difference between a poor and good response. The remarkable response in the patients studied, all nulliparous and younger than age 25, may not be extrapolated to all patients with dysmenorrhea. Treatment of dysmenorrhea by oral contraceptives cannot be advocated, in view of their endocrine and metabolic effects, unless contraception is desired.

▶ [This report represents an expanded version of a preliminary study abstracted in the 1981 YEAR BOOK (pp. 357–358) that we referred to as the "nail in the coffin" regarding the causative relationship between uterine prostaglandin production and primary dysmenorrhea. What is new in this study is the comparison between prophylactic and therapeutic regimens. Theoretically, a prostaglandin synthetase inhibitor should be more effective prophylactically than therapeutically. Yet, there was no apparent difference with respect to whether the medication was started 1 to 3 days before menses or at the onset of flow.] ◀

14–28 **Treatment of Endometriosis: A Study of Medical Management.** A. D. Noble and A. T. Letchworth (Royal Hampshire County

(14–28) Br. J. Obstet. Gynaecol. 87:726–728, August 1980.

Hosp., Winchester) treated 50 patients with endometriosis with hormones: 27 with danazol and 23 with Enovid. These patients had presented with infertility or with symptoms and signs of endometriosis. The diagnosis was confirmed at laparotomy or laparoscopy. Patients were allocated for treatment at random. In each case, treatment was started with a low dose (100 mg of danazol twice daily or 5 mg of Enovid twice daily) and the dose was increased progressively until the patient was amenorrheic. It had been intended to treat each patient for 6 months. In the early part of the study, however unnecessarily high doses of Enovid were given, and in 7 patients who had severe side effects, treatment was discontinued prematurely. Each patient was cautioned to restrict calorie intake but was not warned of other side effects. After 6 months a second laparoscopy was done, and the physical signs at this time were contrasted with the pretreatment grading.

In the group treated with danazol, only 6 of 27 patients needed a dose greater than 400 mg daily. Side effects were a signficant problem. One patient who was taking danazol complained of a hoarse voice, so treatment was stopped. In the Enovid-treated group, 7 of 23 patients failed to complete treatment because of side effects suggesting vascular or clotting dangers. In the danazol-treated group, 44% had side effects, whereas 87% of the Enovid-treated group had side effects. The main symptoms were dyspareunia, dysmenorrhea, and other menstrual abnormalities. Danazol was superior to Enovid in relieving symptoms. Danazol completely relieved or improved symptoms in 20 of 23 patients, whereas Enovid relieved or improved symptoms in 5 of 14 patients.

Thirty patients with fertile husbands complained of infertility. More patients became pregnant after treatment with danazol (9 of 16, 56%) than after Enovid (4 of 11, 29%). Some patients also showed evidence of inadequate progesterone secretion; they subsequently were treated with clomiphene or human chorionic gonadotropin. Treatment with danazol was often successful in ablating or dramatically improving physical signs, especially when the disease was not advanced. There was little change when the disease was associated with dense fibrosis and adhesion formation or when large endometriomas were present. In the Enovid group, only 2 patients had their physical signs ablated. Usually, the plaques changed their appearance, looking edematous and granulomatous rather than smaller in size.

Where endometriosis lends itself to operative excision or destruction, operation should be done. Medical therapy may be considered for patients who do not have discrete localized lesions amenable to surgical extirpation and whose uterus is normally positioned. Medical treatment also may be recommended after an operation if scattered plaques of disease remain.

▶ [In this small series of patients with endometriosis treated medically, danazol got better marks than did a combination oral contraceptive. Medical therapy was not helpful if extensive disease was present.] ◀

14–29 **Dosage Aspects of Danazol Therapy in Endometriosis: Short-Term and Long-Term Effectiveness.** Danazol appears to be the most effective medical treatment for endometriosis. The presently recommended dosage is 400 mg twice daily for 6 months. K. O. Biberoglu and S. J. Behrman (Royal Oak, Mich.) evaluated the efficacy of lower doses of danazol for the relief of surgically confirmed endometriosis in 32 women. Eight patients each received 100, 200, 400, or 600 mg of danazol daily for 6 months. The medication was given twice a day.

Two patients withdrew because of side effects at 3 months. The symptomatic response is shown in Table 1, and the response of positive pelvic findings is given in Table 2. The pelvic findings generally responded more slowly. Both clinical improvement and suppression of the cyclic menstrual pattern were most significant after 4 months of treatment, and a gradual decline in effectiveness ensued. On completion of treatment, 14% of the patients treated with 100 mg, half of those receiving 200 mg, 14% of those receiving 400 mg, and half of those receiving 600 mg were entirely free of endometriosis. When endometriomas were excluded, the respective figures were 14.2%, 62.5%, 57.1%, and 87.5%. Five patients conceived, for a corrected pregnancy rate of 45.4%; 3 had received 600 mg of danazol. Lower doses generally did not cause fewer side effects than the 600-mg dose. The most common side effects were weight gain and increased hair

TABLE 1.—RESPONSE OF SYMPTOMATOLOGY
WITH TIME DURING THERAPY

Percentage of symptomatic relief with danazol

Months	100 mg/day	200 mg/day	400 mg/day	600 mg/day
1	37	61	60	71
2	67	58	63	75
3	66	68	63	85
4	83	77	64	87
5	74	87	72	96
6	54	86	74	96

TABLE 2.—RESPONSE OF POSITIVE PELVIC EXAMINATION
FINDINGS WITH TIME DURING THERAPY

Percentage of improvement in findings with danazol

Months	100 mg/day	200 mg/day	400 mg/day	600 mg/day
1	42	24	32	40
2	46	47	40	62
3	67	67	41	75
4	86	69	58	75
5	80	69	62	88
6	67	79	66	91

(14–29) Am. J. Obstet. Gynecol. 139:645–654, Mar. 15, 1981.

growth. The average symptomatic recurrence rate was 36%, the mean interval being 19 months after completion of treatment.

Lower doses of danazol can produce beneficial effects similar to those obtained with 800 mg daily in the treatment of documented pelvic endometriosis. A dosage of 200 mg daily for 6 months is the lowest possible regimen. A dose of 400 mg daily may be given initially and the dosage adjusted according to the clinical response. Infertile women with mild to moderate endometriosis are the best candidates for danazol therapy. If extensive disease and distortion of pelvic organs are present, danazol may be useful before or after surgery.

▶ [The aim of this study was to evaluate danazol dosages of less than the "standard" 800-mg daily dose in endometriosis. Doses of 100, 200, 400, and 600 mg were compared in a double-blind assessment of both subjective and objective response. In general, the results indicate similar beneficial effects with all doses, although at the lower level (especially 100 mg), symptomatic response was somewhat slower, several patients experienced "rebound" of symptoms during therapy, and symptomatic recurrence after completion was more common. Somewhat curiously, there was no clear relationship between dose and side effects. From these observations, it appears that a starting dose of 200 or 400 mg daily would be reasonable and would result in similar clinical effect, at a substantial cost saving, in comparison with the recommended 800-mg regimen.] ◀

14–30 **Pituitary-Ovarian Function in Normal Women During Menopausal Transition.** As women approach the menopause, their previously regular menstrual cycles suddenly become irregular. In young and old women the interrelation between pituitary and ovarian hormones is well established, but little is known of hormone patterns in perimenopausal women. Mary G. Metcalf, R.A. Donald, and J.H. Livesey (Christchurch, New Zealand) measured concentrations of FSH, LH, estrogens, and pregnanediol in weekly urine samples collected for 14 to 87 weeks (median, 43 weeks) from 31 perimenopausal women aged 36 to 55 years (median, 50 years). The results were compared with those in 22 postmenopausal women (mean age, 55 years) whose last menstrual period had occurred 1 to 14 years previously and in 20 premenopausal women (mean age, 44 years) who had regular, ovulatory, menstrual cycles.

The hormone patterns observed in the perimenopausal women varied widely, both between women and from time to time in the same woman. They ranged from ovulatory cycles with low premenopausal concentrations of FSH, to transient episodes indistinguishable from those found in postmenopausal women with high FSH and LH concentrations. Between these extremes were three patterns rarely seen at other times in reproductive life. (1) In 14 women on 32 occasions lasting 2 to 9 weeks, postmenopausal FSH and LH concentrations occurred in association with high estrogen values. (2) In 18 women on 30 occasions lasting 2 to 8 weeks, there was an elevation of LH (but no elevation of FSH) into the postmenopausal range. (3) In 13 women on 26 occasions lasting 1 to 2 weeks, there was a FSH elevation (but no LH elevation) into the postmenopausal range. These patterns were not seen in any of the premenopausal women.

(14–30) Clin. Endocrinol. 14:245–255, March 1981.

Typically, the approach of the menopause was marked by an increased incidence of high postmenopausal concentrations of FSH and LH. Ovulatory cycles were observed at all stages in the perimenopause and occurred within 16 weeks of the last menstrual period in 7 of the 13 women who became postmenopausal during the study.

The appearance of high FSH and LH concentrations characterizes the perimenopause and often precedes sustained loss of sex hormone secretion by the aging ovary. However, postmenopausal biochemical measurements are no guarantee of the postmenopausal state.

▶ [This extensive study of 31 perimenopausal women makes several interesting points. There is no one typical hormone pattern at this time. Ovulation (as indicated by elevated urinary pregnanediol levels) occurred in most women with cycle lengths of 18 to 35 days and was not rare with longer intervals. Transient elevations of gonadotropins into the menopausal range were common, and these often persisted despite elevated estrogen levels. The authors suggest that gonadotropin release at this time is particularly sensitive to falling estrogen levels and is resistant to inhibition by rising estrogen levels. The fact that apparently ovulatory cycles occurred within 16 weeks of the last menstrual period in 7 of the 13 women who became postmenopausal during the study suggests that we should not be too casual in discussing contraception with perimenopausal women.] ◀

14–31 **Objectively Recorded Hot Flushes in Patients With Pituitary Insufficiency.** Subjective hot flushes have been related temporally to pulsatile secretion of luteinizing hormone (LH) and elevated finger skin temperature. Mulley et al. described two patients with hot flushes that followed hypophysectomy, suggesting involvement of the hypothalamus. David R. Meldrum, Yohanan Erlik, John K.H. Lu, and Howard L. Judd (Univ. of California, Los Angeles) attempted to determine whether patients with pituitary insufficiency have objectively measurable hot flushes similar to those experienced by postmenopausal women, and whether these episodes occur in the absence of augmented LH secretion.

Two young women, aged 23 and 25, with pituitary insufficiency and symptoms of hot flushes were studied. Skin temperature was continuously recorded at the finger and skin resistance over the sternum. Twelve subjective hot flushes occurred during 10 hours of recording. Each was associated with a rise in finger temperature of more than 1 C, and 85% were associated with measurable falls in skin resistance. The changes were identical with those observed in symptomatic postmenopausal women. Circulating gonadotropin concentrations were in the low to low-normal range and indicated minimal pulsatile LH release. Finger temperature changes were not significantly correlated with LH concentrations in either subject.

The findings suggest that the apparent association between pulsatile LH release and the occurrence of hot flushes in postmenopausal women cannot be attributed to augmented LH secretion per se. It instead may be due to hypothalamic factors involved in pulsatile LH release. The limited pulsatile release observed in these two subjects probably represents a maximum response of remaining gonadotrophs to heightened pulsatile secretion of gonadotropin-releasing hormone (GnRH) from the hypothalamus. Some of the hypothalamic neurons

(14–31) J. Clin. Endocrinol. Metab. 52:684–687, April 1981.

that contain GnRH are closely related anatomically to the preoptic-anterior nuclei that regulate body temperature, suggesting that neurotransmitter signals associated with GnRH release may modify thermoregulating neurons and trigger a hot flush.

▶ [Menopausal hot flushes have been found to coincide with gonadotropin pulsations. However, hypophysectomized patients have been reported to experience hot flushes (and this article documents their occurrence by objective skin temperature recording), indicating that LH itself is not involved directly. It must be that something that causes LH release, such as luteinizing hormone-releasing factor, by some manner leads to vasomotor flushing.] ◀

14–32 **Biologic Effects of Various Doses of Conjugated Equine Estrogens in Postmenopausal Women.** In order to determine which estrogen dosage might provide postmenopausal physiologic replacement while avoiding harmful side effects, Flor L. Geola, Anthony M. Frumar, Ivanna V. Tataryn, K. H. Lu, Jerome M. Hershman, Peter Eggena, Mohinder P. Sambhi, and Howard L. Judd conducted a prospective study of the effects of various oral doses of conjugated equine estrogens (0.15, 0.30, 0.625, and 1.25 mg/day for 6 weeks) on biologic and biochemical indicators of estrogenic activity in 21 postmenopausal women. Fifteen premenopausal women with presumably normal physiologic function served as controls.

Both LH and FSH showed decremental decreases with increasing doses of estrogen, though the levels remained significantly higher than control values, even at the highest dosage used. The minimum doses of estrogen that induced significant reductions in the gonadotropins were 0.625 and 0.3 mg for LH and FSH, respectively. Only the 1.25-mg dose caused a change in the vaginal cytology maturation index to values similar to those found in the premenopausal control subjects. The smallest dose that caused a significant decrease in the calcium-creatinine ratio was 0.3 mg. The 0.3-mg dose was the smallest dose that produced a significant increase in renin substrate. The effects of estrogen on sex hormone-binding globulin and thyroid-binding globulin varied widely.

The results indicate that conjugated equine estrogens have variable effects at the sites of action. All of the doses were associated with subphysiologic, physiologic, and pharmacologic responses, but none provided physiologic replacement for all of the functions studied.

▶ [It is a general principle of therapeutics that the minimal effective dose should be used. This article reports a study designed to elucidate the dose-response relationships with respect to conjugated estrogens as hormone replacement therapy postmenopausally. The results indicate, not surprisingly, that the minimal effective dose varies with the variable being measured, and within each variable there is usually a dose response relationship. Gonadotropin levels were suppressed with 0.3 to 0.625 mg, but even with the maximal dose (1.25 mg) there was not suppression to the levels in menstruating women. Restoration of the vaginal epithelium to a normal pattern required 1.25 mg, whereas suppression of the fasting urine calcium-creatinine ratio (an index of bone resorption) was accomplished with as little as 0.3 mg. Two important effects not assessed in this study were endometrial proliferation and relief of hot flushes. The latter, in our experience, usually can be achieved with 0.3 mg, and this amount, again in our experience, usually does not cause bleeding. Thus, we will continue to use 0.3 mg as our "standard" dose.] ◀

(14–32) J. Clin. Endocrinol. Metab. 51:620–625, September 1980.

14–33 Endometrial Findings in Asymptomatic Postmenopausal Women on Exogenous Estrogens: Preliminary Report. Retrospective studies have implicated estrogen replacement therapy as a factor in the increased incidence of endometrial cancer. Donald A. Simsen, Steven R. Shirts, Fred M. Howard, Jerry Sims, and Jay M. Hill (Fitzsimons Army Med. Center, Aurora, Colo.) prospectively studied 94 asymptomatic postmenopausal women who had received exogenous estrogen therapy for 1 to more than 5 years. All patients underwent office endometrial biopsy.

The mean age of 71 patients (75.5%) with negative biopsies was 53.7 years; duration of therapy was less than 3 years in 26 (37%) and 3 years or greater in 45 (63%). Twenty patients (28%) had one or more risk factors (obesity, infertility, diabetes, hypertension, delayed menopause, estrogen-secreting ovarian tumors, and polycystic ovarian syndrome). There were 23 patients (24.4%, mean age, 58.9 years) with abnormal biopsy results confirmed by endometrial curettage: simple or cystic hyperplasia (14%), adenomatous hyperplasia (6.4%), atypical adenomatous hyperplasia (2.1%), and well-differentiated adenocarcinoma (1.1%). Duration of the therapy was less than 3 years in 4 patients (17%) and 3 years or greater in 19 (83%). Curettage specimens showed either no lesion remaining or a lesion similar to the office specimen. Risk factors were present in only 4 patients (17%). None of 9 patients with significant precursor lesions or adenocarcinoma had any standard risk factors. Of 29 other postmenopausal patients receiving estrogen with postmenopausal bleeding, 16 patients (median age, 48.3 years) had benign biopsy findings (55.2%) and 13 (median age, 56.1 years) had abnormal results (44.8%). No curettage specimens showed a more progressive lesion than the office biopsy specimen. Six patients with adenomatous hyperplasia (20.7%) had taken conjugated estrogens for 3 years or more. There were no statistical differences between groups in estrogen dose or regimen. Duration of therapy and risk factors were similar in both groups.

It is not possible to predict which patient receiving estrogen is a higher risk for endometrial hyperplasia, and to avoid missing precursor lesions in endometrial carcinoma, all patients must undergo biopsy. Significant cancer precursor lesions did not appear until patients had been receiving unopposed estrogen replacement therapy for at least 3 years. A safe practice would be to do a pretreatment endometrial biopsy, and if normal, follow with repeated biopsy in 3 years. Office biopsy is believed to be adequate for staging endometrial carcinoma if uterine sounding for depth plus a separate endocervical scraping to rule out cervical involvement are accomplished.

▶ [The results of this study make a convincing case for routine periodic endometrial sampling in patients receiving postmenopausal estrogen replacement.] ◀

14–34 Prevention of Early Postmenopausal Bone Loss: Controlled 2-Year Study in 315 Normal Females. Several therapeutic regimens for osteoporosis are widely used, although their effectiveness has not been established clearly. Recently, controlled trials have dem-

(14–33) Gynecol. Oncol. 11:56–63, February 1981.
(14–34) Eur. J. Clin. Invest. 10:273–279, August 1980.

onstrated that estrogen replacement therapy prevents bone loss in postmenopausal women. Claus Christiansen, Merete S. Christensen, Peter McNair, Clause Hagen, Knud-Erik Stocklund, and Ib Transbøl conducted a controlled, double-blind study of 2 years' duration to assess the effectiveness of various regimens in the prevention of bone loss in menopausal women. Three hundred fifteen healthy women in their early natural menopause were assigned randomly to 7 treatment and 3 placebo groups: 17 β-estradiol, estriol, and sequential norethisterone (hormones); 5 mg of bendroflumethiazide (thiazide) per day; hormones and thiazide; 20 mg of sodium fluoride per day; 2,000 IU of vitamin D_3 (D_3) per day; fluoride and D_3; and 0.25 μg 1α-(OH)-vitamin D_3 (1α-D_3) per day. All subjects received a daily 500-mg calcium supplement. Bone mineral content of both forearms was measured every 3 months using a very precise photon absorptiometric method. Serum mineral concentrations and urinary calcium excretion were determined by standard procedures.

Fig 14–5.—Bone mineral content in early postmenopausal women before and during 2 years' treatment in 8 different groups. Values given as mean ± 1 SEM. *HORM.*, hormone; *THIAZ.*, thiazide; D_3, vitamin D_3; $1\alpha\,D_3$, 1α-(OH)-vitamin D_3. (Courtesy of Christiansen, C., et al.: Eur. J. Clin. Invest. 10:273–279, August 1980; Berlin-Heidelberg-New York: Springer.)

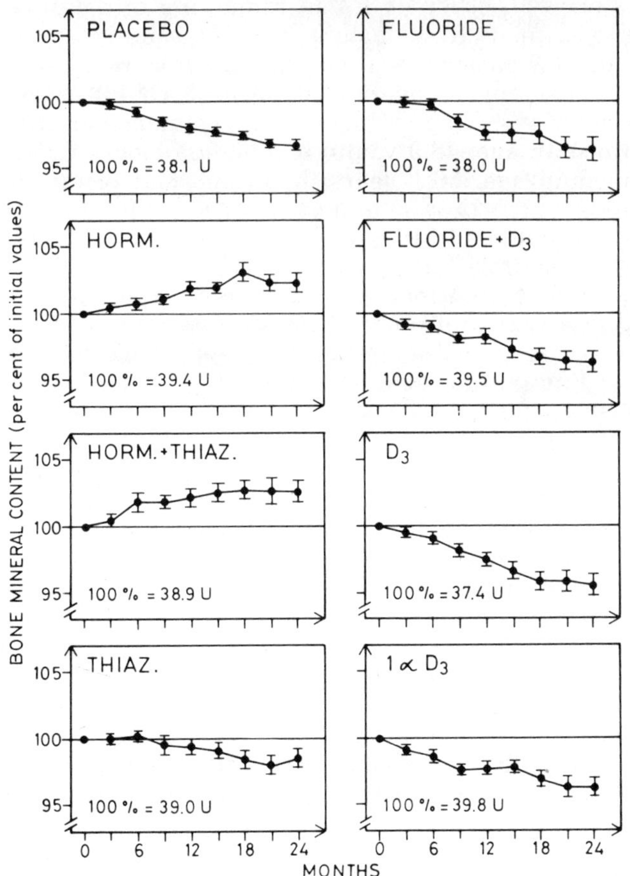

Over the 2-year study period, bone mineral content decreased an average of 3.3% in the combined placebo groups (Fig 14–5). Subjects treated with hormones and hormones plus thiazide showed a 2.5% increase in bone mineral content, with the most pronounced increase occurring in the first year (2%). Treatment with thiazide alone postponed the overall 1.5% decrease in bone mineral content for 6 months. After 2 years, the mean decrease in bone mineral content was 3.6%, 3.7%, and 4.5% for subjects treated with sodium fluoride, sodium fluoride and D_3, and D_3, respectively. The mean decrease in bone mineral content was 3.7% in subjects receiving $1\alpha D_3$.

Hormone treatment established regular withdrawal bleeding in 38 of 43 women. There were no adverse cardiovascular reactions, nor did any cases of endometrial cancer develop.

The results indicate that the early loss of bone mineral after natural menopause was prevented only by combined estrogen-gestagen and calcium treatment, among the regimens tested.

▶ [This study involved the randomized comparison of several methods claimed to prevent postmenopausal bone loss. Only those therapeutic regimens including estrogen were effective; others (thiazide, fluoride, vitamin D) led to bone mineral loss at a rate indistinguishable from placebo. These results seem to indicate that there is no substitute for sex hormones in preventing osteoporosis.

Most previous studies of bone effects of postmenopausal estrogen have focused on peripheral bone. Lindsay and associates (*Lancet* 2:1151, 1980) reported vertebral observations from a controlled study of mestranol-treated women followed for 6 to 12 years after oophorectomy. Estrogen replacement prevented loss of height and vertebral compression, as well as peripheral bone loss.] ◀

14–35 **Bone Mass in Postmenopausal Women After Withdrawal of Estrogen-Gestagen Replacement Therapy.** Postmenopausal administration of estrogens prevents loss of skeletal calcium and thus reduces the fracture rate in elderly women, but it increases the risk of endometrial cancer. The postulated long-term benefit of temporary estrogen therapy on postmenopausal bone mass has been questioned. Claus Christiansen, Merete Sanvig Christensen, and Ib Transbøl (Univ. of Copenhagen) studied the effects of estrogen-gestagen treatment on bone mass in normal women soon after the menopause, with particular emphasis on the rate of bone loss after cessation of treatment.

Of 94 healthy women who had passed a natural menopause 6 months to 3 years before, 43 received estrogen-gestagen treatment for 2 years. Treatment was with 4 mg of 17β-estradiol and 2 mg of estriol on days 1 to 12, 4 mg of 17β-estradiol, 2 mg of estriol, and 1 mg of norethisterone acetate on days 13 to 22, and 1 mg of 17β-estradiol and 0.5 mg of estriol on days 23 to 28. The other 51 women were given placebo. Seventy-seven of the total group were then followed for a third year, during which they were randomized into four subgroups: hormone treatment continued, hormone treatment replaced by placebo, placebo continued, or placebo replaced by hormone treatment. All women received 0.5 gm of calcium daily. Forearm bone mineral content was measured by photon absorptiometry every 3 months for 3 years.

(14–35) Lancet 1:459–461, Feb. 28, 1981.

In the group receiving hormone therapy for all 3 years, mean bone mineral content increased 1.9% after 1 year of treatment, 2.5% after 2 years, and 3.7% after 3 years. In the groups receiving placebo for 2 years followed by hormones for 1 year, bone mineral content increased by 1.4% during the year of hormone replacement. In the group receiving placebo for all 3 years, there was a virtually linear fall in bone mineral content of 1.9% per year. In the group receiving hormone therapy for 2 years followed by placebo for 1 year, withdrawal of hormone replacement induced an annual fall in bone mineral content of 2.3%. The annual rate of bone loss after discontinuance of hormone therapy was identical with that of women receiving only placebo.

Even temporary hormone replacement therapy after menopause has a lasting beneficial effect on bone mass.

▶ [The principal conclusion of this study—that even relatively short-term postmenopausal hormone replacement has lasting benefit on bone density—is in contrast to that of a report abstracted in the 1979 YEAR BOOK (p. 350) in which bone loss seemed to accelerate after hormones were discontinued, implying that indefinite use might be necessary. The question is one of obvious clinical importance.] ◀

14–36 **Decreased Risk of Fractures of the Hip and Lower Forearm With Postmenopausal Use of Estrogens.** Estrogens have been shown to retard the age-related decrease in bone density in postmenopausal women. However, the magnitude of prevention against bone fractures provided by estrogen treatment has not been documented. To assess the preventive effect of estrogens on bone fracture, Noel S. Weiss, Carol L. Ure, Jude H. Ballard, Ann R. Williams, and Janet R. Daling (Univ. of Washington, Seattle) interviewed 327 women, who at the time of their treatment for fracture of the hip or lower forearm were 50 to 74 years of age, as to their use of estrogen preparations. A total of 567 randomly selected women of similar age and from the same region served as controls. Subjects with hip fractures and those with forearm fractures had identical patterns of estrogen use and thus were regarded as one group.

MENOPAUSAL ESTROGEN USE AMONG 320 PATIENTS WITH FRACTURE AND 567 CONTROLS, ACCORDING TO DURATION OF USE

DURATION OF USE	CASES	CONTROLS	RELATIVE RISK *	95 PER CENT CONFIDENCE INTERVAL †
yr		*per cent*		
No use ‡	66	48	1.0	—
1–2	10	9	0.84	0.51–1.4
3–5	9	10	0.89	0.54–1.4
6–9	5	12	0.38	0.22–0.66
≥10	11	21	0.46	0.30–0.69

*Standardized for age group (50–59, 60–69, and 70–74 years), history of hysterectomy, and current versus past use of estrogens, by the method of Mantel and Haenszel.

†Approximate values, by the method of Miettinen.

‡Includes women using estrogens for less than 1 year.

(14–36) N. Engl. J. Med. 303:1195–1198, Nov. 20, 1980.

The estimated risk of fracture during the first 5 years of estrogen use was slightly lower among users than nonusers; however, when the duration of estrogen use was longer than 5 years, the estimated risk of fracture among users was only 40% to 50% that for nonusers (table). The decreased risk of fracture was most pronounced among current users; women who had discontinued use for 3 years or more were at the same risk as nonusers. There was no difference in estimated risk on the basis of dosage (0.625 mg/day vs 1.25 mg/day).

The results support the findings of other studies that estrogens can retard the development of osteoporosis in postmenopausal women and strongly suggest that the decreased risk of hip and forearm fractures should be regarded as a benefit of long-term estrogen use in postmenopausal women.

▶ [This report confirms a previous case-control study (1981 YEAR BOOK, p. 349) and indicates that estrogen use is associated with a decreased risk of hip and forearm fractures in postmenopausal women. This benefit must be viewed alongside the endometrial cancer risk when one is considering estrogen therapy in the menopausal patient. For a thorough discussion of this important topic, see Stanley Birnbaum's special article "Estrogen Therapy in the Menopause," in this edition of the YEAR BOOK.] ◀

14–37 **Increased Incidence of Symptomatic Cholesterol Cholelithiasis in Perimenopausal Women Receiving Estrogen Replacement Therapy: Retrospective Study.** Louis H. Honoré (St. John's, Newfoundland) reviewed data on 262 symptomatic perimenopausal women diagnosed as having cholesterol cholelithiasis to assess the possible association between estrogen replacement therapy and symptomatic cholesterol cholelithiasis. Two hundred ninety women surgically treated for diseases unassociated with estrogen replacement therapy served as controls.

Of the 262 patients with gallstones, 25 had received estrogen replacement therapy for periods of 6 months to 13 years; 23 had received conjugated estrogens and 2, esterified estrogen. Only 8 of the controls had received estrogen therapy. With the use of the Mantel-Haenzel method of analysis, the approximate relative risk of symptomatic cholelithiasis developing in patients who received estrogen replacement therapy was calculated to be 3.72 ($P < .005$). The effect of obesity on the development of cholesterol cholelithiasis also was confirmed. Estrogen therapy and obesity, however, were independent, not additive, factors in the development of cholesterol gallstones, because estrogen therapy increased the risk of cholelithiasis at all weight levels.

Because the risk of cholesterol cholelithiasis developing in perimenopausal women who take estrogens is increased, emphasis should be placed on the prevention and early diagnosis of cholelithiasis.

▶ [In this study, 25 of 262 patients with symptomatic gallstones had been taking estrogen replacement therapy, compared with only 8 of 290 matched controls. The difference is statistically significant, suggesting that estrogen increases the risk of cholesterol cholelithiasis. The study is a retrospective one, with the usual caveat about the appropriateness of matching controls.] ◀

(14–37) J. Reprod. Med. 25:187–190, October 1980.

14–38 **Menopausal Estrogen Therapy and Protection From Death From Ischemic Heart Disease.** Until recently, estrogen replacement therapy in menopause was thought to reduce the risk of coronary artery disease, but several observations have cast doubt on this hypothesis. Ronald K. Ross, Annlia Paganini-Hill, Thomas M. Mack, Mary Arthur, and Brian E. Henderson (Univ. of Southern California, Los Angeles) examined the association between estrogen replacement therapy and death from coronary artery disease, using medical records of a Los Angeles retirement community as the data source for evidence of past estrogen use. Women dying of ischemic heart disease during a 5-year period were compared with living and deceased control groups, matched with the study patients for date of birth, time of entry into the community, race, and socioeconomic status. The deceased cohort was also matched for date of death.

Most well-known risk factors for ischemic heart disease were significant risk factors for death from ischemic heart disease whether comparison was with the living or the deceased control subjects. Patients using conjugated estrogens had a risk ratio for death from ischemic heart disease of 0.43, compared with the living control subjects, and a similar relative risk compared with deceased control subjects. The association could not be attributed to identifiable confounding factors.

These findings suggest that estrogen replacement therapy in postmenopausal women may protect against death from ischemic heart disease, although the mechanism of such an effect is not obvious. Age-adjusted death rates from ischemic heart disease in white women in the United States are more than 4 times the combined mortality from breast and endometrial cancers. If the protective effect of estrogen replacement therapy against fatal ischemic heart disease is confirmed, the benefit would far outweigh any carcinogenic effects of estrogens.

▶ [As we have said many times before, retrospective case-control studies are difficult to interpret. How good are the controls? Do unaccounted-for confounding variables explain the differences in "risk ratios" reported? Even with this uncertainty, the results reported here are encouraging. Estrogen use was associated with a decreased risk of death from ischemic heart disease in these postmenopausal women.] ◀

14–39 **Lipid Metabolic Studies in Oophorectomized Women: Effects Induced by Two Different Estrogens on Serum Lipids and Lipoproteins.** Some studies have indicated a qualitative difference between the effects of synthetic estrogens (17-alkylated) and natural estrogens (nonalkylated) on lipid metabolism. G. Silfverstolpe, A. Gustafson, G. Samsioe, and A. Svanborg (Sahlgrenska Hosp., Göteborg, Sweden) evaluated the effects of orally administered ethinyl estradiol (EE) and estradiol valerianate (E_2V) on lipid metabolism in 11 oophorectomized women. Each estrogen was administered separately for 6 weeks preceded by a minimum of 4 weeks without hormonal replacement therapy. Ethinyl estradiol (20 µg/day) administration was begun 6 weeks after hysterectomy and E_2V (2 mg/day)

(14–38) Lancet 1:858–860, Apr. 18, 1981.
(14–39) Gynecol. Obstet. Invest. 11:161–169, 1980.

was given 6–12 months later. Blood samples were obtained before and after the course of estrogen therapy and 3 fractions of lipoproteins were isolated: very low-density lipoproteins (VLDL), low-density lipoproteins (LDL), and high-density lipoproteins (HDL). Serum levels of phospholipids, cholesterol, and triglycerides were measured.

Ethinyl estradiol caused an increase in total serum triglyceride and phospholipid levels as well as LDL triglyceride levels. Estradiol valerianate caused a decrease in total serum triglyceride levels as well as levels of VLDL total lipids and phospholipids, total and free cholesterol, and triglycerides. Estradiol valerianate also decreased levels of LDL total lipids and phospholipids, total and free cholesterol, and triglycerides. High-density lipoprotein total lipid levels were increased by E_2V as a result of increases in levels of phospholipids and total cholesterol. A positive correlation was observed between plasma insulin values during oral glucose tolerance tests and VLDL triglyceride levels after administration of E_2V. This supports the contention that insulin influences the production rate of hepatic triglyceride.

The results indicate that the most marked difference between EE and E_2V is in triglyceride metabolism. The fact that E_2V increased HDL cholesterol levels but not triglyceride levels suggests that the effect of E_2V is more physiologic than that of EE.

▶ [This study compares the effects of estrogen replacement with "natural" and "synthetic" agents on serum lipids. The major difference was seen in triglycerides (mainly VLDL portions), which were increased with ethinyl estradiol and decreased with estradiol valerianate. The authors speculate that the EE-related increase in VLDL triglyceride production rate is mediated through insulin.] ◀

14–40 **Effects of Different Progestogens on Lipoproteins During Postmenopausal Replacement Therapy.** The menopause is associated with a striking increase in the low-density lipoprotein (LDL) cholesterol concentration, a major risk factor in the development of coronary heart disease. Estrogen-replacement therapy reduces LDL cholesterol levels and increases high-density lipoprotein (HDL) cholesterol levels, whereas androgens have the opposite effect. Because the presence of HDL cholesterol has been negatively correlated with coronary heart disease, both effects of estrogen should protect against the development of coronary disease. However, because unopposed estrogen treatment increases the risk of endometrial carcinoma developing, a cyclic progestogen is often added to offset that effect. Progestogens may increase the risk for development of coronary heart disease and other atherosclerotic complications. To study the effect of different types of progestogens on lipoprotein metabolism, Erkki Hirvonen, Marjatta Mälkönen, and Vesa Manninen (Univ. of Helsinki) treated three groups of postmenopausal women (6 patients each) for 3 weeks with estradiol valerate, 2 mg/day, and continued the treatment with different sequential estradiol-progestogen regimens, from day 15 to day 24 of the cycle as follows: group A received norethindrone acetate, 10 mg/day; group B, medroxyprogesterone acetate, 10 mg/day; and group C, norgestrel, 0.5 mg/day. These regimens were followed for two consecutive cycles.

(14–40) N. Engl. J. Med. 304:560–563, Mar. 5, 1981.

Estradiol valerate alone tended to decrease total and LDL cholesterol levels and to increase the HDL cholesterol concentration in some patients. After subsequent combined treatment, total cholesterol levels decreased in all groups by 10% to 18% from baseline values ($P < .05$). The greatest absolute decrease in the total cholesterol level occurred in women with initially high concentrations. The levels of HDL cholesterol decreased by 20% from baseline after 1 month of combined treatment in groups A ($P < .05$) and C ($P < .01$); no significant change occurred in group B. The magnitude of decrease in the HDL cholesterol concentration was not related to initial values. There was a slight (not statistically significant) decrease in the LDL cholesterol level during treatment. Triglyceride values decreased significantly only in group C.

These results suggest that the androgenic progestogens of the 19-nortestosterone series reverse the beneficial effect of postmenopausal treatment on HDL cholesterol levels, whereas the hydroxyprogesterone derivative medroxyprogesterone acetate (which has neither androgenic nor estrogenic properties) has no such effect; although it prevented the estrogen-induced increase in HDL cholesterol concentration, the drug did not cause a significant drop from the initial level. In this context, medroxyprogesterone acetate appears to offer some limited advantage over other progestogens thus far investigated.

▶ [Life does get more complicated! In the 1980 YEAR BOOK, we noted that the increase in high-density lipoproteins (HDL) as a result of estrogen therapy in postmenopausal women might have a beneficial effect concerning the development of atherosclerosis. The use of intermittent progestin therapy along with estrogens in treating menopausal symptoms is becoming more common. The hope, of course, is to limit stimulation of the endometrium. The present study suggests that adding the progestin has the additional effect of *lowering* HDL levels. This (in theory, at least) is not what we want to do. More study is needed to know what dose of what progestin at what frequency is sufficient to protect the endometrium while at the same time not affecting the plasma lipoprotein pattern adversely. In fairness, the clinical significance of altering lipoprotein levels remains speculative.] ◀

14–41 **Hormones and Sexuality: Effect of Estrogen and Progestogen.** Lorraine Dennerstein, Graham D. Burrow, Carl Wood, and Graeme Hyman (Univ. of Melbourne) investigated the effects of estrogen and progestogen on female sexual behavior in 49 women who had undergone hysterectomy and bilateral salpingo-oophorectomy in a double-blind placebo-controlled crossover study. Over a 12-month period, each woman received 3 months each of ethinyl estradiol, 50 µg/day; levonorgestrel, 250 µg/day; a combination of these two substances (Nordiol); and a placebo.

Previous reports have detailed some of the findings of this study. After the study, women rated their preferences. Ethinyl estradiol was most preferred, followed by the combination of ethinyl estradiol and norgestrel, then norgestrel, and placebo. Only women who had stable satisfying heterosexual relationships with a coital frequency of at least twice per month were accepted for this study. Changes in sexual behavior were reported in monthly interviews. Sexual desire, sexual enjoyment, vaginal lubrication, and orgasmic and coital frequency

(14–41) Obstet. Gynecol. 56:316–322, September 1980.

were reported. A written analogue rating scale of sexual response was also completed. A total of 13 women ceased participation in the study without receiving four treatment regimens because of psychologic symptoms (depression, irritability, etc.), hospitalization, and other reasons not related to the study. Interview reports were recorded on an ordinal scale and drugs were ranked.

After the first month, no statistically significant findings were evident, but after the second month, there was a significant difference between estrogen-containing compounds and non-estrogen-containing compounds for both sexual desire and enjoyment. More vaginal lubrication was reported after ethinyl estradiol than after placebo. After the third month, ethinyl estradiol was associated with significantly more sexual enjoyment and desire than placebo. Frequency of orgasms was greatest with ethinyl estradiol, then Nordiol, then norgestrel, and lastly, with placebo. There was also significant patient-drug interaction, indicating that some women responded to different drugs in different ways. The hormones studied were known to have differential effects on hot flushes, but drugs appeared not to affect orgasmic frequency by alleviation of hot flushes alone. Frequency of coitus was not significantly affected by the drugs administered. While ethinyl estradiol had beneficial effects in the areas cited, norgestrel appeared to be inhibitory in the area of sexual enjoyment (i.e., lower than placebo).

Results suggest that there were other factors influencing sexual response, because of the highly significant patient-drug interaction, and that hormones have a direct influence on certain aspects of sexuality, apart from their influence on hot flushes. The large interpatient variability suggests that in studies of the effects of hormones, use of a crossover design is highly desirable. Larger numbers of women may be necessary to overcome patient variability. Analogue scales used in the study showed no significant effects of drugs. These scales may not have been appropriate for the measurement of sexual behavior in the present study.

The findings have implications for women both with regard to variations in endogenous hormones and for the many women receiving exogenous hormones.

▶ [This study is well designed to assess the effects of ethinyl estradiol and levonorgestrel on human female sexuality—so well designed, in fact, that the data seem to have been used as the basis of four previous articles dealing with drug preferences, hot flushes, headache, and affect. This report addresses the effect of the drugs on sexual behavior, and the results indicate that the estrogen had generally greater effect on desire, enjoyment, and orgasmic frequency, but not on coital frequency, suggesting that the last may reflect partner's wishes. The "beneficial" effects of estrogen were lessened by addition of progestogen. Though these findings are of interest, their applicability to the clinical situation, in particular the selection of types of oral contraceptive, is more problematic.] ◀

14–42 **Intravaginal Administration of Progesterone: Enhanced Absorption After Estrogen Treatment.** Cyclic progesterone administration to women on long-term estrogen replacement may protect against the development of endometrial hyperplasia and neoplasia.

(14–42) Fertil. Steril. 35:433–437, April 1981.

The vaginal route has been found to be most efficient for absorption of estrogen. Benito Villanueva, Robert F. Casper, and Samuel S. C. Yen (Univ. of California, San Diego, at La Jolla) evaluated the vaginal and sublingual routes of progesterone administration in postmenopausal women. Intravaginal administration of 50 mg of progesterone in suspension, in the posterior vaginal vault, was carried out in 4 estrogen-deficient women receiving Premarin and in 5 not given any hormone for at least 6 months. Eight postmenopausal women, 5 of them taking Premarin, received 50 mg of progesterone intramuscularly. Five postmenopausal women receiving no hormone therapy were given the same dose sublingually.

Progesterone was absorbed rapidly through the vaginal mucosa, with more than a 10-fold rise in circulating concentrations 15 minutes after administration. Peak values were reached within 1 to 2 hours and persisted during the 7 hours of frequent sampling. Peak values were lower in women receiving no estrogen therapy. Intramuscular injection led to somewhat slower appearance of the hormone in the serum. Sublingual administration resulted in rapid appearance of progesterone in serum, but much lower values were observed. Estimates of the area under the curve indicated that subjects given progesterone vaginally after estrogen treatment absorbed as much as the patients given injections, whereas those given progesterone vaginally without estrogen pretreatment absorbed only half as much. Much longer absorption resulted from injection of progesterone. The time to peak values was by far the longest in this group.

The vaginal mucosa is an efficient site of absorption of progesterone into the circulation. Postmenopausal women receiving estrogen replacement would benefit most from this route of administration. Although it is less convenient than the oral route, natural progesterone rather than orally active synthetic progestin can be used. Vaginal application appears to be potentially more convenient than injections, especially for long-term treatment.

▶ [Several reports have noted that estrogen is absorbed rapidly and to a great extent from the vagina, and this study finds a similar situation with respect to progesterone. If it is desirable to give progesterone to "protect" against the effects of unreported estrogen treatment, as most authorities think it is, perhaps a vaginal cream containing both hormones would be worth considering. Another means of "protecting" the endometrium is considered in the following article.] ◀

14-43 Cyclic Clomiphene Citrate Treatment Lowers Cytosol Estrogen and Progestin Receptor Concentrations in Endometrium of Postmenopausal Women on Estrogen Replacement Therapy. Studies have indicated that a nonsteroidal antiestrogen, clomiphene citrate, might prevent the stimulatory action of estrogens on human endometrium. E. Kokko, O. Jänne, A. Kauppila, and R. Vihko (Univ. of Oulu) investigated the mechanism of this effect in 19 postmenopausal patients. Nine women were treated with conjugated estrogens, 1.25 mg/day for 6 months, supplemented cyclically with clomiphene citrate, 50 mg/day, for 10 days after every 7 weeks without interruption of estrogen treatment; 10 patients took clomiphene citrate alone

---

(14–43) J. Clin. Endocrinol. Metab. 52:345–349, February 1981.

(without estrogens) during the same 10-day periods. Estrogen and progestin receptors were measured from the endometrial cytosol after the first estrogen period and after the first and third clomiphene treatments.

Estrogen treatment produced endometrial estrogen and progestin receptor concentrations comparable to the respective receptor levels in premenopausal women. The estrogen receptor concentration in atrophic endometrium was significantly higher than that in hyperplastic endometrium after the initial estrogen period, whereas corresponding progestin receptor levels were independent of tissue histology. The first clomiphene citrate treatment reduced the estrogen receptor content to below the limit of detection in all but 2 patients. This change was statistically significant in both the presence and absence of simultaneous estrogen administration ($P < .01$). After the next 2 treatment cycles, the estrogen receptor concentration was detectable in 2 patients receiving clomiphene alone and in 3 patients given clomiphene and estrogen. Mean levels in both groups remained significantly lower than the respective values after the initial estrogen treatment period ($P < .05$). Compared to values at the end of the preceding estrogen period, progestin receptor concentrations were significantly lower only after the first clomiphene period in both groups. After the following 2 treatment cycles, progestin receptor concentrations tended to increase over those noted after the first clomiphene period. The effect of clomiphene was independent of the initial histologic appearance of the endometrium and led to endometrial atrophy in most patients.

Because the effect of clomiphene was independent of simultaneous estrogen administration, the drug acted as a pure antiestrogen in this treatment modality. The observation that receptor concentrations were somewhat higher after the third clomiphene treatment than after the first may be explained by the estrogen treatment given in between. The present treatment resulted in more pronounced depression of estrogen receptor levels in relation to those of the progestin receptor than occurs during progestin treatment. This finding suggests that the mechanisms leading to depletion of such receptors during these two regimens differ. It is not known whether the two types of treatment have additive effects.

▶ [The antiestrogen effects of clomiphene resulted in endometrial atrophy and a decrease in endometrial estrogen receptors in these postmenopausal women. Whether clomiphene has a role in place of or in addition to progestins, either cyclicly with estrogen in the treatment of menopausal symptoms or continuously in the treatment of recurrent endometrial cancer, remains to be seen.] ◀

14–44 **Use of Medroxyprogesterone Acetate for Relief of Climacteric Symptoms.** John C. Morrison, Dan C. Martin, Richard A. Blair, Garland D. Anderson, Bradford W. Kincheloe, G. William Bates, James W. Hendrix, Michel E. Rivlin, Evelyn K. Forman, Maureen G. Propst, and Robert Needham assessed the effectiveness of medroxyprogesterone acetate (Depo-Provera, DMPA) in a double-blind, randomized, placebo-controlled study involving 48 perimenopausal and postmeno-

(14–44)   Am. J. Obstet. Gynecol. 138:99–104, Sept. 1, 1980.

pausal women. All experienced daily hot flashes and night sweats for at least 4 weeks prior to starting the program. Three dosage schedules (50 mg, 100 mg, and 150 mg) of DMPA were investigated. After a 2-week observation period to establish a baseline, each participant was given one injection of either DMPA or placebo. Patients were evaluated historically at 2, 4, 6, 8, 10, and 12 weeks after injection.

Age, parity, and incidence of hysterectomy in the treatment group were different from those findings in the placebo group. Patients in the treatment group were considerably younger, and a significant number had prior hysterectomy at an early age. Other criteria (e.g., onset and length of symptomatology, gravidity, incidence of prior estrogen therapy) were not significantly different between the groups. However, significant differences were found between the treatment and placebo groups in patient dropout rate, subjective improvement, and satisfaction with therapy, as well as diminution in number of hot flashes and night sweats. Among 24 patients in the 100-mg and 150-mg DMPA groups, none discontinued the study because of treatment failure; in the 50-mg DMPA group, 2 patients discontinued the study at 6 and 8 weeks, respectively. In the placebo group, 75% (9 women) dropped out of the study between 6 and 10 weeks (average 6.5 weeks). Only 3 of 12 patients receiving placebo completed the course, whereas only 2 of 35 women in the DMPA groups dropped out because of treatment failure. Placebo patients experienced an improvement of 15% to 20% in symptomatology during the course of therapy, but this effect varied widely among patients at each assessment period. Treatment groups reported 75% to 100% relief of symptoms between the second and fourth weeks after treatment was begun.

Differences between the three dosage levels of DMPA did not produce the expected dose-response curve. There appeared to be stratification in satisfaction based on the amount of DMPA administered, but the trend was not statistically significant. All patients receiving DMPA evidenced a 25% to 45% reduction in frequency of vasomotor symptoms which continued through the fourth week and then plateaued between 5% and 50% of the original level. The differences in response among patients receiving various dosages were not statistically significant. Side effects included irregular bleeding, emotional lability, depression, and weight gain. Only 3 patients had irregular bleeding; surgical intervention was not required. Other symptoms tended to resolve by the third week of treatment.

The data confirm the efficacy of DMPA in reducing the number of climacteric symptoms in perimenopausal and postmenopausal patients, and in providing a subjective increase in the sense of well-being. It is thus a logical treatment choice in women who are intolerant of estrogen compounds or who do not receive relief from hormone therapy. The question of the smallest effective dose of DMPA remains undetermined.

▶ [This study indicates that parenteral medroxyprogesterone acetate is quite effective in alleviating menopausal hot flushes. There was a slight tendency toward a dose-response relationship, with 100-mg and 150-mg monthly doses marginally superior to the 50-mg dose level. Patients with severe enough hot flushes to require treatment sometimes have a contraindication to estrogen (e.g., previous breast or endometrial cancer), and in such instances medroxyprogesterone may be of great help. In a limited experience, we have been less impressed with oral medroxyprogesterone in relieving menopausal symptoms. A different view follows. Read on.] ◄

14–45 Oral Medroxyprogesterone in Treatment of Postmenopausal Symptoms. Isaac Schiff, Dan Tulchinsky, Daniel Cramer, and Kenneth J. Ryan (Boston) conducted a double-blind crossover study to compare the effects of placebo and medroxyprogesterone acetate (20 mg daily) on vasomotor flushes and blood hormones in 32 postmenopausal women. Sixteen were 1–24 years postmenopausal, and 16 had previously undergone hysterectomy and oophorectomy for benign gynecologic disese. After 1 week of establishing baseline symptoms, the women were randomly assigned to a drug or placebo group for 12 weeks, after which they were crossed over to the other regimen. Five of the women dropped out of the study during a placebo period and were not considered in the final analysis. Four 20-ml blood samples were drawn before initiation of treatment and at the end of each 12-week period.

The mean number of vasomotor flushes occurring weekly, shown as a percentage change from the control period, is seen in Figure 14–6. In women initially receiving placebo, a decreased number of flushes was noted at the second week of treatment; improvement continued until a total decrease of 25.9% was achieved between week 9 and 12 of placebo treatment. A further 34.5% reduction was observed after this group switched to the active drug regimen. In patients first taking medroxyprogesterone, a significant reduction in vasomotor

Fig 14–6.—Graph depicts weeks of treatment in postmenopausal patients. (Courtesy of Schiff, I., et al.: JAMA 244:1443–1445, Sept. 26, 1980; copyright 1980, American Medical Association.)

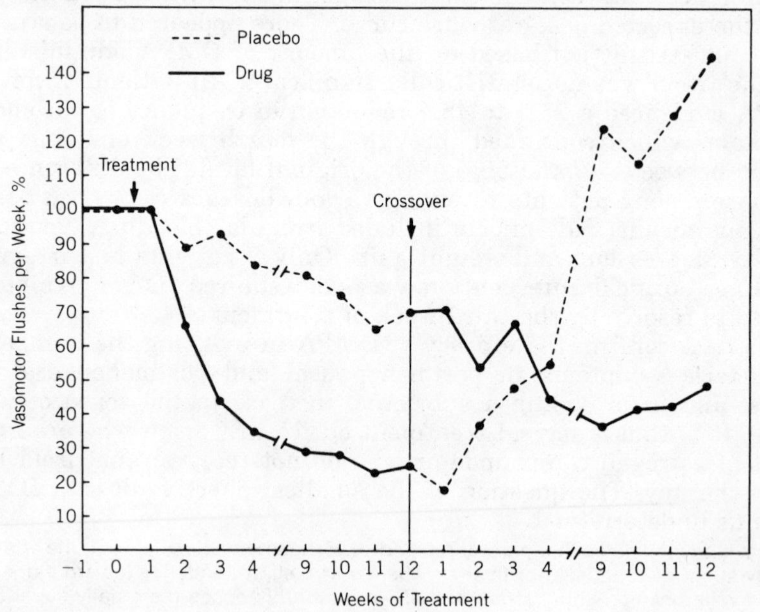

(14–45) JAMA 244:1443–1445, Sept. 26, 1980.

flushes was observed at the second week; overall, a reduction of 73.9% was noted by 9–12 weeks. When these patients switched to placebo, marked worsening of symptoms occurred. By the 12th week of each cycle the drug completely abolished vasomotor flushes in 9 of 27 patients and reduced the frequency in 11, but 7 patients continued to experience two or more flushes daily. Placebo produced complete relief in 4 patients. Medroxyprogesterone produced a significant 27% and 29% decline in both follicle-stimulating and luteinizing hormone levels, respectively; placebo had no effect. In addition, the drug produced a small but significant elevation in prolactin levels as compared with placebo. No changes in basal cortisol concentrations or in response to corticotropin were noted with the drug, nor did it have any effect on vaginal cytology.

These results suggest that placebo is effective only when used initially. Vaginal bleeding occurred in 5 patients receiving the active drug, a progestin effect disclosed by endometrial biopsy. The active drug can presumably reduce endometrial hyperplasia, but cannot substitute totally for estrogen therapy. The findings suggest that medroxyprogesterone may be used to treat symptomatic women when estrogen administration is undesirable.

▶ [A beneficial effect of oral Provera on menopausal vasomotor symptoms is demonstrated here. The drug is probably worth a try in those patients with severe symptoms for whom estrogen therapy is contraindicated. The authors rightly point out that medroxyprogesterone will not improve vaginal atrophy and will probably not prevent osteoporosis.] ◀

15. Infertility

15–1 **Arcuate and Bicornuate Uterine Anomalies and Infertility.**
Togas Tulandi, George H. Arronet, and Robert A. McInnes (Royal
Victoria Hosp., Montreal) found uterine anomalies in 23 of 2,240
women (1.03%) seen at an infertility clinic during 1960 to 1976. The
23 patients were aged 21 to 41 years (mean, 30); 18 had primary infertility an average of 2 years in duration (range, 1½ to 11) and 5
had repeated pregnancy wastage. No case of septate uterus was
found.

Of 7 patients with arcuate uterus, 6 (86%) achieved a term pregnancy. The other patient had an azoospermic husband and declined
artificial insemination. Of these 7 women, 6 had primary infertility.

Of 13 patients with bicornuate uterus (unicollis), 6 underwent metroplasty and 4 of these 6 (67%) achieved a term pregnancy. Of the
other 7 women, 1 achieved pregnancy during investigations, 1 refused
surgery, and 5 were not operated on because of uncorrected nonuter-
ine factors.

The 1 patient with didelphys uterus had a severely oligospermic
husband and did not achieve pregnancy. Of 2 women with unicorn-
uate uterus, 1 conceived while being investigated and the other had,
in addition, bilateral tubal obstruction.

▶ [Conventional teaching holds that müllerian duct abnormalities may lead to pregnancy wastage but are unlikely causes of infertility. This report suggests otherwise, for
4 of 5 patients with an arcuate uterus and 4 of 6 with a bicornuate uterus conceived
after metroplasty. However, in the absence of any controls it is difficult to interpret
such results. In our opinion, surgical repair of a uterine malformation in a patient com-
plaining of infertility is a last resort, to be done only after a thorough investigation and
with the patient's full understanding of the situation.] ◀

15–2 **Triple Evaluation of Tubal Patency.** José A. Portuondo, Abel D.
Echanojauregui, J. Peña Irala, and J. Calonge (Univ. of Bilbao,
Cruces-Bilbao, Spain) evaluated 336 infertile women by tubal insuf-
flation, hysterosalpingography, and laparoscopy.

Results with the three methods agreed in 219 patients (65%). The
rate of false results of tubal insufflation was 18.4% (9.8% false negative and 8.6% false positive). The rate of false negative results by
hysterosalpingography was 9.5%. Peritubal and periovarian adhesions were suspected by hysterosalpingography in 9 patients (2.7%),
which subsequent laparoscopy did not confirm.

The rate of false negative results of laparoscopy was only 6.8%, and
additional pelvic pathologic features were detected by laparoscopy in
60 patients (17.8%). Pelvic adhesions (36 patients) and endometriosis

---

(15–1) Fertil. Steril. 34:362–364, October 1980.
(15–2) Int. J. Fertil. 25:307–310, 1980.

(24 patients) were the pathologic processes most commonly missed by hysterosalpingography.

Tubal patency findings by laparoscopy and hysterosalpingography did not coincide in 16.3% of the patients, and both tests were needed in 30% of the infertile patients.

It is concluded that hysterosalpingography and laparoscopy should be considered supplementary and that when both of these can be performed, tubal insufflation can be abandoned or its discrepant results rejected, because it gives no further information and has a high rate of false results.

▶ [Most infertility experts nowadays seem to agree that tubal insufflation or the Rubin test is without much value as an index of tubal patency. The conclusion seems supported by this study, which indicates further that there is little apparent advantage one way or the other with respect to hysterosalpingogram versus laparoscopy-chromotubation. It is a little disquieting that these two procedures yielded discordant results in one sixth of the subjects. Laparoscopy is generally a more involved procedure (anesthesia, perhaps hospitalization, etc.), but does provide the opportunity for making ancillary diagnoses (17.8% of the patients in this series had additional unsuspected pelvic disease diagnosed laparoscopically). The authors conclude that many patients require both studies.] ◀

15–3 **Tubal Intramural Polyps and Their Relationship to Infertility.** Menachem P. David, David Ben-Zwi, and Leah Langer (Tel-Aviv) examined the role of fallopian tube polyps in infertility in a retrospective study of 2,156 hysterosalpingograms obtained between 1969 and 1979 and correlated the findings with the case histories of the patients. Fifty-four cases (2.5%) of intramural polyps were identifed and classified into four groups according to the size (small and/or large) and location (unilateral, bilateral) of the polyps (Fig 15–1). An additional 34 cases of small unilateral filling defects were also seen but were excluded from this series to minimize the possibility of false positive results.

After hysterosalpingography, 25 patients (54%) had conceived at the time of follow-up and 21 (46%) had not. The conception rates be-

Fig 15–1.—Bilateral, large polyps. (Courtesy of David, M. P., et al.: Fertil. Steril. 35:526–531, May 1981.)

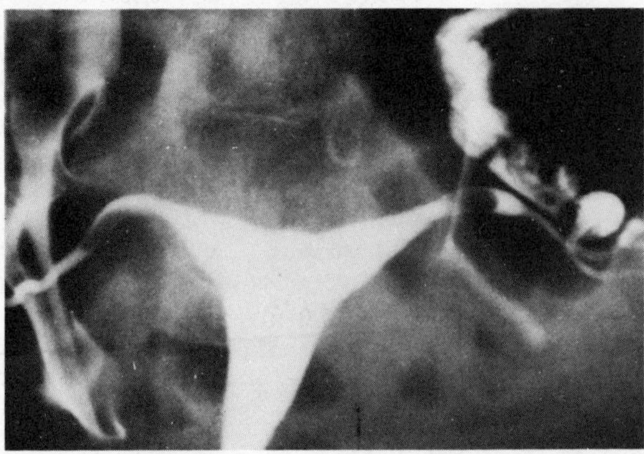

(15–3) Fertil. Steril. 35:526–531, May 1981.

fore and after hysterosalpingography were almost identical. The highest conception rate was among women who had undergone hysterosalpingography for reasons other than infertility. The conception rate was 50% in 28 women whose infertility could be explained by a detectable disturbance (not polyps) and who were treated accordingly. The cause of infertility could not be explained in 17 women, yet 11 conceived despite no treatment. Anovulation was the most common diagnosis in the patients with detectable disorders. Except for a lower incidence of infertility in patients with large unilateral polyps, there were no significant differences between the groups with polyps.

The results suggest that women with intramural fallopian tube polyps should be considered to be relatively subfertile and should be treated for other causes of infertility, if present. In patients with unexplained infertility and in those where treatment fails, the presence of a tubal polyp should be viewed as a possible cause of infertility, and surgical treatment should be considered.

▶ [In this large series of hysterosalpingograms, tubal intraluminal polyps were found in 2.5% of studies. Among those women who had other potential reasons for infertility concomitantly, half (14 of 28) conceived after treatment of the other condition. Surprisingly, among 17 women without any other cause for sterility, 11 (65%) conceived with no treatment at all. This is hardly strong evidence of a relationship between tubal polyps and infertility!

Stangel and associates (*Fertil. Steril.* 35:580, 1981) reported a case of microsurgical resection of bilateral tubal polyps that was successful in terms of restoring a normal hysterosalpingography pattern. However, conception did not occur during more than a year postoperatively, and the patient was then lost to follow-up.] ◀

15–4 **Laparoscopic Sperm Recovery in Infertile Women.** A. A. Templeton and D. Mortimer (Univ. of Edinburgh) studied women infertile for no known cause to determine whether they had abnormalities of sperm migration to the site of fertilization.

Forty-four couples were selected on the basis of infertility lasting at least 2 years, normal histories and findings on examinations, normal ovulatory menstrual cycles, and semen showing normal volume, motility, density, morphology, agglutination, and physical features. Intracervical insemination with husband's ejaculate was carried out at midcycle. A sample of cervical mucus was then aspirated and examined for sperm numbers and characteristics. Laparoscopy was performed 5 to 6 hours after insemination. The peritoneal fluid lying in the pouch of Douglas was aspirated. The fimbriated end of each fallopian tube was then rinsed with flushing fluid and the flushings were aspirated from the pouch of Douglas. Tubal patency then was checked and an endometrial biopsy specimen was taken.

Of the 44 couples recruited for the study, 20 were excluded because of pelvic abnormalities seen at laparoscopy (9), semen not normal on day of laparoscopy (6), in luteal phase (4), or slides damaged (1). In 15 of the other 24 women, spermatozoa were identified in the peritoneal fluid, and so far (follow-up, 7 to 16 months), 7 of these have conceived spontaneously. None of the 9 women from whom spermatozoa were not recovered have become pregnant, There was no corre-

---

(15–4) Br. J. Obstet. Gynaecol. 87:1128–1131, December 1980.

lation between sperm recovery and the quality of the postinsemination cervical mucus examination.

The finding, at laparoscopy, of spermatozoa in peritoneal fluid of some infertile women may be important in their subsequent management because it shows that the sperm have the ability to reach the site of fertilization. The technique is easy to learn and adds only a few minutes to a routine laparoscopic examination of the pelvis. As sperm migration does not usually occur in the early follicular and luteal phases of the menstrual cycle, timing of the procedure is important. The test also has some prognostic value—pregnancy occurred in 47% of patients where spermatozoa were identified in the peritoneal fluid but in none of those where sperm were not found. When spermatozoa are identified but pregnancy does not occur, the fertilizing ability of the spermatozoa should be investigated.

▶ [The findings of the postcoital test did not predict the recovery of spermatozoa from the peritoneal cavity in these infertile women with patent tubes. Half of the patients with spermatozoa identified have conceived versus none in the group (N = 9) in which sperm were not recovered. This study suggests a possible benefit in performing laparoscopy about the expected time of ovulation in infertile patients. Those interested in the luteinized unruptured follicle (1979 YEAR BOOK , p. 387) recommend performing laparoscopy 3 to 5 days after the thermal shift, however, and we suspect that on a routine basis most of these procedures are done relatively early in the follicular phase. Could one obtain this sort of information on sperm transport by performing a postcoital culdocentesis at midcycle?] ◀

15–5 **Some Properties of Rectum and Vagina as Sites for Basal Body Temperature Measurement.** The choice of site for body temperature measurement and consistency in positioning the thermometer are important in achieving reliable and interpretable basal body temperature graphs in women. Robert M. Abrams and J. Patrick Royston studied the distribution of temperatures in vagina (T_V) and rectum (T_R) measured in women on awakening.

There were no significant differences between T_R and T_V at insertion depths of 5, 9, or 13 cm. Estimation of deep body temperature was not improved by inserting a thermojunction beyond 5 cm in the vagina or rectum. Rates of change in T_V after ingestion of a 300-ml iced drink were significantly greater than rates of change in T_R.

▶ [This study indicates that the vagina is a perfectly acceptable site for measuring basal body temperature, provided the thermometer is inserted at least 5 cm.] ◀

15–6 **Adjustment of Basal Body Temperature Measurements to Allow for Time of Waking.** Variability in the daily measurement of basal body temperature (BBT) introduced by differences in the time of day at which the temperature is taken and the so-called weekend effect can make interpretation of the BBT shift difficult or impossible. To determine whether an adjustment factor could be found to simplify the interpretation of BBT charts, J. P. Royston, R. M. Abrams, Mary P. Higgins, and Anna M. Flynn studied 18 BBT charts obtained from student nurses with variable waking-sleeping schedules and 18 BBT charts from women with very regular waking habits.

Waking times among the student nurses varied between 0530 and

(15–5) Fertil. Steril. 35:313–316, March 1981.
(15–6) Br. J. Obstet. Gynaecol. 87:1123–1127, December 1980.

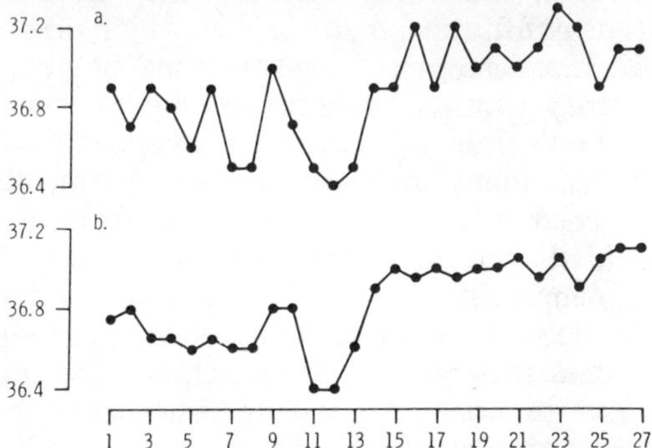

Fig 15–2.—Relationship between recorded postmenstrual temperature and time of waking in a chart from a student nurse. The inscribed line, fitted by least-squares linear regression, represents a slope of 0.08 C/hour. (Courtesy of Royston, J. P., et al.: Br. J. Obstet. Gynaecol. 87:1123–1127, December 1980.)

1100 hours. Analysis of their BBT charts by linear regression showed a clear association between BBT and time of waking, with a slope of 0.084 C/hour. Analysis of covariance of postmenstrual, preshift BBTs revealed a highly significant (P <.001) temperature-time common regression slope of 0.086 C/hour. A variation in individually estimated slopes of between 0.05 and 0.15 C/hour was not sufficient to dismiss the validity of a single representative slope. Based on the pooled slope of the linear regression of temperature at time of waking, a round adjustment factor of 0.1 C/hour was adopted. Application of this adjustment factor reduced the variability of postmenstrual temperatures as measured by their standard deviation from a baseline waking time temperature (Fig 15–2). Regression analysis of premenstrual temperatures gave an adjustment factor of 0.05 C, which was not sufficiently different from the postmenstrual adjustment factor to introduce significant overcorrection in temperatures around the shift point.

The adjustment factor is very easy to apply. It simply involves counting down one square on a BBT chart for each hour later than usual that the woman takes her temperature or one square up for each hour earlier than usual.

▶ [The "basal" vaginal temperature increases 0.1 C/hour during the morning. Presumably, oral temperature readings would vary in a similar fashion. This information will help us answer questions from infertility patients concerning the effects of different times of awakening on their basal body temperatures. Figure 15–2 nicely demonstrates how adjusting the temperature for the waking time makes the chart easier to interpret.] ◀

15–7 **Maturation Value as an Indicator of Serum Estrogen Concentration During Treatment With Gonadotropins.** Treatment with human menopausal gonadotropins (hMG) must be monitored carefully so that human chorionic gonadotropins are given at the proper time to induce ovulation. Daily estrogen determinations are expensive, complex, and inconvenient. Merete R. Jensen, Barbara J. Kap-

---

(15–7) Acta Cytol. 25:251–254, May–June, 1981.

lan, Richard P. Marrs, and Charles M. March (Univ. of Southern California) evaluated exfoliative cytology as a means of estimating fluctuations in serum estrogen concentrations during hMG therapy. Fourteen anovulatory women, aged 20 to 33 years, who had failed to respond to clomiphene therapy with hCG were studied. Two had primary and 8 had secondary amenorrhea and 4 had oligomenorrhea. Treatment consisted of hMG for 5 to 15 days. Smears were obtained from the middle third of the lateral vaginal wall, and serum was sampled for determination of total immunoreactive estrogens.

An exponential rise in serum estrogen concentration was observed as full follicular maturation was approached. Human chorionic gonadotropin was given when the estrogen concentration rose to 500 to 1,000 pg/ml; all 23 courses resulted in ovulation, and 5 patients conceived. Four patients showed an increase in maturation values corresponding to the rise in serum estrogen concentration; no correlation was evident in the other 10 patients. Only 1 of 7 patients given repeated treatment showed correlation between maturation values and serum estrogen concentrations in each course of treatment. Changes in maturation values lagged behind the rise in serum estrogen concentrations. Overall correlation between serum estrogen and maturation values was poor.

Vaginal smears cannot be used to monitor circulating estrogen concentrations during treatment with hMG to induce follicular maturation. The rapid rise in hMG-induced estrogen concentration probably does not allow time for vaginal epithelial changes to occur, and progesterone secretion after ovulation blocks vaginal epithelial changes secondary to estrogen secretion.

▶ [Some type of daily estrogen assessment is essential in gonadotropin treatment of anovulation if hyperstimulation and multiple ovulation are to be minimized. If vaginal cytology were sufficiently precise, it would be much simpler (and therefore much more useful) than blood or urine assays. Unfortunately, as indicated in this comparative study, it is not good enough. Estrogen effects on the vaginal epithelium apparently lag too far behind blood levels.] ◀

15–8 **Combined Use of Clomiphene and Intranasal Luteinizing Hormone-Releasing Hormone for Induction of Ovulation in Chronically Anovulatory Women.** A limiting factor in a trial of luteinizing hormone-releasing hormone (LHRH) therapy in patients requiring ovulation induction has been the need to administer the substance parenterally. Shaila A. Phansey, Mary A. Barnes, H. Oliver Williamson, Julius Sagel, and R. M. G. Nair (Charleston, S.C.) used combined therapy with clomiphene and intranasal LHRH to induce ovulation in 8 chronically anovulatory, normoprolactinemic women with secondary amenorrhea or oligomenorrhea under treatment for infertility. In all patients, withdrawal bleeding could be induced with medroxyprogesterone acetate (Provera), 50 mg orally. Previous treatment with increasing daily clomiphene doses from 50 mg to 150 mg for 5 days had failed to induce ovulation in all patients even when combined with subsequent human chorionic gonadotropin therapy; this failure suggested follicular dysfunction. Clomiphene ci-

(15–8) Fertil. Steril. 34:448–451, November 1980.

trate, 100 mg daily, was given from day 5 to day 9 of a spontaneous or Provera-induced cycle. Synthetic LHRH (concentration, $3\mu g/\mu l$ of normal saline) was administered intranasally in varying doses from day 11 to day 14 in an attempt to induce late follicular development and ovulation. The initial dose, administered between 9 AM and 10 AM, was repeated every 2 hours for a total of 3 doses daily.

Five patients ovulated and 3 conceived. Ovulation was documented in 7 of 10 treatment cycles. Two patients conceived during the first treatment cycle and the third patient, during the second treatment cycle. Ovulation was delayed 8–10 days after LHRH therapy in 2 of the ovulatory patients. Of the 3 patients who remained anovulatory, 2 had spontaneous menses 7–14 days after therapy; this had not occurred for several years. On the first day of LHRH therapy, there was a small increase in the luteinizing hormone concentration at 30 minutes, and a maximal response at 150 minutes, in 3 patients who showed evidence of ovulation. Luteinizing hormone response was inadequate in 2 patients who failed to ovulate. Plasma estradiol levels in 3 patients who ovulated were in the midfollicular phase range. In those who failed to ovulate, estradiol levels were comparable to those noted in the early follicular phase. The mean plasma prolactin level was 6.75 ± 1.76 ng/ml. No side effects or complications were noted.

The success achieved with combined clomiphene and intranasal LHRH administration suggests a therapeutic potential for this approach in the management of anovulatory infertility.

▶ [Though this is a small series, the results are extremely encouraging. Of 8 women with anovulation resistant to clomiphene-human chorionic gonadotropin treatment, 5 ovulated and 3 conceived with sequential clomiphene-nasal LHRH. Although success with parenteral LHRH has been reported, this is the first indication that the nasal route can be used effectively. An approach such as this may be preferable to therapy with menopausal gonadotropins if it avoids the problems of hyperstimulation and multiple gestation. A series as small as this cannot tell us much about complications, but it is encouraging that the luteinizing hormone levels in responsive patients increased by 50% to 150%, which is about that occurring in normal cycles.] ◀

15-9 **Diagnosis of the Luteinized Unruptured Follicle Syndrome by Steroid Hormone Assays on Peritoneal Fluid.** The formation of a corpus luteum without subsequent ovulation (luteinized unruptured follicle syndrome) is an apparently frequent occurrence in women with regular biphasic menstrual cycles and infertility. Because laparoscopy may not detect an ovulation stigma and because patients cannot be subjected to repeat laparoscopies during successive menstrual cycles, the diagnosis of this syndrome is difficult. To determine whether assays of steroid hormones in peritoneal fluid could distinguish between a ruptured follicle with subsequent corpus luteum formation and a luteinized unruptured follicle, P. R. Koninckx, P. De Moor, and I. A. Brosens (Leuven, Belgium) assayed progesterone and estradiol-17β concentrations in peritoneal fluid. The fluid was aspirated from the pouch of Douglas during the luteal phase in 77 women with regular biphasic menstrual cycles and primary or secondary infertility. Concentrations of total protein, transcortin, and sex hor-

(15–9) Br. J. Obstet. Gynaecol. 87:929–934, November 1980.

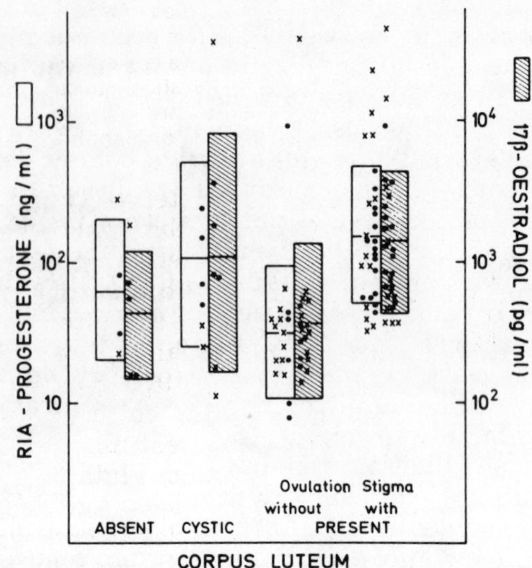

Fig 15–3.—Concentration of progesterone and estradiol-17β in peritoneal fluid of women according to laparoscopic appearance of corpus luteum; *x* indicates absence and *solid circle* indicates presence of pelvic endometriosis. The mean$_{log}$ ± SE is indicated. (Courtesy of Koninckx, P. R., et al.: Br. J. Obstet. Gynaecol. 87:929–934, November 1980.)

mone-binding globulin (SHBG) also were assayed. The ovaries were examined by laparoscopy for the presence or absence of a corpus luteum and of an ovulation stigma.

Macroscopically, an ovulation stigma was observed in 43% of the women, was difficult to evaluate in 14%, and was absent in 43%. Concentrations of total protein, transcortin, and SHBG were similar for those with and without an ovulation stigma. Progesterone and estradiol-17β peritoneal fluid concentrations were significantly higher in those women with an ovulation stigma than those without one between day 15 and 20 of the cycle. However, individual women with a cystic corpus luteum or without an ovulation stigma on occasion had high peritoneal fluid concentrations of progesterone and estradiol-17β (Fig 15–3). Nonetheless, the range of progesterone and estradiol-17β concentrations was sufficiently different in the early luteal phase to allow for an accurate diagnosis of ovulation, the only limitation being the presence of a cystic corpus luteum.

The findings demonstrate that the use of both hormone determinations could lead to an accurate diagnosis of ovulation in 92% of women with an ovulation stigma and 80% of those without an ovulation stigma. It is recommended that assays of peritoneal fluid concentrations of progesterone and estradiol-17β be performed in all women with biphasic menstrual cycles and primary or secondary infertility.

▶ [The luteinized unruptured follicle syndrome as a cause of infertility was considered in the 1979 YEAR BOOK (p. 387); the authors of the present paper speculated in a report abstracted in the 1981 YEAR BOOK (pp. 369–370) that it may be etiologic in endometriosis. Koninckx and colleagues consider this entity to be a common cause of unexplained infertility. The present study is an attempt to make the diagnosis more easily than with laparoscopic visualization of the stigma. Cul-de-sac fluid estradiol and progesterone levels were (not surprisingly) higher in cases in which a stigma was present, but there was some overlap. Confirmatory work from other investigators is needed in order to put this entity into proper perspective. If this is a common problem and if the peritoneal fluid hormone levels are generally diagnostic, then culdocentesis in the few days after "ovulation" may become part of the standard infertility workup. Others have found ovulation induction therapy with clomiphene or menotropins to be efficacious in the relatively small number of patients so treated.] ◄

15–10 **Spermatogenesis Before and After Renal Transplant.** Nelson Rodrigues Netto, Júnior, Giglio Pecoraro, Emil Sabbaga, and Gilberto Menezes de Góes (Univ. of São Paulo) investigated the relationship of fertility and renal transplantation through quantitative analysis of testicular biopsy specimens obtained before and after renal transplantation from 9 patients with chronic renal failure who underwent renal transplantation between 1974 and 1976. Studies included urinalysis (with sediment and quantitative culture), complete blood count, determination of serum urea and creatinine levels, and creatinine clearance, and measurement of serum glutamic oxalacetic and glutamic pyruvic transaminase concentrations. Age range was 18–51 years, the median being 36 years. Testicular biopsy was carried out simultaneously with transplant: a scrotal incision 1–2 cm in length exposed the testicular surface, allowing removal of a small fragment of the testicular tunica albuginea and parenchyma. Posttransplant testicular biopsy was performed 10.4 months later, on average. The biopsy was always done on the side opposite to the transplant. Six patients had ligation and section of the spermatic cords during transplant. No testicular atrophy or hydrocele resulted.

All patients were impotent before transplant. Sexual activity after transplant returned to levels of the initial stages before nephropathy. None of the patients' wives became pregnant during the study period. Tubular cell counts (means and standard deviations) are shown in the table. A significant improvement in spermatogenesis was observed after renal transplantation, although spermatogenesis did not quite return to normal levels, perhaps due to residual testicular lesions or to the side effects of immunosuppressive drugs (azathioprine and prednisone). Both Sertoli cells and spermatogonia continued to be found in reduced numbers after renal transplant, perhaps because the

TUBULAR CELL COUNT: MEANS AND STANDARD DEVIATIONS

Cell type	Pretransplant	Posttransplant	Calculated t
Sertoli	9.3 ± 4.7	8.4 ± 4.2	0.67 NS[a]
Spermatogonia	0.0 ± 6.5	14.5 ± 6.6	1.81 NS[a]
Spermatocytes	7.0 ± 6.2	17.5 ± 7.3	2.96 S[b] ($P < 0.02$)
Spermatids	1.8 ± 2.5	8.6 ± 5.8	3.92 S[b] ($P < 0.01$)
Spermatozoa	0.33 ± 0.68	3.4 ± 4.11	2.30 S[b] ($P < 0.05$)
Total germinative cells	18.4 ± 14.2	43.7 ± 24.2	25.31 S[b] ($P < 0.001$)

[a]NS = not significant.
[b]S = significant.

(15–10) Int. J. Fertil. 25:131–133, 1980.

Sertoli cells, given their topographic relations, are the metabolic support for the germinative cells. These cells also are believed to exert control on differentiation of germinative cells. Large liposoluble molecules and proteins can cross the cell membranes separating these cells. This transfer occurs mainly between the Sertoli cells and the spermatogonia. Testicular histometry showed that the Sertoli cells and spermatogonia mainly were involved and that there was no significant improvement after transplant. Possibly, the lesion of these cells in chronic renal failure may explain the failure to reach full normal values.

▶ [In this study, there was a distinct and substantial improvement in spermatogenesis with renal transplantation, presumably reflecting correction of uremia. More impressive, perhaps, is the statement that impotence, which was present in all before the transplant, disappeared and sexual activity returned to its predisease level.] ◀

15–11　**Sperm Penetration Assay: Useful Test in Evaluation of Male Fertility.** Apart from production of a pregnancy, there has never been a satisfactory test of male fertility. Variables of semen analysis do not correlate well with demonstrated fertility. Yanagimachi et al. suggested that the zona pellucida-free hamster egg might serve as a

Fig 15–4 (top).—Unpenetrated egg with sperm on surface. White areas *(arrow)* are typical when attachment occurs without subsequent penetration.

Fig 15–5 (bottom).—Egg penetrated by sperm. Arrows indicate enlarging sperm heads with tails.

(Courtesy of Karp, L. E., et al.: Obstet. Gynecol. 57:620–623, May 1981.)

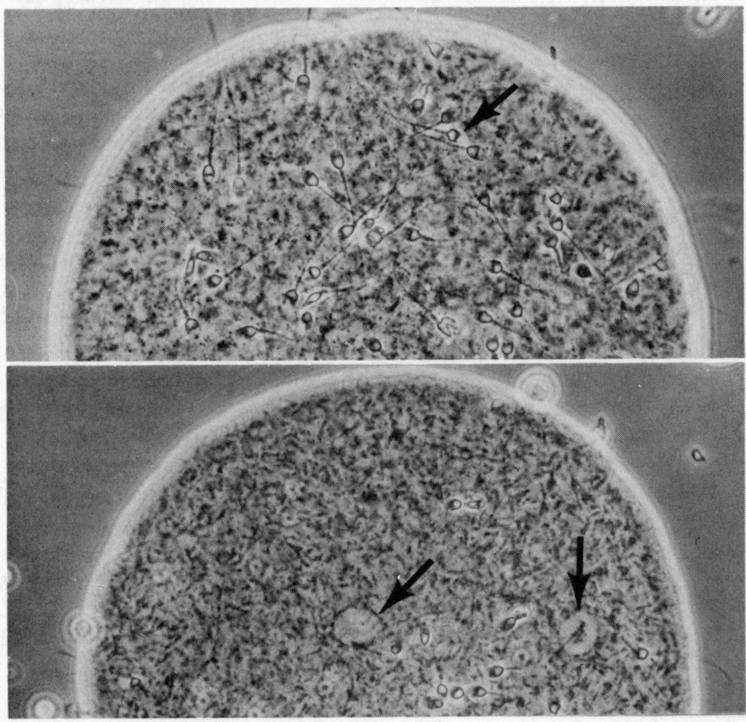

TABLE 1.—Comparison of SPA and SFA in 108 Infertile and 25 Fertile Couples*

	N	+SPA/+SFA[†]	+SPA/−SFA	−SPA/+SFA	−SPA/−SFA	McNemar's χ^2 (P)
Fertile couples	25					
Controls, wife currently pregnant	25	21	4	0	0	2.25 (> .1)
Infertile couples	108					
Controls, wife previously pregnant by different spouse, no female infertility factor	19	0	0	10	9	8.10 (< .01)
Wife never pregnant, no female infertility factor	41	2	2	20	17	13.1 (P < .001)
Wife previously pregnant by different spouse, female infertility factor now present	8	4	1	2	1	0 (P > .975)
Wife never pregnant, female infertility factor	40	26	2	2	10	0 (P > .975)

*Criteria for normal SFA: count, $>20 \times 10^6$/ml; motility, >60%; morphology, >60% normal forms. Criteria for normal SPA: normal, ≥15% to 100%; abnormal, ≤12% (no scores in 12% to 14% range).
†Positive test (+) had normal result, and negative test (−) had abnormal result.

surrogate for the human egg in predicting the fertilizing capacity of human men, and Rogers et al. found that this test discriminates between fertile and infertile men much more clearly than does semen analysis. Laurence E. Karp, Roger A. Williamson, Donald E. Moore,

TABLE 2.—SENSITIVITY AND SPECIFICITY* OF SPA AND SFA

	Sperm penetration assay		Seminal fluid analysis	
	No.	Percent	No.	Percent
Sensitivity	19/19	100	9/19	47
False positives	0/19	0	10/19	53
Specificity	25/25	100	21/25	84
False negatives	0/25	0	4/25	16

*Sensitivity: percentage of patients with infertility who were classified correctly; specificity: percentage of patients without infertility who were classified correctly.

Kirkwood K. Shy, Stephen R. Plymate, and W. Dianne Smith compared the sperm penetration assay (SPA), for predicting male fertility and infertility, with seminal fluid analysis (SFA) in 133 men, 108 of whom were from infertile couples who had had complete workups. In 60 instances no abnormality was found in the wife. Tests were done with eggs from golden hamsters treated with pregnant mare's serum and human chorionic gonadotropin (Figs 15–4 and 15–5).

The results of the SPA and SFA are compared for the 108 infertile and 25 fertile couples in Table 1. A positive SPA consisted of 15% or more penetrated eggs. A value of 11% or less correlated with a clinical history of infertility and was considered to be a negative test. The sensitivity and specificity of the SPA and of SFA are compared in Table 2. The clinically fertile and infertile groups were distinct; no test results were in the 12% to 14% range. The difference between the predictive abilities of the SPA and SFA was significant only in predicting infertility. In cases in which the wife had had a pregnancy and there was no female infertility factor, the test was 100% sensitive. Where the wife was currently pregnant, the test was 100% specific.

Male fertility may not remain as constant over long periods as had been thought. Apart from many research applications, the SPA should be useful to clinicians who investigate infertile couples. Decisions about varicocele surgery may be facilitated by the SPA, and both husbands and donors might be screened before artificial insemination.

▶ [This test uses sperm penetration of hamster eggs as a "dynamic" index of male fertility. The results are almost too good to be true—100% sensitivity and specificity and no false positive or false negative results. Clearly, confirmatory studies are needed. In addition, one wonders what (if any) therapy might be appropriate for persons with negative tests.

Hall (*Fertil. Steril.* 35:457, 1981) also studied the sperm penetration assay and found about one fourth of infertile men with normal semen analysis but negative penetration tests. Dor and associates (ibid., p. 535) noted a correlation between the hamster egg penetration test and the Franklin-Dukes slide test.] ◀

15–12 Possible Relationship Between In Utero Diethylstilbestrol Exposure and Male Fertility. Women exposed to diethylstilbestrol

(15–12) Am. J. Obstet. Gynecol. 140:186–193, May 15, 1981.

SUMMARY OF RESULTS OF SPA AND SFA IN THE THREE GROUPS STUDIED

	DES-exposed (No.-17)	*Non–DES-exposed (No.-12)*	*Fertile controls (No.-11)*
SPA:			
$\geq 15\%$	3	10	11
$\leq 14\%$	14	2	0
SFA:			
Count			
>20 m/ml	16	11	11
<20 m/ml	1	1	0
Morphology			
>60% Oval forms	16	11	11
<60% Oval forms	1	1	0
Motility			
>60% Motile	10	11	11
<60% Motile	7	1	0

(DES) in utero have no apparent difficulty conceiving, but their relative risk of an unfavorable pregnancy outcome is increased. Recent data suggest that in utero DES exposure also may be harmful to male fetuses. M. A. Stenchever, R. A. Williamson, J. Leonard, L. E. Karp, B. Ley, K. Shy, and D. Smith (Univ. of Washington, Seattle) studied 17 men exposed prenatally to DES, along with 12 nonexposed subjects and 11 husbands of pregnant women. The study men had an average age of 25 years. Four had unsuccessfully attempted to impregnate their wives for 1–4 years. Thirteen subjects had never had unprotected coitus. The sperm penetration assay (SPA) was performed using eggs from golden hamsters.

None of the 17 DES-exposed men had produced a conception. All but 1 had sperm counts of more than 20 million/ml. Seven had motilities of less than 60%, and 1 had only 58% oval forms. Only 3 subjects had an SPA in the fertile range; none had yet attempted a pregnancy. All 4 subjects who had failed to impregnate their wives had subnormal SPAs. Eight subjects had a varicocele, and 7 had epididymal cysts. Two had a soft prostate. One subject had a congenitally absent testis. Only 2 of 12 non-DES-exposed subjects had abnormal SPAs. Four of these subjects had varicoceles. The findings are summarized in the table. Genital anomalies were significantly more frequent in DES-exposed men than in non-DES-exposed subjects.

Those findings suggest a relationship between in utero DES exposure and male infertility. Definite conclusions cannot be drawn until a larger study with adequate control subjects is carried out and DES-exposed subjects are followed up over the long term with respect to fertility. It is not clear that male fertility as predicted by the SPA is constant over time. The DES-exposed men are quite young, and maturation of the genital tract may have an effect in changing their fertilizing capacity as they become older.

► [Many papers have been written on the effect of DES exposure during intrauterine life on female offspring but male offspring have received little attention. Some morphological effects (such as epididymal cysts) have been suggested, but this is the first indication of functional sequelae. The findings are dramatic—only 3 of 15 DES-exposed men had normal (i.e., fertile) sperm penetration assay results, compared with 10 of 12 controls.

In an experimental study involving DES administration to pregnant rhesus monkeys, Thompson and associates (*J. Reprod. Med.* 26:309, 1981) noted that 3 of 5 male offspring followed to age 7 years exhibited genital abnormality (testicular hypoplasia, preputial adhesions, and/or undescended testes).] ◄

15–13 **Artificial Insemination With Husband's Semen: Prognostic Factors.** William H. Pfeffer, Edward E. Wallach, William W. Beck, and Anne T. M. Barrett (Univ. of Pennsylvania) reviewed the records of the 38 couples treated with artificial insemination with the husband's semen (AIH) during 1976 to 1980 as the initial treatment of infertility that had lasted more than 12 months and during which postcoital test results revealed less than 15 motile sperm per high-power field of endocervical mucus. Couples treated with AIH for other indications were excluded, but couples with additional infertility factors were not. On the days prior to and after the expected thermal nadir, 0.5 ml of semen (produced by masturbation within 1 hour of insemination) was placed in the endocervical canal by means of a blunt-tipped metal cannula. The remaining 1.5–5.0 ml of semen was placed in a Silastic cup that was positioned over the cervix and left in place for 6 to 8 hours.

Conception occurred in 12 of 148 AIH cycles and in 1 of 178 natural insemination (NIH) cycles. The conceiving and nonconceiving couples had had a similar period of prior infertility. Semen parameters were not very helpful in predicting which couples would be successful, although there was some indication that men with both density less than 25 million sperm/ml and motility less than 50% were unlikely to establish a pregnancy through AIH. Couples that demonstrated more than 15 motile sperm per high-power field on a postcoital test performed 2 hours after AIH were more likely to conceive through AIH than couples who demonstrated less than 15 motile sperm. Infertility factors in addition to suboptimal postcoital test results were found in 4 of 12 couples who conceived by AIH and in 12 of 24 couples who did not.

Artificial insemination with the husband's semen may be useful in the treatment of infertile couples who have suboptimal postcoital test results. The postcoital test performed after AIH appears to have value in predicting which couples will succeed with AIH.

► [This retrospective study addresses the question of whether artifical insemination with the husband's semen (AIH) is of benefit in the infertile couple with a poor postcoital test result. The technique of AIH involved injecting 0.5 ml of fresh semen in the endocervical canal and placing the remainder in a cup over the exocervix to be left in place for 6–8 hours. Conception occurred in 32% of patients and 8.1% of cycles with AIH, compared with 3% and 0.6%, respectively, with "natural" insemination. Not surprisingly, instances in which a 2-hour postinsemination examination of the cervical mucus indicated more than 15 motile sperm per high-power field were more likely to result in conception than those in which the findings were less favorable. From these results, it appears that AIH may be of some value in the infertile couple with a suboptimal postcoital test result and perhaps might be tried prior to immunologic testing or extensive studies of sperm-mucus relationships.] ◄

15–14 **Homologous Artificial Insemination After Long-Term Semen Cryopreservation.** Stanley Friedman and Stephen Broder (Univ. of

(15–13) Fertil. Steril. 34:356–361, October 1980.
(15–14) Ibid. 35:321–324, March 1981.

California, Los Angeles) report that from 1969 through 1979, 475 men deposited semen specimens prior to vasectomy or therapeutic sterilization. Prefreeze sperm counts and motility were significantly higher in the prevasectomy group. Semen specimens sufficient in number to provide a realistic chance of success for future conception (12 or more inseminations) were not usually obtained. Later, 5 wives of 177 vasectomized men and 16 wives of 183 therapeutically sterilized men returned for artificial insemination (AI) with their husbands' semen.

Only 1 conception, with subsequent birth of a normal female infant, resulted among the 21 women; this conception occurred after a single AI of a 7-year-old specimen obtained before vasectomy. The postthaw motility of this specimen (45%) was better than that of most other thawed specimens. Postthaw motilities were unpredictable despite comparable prefreeze motilities. Postthaw motilities for vasectomized men varied from 10% to 45% and for therapeutically sterilized men from 10% to 40%.

Due to the unpredictability of postthaw motility, semen cryopreservation is no guarantee of "fertility insurance." Increased awareness of the availability and requirements of optimal semen banking could result in a greater number of specimens being deposited. By referral to the semen bank as soon as possible after diagnosis, harmful effects of disease and therapy on sperm quality might be mitigated. It is important not to oversell the concept of "fertility" or "vasectomy insurance" when semen is deposited for this purpose.

▶ [This report, although the number of cases is not large, suggests that cryopreservation of semen may not be such hot "vasectomy insurance!" The authors make the point that if semen is stored for this purpose, there should be enough for 12 inseminations so as to provide a realistic chance of success.] ◀

15–15 **Laparoscopic Findings in Twenty-five Failures of Artificial Insemination.** In the artificial insemination donor program at the University of Wisconsin Hospital, Madison, pretreatment evaluation is limited to history, physical examination, erythrocyte sedimentation rate, VDRL results, *Mycoplasma* culture, gonococcal culture, biphasic body temperature charts, secretory phase endometrial biopsy, and rubella antibody titer. In this program, a pregnancy rate of 52% has been achieved, with 92% of conceptions occurring in the first 6 treatment cycles. Fredrik F. Broekhuizen, Ray V. Haning, Jr., and Sander S. Shapiro retrospectively evaluated the laparoscopic findings, treatment, and follow-up of 25 patients in whom artificial insemination was unsuccessful.

The laparoscopic findings were abnormal in 18 (72%) patients, whereas the other 7 patients had a normal pelvis with patent fallopian tubes. Laparoscopy showed only endometriosis in 15 patients and pelvic adhesions in 3 patients, 2 of whom had had pelvic surgery. In the 15 patients with mild to severe endometriosis only, surgical or medical treatment preceded artificial insemination in 12 and ovulatory disorders requiring treatment were found in 6 (table). Two of the

---

(15–15) Fertil. Steril. 34:351–355, October 1980.

ENDOMETRIOSIS IN 15 ARTIFICIAL INSEMINATION
DONOR (AID) FAILURES

	Mild	Moderate	Severe
No. of patients	8	5	2
Ovulatory disorders	5	0	1
No subsequent AID	2	0	1
Surgical or medical treatment followed by AID	6	5	1
Pregnancies	2	0	0

patients in this group with mild endometriosis subsequently conceived after either surgical or medical (danazol) treatment only. The incidence of endometriosis and pelvic adhesions in this series did not differ significantly from the incidence of these entities in a randomly chosen group of 50 women being treated at the same institution for unexplained infertility. The overall pregnancy rate after surgical or medical treatment was 22.2% for those with positive laparoscopic findings and 20% for those with negative findings.

The use of diagnostic laparoscopy in patients who fail to conceive with artificial insemination is justified only if the patient is committed to continue attempts after laparoscopy and disease-oriented therapy.

▶ [Among 25 patients who failed to conceive with at least 6 cycles of donor insemination, laparoscopy diagnosed previously unsuspected disease in 18. Not surprisingly, the most common finding (15 patients) was endometriosis, usually mild but sometimes more extensive (see the table). The pregnancy rate of 16.6% after medical or surgical treatment (not otherwise specified) of endometriosis is not especially encouraging.] ◀

15–16 Immunologic Infertility: Identification of Patients With Antisperm Antibody. Antisperm antibodies have been implicated as a cause of infertility, yet there is some question about the reliability of the assays used to detect antisperm antibodies. Gilbert G. Haas, Jr., Douglas B. Cines, and Alan D. Schreiber (Univ. of Pennsylvania) used a modification of the radiolabeled Coombs antiglobulin test to detect circulating antisperm antibodies in 614 patients, including 257 couples, with unexplained infertility. For the assay, radiolabeled rabbit anti-IgG was adsorbed with normal human erythrocytes to eliminate nonspecific binding of IgG to cell surfaces.

Forty-two female and 21 male patients had positive test results for plasma IgG antisperm antibodies. In 3 couples, both partners showed positive results. Three male and 3 female patients with more marked antisperm-antibody activity had follow-up studies. Of these, 3 men and 1 woman were treated with systemic corticosteroids (table). Pregnancy occurred in 2 couples showing a spontaneous decrease in plasma sperm antibodies and in 2 couples in which a partner had been treated with corticosteroids (table). Plasma IgG antisperm-antibody activity became undetectable in all 6 couples.

This radiolabeled-antiglobulin test for antibodies against sperm is

(15–16) N. Engl. J. Med. 303:722–727, Sept. 25, 1980.

Follow-up of Six Infertile Patients With Raised Levels of
Antisperm Antibody

PATIENTS	AGE/SEX	TITER *	FOLLOW-UP TITER	RESULT
Corticosteroid-treated				
Patient 1	28/M	1:20	Undetectable	Continued infertility
Patient 2	31/M	1:280	Undetectable	Partner became pregnant
Patient 3	35/M	1:20	Undetectable	Continued infertility
Patient 4	31/F	1:32	Undetectable	Pregnancy
Untreated				
Patient 5	33/F	1:320	Undetectable	Pregnancy
Patient 6	32/F	1:20	Undetectable	Pregnancy

*Maximal dilution of plasma that resulted in a positive radiolabeled antiglobulin test.

objective and is clinically useful for identification and management of patients with suspected antibody-mediated infertility.

▶ [A new wrinkle in testing for possible immunologic infertility! A modified Coombs test was used to identify antisperm IgG in the serum of patients with unexplained infertility. Six patients with high levels of antibody activity were studied further. Four pregnancies occurred. These were associated with undetectable antibody activity on follow-up testing. Two patients had been treated with corticosteroids; 2 had had spontaneous remission of their antibody.

Only a very small percentage of patients had high levels of antisperm antibody. The importance of immunologic factors in unexplained infertility and the role of this particular testing procedure have not yet been clearly defined. Read on.] ◀

15–17 **Spermagglutinating Antibodies and Sperm Penetration of Cervical Mucus From Infertile Women With Spermagglutinating Antibodies in Serum.** Hans Jakob Ingerslev (Univ. of Aarhus) demonstrated spermagglutinins by the tray agglutination technique in cervical mucus collected during presumably ovulatory cycles in 8 of 21 women with serum spermagglutinating antibodies; the patients were being treated for infertility. The spermagglutinin titer in cervical mucus was (with 1 exception) equal to or one to three steps lower than that in serum. A "poor" sperm penetration test was recorded exclusively in 2 of the 8 women with spermagglutinins in cervical mucus. A "good" sperm penetration test was recorded in a similar fraction of those with and without spermagglutinins in cervical mucus; no correlation was observed between migration distance of the foremost spermatozoon and mucus spermagglutinin titers. Results of the sperm-cervical mucus contact (SCMC) test were significantly correlated to cervical mucus spermagglutinin titers. A positive SCMC test was recorded in 3 of 8 patients with mucus spermagglutinating antibodies, but in none of the 13 women without these antibodies. A close association was observed between SCMC test and sperm pene-

(15–17) Fertil. Steril. 34:561–568, December 1980.

tration test results. None of 6 women who gave birth to a child during the interval from initial detection of serum sperm antibodies to the cervical mucus studies had a positive SCMC test, and all had a "good" or "fair" sperm penetration test. The decrease in spermagglutinin titers in preovulatory cervical mucus observed during treatment with 50 µg of ethinyl estradiol daily from day 5 to day 25 in 6 of 7 patients was significantly associated with improved sperm penetration in vitro. In 3 patients the SCMC test improved during estrogen treatment.

Based on the results of this study, the incidence of spermagglutinating antibodies in cervical mucus from infertile women is estimated to be 2.2%. However, an inhibiting effect on sperm penetration in cervical mucus by spermagglutinins is expected to occur in less than 1% of women from infertile couples. It seems possible that patients with circulating antibodies, but not cervical mucus sperm antibodies, may have had a period of sperm antibody production in the cervix which impaired spermatozoal penetrability of the mucus, reducing the chance of conception. Optimal evaluation of the migration-inhibiting effect of spermagglutinins in cervical mucus is obtained by the SCMC test; the sperm penetration test seems to yield comparable results when both migration distance and migration density are determined. The pronounced reduction of cervical mucus sperm antibody content during estrogen medication was probably due to dilution of immunoglubulins in the mucus caused by increased secretory activity during estrogen treatment. These observations may indicate a new possibility for estrogen treatment of infertility caused by spermagglutinating antibodies in the cervical mucus.

▶ [Although the final sperm antibody story remains to be told, this study adds useful information. Only a minority of women with spermagglutinating antibodies in serum will have them in cervical mucus. The presence of the latter is correlated in a general way with the results of in vitro sperm-mucus interaction tests, although exceptions to what would be predicted are not rare. Finally, estrogen treatment results in improved interaction tests and declining antibody levels in the cervical mucus.] ◀

15–18 **Pregnancies in Humans by Fertilization In Vitro and Embryo Transfer in the Controlled Ovulatory Cycle.** Fertilization and early preimplantation development of the human ovum in vitro have been proposed as a treatment for infertility due to occluded or damaged fallopian tubes and as a diagnostic test for infertility of unknown cause. Both documented successes were in women with natural or spontaneous ovulatory cycles. A. O. Trounson, J. F. Leeton, C. Wood, J. Webb, and J. Wood (Monash Univ.) studied 50 women whose long-term infertility was considered to be primarily tubal in origin. Twenty patients (group 1) remained on their natural ovulatory cycles, and laparoscopy for oocyte collection was timed for $25\frac{1}{2}$ to $27\frac{1}{2}$ hours after the luteinizing hormone surge. Ten patients (group 2) received 150 mg of clomiphene citrate daily on cycle days 5 to 9. Twenty patients (group 3) received both clomiphene and, on day 12, 13, or 14, 4,000 IU of human chorionic gonadotropin (hCG) given intramuscularly 35 to 36 hours before planned laparoscopy. Mature oocytes were mixed with the husband's sperm in Ham's F10 medium. Embryos de-

---

(15–18) Science 212:681–682, May 8, 1981.

TABLE 1.—RECOVERY OF OOCYTES FROM PATIENTS WITH TUBAL INFERTILITY AND DEVELOPMENT OF EMBRYOS TO AT LEAST FOUR-CELL STAGE AFTER FERTILIZATION IN VITRO

Group and treatment	Ovarian response at laparoscopy			Patients from whom mature oocytes were obtained	Embyro development	
	Total number of patients	Patients who had ovulated	Patients with no large follicle		Number of mature oocytes	Number of embryos developed
1. Natural cycle	20	4	1	13	13	12
2. Clomiphene and natural ovulation	10	1	1	7	11	10
3. Clomiphene and hCG	20	0	0	20	31	27
Total	50	5	2	40	55	49

TABLE 2.—RESULTS OF EMBRYO TRANSFER AFTER IN VITRO FERTILIZATION

Group and treatment	Number of			
	Patients with transferred embryos	Embryos transferred to each patient	Patients with increased elevated βhCG	Normal pregnancies
1. Natural cycle	11	1	1	0
2. Clomiphene and natural ovulation	5	1	0	0
	2	2	1	1*
3. Clomiphene and hCG	7	1	3	2
	9	2	3	1
Total	34		8	4

*Twin fetuses present.

veloping to the four- or eight-cell stage after 45 to 76 hours in vitro were transferred to the uterine cavity.

The results are given in Tables 1 and 2. At least 1 mature oocyte was obtained from all group 3 patients, and 87% of 31 oocytes developed to embryos of at least four cells. Embryos were transferred to 11 group 1 patients, but increased β-hCG was found in only 1 patient. Embryos were transferred to 7 group 2 patients. One patient received 2 four-cell embryos, and ultrasonic examination showed normal twin fetuses. Embryos were transferred to 16 group 3 patients, 3 of whom showed increases in β-hCG. Another 3 patients had ultransonically normal single fetuses. Two pregnancies have progressed normally to at least 7 months' gestation. Two of the 3 patients received hydroxyprogesterone for the first 12 weeks of gestation.

It is definitely feasible to use hormones to control the ovulatory cycle for fertilization in vitro. The success rate in this series is encouraging, but for clinical purposes it is unsatisfactory. Either the embryos have reduced viability, or the transfer procedure and subsequent treatment of the patient could be improved.

▶ [Most of us are not into in vitro fertilization and embryo transfer and, therefore, this abstract is not immediately relevant to our daily practice. Nevertheless, the topic has generated such widespread public interest that it is probably a good idea for all of us to be aware of what is going on in this fascinating area.

This same group has published another paper (*Fertil. Steril.* 35:502, 1981) in which they analyzed nine pregnancies resulting from in vitro fertilization and embryo transfer.] ◄

16. Contraception

16–1 **Oral Contraceptives and the Decline in Mortality From Circulatory Disease.** Richard A. Wiseman (Burgess Hill, England) and Kenneth D. MacRae (London) report that many publications have claimed that oral contraceptives (OCs) are associated with an increased risk of circulatory disease, in particular, thromboembolism, subarachnoid hemorrhage, and myocardial infarction; yet between 1962 and 1976, when OCs became widely used in the United Kingdom, death rates from circulatory disease in women of reproductive age fell steadily, by 34% (Figs 16–1 and 16–2). This decreased mortality was greater in young women than in men of comparable age and did not occur in older women. The mortality attributable to nonrheumatic circulatory disease for the 4 or 5 years before the introduction of the pill was fairly static.

These data tend strongly to refute the belief that OCs are causative of circulatory disease. A plausible mechanism explaining a direct protective effect of OCs is that increased high-density lipoprotein cholesterol levels are protective against coronary heart disease; estrogens have been reported to increase such levels, whereas progestogens tend to decrease them. All the early combined OCs were estrogen-dominated; only in 1973 was a low-estrogen OC introduced. If this hypothesis is correct, a gradual removal of the protective effect might be seen in the future.

It was concluded that OCs could not be completely responsible for the decreased mortality, although a partial protective effect could not be ruled out. The findings on circulatory mortality are not confined to

Fig 16–1.—All circulatory disease. Mortality in women per 100,000 population in England and Wales, aged 15–44 years inclusive. (Courtesy of Wiseman, R. A., and MacRae, K. D.: Fertil. Steril. 35:277–283, March 1981.)

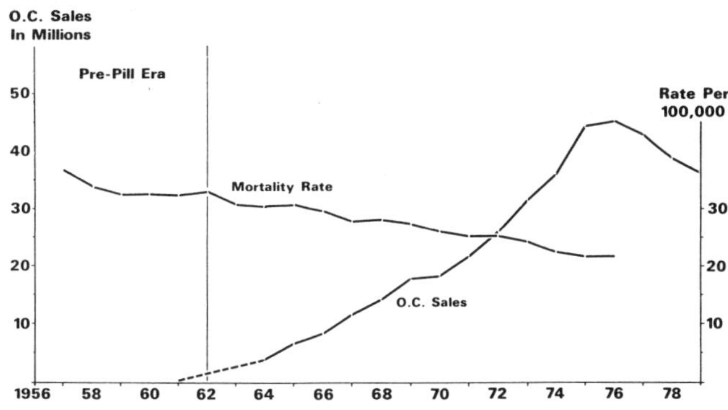

(16–1) Fertil. Steril. 35:277–283, March 1981.

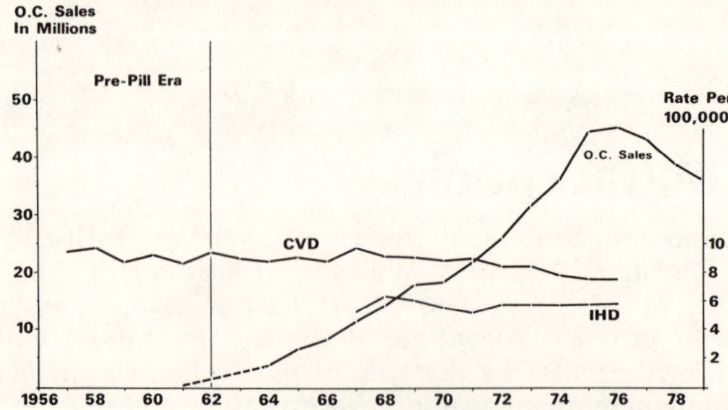

Fig 16–2.—Cerebrovascular *(CVD)* and ischemic heart disease *(IHD)*. Mortality in women per 100,000 population in England and Wales, aged 15–44 years inclusive. (Courtesy of Wiseman, R. A., and MacRae, K. D.: Fertil. Steril. 35:277–283, March 1981.)

the United Kingdom. It is suggested that when mortality trends are opposed to results of case-control or cohort studies, doubts are cast on the conclusions about causal relationships.

▶ [Because of several case-control epidemiologic studies, there is a general view that oral contraceptives predispose a patient to thromboembolism, ischemic heart disease, and perhaps to stroke as well (the latter issue is confused by an association in some, but not all, studies with subarachnoid hemorrhage rather than with thrombosis). If that general view reflects reality, one might predict an increase in cardiovascular mortality in a population of women in association with the introduction of oral contraceptives on a large scale. Not so, according to this report. The declining incidence of rheumatic heart disease largely explains the falling mortality rate, but deaths from those conditions allegedly associated with an increased risk in oral contraceptive users have not increased despite the use of oral contraceptives by one third of British women of reproductive age. Other factors are probably operative here, and this death certificate study should not be regarded as the final word; however, these results may make oral contraceptive users and their gynecologists a little more comfortable.] ◀

16–2 **Fibrinolytic Response and Oral Contraceptive-Associated Thromboembolism.** Salvatore V. Pizzo, James G. Lewis, Elizabeth E. Campbell, and Nancy A. Dreyer studied fibrinolytic activity in 12 women with a recent history of thromboembolism while taking oral contraceptives and in 28 age-matched controls with no history of thromboembolism. All women had stopped using oral contraceptives at least 12 months before study. A new, sensitive, and highly quantitative assay was used to evaluate the mean fibrinolytic response to venous occlusion.

The fibrinolytic response of all subjects was stratified into quartiles. The control subjects segregated as expected (9, 6, 7, and 6 subjects in the first, second, third, and fourth quartiles, respectively). The fibrinolytic responses of all 12 study patients fell into the first two quartiles (8 in the first and 4 in the second). Mean fibrinolytic responses were 12.3 units for control subjects and 3.9 units for study patients.

The findings suggest that a low fibrinolytic response may signal a natural predisposition to venous thromboembolism, which could be

---

(16–2)   Contraception 23:181–186, February 1981.

triggered by use of synthetic estrogens. However, the assay cannot be used as a screening test for oral contraceptive-related risk of thromboembolism, because at least 50% of the control subjects also segregated into the first two quartiles.

▶ [Using a sensitive test of extrinsic plasminogen activator, the authors of this report found that women with a past history of venous thromboembolism while taking oral contraceptives had a much lower "fibrinolytic response" than did age-matched control subjects. Although the overlap with control subjects was too great to advocate the clinical use of this test as a screen in prospective pill takers, the findings are interesting and, if confirmed, might help explain why certain women develop the rare "idiosyncratic" thrombotic complications of oral contraceptive use.] ◀

16–3 **"Escape" Ovulation in Women due to Missing of Low-Dose Combination Oral Contraceptive Pills.** It is generally held that in women taking combination oral contraceptives, the risk of pregnancy increases if a pill is missed, but there are no published data to support this clinical impression. V. Chowdhury, U. M. Joshi, K. Gopalkrishna, S. Betrabet, S. Mehta, and B. N. Saxena (Bombay, India) studied the effect of deliberate omission of one or two pills in normal women.

In a pretreatment cycle, blood samples were obtained between days 22 and 25 for estimation of serum progesterone levels. Cervical mucus samples and lateral vaginal wall smears were collected and examined 3 times a week, and an endometrial biopsy sample was taken between days 21 and 25 for histologic study. All women were then given low-dose combination oral contraceptives containing 1 mg of norethisterone acetate and 30 μg of ethinyl estradiol. Ten normally menstruating control women were told to take the pills daily for 21 days starting on day 5 of the cycle. Thirty-five women who had been sterilized were asked to "miss" pills on 2 consecutive days anywhere between day 7 and day 17 of the first treatment cycle. Nineteen sterilized women were asked to similarly "miss" pills in the fourth treatment cycle. Studies of blood, cervical mucus, lateral vaginal wall smears, and endometrial biopsy were repeated.

Only 1 control woman had serum progesterone levels suggestive of an ovulatory cycle. Endometrial biopsy tissue, available in 8 of the subjects, showed no secretory effect. "Escape" ovulation, as indicated by serum progesterone levels above 4 ng/ml, was observed in 10 of 35 women in the first treatment cycle group and in 5 of 19 in the fourth treatment cycle group. However, in all these women, the endometrial biopsies showed a hormone effect, as reflected by atrophic glands with excessively stimulated stroma, but no secretory effect. In 5 of 35 women in the first cycle treatment group and in 7 of 19 in the fourth cycle treatment group, the endometrium was so scanty that a suitable biopsy specimen could not be obtained. In all women who missed pills, the cervical mucus remained thick and scanty with impaired spinbarkeit and poor or no ferning pattern.

Although missing one or two low-dose combination pills may result in escape ovulation in some women, the continuing pharmacologic effects on the endometrium and cervical mucus may provide contracep-

---

(16–3) Contraception 22:241–247, September 1980.

tive protection in a manner similar to that reported in women using low-dose gestagen-only pills. The relative degree of contraceptive protection in women occasionally missing the low-dose combination pills is probably reduced compared with that seen in women taking the pills daily.

▶ [These results indicate that missing pills on 2 consecutive days during the first half of a cycle of low-estrogen combination pills is associated with a 25% to 30% frequency of breakthrough ovulation as indicated by plasma progesterone levels. However, in all instances tested, both the endocervical mucus and the endometrial biopsy were unfavorable for conception and implantation, respectively. Thus, it appears that the contraceptive efficacy of low-estrogen oral contraceptives is maintained by the cervix and endometrium in the face of fairly frequent ovulation when pills are missed.] ◀

16–4 **Prospective Studies of Carbohydrate Metabolism in "Normal" Women Using Norgestrel for 18 Months.** William N. Spellacy, William C. Buhi, and Sharon A. Birk (Univ. of Illinois, Chicago) studied carbohydrate metabolism before and after 18 months of daily use of norgestrel, 0.075 mg, by 50 "normal" women. Studies involved a 3-hour oral glucose tolerance test.

There was a significant increase in the women's weights, from a mean of 138.6 lb ± 3.8 SEM to 146.5 lb ± 4.7 SEM; all plasma insulin and all blood glucose values were significantly elevated at the 18-month test. All initial glucose tolerance tests were normal, but 8 (16%) of the glucose curves were abnormal at the 18-month test.

The data suggest a systemic metabolic effect of norgestrel that may play a role in accelerating atherogenesis. The increased weight might produce the insulin resistance and hyperglycemia, or might be a result, or both.

16–5 **Lipoprotein Changes May Be Minimized by Proper Composition of a Combined Oral Contraceptive.** Women of fertile age seem to be protected from ischemic cardiovascular disease. One reason may be that they have lower triglyceride levels and higher high-density lipoprotein (HDL) levels than men. During oral contraceptive treatment, the incidence of cardiovascular disease increases in women; this has mainly been believed to be an effect of estrogen. Ulf Larsson-Cohn, Lars Fåhraeus, Lars Wallentin (Univ. Hosp., Linköping, Sweden), and Göran Zador (Stockholm) determined levels of lipids, HDL cholesterol, and sex hormone-binding globulin (SHBG) in 98 healthy women treated with combined OC containing ethinyl estradiol (EE) and levonorgestrel (NG) in the following combinations: 20/250 (20 μg EE + 250 μg NG), 30/250, 30/150, and a so-called three-phase or step-up drug (6 days of 30/50 followed by 5 days of 40/75 and 10 days of 30/125). Ethinyl estradiol and NG ratios were 0.08, 0.12, 0.20, and 0.35, respectively. Tablets were taken daily for 3 weeks, followed by 1 week without medication.

After 6 months, there was a mean reduction of 41% of SHBG in the 20/250 group (P <.01), but there was no change in the 30/250 group. Mean SHBG levels tended to be increased by 30/150 at all treatment intervals (not statistically significant). There was marked increase (202%) in the group given the three-phase drug (P <.01). The coeffi-

(16–4) Fertil. Steril.35:167–171, February 1981.
(16–5) Ibid., pp. 172–178.

cient of correlation between EE/NG and mean percentage alteration of SHBG in each group was 0.977.

Mean cholesterol concentration was significantly lowered in groups treated with 20/250, 30/250, and 30/150 after 1 month but not after 3 or 6 months. After the first cycle, mean HDL cholesterol levels were changed and stable in all groups. High-density lipoprotein cholesterol and HDL cholesterol-to-cholesterol ratios were reduced markedly by 20/250 and 30/250, but 30/150 and the three-phase drug caused only minor reductions. Mean change in HDL cholesterol levels showed a good correlation with mean changes in SHBG and EE/NG ratios. Mean phospholipid levels were unchanged in three groups, but there was a significant mean increase in the three-phase group after 3 and 6 months. Mean changes in HDL phospholipid levels were similar to those of HDL cholesterol, but were less marked. The coefficient of correlation between EE/NG ratios and mean percentage change in HDL phospholipid levels was 0.996. The mean triglyceride concentration was significantly increased after 3 or 6 months, or both, in all groups. After 6 months, coefficients of correlation between mean percentage change in SHBG levels and HDL phospholipids or triglycerides were 0.956 and 0.746, respectively.

It is concluded that SHBG may be used as an index of estrogenicity of a combined oral contraceptive and that EE and NG may be balanced to minimize undesirable effects on lipid metabolism. It is likely that the linear relationship found between EE/NG ratios and mean change in SHBG values is valid only within a fairly limited dose range. As progesterone-derived progestogens are less antiestrogenic than those derived from testosterone, they may have a lower tendency to reduce HDL levels. Changes in HDL levels are probably related not only to type of treatment but also to pretreatment lipoprotein pattern. The slow increase in triglyceride levels (3–6 months) contrasts with the rapid reduction of HDL apparent after 1 month of treatment. Therefore, reduction of HDL levels and increase in triglycerides apparently occur by different mechanisms. The initial transitory cholesterol reduction could be related to rapid decrease of cholesterol levels in HDL; later cholesterol return could be caused by its increase in very low-density lipoprotein or low-density lipoprotein as reflected in the later increase in triglyceride concentration. Since 30/150 and the three-phase drug had the least influence on HDL levels and HDL cholesterol-to-cholesterol ratios, it seems unlikely that these two drugs might affect development of atherosclerosis.

▶ [This article and the preceding one, both reports on the metabolic effects of oral contraceptive steroids, add information, but no final answers. In the preceding study, a very low dose of norgestrel (given as a "minipill") was associated with a decrease in glucose tolerance. Interpretation is hampered by the fact that the subjects gained weight during the period of observation. Whether the weight gain was related to the medication or, on the contrary, was independent of the medication but related to the glucose intolerance, is unknown.

In this study by Larsson-Cohn et al., HDL cholesterol levels were best maintained with the most estrogenic ethinyl estradiol-levonorgestrel combinations. High-density lipoprotein is thought to be protective against the development of atherosclerosis, so an oral contraceptive that did not lower HDL levels "should" be advantageous. Yet, a few years ago, because of the alleged connection between high-estrogen preparations and thromboembolic problems, the rush was on to prescribe oral contraceptives with ever lower amounts of estrogen. It makes sense that the type and dose of both estrogen and progestin and their interaction should be important in the sum of effects of an oral contraceptive on the female organism. What we don't know is what is best!] ◄

16–6 **Study of Interaction of Low-Dose Combination Oral Contraceptive With Ampicillin and Metronidazole.** J. V. Joshi, U. M. Joshi, G. M. Sankholi, U. Krishna, A. Mandlekar, V. Chowdhury, K. Hazari, K. Gupta, U. K. Sheth, and B. N. Saxena (Bombay) studied plasma levels of norethisterone (NBT), ethinyl estradiol (EE), ampicillin, and metronidazole in 16 healthy women who were taking low-dose oral combination contraceptive pills (containing NET acetate, 1 mg, and EE, 30 μg). Six of them, concurrently, received ampicillin, 500 mg twice daily for 5–7 days, and 10 received metronidazole, 400 mg 3 times a day for 6–8 days.

Neither ampicillin nor metronidazole therapy altered the "peak" or 24-hour plasma levels or the area under the plasma concentration-time curve for NET or EE. Ampicillin had a plasma level of 4–21 μg/ml at 2 hours and was still detectable at 6 hours. Metronidazole had a peak level of 12–38.5 μg/ml and was detectable even at 24 hours. Oral contraceptive treatment did not alter peak ampicillin or metronidazole levels. Progesterone levels were in the anovulatory range in all ampicillin treatment cycles. In the metronidazole group, in 2 of 10 women progesterone rose more than 4 ng/ml; in another group of 15 women treated with metronidazole, only 1 women showed a rise of more than 4 ng/ml.

The occurrence of "escape ovulation" as suggested by the progesterone rise in 3 of 25 metronidazole-treated women was either a chance incidence due to a different pharmacologic response in them, or most probably was due to default in their regular pill intake. This is supported by the observation that 1 of these 3 women also showed ovulatory progesterone values when oral contraceptive alone was given, without metronidazole therapy. In the control group also, 1 of 10 women had ovulatory progesterone values in oral contraceptive-treated-only cycles. Even though there may be an "escape ovulation" in some women taking combination oral contraceptives concurrently with metronidazole, it is likely that these women may continue to have contraceptive protection, although relatively reduced in efficacy, due to the peripheral combined action of NET and EE at the endometrial and cervical mucus levels.

In vitro studies indicate that concentrations of ampicillin and metronidazole above 2 μg/ml are effective to kill pathogenic organisms. Thus, the present study suggests that the therapeutic efficacy of these drugs is not reduced by concurrect intake of combination oral contraceptives.

► [Antibiotic treatment of pregnant women can affect estrogen levels in blood and urine. Presumably, the alteration of gut flora due to the antibiotic interferes with the normal enterohepatic circulation of estrogens. Occasional cases of accidental pregnancy in users of oral contraceptives who are also being treated with antibiotics have

(16–6) Contraception 22:643–652, December 1980.

been reported (1981 YEAR BOOK, p. 384). The present study in a small number of pill users treated with ampicillin or metronidazole suggests that blood levels of norethisterone and ethinyl estradiol are not lowered by concomitant administration of the antibiotics. While this is reassuring, it doesn't really establish that the risk of accidental pregnancy in pill users is not increased by antibiotic administration. This is a separate question. In this light, the relatively frequent presumptive escape ovulations with metronidazole treatment (in 3 of 25 patients) cause concern. The jury is still out.] ◄

16–7   A Study of Interaction of a Low-Dose Combination Oral Contraceptive With Antitubercular Drugs. Rifampicin has been associated with menstrual irregularities and unplanned pregnancy in women taking combined oral contraceptives (OC). To investigate a possible interaction between low-dose combined OCs and antitubercular drugs, J. V. Joshi, U. M. Joshi, G. M. Sankolli, K. Gupta, A. P. Rao, K. Hazari, U. K. Sheth, and B. N. Saxena (Bombay) studied 39 women receiving a low-dose OC containing 1 mg of norethisterone acetate (NET) and 30 μg of ethinyl estradiol (EE). Nine of these women were concurrently treated with a "triple" antitubercular treatment consisting of paraaminosalicylic acid (PAS), isonicotinic acid hydrazide (INH), and streptomycin. Plasma levels of NET, EE, PAS, and INH were measured and the area under the curve for NET and EE was calculated by the trapezoid rule.

Women concurrently treated with the "triple" antitubercular regimen showed no significant changes in plasma levels of NET and EE and their area under the curves when compared with control subjects. Only 1 woman reported menstrual irregularities, and plasma levels of PAS and INH were not altered by OC use. Rifampicin therapy resulted in a significant reduction in 24-hour plasma levels of NET. Although there were individual reductions in plasma EE levels, they were not statistically significant. Of 7 regularly menstruating women receiving rifampicin, 2 had a premenstrual increase in progesterone levels (greater than 4 ng/ml) suggestive of ovulation and 3 reported menstrual irregularities.

The results confirm that rifampicin reduces NET levels and suggest that rifampicin reduces the effectiveness of OCs and increases the incidence of menstrual irregularities.

► [The antitubercular drug rifampicin has been observed apparently to lower the efficacy of oral contraceptives, presumably by inducing enzymes involved in drug metabolism. This study compares plasma levels of norethisterone and ethinyl estradiol in patients using low-dose oral contraceptives who are treated with rifampicin or a combination of three other antitubercular drugs (INH, PAS, and streptomycin). Whereas those in the latter group exhibited no alteration from normal, patients taking rifampicin had significantly lower norethisterone levels and a (nonsignificant) tendency toward lower ethinyl estradiol values, indicating that the effect is due to the drug rather than to disease. Moreover, 2 of 7 rifampicin-treated subjects had plasma progesterone levels indicating breakthrough ovulation. Clearly, patients on rifampicin therapy cannot rely on low-dose oral contraceptives and should use another method.] ◄

16–8   Interaction of Phenobarbital and Other Anticonvulsants With Oral Contraceptive Steroid Therapy was studied by D. J. Back, M. Bates, A. Bowden, A. M. Breckenridge, M. J. Hall, H. Jones, M.

(16–7) Contraception 21:617–629, June 1980.
(16–8) Ibid., 22:495–503, November 1980.

MacIver, M. Orme, E. Perucca, A. Richens, P. H. Rowe, and E. Smith (Univ. of Liverpool). In 5 women with grand mal epilepsy on long-term anticonvulsant and oral contraceptive therapy (ethinyl estradiol [EE], 50 µg, plus levonorgestrel, 250 µg daily) studied, the plasma EE concentration was 11.1 ± 4.5 pg/ml. These values were at the lower end of the range found in the same laboratory in normal women taking 30 µg EE daily (6–190 pg/ml). Plasma norgestrel concentrations in the 5 women studied (mean 0.83 ± 0.19 ng/ml) were also at the lower limit of the range for the laboratory. The sex hormone-binding globulin (SHBG) capacity (mean 206.4 ± 32.1 nmoles/L) was higher than that reported in another group of control women taking only oral contraceptive steroids in a similar dose (140.1 ± 22.1 nmoles/L). Anticonvulsant drugs taken by the 5 women studied included (mg/day) phenytoin (250–350), carbamazepine (200–800), primidone (250), sodium valproate (1,200), methsuximide (900), and ethosuximide (750).

Four women were studied prospectively for 3 months, over 1 cycle before and 2 cycles during phenobarbital therapy, 30 mg twice daily. In 2 of these, significant falls in the plasma EE concentration occurred (from 104.8 ± 13.4 to 37.7 ± 2.0 pg/ml and from 125.6 ± 23.8 to 34.8 ± 6.7 pg/ml); there was breakthrough bleeding in both women. Plasma phenobarbital concentrations ranged from 5.5 to 6.5 µg/ml in these 2 women. The EE plasma concentration was not reduced significantly in the group as a whole. No significant changes in plasma concentrations of follicle-stimulating hormone, progesterone, norethindrone, or norgestrel were seen. There was a significant increase in the SHBG capacity in all 4 women (mean 215.8 ± 52.0 nmoles/L to 275.0 ± 56.5 nmoles/L).

These changes are consistent with the known microsomal enzyme-inducing effect of phenobarbital. The failure of 2 patients to show enzyme induction with phenobarbital, 30 mg twice daily, is not surprising since interindividual variation is known. If a larger dose of phenobarbital had been used, it is likely that EE plasma concentration changes would have been seen in all patients. The lack of change in norethindrone and norgestrel plasma concentrations in the 4 patients taking phenobarbital may have been because of the small dose. The increase in the SHBG capacity of plasma was probably due to increased protein synthesis by phenobarbital. Norethindrone and norgestrel bind with high affinity to SHBG, and the effect of phenobarbital to further increase this binding will decrease the free circulating concentration of these steroids.

It is suggested that women requiring oral contraceptive steroids and receiving long-term phenobarbital therapy should initially receive 50 µg EE. If breakthrough bleeding occurs, this dose may need to be increased to 80 or 100 µg daily.

▶ [These results suggest that anticonvulsant drugs, particularly barbiturates, may affect metabolism of ethinyl estradiol (EE) in some patients so as to lower plasma levels. It is interesting that the 2 (of 5) patients in the prospective study who demonstrated the steepest declines in EE levels experienced concomitant vaginal bleeding. These observations imply that we should be cautious about putting women on ultra-low-dose estrogen oral contraceptives when they are taking anticonvulsants.] ◀

16–9 **Bacteriologic Colonization of Uterine Cavity: Role of Tailed Intrauterine Contraceptive Device.** Intrauterine contraceptive devices (IUDs) and cervicouterine devices have been implicated as causes of pelvic inflammatory disease, with vaginal bacteria gaining entry to the upper genital tract through the projection of part of the device through the cervical canal. Richard A. Sparks, Bernard G. A. Purrier, Peter J. Watt, and Max Elstein examined the effects of various types of tailed and tail-less IUDs on the bacteriologic state of the uterus in 22 women with a variety of IUDs in place who underwent hysterectomy. Fourteen women were using devices having a monofilamentous tail. Eight used Dalkon shields, 3 with multifilamentous tails and 5 with no tails. The mean age was 35 years. The chief indication for hysterectomy was menorrhagia, often coupled with a request for sterilization.

All 5 uteruses with a tail-less IUD were sterile, while 15 of 17 with a tailed device contained bacteria. The organisms had not reached the fundus. Most were commensals. Surface bacterial counts decreased as the cervical canal was ascended, with few organisms present in the uterine cavity. There were no differences between monofilamentous and multifilamentous tails. The bacteria were not introduced by device insertion, because they were present long after insertion in several cases. Bacteria were cultured from only 4 devices.

The findings support the view that tailed IUDs predispose to the ascent of organisms in the genital tract. In nulliparas, who probably have an increased risk of acquiring pelvic inflammatory disease, careful consideration should be given to whether an IUD should be used at all. If it is, the cervical appendage might be removed or cut short within the cervical canal. Further study is needed of the protective mechanisms of the uterus, with which the tail of the IUD interferes.

▶ [The interpretation of this study is hampered by the fact that the devices without tails were present for a mean of 3 months' duration versus a mean duration measured in years for the tailed devices. Nevertheless, the suggestion that the tail, by interfering with the normal protective function of the cervical mucus, predisposes to bacterial colonization (albeit with small numbers of bacteria) is certainly plausible. If this colonization helps explain pelvic infection associated with IUDs, then Grafenberg's advice of more than a half century ago to use devices without tails may have been on target. Our standard teaching has been that, although bacterial contamination occurs at the time of IUD insertion, the endometrium in IUD users is sterile. We hope others will attempt to confirm the observations reported here. We may be misleading our medical students—again!] ◀

16–10 **Intrauterine Contraception With Levonorgestrel: A Comparative Randomized Clinical Performance Study.** Carl Gustaf Nilsson, Tapani Luukkainen (Univ. of Helsinki), Juan Diaz (Campinas, Brazil), and Hannu Allonen (Univ. of Turku) compared a nova-T copper-releasing intrauterine device (IUD) inserted postmenstrually (156 women) with two levonorgestrel-releasing IUDs consisting of a plain nova-T device carrier to which was attached a Silastic rod impregnated with 50% levonorgestrel; one IUD was estimated to release 20 µg of levonorgestrel daily (164 women) and the other, 30 µg daily (163 women).

(16–9)   Br. Med. J. 282:1189–1191, Apr. 11, 1981.
(16–10) Lancet 1:577–580, Mar. 14, 1981.

No statistically significant differences in reasons for termination of the three IUDs were found within 12 months. Continuation rates for the levonorgestrel IUDs were 84.1 and 81.4 and for the nova-T device, 87.5. There were no infections. Expulsion rates were lower with the levonorgestrel IUDs than with the control IUD, but the difference was not statistically significant. Amenorrhea was a reason for removal only with the levonorgestrel IUDs; studies suggest it was not associated with deterioration in hormone function of the subjects. Removal rates for the levonorgestrel IUDs were accounted for mainly by removals for intermenstrual spotting; there were none for heavy bleeding. However, most removals of nova-T IUDs were for heavy bleeding. Four terminations because of accidental pregnancy (rate, 2.6) were recorded with the nova-T IUD; one accidental pregnancy, which turned out to be ectopic, occurred with the lower-dose levonorgestrel-releasing IUD (rate, 0.6) and none with the other. During all four 90-day periods, there was a significantly larger number of days of menstrual bleeding with the nova-T IUD than with either levonorgestrel IUD (Fig 16–3). The number of days of menstrual bleeding and spotting remained the same during all four periods with the nova-T IUD, whereas a highly significant fall in days of menstrual bleeding and spotting began after the first 90 days with both levonorgestrel IUDs and continued to the end of the first year. The total number of days of menstrual bleeding and spotting together was significantly greater with the levonorgestrel IUDs than with the nova-T IUD during the first 90 days after insertion. Thereafter and up to a year after insertion the number of days of menstrual bleeding and spotting together was significantly lower with both levonorgestrel IUDs than with the nova-T IUD. During the last two 90-day periods there was no significant difference between the devices in number of days of spotting.

As the levonorgestrel IUDs were inserted with the same technique

Fig 16–3.—Total number of days of bleeding and days of spotting for two levonorgestrel IUDs and a nova-T device during four 90-day periods starting from the day of insertion. (Courtesy of Nilsson, C. G., et al.: Lancet 1:577–580, Mar. 14, 1981.)

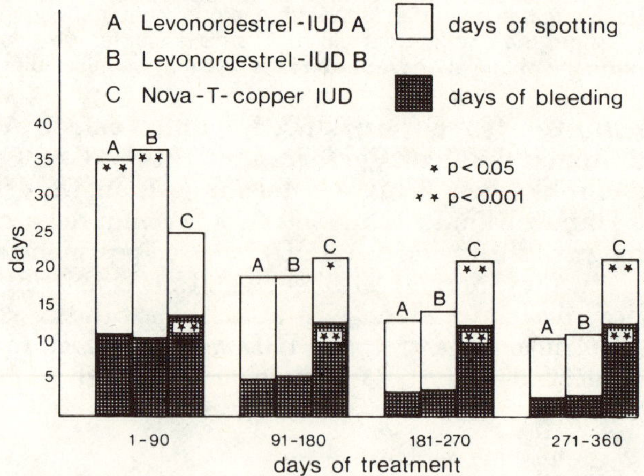

as the nova-T device, the low pregnancy rate associated with the former suggests that correct fundal insertion is not crucial for good protection against pregnancy, the local steroid release effect giving sufficient protection. The levonorgestrel IUD used by the subject who became pregnant was analyzed after removal and was found to have released an average of 6 μg of levonorgestrel daily—far less than was intended; no explanation was found. The levonorgestrel IUDs in this study have been calculated to have a life span of at least 7 years. The fewer days of bleeding associated with the levonorgestrel IUDs protect against pelvic inflammatory disease. Use of levonorgestrel for intrauterine release seems to be promising for achieving a long-lasting intrauterine contraceptive device.

▶ [The progesterone-containing IUD commercially available in the United States has the significant disadvantage of required yearly replacement. The experimental device studied by Nilsson et al. contains the potent agent levonorgestrel and has been calculated to have a life span of 7 years. Although the 12-month figures don't indicate a continuation rate superiority for the progestin device over the copper-T, the trend toward decreased bleeding with continued use suggests there may be an advantage of the progestin IUD related to this factor. Long-term follow-up studies should provide useful information in this regard.] ◀

16–11 ***Actinomyces*-Like Organisms in Cervical Smears From Women Using Intrauterine Contraceptive Devices.** Helen L. D. Duguid, David Parratt, and Robert Traynor (Dundee, Scotland) used an Ayre spatula, modified to enable its tip to be inserted into the endocervical canal, to obtain cervical smears from 293 users of intrauterine contraceptive devices and from 300 randomly selected women who were taking oral contraceptives. The smears were stained by the Papanicolaou and Gram methods and examined for *Actinomyces*-like organisms.

Smears positive for *Actinomyces*-like organisms were found in 40 (31.3%) of 128 women using plastic devices, usually the Saf-T-coil, in 2 (1.2%) of 165 women using copper-containing devices, usually the Gravigard, and in none of the 300 control women. Colonization was more common in women whose plastic devices had been in situ for more than 2 years. Of the 42 women with positive smears, 38 had been using a plastic device for more than 2 years. There were strong correlations between the presence of the organisms and recorded incidences of pain and both clinical and cytologic evidence of inflammation of the lower genital tract.

Plastic intrauterine devices apparently predispose to colonization by *Actinomyces*-like organisms, particularly after long-term use. Because of their apparent bacteriostatic action, copper devices should probably be used more widely.

▶ [Several reports in recent years (e.g., 1979 YEAR BOOK, pp. 264 and 419; and 1980 YEAR BOOK, p. 430) have called attention to an association between prolonged use of intrauterine devices (IUDs) and genital or urinary colonization with *Actinomyces* organisms, specifically *Actinomyces israelii*. This paper is the first to suggest a correlation with the type of IUD. Nearly one third of subjects with plastic IUDs had *Actinomyces*-like organisms demonstrated by gram staining of cervical smears, compared with 1.2% of women with copper IUDs and none of the control women. Copper has been shown

---

(16–11) Br. Med. J. 281:534–537, Aug. 23, 1980.

to have some weak antimicrobial activity in vitro, which may be the explanation for these results. In any event, this is yet another argument in favor of copper IUDs.] ◄

16–12 **Elective Sterilization in Childless Women.** Lloyd Benjamin, Lidia M. Rubinstein, and Vicki Kleinkopf (Univ. of California, Los Angeles) analyzed follow-up data on a series of 35 nulliparous women sterilized by laparoscopic tubal ligation for changes in menstrual pattern, motivation, and poststerilization adjustment problems, with particular interest in feelings of regret. Women requesting sterilization were counseled in individual sessions by specially trained personnel. Patients were scheduled for surgery approximately 2 months after the initial visit, providing them with additional time to consider the decision. The procedure used was laparoscopic sterilization by electrocautery or the application of Silastic Falope-Rings. With the patient under general anesthesia, surgery was performed by the resident staff, with direct supervision of a faculty member. Patients were contacted 18–48 months after the 2-week postoperative visit and requested to complete a questionnaire. Mean age of patients was 28.3 years (range, 18–42); 48% were single and 23%, married. Reasons for sterilization included medical indications (severe diabetes, malignant hypertension, genetic disease carrier state), 17%; inability to tolerate other contraceptive methods, 23%; and a strong commitment to remain childless, 60%.

Postoperative complications included wound infection (2 patients) and severe pain lasting more than 48 hours (2 patients). There was 1 failure, resulting in ectopic pregnancy. The range and mean values of the duration of menses as well as the length of the cycle were not changed significantly after surgery. Most women reported no changes in the amount of menstrual flow. The majority of women stated that tubal ligation did not elicit changes in either their sex lives (77%) or partner relationships (80%). None of the women considered that sterilization resulted in a worsened sex life. Feelings regarding surgery roughly paralleled those regarding sterility; however, incidence of unhappiness related to surgery (20%) was higher than incidence of unhappiness related to sterilization (11.4%). Four women (11.4%) expressed unhappiness about sterilization and an equal number expressed ambivalence. Of the unhappy women, 3 gave medical reasons prompting their sterilization; only 1 of the ambivalent group gave such reasons. At the time of follow-up, 80% were willing to repeat the operation; none had sought reversal. Of 2 women not willing to repeat the operation, 1 reported a severely painful surgical experience and the other reported severe dysmenorrhea after surgery.

The dissatisfaction rate of 11.4% in this study is consistent with figures reported in long-term studies of mostly parous women. This study indicates that nulliparous women choosing sterilization for medical reasons were at a higher risk for future unhappiness about their sterility, but true regret was not expressed in all cases. Furthermore, individual counseling may have accounted for the low rate

(16–12) Fertil. Steril. 34:116–120, August 1980.

of regret. Age was less a risk factor for regret than medical indications for the procedure.

▶ [Many gynecologists, particularly those of us older than age 40, have difficulty dealing with the recent increase in requests for elective sterilization by nulliparous women. We know that a certain proportion of sterilized women later regret, for various reasons, having had the operation, and the assumption is that the childless woman is at particular risk for some such change in her life situation. The results of this survey of 35 nulliparous women 1½ to 4 years after sterilization do not seem to support this concern. Adverse effects on relationships were infrequent, and relatively few patients expressed regret at having been sterilized. Moreover, changes in menstrual function were not reported with any greater frequency than that in surveys of sterilized parous women. Individualized preoperative counseling and a 2-month waiting period may have been factors in the generally sanguine results reported.] ◀

17. Abortion

17–1 **Fetal Loss After Implantation: Prospective Study.** The true rate of spontaneous abortion in early pregnancy is unknown. J. F. Miller, E. Williamson, J. Glue, Y. B. Gordon, J. G. Grudzinskas, and A. Sykes prospectively studied the rate of spontaneous abortion after nidation in 197 women, representing 623 menstrual cycles. The diagnosis of pregnancy was based on the presence of elevated urinary human chorionic gonadotropin (hCG) during the luteal phase of the menstrual cycle.

Of the 623 menstrual cycles studied, 152 (24.4%) showed evidence of conception. Only 87 (57%) of these conceptions advanced beyond 20 weeks' gestation. Of the conceptions that did not reach 20 weeks' gestation, 50 were diagnosed by elevated β-hCG levels and 15 showed both biochemical and clinical evidence of pregnancy. Spontaneous abortion was apparent in 14 (13.7%) of 102 recognized pregnancies. The conception rate during the first cycle after removal of an intrauterine device was 36.7%; this was similar to the conception rate for women studied during the fourth cycle after discontinuation of hormonal contraception (32%).

The major advantages of this study over previous studies are that the data were obtained prospectively and that the diagnosis of pregnancy was based on both clinical and biochemical criteria.

▶ [This prospective study nicely demonstrates how often early unrecognized pregnancies are lost. Of the lost conceptions, only one fourth were clinically recognized abortions; the others were identified only by raised β-hCG levels. The authors suggest that implantation is necessary for measurable production of hCG and that they were identifying postimplantation conceptions. If this is so, one would predict that certain fertilized ova do not implant and that the total conception loss rate therefore exceeds the reported 43%.] ◀

17–2 **Serial β-Subunit Human Chorionic Gonadotropin Doubling Time as a Prognosticator of Pregnancy Outcome in an Infertile Population.** With the β-subunit human chorionic gonadotropin radioimmunoassay (β-hCG RIA), hCG can be detected for pregnancy diagnosis as early as days 8 to 11 after ovulation, shortly after implantation. The exponential increase in hCG levels that follows in the first 20 to 30 days of gestation has been correlated with the doubling time of trophoblastic cell number. Frances R. Batzer, Sheldon Schlaff, Alvin F. Goldfarb, and Stephen L. Corson (Univ. of Pennsylvania, Philadelphia) prospectively evaluated β-hCG by RIA in blood samples obtained during the first 30 days of gestation from an asymptomatic, infertile population at high risk for pregnancy loss (414 samples in 281 pregnancies analyzed).

(17–1) Lancet 2:554–556, Sept. 13, 1980.
(17–2) Fertil. Steril. 35:307–312, March 1981.

With single, random β-hCG samples, 77% of successful pregnancies and 59% of abortions were correctly identified. With the use of β-hCG doubling time (mean 2.2 days ± 1.0 [2 SD], calculated by dividing the slope of the line derived from serial hCG values by the logarithm of 2), 88% of successful pregnancies and 76% of abortions were identified correctly. Of 78 successful pregnancies studied, 14 that progressed had a delayed hCG rise on the basis of doubling time, whereas 64 had normal doubling times. Although an early hCG value in a case of sextuplets was more than 6 times the mean value for that day, 7 of the remaining 8 multiple pregnancy samples had normal random hCG values; doubling times were normal in all.

Dating of random hCG samples based on ovulation is necessary to avoid false identification of low-for-date values; the use of hCG doubling time eliminates this error by making each patient her own control. This is especially useful in an infertile population with erratic ovulation. Availability within the first 30 days of pregnancy makes this method desirable for pregnancy assessment. Although doubling time appears to offer little advantage over random hCG sampling for identification of successful outcome in association with normal values, it is a significantly better predictor for pregnancy associated with low-for-date values ($P < .05$) because of the normal wide daily range of hCG values. The range of doubling time in aborters (0.34–20.06 days) was too great to generate a mean of significance. Frequency of doubling time in aborters appeared to be constant over 0.5–10 days, probably indicating multiple causes of pregnancy wastage. Several repetitive patterns of abnormal early hCG rise were observed. A negative doubling time or hCG slope was noted in 26 patients—a pattern associated with occult pregnancy and/or early subclinical abortion. A normal slope in doubling time was seen in patients who aborted in the second trimester (5 of 9), when other than placental abnormalities are thought to be etiologic. A persistently low slope (slow doubling time) occurred often several weeks before clinical abortion. The necessity for therapeutic manipulation in the infertile population in this study may make extrapolation of data to normal women less accurate. The 5% multiple gestations were also reflective of therapeutic manipulation. Closer evaluation of early hCG patterns and doubling time may prove diagnostic of specific problems, some of which may be amenable to therapeutic intervention.

▶ [It makes sense that the ability of early pregnancy hCG determinations to predict spontaneous abortion is improved if serial values are obtained. The normal doubling time presumably reflects a normal amount of functioning trophoblast and a continuing pregnancy. We remain generally unenthusiastic about this sort of attempt to predict the outcome of early pregnancy. In the absence of a *perfect* predictor, a "wait and see" approach is the one we favor.] ◀

17–3 **Fatal Septic Abortion in the United States, 1975 to 1977.** Abortion-related deaths have declined dramatically since 1940, but sepsis remains the most common cause of death from abortion in the United States. David A. Grimes, Willard Cates, Jr., and Richard M. Selik (Center for Disease Control, Atlanta) reviewed 36 deaths from septic

---

(17–3) Obstet. Gynecol. 57:739–744, June 1981.

abortion occurring in the United States between 1975 and 1977. Twelve deaths occurred after legal and 8 after illegal abortion, and 15 followed spontaneous abortion. One case was unclassified. The estimated death-to-case rates for septic abortion were 0.4 and 0.6 deaths per 100,000 legal and spontaneous abortions, respectively. Unmarried teenagers having incomplete abortion at 16 weeks' gestation or later by placement of an intrauterine foreign body had the highest mortality risk from infection after legal abortion. Seven women in the spontaneous abortion group had preexistent medical or surgical conditions. Predominantly aerobic organisms were isolated from 23 women. Instillation procedures appeared to be more hazardous than curettage techniques. Uterine perforation was a strong risk factor for death from sepsis after legal abortion.

Much can be done to prevent deaths from septic abortion. Wider availability of legal abortion services may further reduce the number of hazardous illegal abortions performed. Minimizing delays associated with abortion services can reduce deaths from infection. Young single women in particular should be told of the signs and symptoms of infection and urged to obtain treatment promptly should infection develop. Early curettage for possible incomplete abortion, whether induced or spontaneous, can aid both diagnosis and treatment. Routine removal of intrauterine devices (IUDs) from pregnant women appears to have reduced the risk of death from IUD-associated septic spontaneous abortion. The usefulness of antibiotic prophylaxis in reducing the risk of sepsis after abortion is unclear. Selection of the safest abortion method at each gestational age can reduce deaths from sepsis. If more curettage procedures are done, fewer of the more hazardous instillation techniques may be used. Thorough evacuation of the uterine contents and avoidance of perforation at abortion can minimize infection.

▶ [The real lesson here is to be certain that patients, especially young single women whose families may be unaware of the abortion procedure, understand the signs and symptoms of infection after abortion and the importance of prompt medical evaluation should these signs and symptoms develop.] ◀

17–4 **Prevention of Infection After Abortion with Supervised Single Dose of Oral Doxycycline.** Pelvic infection, which follows about 1.5% of induced abortions, may permanently impair fertility. Doxycycline (Vibramycin) is a long-acting tetracycline, and a single oral dose of 500 mg usually gives effective blood concentrations for at least 4 days. The drug has the low toxicity of tetracyclines, but its absorption is unimpaired by food and it is effective against gonococci and *Chlamydia*. Colin Brewer (British Pregnancy Advisory Service, Wootton Wawen, West Midlands) reviewed the results of a controlled trial of doxycycline.

During the study, all patients having an abortion (other than those having simultaneous sterilization) were given, with supervision, either five 100-mg doxycycline capsules or five placebo capsules. Patients were asked to report any complications occurring after the abortion procedure. Doxycycline was given to 1,519 patients and pla-

(17–4) Br. Med. J. 281:780–781, Sept. 20, 1980.

cebo to 1,431. In the placebo group, 8 reports of complications seemed to include pelvic infection, compared with 1 such report in the doxycycline group; this difference was significant.

It is suggested that 500 mg of doxycycline considerably reduced the incidence of infection after abortion chiefly because single-dose supervised administration virtually eliminated the problems of compliance and poor absorption. Though nausea is a recognized side effect of doxycycline, especially when the drug is given in high dosage, nausea rarely occurred and hardly ever led to vomiting. Resultant savings on the cost of treating pelvic infections would probably exceed the cost of the antibiotic. The benefits of avoiding infertility after abortion are difficult to quantify, but they must justify routine use of this prophylactic treatment. The regimen should probably be adopted without delay. The treatment may also be suitable for prophylaxis in other operative procedures.

▶ [This study suggests that a single oral dose of doxycycline (a long-acting tetracycline) gives effective prophylaxis against infection after induced abortion. Infectious morbidity is uncommon after this procedure, however, and the case for any sort of antibiotic prophylaxis is therefore a hard one to make. We do not advocate the routine use of antibiotics in this situation.] ◀

17–5 **Fatal Ectopic Pregnancy After Attempted Legally Induced Abortion.** From 1973 through 1978, the Center for Disease Control's abortion mortality surveillance program identified 10 deaths in the United States caused by ruptured ectopic pregnancy after attempted legally induced abortion. George L. Rubin, Willard Cates, Jr., Julian Gold, Roger W. Rochat, and Carl W. Tyler, Jr. (Center for Disease Control, Atlanta) discuss the clinical and epidemiologic characteristics of these cases and offer suggestions to prevent fatal ectopic pregnancies in young women who seek abortions.

The women ranged in age from 18 to 31 years (median age, 23); 6 had had a previous abortion. The estimated gestational age ranged from 4 to 14 menstrual weeks (median, 8.8). Clinical symptoms suggestive of ectopic pregnancy were noted at the preabortion examination in 4 of the women. In 7 cases the presumed products of conception were sent to an outside pathologist for microscopic examination; 3 of the women died before the pathology reports were received, and attempts to locate the other 4 women, for whom no products of conception were identified, were unsuccessful.

The identification of the products of conception at the time of abortion while the patient remains available for re-examination, recurettage, and other procedures is important for the prevention of fatal ectopic pregnancy after abortion. If grossly identifiable chorionic villi are not detected, additional clinical and pathologic examinations should be carried out. Patients should be informed of possible complications and followed closely.

▶ [The point is reemphasized that presumed products of conception should be examined macroscopically at the time of the suction curettage for elective abortion. If villi are identified, the presence of an intrauterine pregnancy is confirmed. If villi cannot be identified, the patient should be reevaluated. If the index of suspicion of ectopic

(17–5) JAMA 244:1705–1708, Oct. 10, 1980.

pregnancy is high, laparoscopy should be performed. If not, arrangements for both a quick pathology report and careful patient follow-up can be made right on the spot.] ◄

17–6 Midtrimester Abortion by Dilatation and Evacuation Versus Intra-amniotic Instillation of Prostaglandin $F_{2\alpha}$: A Randomized Clinical Trial. The safety of midtrimester abortion by dilatation and evacuation (D-E) has been reported recently. David A. Grimes, Jaroslav F. Hulka, and Mary E. McCutchen (Univ. of North Carolina, Chapel Hill) conducted a randomized clinical trial of 100 women judged to be 13 to 18 menstrual weeks' pregnant to compare the safety and feasibility of midtrimester abortion by outpatient D-E with that for inpatient intra-amniotic instillation of prostaglandin $F_{2\alpha}$ ($PGF_{2\alpha}$).

Patient characteristics were not significantly different between the groups. The interval between clinical evaluation and abortion was significantly shorter for those subjects assigned to abortion by D-E ($P<.001$; mean, 3.7 versus 10.1 days). Subjects slated for abortion by $PGF_{2\alpha}$ discontinued participation in the study more often than those assigned to D-E abortion ($P<.05$; 12% versus 0). Subjects undergoing abortion by $PGF_{2\alpha}$ had a relative risk of sustaining a complication that was 5.7 times that of subjects undergoing D-E abortion ($P<.001$) (table). The incidence of vomiting and diarrhea was significantly higher among subjects receiving $PGF_{2\alpha}$.

Even though midtrimester D-E abortion requires more technical facility than instillation techniques, it appears to be more acceptable to women and is faster and safer than instillation of $PGF_{2\alpha}$.

► [A number of enthusiasts for dilation and evacuation (D-E) as a means of second-trimester abortion have contended that this surgical procedure is simpler and safer than amnioinfusion techniques. This report describes the first truly randomized study, and the results seem to confirm that D-E is more acceptable and associated with fewer side effects than intra-amniotic instillation of prostaglandin $F_{2\alpha}$. The greater degree of "compliance" in the D-E group is actually an artifact of the local situation, because

COMPLICATIONS BY METHOD

	D-E (*n* = 50)	$PGF_{2\alpha}$ (*n* = 44)
Major complications		
Grand mal seizure	0	1
Hemorrhage requiring transfusion	0	2
	0	3 (7%)
Minor complications		
Hemorrhage (not requiring transfusion)	0	5
Febrile morbidity	1	4
Trauma to cervix or vagina	2	2
Prostaglandin reaction	0	1
	3 (6%)	12 (27%)
Total	3 (6%)	15 (34%)*

*$P<.001$.

(17–6) Am. J. Obstet. Gynecol. 137:785–790, Aug. 1, 1980.

patients randomized to amnioinfusion had to wait until a hospital bed was available. In this regard, it is of interest that 10% of them decided to carry their pregnancies to term during this longer wait; some would not regard this as a disadvantage! Whereas D-E may well be the method of choice for pregnancy termination during the early second trimester, the procedure does require technical skills and some degree of experience. It is not, in our opinion, to be undertaken by the "casual" operator.] ◄

17-7 Study on the Effects of Induced Abortion on Subsequent Pregnancy Outcome. Induced abortion is prevalent today, and serious questions have arisen concerning its long-term effects on subsequent pregnancies. Carol Madore, Warren E. Hawes, Frank Many, and Alfred C. Hexter (Univ. of California, Berkeley) have reported evidence that a prior induced abortion is associated with a small but statistically significant increase in the risk of subsequent pregnancy failure. Pregnancy outcome was assessed in 2,081 women who had had one or more previous induced abortions and in 4,098 control subjects matched for race, age, and hospital of delivery. Data were obtained from women delivering spontaneously at nine California hospitals in a 16-month period in 1976–1978. The study and control groups had similar educational levels and first-trimester prenatal care. About 8% of each group had had a previous spontaneous abortion. There were no significant differences in prenatal medical risk factors.

Most pregnancy complications were similar in the study and control groups, with no difference in rates of spontaneous abortion, ectopic pregnancy, congenital anomalies, or low birth weight infants individually. A small but significant increase in incidence of pregnancy failure (i.e., all outcomes taken together) was observed in the study group, but the increased risk was substantially smaller than that associated with several social, economic, and behavioral indicators. Previous elective abortion increased the risk of pregnancy failure by about 45%, with other factors held constant. Mothers who had never practiced contraception had more than double the risk of mothers who had used some method of contraception. Prior therapeutic abortion was not predictive of low birth weight.

Induced abortion appears to have a small adverse effect on subsequent pregnancy outcome. The finding that contraception was the chief variable in this study may indicate that it is a surrogate for self-care. Any effect of prior abortion may reflect unmeasured variables for which prior abortion acts as a surrogate, rather than being a result of the physiologic action of abortion.

► [Few questions are as important as that of whether or not induced abortion affects the outcome of subsequent pregnancies. Previous studies have come down on both sides of the issue. The problem is that of separating confounding and intervening variables from the variable of induced abortion. In other words, is an unfavorable outcome a reflection of prior abortion or something(s) about patients who have elected abortion? This study attempted to sort some of the problems out by statistical methods taking into account other factors influencing pregnancy outcome (socioeconomic status, prenatal care, smoking, etc.). The results suggest a modest effect; risk of pregnancy failure (ectopic, spontaneous abortion, and perinatal death) was increased 45% in cases over controls, whereas six other variables carried higher risk. The question

(17-7) Am. J. Obstet. Gynecol. 139:516–521, Mar. 1, 1981.

can only be answered definitively by a prospective randomized study, but that, of course, is impossible.] ◄

17–8 **Attitudes of Patients After "Genetic" Termination of Pregnancy.** Early termination of unwanted or unplanned pregnancies rarely is followed by severe or persistent adverse psychiatric or social events, but "genetic" terminations end planned, or at least wanted, pregnancies. They are associated with intense anxiety surrounding prenatal diagnosis of fetal abnormality, and the surgical methods used are more radical. P. Donnai, N. Charles, and R. Harris (Manchester, England) interviewed 12 of 15 women with abnormal fetuses who underwent termination in 1976 to 1979. Four patients reported that family and friend support had been poor. Three patients were considered to have made only a fair emotional recovery from the experience, whereas 2 others had continued to have a distressing reaction. All the patients exhibited emotional strain while talking about the event. One very distressed patient felt that the pregnancy should have continued.

Women must understand the nature of and reasons for prenatal tests. Most women, having learned about the nature of a fetal malformation, are anxious for termination to be effected as soon as possible. The mode of termination must be discussed with the patient. Several of the present patients elected hysterotomy so as to be unaware of the event. Careful counseling and support for patients undergoing termination are essential, not only at the time of termination but in the following weeks. A follow-up home visit could be made by a health visitor in liaison with the general practitioner. These women are vulnerable to depression and social disruption. A prospective study is planned that will include psychiatric collaboration in assessing patients undergoing genetic abortions with the goal of identifying factors contributing to prolonged depression after the procedure.

► [One might assume that the patient who has a pregnancy terminated for what she regards as good and sufficient reason (i.e., a serious congenital defect) would be in a better position to handle the attendant psychological stresses than one whose termination was more purely elective. This report suggests otherwise, however. To be sure, the number of subjects is small, the study is descriptive or anecdotal, and there is no comparison group. But the findings suggest that patients undergoing abortion for genetic reasons need specialized and intensive counseling, particularly over the weeks or months after the abortion.] ◄

(17–8) Br. Med. J. 282:621–622, Feb. 21, 1981.

18. Breast Diseases and Primary Care

18–1 **Value of Breast Self-Examination.** Self-discovery of a breast lump, either accidentally or by deliberate breast self-examination (BSE), is the most common event leading to the diagnosis of breast cancer. Charles M. Huguley, Jr., and Robert L. Brown (Georgia Cancer Management Network, Inc., Atlanta) examined the influence of self-examination on the stage of diagnosed breast cancer in 2,092 women seen with breast cancer from 1975 to 1979. The presence or absence of node involvement and the number of involved nodes were recorded in 89% of cases. Two thirds of the women reported practicing BSE, one-third once a month and the rest less often. More women younger than age 50 years than older women practiced BSE, and the proportion increased with educational level and with personal experience with breast cancer in the family. The largest number of women learned BSE from physicians. Nurses believed that 57% of the patients evaluated practiced BSE correctly.

The practice of BSE is related to the stage of disease in the table. About 80% of cancers were found by the women themselves, 21% by BSE. Of 719 women who practiced BSE monthly, 45% found their cancers in this way. Patients who practiced BSE had earlier cancers than the others. This was true for both blacks and whites, for all educational and economic levels, and for all age groups. It also was true within each period of delay between first symptoms and medical consultation. There was little difference in stage of disease in relation to overall frequency of BSE.

The data clearly show a correlation between performance of BSE and early discovery of breast cancer, although a causal relationship cannot be proved. Although BSE is not the final answer, it is a significant advance in the continuing fight against breast cancer. It has the potential for helping more women find their cancers early than any other method presently available and feasible for widespread use. Breast self-examination is safe and involves no cost.

▶ [Most breast cancers are discovered by the patient. Even in those who practice breast self-examination, an accidental discovery between "self-examinations" is the usual story. Nonetheless, the association between the performance of breast self-examination and the early detection of breast cancer is clear. Whether this is causal or whether breast self-examination and early detection simply both reflect a heightened health consciousness on the part of the patient is unknown. In the absence of a prospective randomized trial (which we are unlikely to see), the prudent thing for us to do is to teach our patients breast self-examination and to encourage them to practice it regularly.] ◀

18–2 **Breast Self-Examination, Relationship to Stage of Breast Cancer at Diagnosis.** Periodic breast self-examination is an inex-

(18–1) Cancer 47:989–995, Mar. 1, 1981.
(18–2) Ibid., pp. 2740–2745, June 1, 1981.

RELATION OF PRACTICE OF BSE TO TNM PATHOLOGIC STAGE OF DISEASE WITHIN METHODS OF DETECTION

Method of detection	No.	% in Stage 0, I	% in Stage II	% in Stage 0, I, II	% in Stage III, IV
BSE	431	27.4	56.8	84.2	15.7
Self—accidentally					
BSE practitioners	710	25.4	56.2	81.6	18.4
No BSE	481	17.5	46.4	63.9	36.2
Total	1191	22.2	52.2	74.4	25.6
Physician's examination					
BSE practitioners	190	37.9	47.4	85.3	14.8
No BSE	168	22.1	39.9	62.0	38.1
Total	358	30.4	43.9	74.3	25.7
Mammography & screening					
BSE practitioners	71	61.9	32.4	94.3	5.6
No BSE	14	57.1	28.6	85.7	14.3
Total	85	61.2	31.7	92.9	7.1
Other					
BSE practitioners	2	0	100.0	100.0	0
No BSE	16	18.7	50.0	68.7	31.3
Total	18	16.7	55.5	72.2	27.8
All methods					
BSE practitioners	1404	29.5	54.0	83.5	16.5
No BSE	679	19.4	44.5	63.9	36.1
Total	2083	26.2	50.9	77.1	22.9

pensive and noninvasive approach for achieving earlier diagnosis of breast cancers. Joseph G. Feldman, Anne C. Carter, Anthony D. Nicastri, and Susan T. Hosat (SUNY, Downstate Med. Center, Brooklyn) examined the relation between periodic self-examination and the pathologic stage of disease in 996 newly diagnosed patients with breast cancer who were treated at 13 hospitals in Brooklyn during $3^1/_2$ years (1975–1979). The population reflected mixed socioeconomic characteristics. The distribution of stage of disease was similar to that reported in the National Cancer Institutes's SEER study.

The reported practice of self-examination was clearly related to stage of disease at diagnosis. Over 48% of women with invasive disease who practiced self-examination at least several times a year were diagnosed before nodal involvement, compared with 38% of those who rarely and 33% of those who never practiced self-examination. The rate of distant metastasis at diagnosis rose from 2.7% for women who practiced self-examination monthly to 14.6% for those who never practiced it. There were few differences in stage of disease between women who practiced self-examination monthly and those who performed it several times a year. Larger tumors were significantly more frequent in women who rarely or never practiced self-examination.

Highly educated women, younger women, those who were married, and those who had used oral contraception were more likely to practice self-examination. Little difference in the practice of self-examination was found with respect to race or delay between initial symptoms and treatment.

Regular periodic breast self-examination is associated with the diagnosis of breast cancer at an earlier stage and with a reduction in mortality: a 10% decline in 5-year mortality for white women and a 17% reduction for nonwhite women. These effects are observed in a wide range of population subgroups.

▶ [Although a different staging system was utilized here, these results are consistent with those of Huguley and Brown presented above.] ◀

18-3 **Comparison of Breast Tumors Evaluated by Ultrasound, Mammography, and Clinical Investigation.** H. De Gezelle, A. Vanpeperstraete, P. Defoort, R. Serreyn, and D. Vandekerckhove (Ghent State Univ.) evaluated by clinical examination, mammography, and ultrasound 111 women admitted for biopsy of a breast tumor. The biopsy results were not known by the echographist.

Histologic examination showed that 51 of the 111 tumors were malignant. In the 60 benign lesions, the diagnostic accuracy was 88.3% for ultrasound, 85% for mammography, and 91.7% for clinical examination (Table 1). For the 51 malignant tumors, the diagnostic accuracy was 86.3% for ultrasound, 80.4% for mammography, and 78.4% for clinical examination (Table 1). Ultrasound provided the most accurate diagnosis of the widest range of tumor sizes (Table 2). There were 7 false negative ultrasound studies and 10 false negative mammograms. When the three diagnostic methods were combined, 5 of 51 malignant tumors were considered benign, 4 of which were less than 2 cm in diameter. In 36 cases in which enlarged axillary lymph nodes were found at operation, 32 were detected by ultrasound, while only

(18–3) Arch. Gynecol. 230:219–223, May 1981.

TABLE 1.—CORRELATION AMONG ULTRASOUND, MAMMOGRAPHY, AND CLINICAL FINDINGS IN BREAST TUMOR DIAGNOSIS

Histology	Evaluation	Echography	(%)	Mammography	(%)	Clinical diagnosis	(%)
Malignant 51	Malignant	32	–	25	–	24	–
(46%)	Suspicious	12	86.3	16	80.4	16	78.2
	Benign	7	13.7	10	19.6	11	21.6
Benign 60	Benign	53	88.3	51	85.0	55	91.7
(54%)	Suspicious	6	–	7	–	4	–
	Malignant	1	11.7	2	12.0	1	8.3

TABLE 2.—ULTRASOUND, MAMMOGRAPHIC, AND CLINICAL FINDINGS ACCORDING TO SIZE OF MALIGNANT BREAST TUMORS

Size of tumour	Echography	Positive diagnosis (%)	Mammography	Positive diagnosis (%)	Clinic.	Positive diagnosis (%)
Less than 2 cm	11	7	63.6	7	63.6	6	54.5
2–5 cm	36	32	88.9	31	86.0	30	83.3
More than 5 cm	4	4	100.0	3	75.0	4	100.0

18 were detected by clinical examination. The tumor was localized more precisely by ultrasound than by mammography. In 2 patients with tumors larger than 5 cm in diameter, the results of the first biopsy were negative, whereas carcinoma was found in the second biopsy specimen taken from a site that appeared most suspicious on ultrasound.

It is concluded that ultrasound scans are safe, efficient, and reasonably reliable in detecting malignant characteristics of breast tumors and lymph node enlargement. Greater diagnostic accuracy for small tumors may be available with technical improvements.

▶ [From these observations, it appears that ultrasound, mammography, and clinical examination of breast masses have similar rates of diagnostic accuracy. With all three techniques, the accuracy varies inversely with the size of the tumor.

In a similar study, Cole-Benglet and associates (*Radiology* 139:693, 1981) compared results with ultrasound and radiographic mammography; the two techniques gave similar results.] ◀

18–4 **The Click-Murmur Syndrome: A Clinical Problem in Diagnosis and Treatment** is discussed by Melvin D. Cheitlin and Randolph C. Byrd (Univ. of California, San Francisco). Patients with an abnormally prolapsing mitral valve now can be recognized echocardiographically even in the absence of typical auscultatory findings. Some patients with a click or murmur have no echographic or angiocardiographic abnormalities. From 5% to 10% of the population may have the auscultatory findings of the click-murmur syndrome. They presumably are a result of abnormal mitral valve support during ven-

---

(18–4) JAMA 245:1357–1361, Apr. 3, 1981.

MANAGEMENT OF CLICK-MURMUR
SYNDROME

Techniques

Asymptomatic patient
  Reassure
Symptomatic patient
  Reassure
  Treat symptoms (propranolol hydro-
    chloride)
Patient with abnormal ECG findings,
  arrhythmias, syncope, or family history
  of sudden death
      Ambulatory ECG monitoring for
        24-48 hr
      Treadmill exercise test if symptoms
        present on exertion
      Antiarrhythmic drugs
Patient with mitral insufficiency
  Endocarditis prophylaxis
Patient with severe mitral insufficiency
  Medical treatment
  If class III on adequate treatment,
    surgery
Thromboembolism
  Anticoagulation with warfarin sodium or
    antiplatelet drugs
All Patients Should Be Reevaluated
  Periodically for Change

---

tricular contraction, with abnormal slippage and prolapse of the valve into the left atrium. The basic cause may be redundant valve tissue and elongated chordae, poor left ventricular contraction, or an abnormal left ventricular diastolic shape. Severe mitral insufficiency occasionally develops. Other complications include infective endocarditis, various arrhythmias and sudden death, and thromboembolism. However, the vast majority of patients have no complications.

Management of patients with the click-murmur syndrome is outlined in the table. The asymptomatic patient with a nonejection click, with or without a murmur, merely requires reassurance if there is no family history of sudden death and the ECG is normal. Antibiotics may be used at the time of dental or surgical procedures. It is most important to avoid frightening the patient. Symptomatic patients should be evaluated for arrhythmias by ambulatory ECG monitoring, especially if ECG changes are present. If frequent or multiform premature ventricular contractions are present or there are premature ventricular contractions in runs, antiarrhythmic therapy should be instituted. Mitral insufficiency, if severe, should be managed medically, or surgery advised if functional class III features are present. Any patient with thromboembolism is a candidate for anticoagulation or antiplatelet therapy with aspirin or dipyridamole. At present, there is insufficient evidence to warrant antiplatelet drug therapy for all patients with the click-murmur syndrome.

▶ [This review was abstracted because the diagnosis of the click-murmur syndrome (mitral valve prolapse) is common these days. Physical findings include a click and late systolic murmur heard best at the apex. The condition may occur in patients with underlying connective tissue disorders or other cardiac pathology or may present as an isolated finding. Persons with the syndrome generally do well, but symptomatic mitral insufficiency, thromboembolism, arrhythmias, and endocarditis are occasional complications. Because of the last, we give these individuals standard bacterial endocarditis prophylaxis in labor. (A contrary view concerning standard bacterial endocarditis prophylaxis in labor in general is expressed elsewhere in this edition.)] ◄

Subject Index

A

Abdominal
circumference
measurements, sonar fetal, 27
ultrasound of, 126
wound disruption prevention, Smead-
Jones closure technique in, 273
Abnormalities (*see* Anomalies)
Abortion, 456 ff.
"genetic," attitudes after, 461
induced, pregnancy outcome after, 460
infection prevention by doxycycline
after, 457
legal, fatal ectopic pregnancy after,
458
midtrimester, by dilatation and
evacuation vs. prostaglandin $F_{2\alpha}$,
459
septic, fatal, in U.S., 456
spontaneous, 213 ff.
alcohol and, 213
drinking during pregnancy and, 214
smoking and, 213
Acetonuria: maternal, children's
psychomotor development after,
35
ACTH: maternal, relationship to cortisol
throughout pregnancy, 20
Actinomyces-like organisms: and IUD,
451
Adenocarcinoma
cervix, evaluation and pathology, 303
endometrium, 316 ff.
in adenomyosis, 317
estrogena and, conjugated, 308
positive tubal cytology in, 316
uterus, after radiotherapy in cervical
cancer, 318
Adenoma: pituitary, prolactin-secreting,
evaluation, 380
Adenomyosis: endometrial
adenocarcinoma in, 317
Adolescent menorrhagia, 395
Adrenal, 388 ff.
androgen function and DHEAS, 389
-pituitary function after prednisone,
388
β-Adrenergic stimulation: in cesarean
section, 171
Adrenocorticotropin: maternal,
relationship to cortisol throughout

pregnancy, 20
Age: and survival in carcinoma of
cervix, 304
Aggression: increased by prenatal
exposure to progestins, 208
Alcohol
abortion incidence and, spontaneous,
213
fetal alcohol syndrome, immune
deficiency in, 216
Alcoholism
maternal, with abstinence during
pregnancy, birth weight decrease
after, 215
zinc status during pregnancy and, 30
Alpha-fetoprotein (*see* Fetoprotein)
Ambulation: vs. oxytocin for labor
enhancement, 162
Amenorrhea, 375 ff.
bromocriptine in, 378
-galactorrhea syndrome
hyperprolactinemic, regression after
bromocriptine, 375
after pituitary tumor removal, 379
ovulation induction in, with
bromocriptine and clomiphene,
377
Amniocentesis
genetic, in twin pregnancy, 187
-induced rises of α-fetoprotein
concentrations, 135
in premature labor, 144
Amnion rupture: early, causing
compression-related defects, 211
Amniotic fluid, 128 ff., 191 ff.
α-fetoprotein in, relation to glucose,
191
blood in, and phosphatidylglycerol
detection, 130
cells, adhering, glial origin of, 192
C-peptide as index to intrauterine
fetal growth, 25
creatine kinase in fetal death
diagnosis, 133
meconium-stained, in perinatal
outcome prediction, 164
MUGB proteases in, 194
phosphatidylglycerol predicting
intrauterine growth retardation,
129
phospholipid profile as index of fetal
lung maturation, 128

precursors in placental membranes,
139
Proteases: MUGB, in amniotic fluid, 194
Protein(s)
C-reactive (*see* C-reactive protein)
intake, effect on breast milk, 225
placental, in trophoblastic tumors, 334
values in breast milk in induced
lactation, 226
Pseudohermaphroditism: female, due to
danazol, 209
Psychomotor development: in children
after maternal acetonuria and low
pregnancy weight gain, 35
Puerperal, 230 ff.
fever, *Mycoplasma hominis* infection
in, 231
infectious morbidity, 232
lymphocytic thyroiditis, 230
Pulmonary
(*See also* Lung)
bronchopulmonary dysplasia, growth
and development after, in
children, 243
Purpura: thrombotic thrombocytopenic,
during pregnancy, 50

Q

Quadruplet pregnancy: management,
102

R

Radiation (*see* Radiotherapy)
Radiotherapy, 306 ff.
of cervical cancer, adenocarcinoma of
uterus after, 318
of cervical carcinoma, 303
ovarian endocrine function after,
306
in endometrial carcinoma,
postoperative, 312
ureteral obstruction after, 307
Rape: HLA typing after, 196
Reanastomosis: microsurgical tubal, 271
Rectum: as site for basal body
temperature measurement, 424
Reproductive
endocrine system, in cystic fibrosis,
384
potential, female, after Hodgkin's
disease treatment, 62
Respiratory distress: dexamethasone to
prevent, in newborn, 237
Retardation (*see* Intrauterine, growth
retardation)
Retinopathy: diabetic, and pregnancy, 39
Rh
immunoglobulin after ectopic
pregnancy, 260

isoimmunization, fetal transfusion by
fectoscopy in, 98
-negative women, fetomaternal
hemorrhage in, 163
Ritodrine
metabolic effects during pregnancy,
149
in premature labor, 145 ff.
comparison with cortisol and 17α-
hydroxyprogesterone, 146
three regimens, 145
Rubella: congenital, in maternal rubella
antibodies, 197
Rupture: amnion, early, compression-
related defects from, 211

S

Saline solution: in vaginal preparation
for surgery, 265
Salpingitis, 350 ff.
Chlamydia trachomatis in, 348
gonococcal, recurrence and *Neisseria
gonorrhoeae*, 350
microbiology and pathogenesis, 350
Sarcoma
fibrosarcoma of ovaries, 323
leiomyosarcoma of uterus,
clinicopathology, 319
Scalene node biopsy: in carcinoma of
cervix, 305
School achievement: after small-for-
dates birth, 237
Scoliosis: idiopathic, effect of pregnancy
on, 61
Semen (*see* Sperm)
Sepsis: genital tract, clindamycin,
chloramphenicol, ticarcillin and
gentamicin in, 352
Septic abortion: fatal, in U.S., 456
Sex
differences in fetal lung maturation,
24
hormone-binding globulin, and
endometrial carcinoma, 311
prediction, fetal, and maternal
chorionic gonadotropin, 18
steroid(s)
bromocriptine in early pregnancy
and, 15
levels in cystic fibrosis, 384
Sexual dysfunction: and incontinence,
283
Sexuality: estrogen and progestogen, 413
Sickle cell anemia: during pregnancy,
erythrocytopheresis for, 51
Skin-fold thickness: after maternal
smoking, 218
Small-for-dates birth: school
achievement and behavior after,
237

You already have enough to read—
So why are we suggesting you read these, too?

Because nowhere else can you find periodicals offering these special advantages—

- ✔ *original* articles on a *single* topic
- ✔ written by experts in the field
- ✔ convenient *pocket–size* format

← more

except in these—

- Current Problems in Surgery®
- Current Problems in Pediatrics®
- Current Problems in Cancer
- Current Problems in Cardiology
- Current Problems in Obstetrics and Gynecology
- Current Problems in Diagnostic Radiology
- Disease–a–Month®
- Year Book of Pediatrics Newsletter